Researches in Epidemiology

Researches in Epidemiology

Edited by **Tony Andrew**

hayle
medical

New York

Published by Hayle Medical,
30 West, 37th Street, Suite 612,
New York, NY 10018, USA
www.haylemedical.com

Researches in Epidemiology
Edited by Tony Andrew

International Standard Book Number: 978-1-63241-342-0 (Hardback)

Printed in China.

Contents

Preface

Epidemiology is the branch of medicine which is concerned with the distribution, incidence and possible control of diseases and other factors relating to health. This book gives an overview on the diverse aspects of epidemiological research, brings together the expertise and enthusiasm of an international panel of leading researchers to provide a coherent overview of the field. The topics included in this book are epidemiology of varied manifestations of neuro-psychiatric disorders, virology and epidemiology, the epidemiology of dermatomycoses and Candida spp. infections, epidemiology of wildlife tuberculosis, epidemiologic access to the course of microbial nature of milk and milk products, Cox proportional hazards paradigm, epidemiology of primary immunodeficiency diseases, family-based genetic epidemiology and many more. This book includes writings of international experts and is a worthy resource for clinicians, researchers and students; who intend to address these issues.

This book is a result of research of several months to collate the most relevant data in the field.

When I was approached with the idea of this book and the proposal to edit it, I was overwhelmed. It gave me an opportunity to reach out to all those who share a common interest with me in this field. I had 3 main parameters for editing this text:

1. Accuracy - The data and information provided in this book should be up-to-date and valuable to the readers.
2. Structure - The data must be presented in a structured format for easy understanding and better grasping of the readers.
3. Universal Approach - This book not only targets students but also experts and innovators in the field, thus my aim was to present topics which are of use to all.

Thus, it took me a couple of months to finish the editing of this book.

I would like to make a special mention of my publisher who considered me worthy of this opportunity and also supported me throughout the editing process. I would also like to thank the editing team at the back-end who extended their help whenever required.

Editor

Section 1

Epidemiology of Dermatomycoses and *Candida* spp. Infections

1

Epidemiology of Bloodstream *Candida* spp. Infections Observed During a Surveillance Study Conducted in Spain

R. Cisterna, G. Ezpeleta and O. Tellería
Clinical Microbiology and Infection Control Department
Basurto Hospital, Avenida Montevideo – Bilbao
Spain

1. Introduction

Candida bloodstream infections (BSI) have become a major healthcare problem, specially in tertiary- care hospitals worldwide (Al-Jasser & Elkhizzi, 2004, Almirante et al., 2005, Alonso-Valle et al., 2003, Atunes et al., 2004 Asmundsdottir et al., 2002, Costa et al., 2000, Fraser et al., 1992, Garbino et al., 2002, Luzzati et al. 2000, Marchetti et al., 2004, Pappas et al., 2003, Viudes et al., 2002). Several risk factor identified among patients hospitalized for long periods such as the exposition to broad spectrum antimicrobial and/or immunosuppressive chemotherapy, parenteral nutrition, and invasive medical procedures have contributed to this fact (Blumberg et al., 2001, Fraser et al., 1992). Despite some improvements in fungal BSI diagnosis during last years, candidemia diagnosis remains difficult. Besides, following the data appeared in the classical study from Berenguer and colleagues, only 50% of patients with disseminated candidiasis will have positive blood cultures and even fewer will have an antemortem diagnosis (15% to 40%) (Berenguer et al., 1993). Therefore, invasive candidemia is not easy to diagnose, has an expensive treatment and finally is a serious, often life-threatening infection (Girmenia et al., 1996, Messer et al., 2009).

Although the incidence of candidemia has increased steadily among hospitalized patients during the eighties and nineties, recent series suggest that This increase has stabilized, but with great variations between different geographical locations with similar socio-economical development even in the same continent. For instance, in The Netherlands an increasing incidence of candidemia has been reported during the period between eighties and nineties (Voss et al., 1996) but on the other hand, in a neighbouring country such as Switzerland the incidence of *Candida* BSI infections remained unchanged during the same period (Marchetti et al., 2004). Therefore, it seems that there are some differences in the epidemiology of candidemia between different countries.

Besides, in recent years, a trend towards increasing resistance to both traditional and more recently introduced antifungal agents has been observed amongst invasive *Candida* infections, underscoring the need for continuous surveillance to monitor trends in incidence, species distribution, and antifungal drug susceptibility profiles.

The epidemiology of candidemia has been extensively studied in many countries and there are some large series published in this field (Alonso-Valle et al., 2003, Atunes et al., 2004, Banerjee et al., 1991, Colombo et al., 2006, Diekema et al., 2002, Kao et al., 1999, Messer et al., 2009, San Miguel et al., 2005, Silva et al., 2004, Tortorano et al., 2004, Trick et al., 2002). But, most of the data on candidemia in Spain until recent days are limited to retrospective reviews of medical records or observational studies conducted in a limited geographical area (Almirante et al., 2005, Alonso-Valle et al., 2003, Pemán et al., 2002, Pemán et al., 2011). Regarding the Spanish data available on antifungal resistance is often assessed by occasional surveys or reported in summaries of sporadically occurring cases of treatment failures. The purpose of such investigations is to monitor levels of susceptibility to different agents. However, long-term prospective studies of antifungal susceptibility have the advantage of eliminating a number of variable factors which may affect these assessments. Some of these factors include temporary changes in patterns of Invasive Candida infections (as stated before) and transient alterations in antifungal resistance due to special conditions (e.g. candidemia outbreaks in ICUs). Consequently, the epidemiological data about candidemia and its impact in the healthcare system is unknown, and no reliable nationwide data are available. In order to make a realistic global perspective of invasive Candida BSI, we designed a prospective laboratory-based surveillance study comprising 40 tertiary care hospitals across the country, to assess the incidence, species distribution, frequency of antifungal resistance, and risk factors for candidemia.

2. Materials and methods

Study design

A prospective laboratory-based surveillance was established to monitor the predominant *Candida* species and antifungal resistance patterns of nosocomial and community-acquired invasive *Candida* infections via a network of sentinel hospitals distributed by geographic location across the country.

The participating institutions include 40 medical centers which provide medical care either to adults and children in several medical specialties. Each participant hospital contributed prospectively clinical and epidemiological results (organism identification, date of isolation, hospital location, intrinsic and extrinsic risk factors for candidemia) on clinically significant consecutive blood culture isolates of Candida spp. (one isolate per patient) detected during the 12-month period from June, 2008 through June, 2009. All isolates were saved on agar slants and were sent on a trimestral basis to the Mycology Laboratory at Basurto Hospital for storage, further characterization and reference susceptibility testing.

Clinical definitions

Clinical and case definitions were according the NHSN (formerly NNISS) methodology. Statements defining a case and other clinical conditions are summarized in Table 1.

Quality control measures of clinical data

The clinical case report list of each hospital was compared with the isolates received at Basurto Hospital to perform the antifungal susceptibility in order to verify that neither cases nor isolates were missed. Audits of medical records to verify accuracy of data and completeness were performed on 25% of cases.

Incident case of candidemia:	The incident isolation of *Candida spp.* from a blood culture.
New incident case of candidemia:	An episode of candidemia occurring more than 30 days after the initial incident isolation.
Breakthrough candidemia:	The incident isolation of *Candida* spp. from a blood culture from a patient receiving systemic antifungal therapy for any reason.
Fever:	Peripheral body temperature equal or higher than 37.8°C
Neutropenia:	An absolute neutrophil count of less than 500 cells / mm^3.
Adult patients:	All patients whose age was over 14 years old.

Table 1. Definitions according to NHSN (formerly NISS) used in this study

In vitro susceptibility testing

Antifungal susceptibility tests were performed by using the broth microdilution assay according to the methodology recommended by the CLSI (formerly known as NCCLS), document M27-A2 (NCCLS, 2002) using a microtiter plate. Each isolate was tested against different antifungal drugs at the indicated concentration range suggested in the CLSI document. Quality control (QC) was ensured by testing the CLSI recommended QC strains, *C. krusei* ATCC 6258, and *C. parapsilosis* ATCC 22019.The MIC endpoint for amphotericin B, azoles and echinocandins and interpretative MIC breakpoints for azoles and echinocandins were those suggested by the CLSI document M27-A2, but for the definition of the amphotericin B MIC breakpoints we used the values suggested from a previous study published by Nguyen *et al.* (Nguyen et al., 1998).

Statistical analysis

The numbers of admissions and patient-days were collected to calculate incidence rates. The incidence rate for each hospital was calculated as the number of candidemias per 1,000 admissions, whereas the overall incidence was determined using summed denominators of patient-days and admissions to calculate pooled mean rates. The data generated during the year of the surveillance on the different risk factors, underlying diseases, morbidity and mortality were recorded in a Microsoft Access 2003 (Microsoft Corporation, Redmond, WA) based case report database. Categorical data were analyzed using Chi-square or Fisher's exact tests as appropriate, and continuous variables were compared using the t-test or Wilcoxon test according to the significance of the normality test. Spearman rank-order correlation was used to measure the relationship between the MICs of fluconazole and voriconazole. We performed univariate and multivariate analysis of factors associated with candidemia caused by isolates with decreased susceptibility to fluconazole. Variables significant at *p*-values of less than 0.05 by univariate analysis were included in a multivariate model using a repeated measures logistic regression model (backward and forward). Data were analyzed using the SPSS 11.0.1 software (SPSS, Inc. Chicago, IL) and Stata 8.0 (Stata Corporation, Lenexa, TX).

3. Distribution of Candida blodostream infections

During the 12-month study period a total of 984 Candida BSIs were reported. The calculated overall incidence was 1.09 cases per 1,000 admissions, however the incidence rate changed a lot between the 40 centers enrolled in this study and ranged from 0.76 to 1.49 cases per 1,000 admissions.

Among the invasive Candida BSIs, 45.3 % occurred in patients in an medical service, 23.5% in patients hospitalized in an intensive care unit, 17.6% in patients in a surgical ward, 7.41% in a pediatric ward and finally 4.06% in other services. Most of the patients (98.7%) were hospitalized and only nine of them were outpatients at the time of diagnosis.

Candidemia incidence was slightly higher in males (64.02% of the case patients) and the global average age at the onset of the episode was 41 years with a median age was 53 years among adult patients and 7 months among children.

The frequency of BSIs due to the most frequently isolated species of *Candida* in the study sites are presented in Table 2.

Species	No. (%) of cases	Range (in %) between clinical settings
C. albicans	483 (49.08%)	27 - 54
C. parapsilosis	204 (20.73%)	7 - 40
C. glabrata	134 (13.61%)	2 - 14
C. tropicalis	106 (10.77%)	16 - 29
C. krusei	21 (2.13%)	0 - 9
Other species [a]	36 (3.65 %)	0 - 4

[a] Species with less than 10 isolates are included in this category. This category includes *C. famata, C. lusitaniae, C. pelliculosa* and *Candida spp.*

Table 2. Species distribution and incidence among 984 cases of candidemia detected during prospective sentinel surveillance in Spain from June 2008 to June 2009

Overall, the 49.08% of the cases were attributable to *C. albicans*, 20.73% were attributable to *C. parapsilosis*, 13.61% were attributable to *C. glabrata*, 10.77% were attributable to *C. tropicalis*, 2,13% to *C. krusei* and the rest of the cases (3.65%) were attributable to other species. The distribution of Candida species among adult population was similar to the one found in pediatric cases, however, the distribution of species varied considerably when analyzed between centers as it has been reflected in the ranges specified in Table 2. The species distribution among our study isolates is similar to that described by Pfaller et al. (Pfaller et al., 1998) in Latin America with data collected by the Sentry Antimicrobial Surveillance Program. As Pfaller and colleagues described previously, the proportion of species isolated varies considerably among medical centers beign unclear the reasons for such differences and they could be attributed to many different influences.

Table 3 summarizes the overall clinical characteristics and outcome of the 984 candidemia cases identified.

At the time of candidemia diagnosis, neoplasia was documented for 195 (19.84%) patients, 35 of which (17.94%) were affected with hematologic malignancies Prior surgery was recorded from 311 (31.6%) patients (311 of a total of 984), being most of them abdominal surgeries (64% of total surgical patients). Two third of the patients (66.97%) had a central venous catheter and one quarter (26.93%) of them were under mechanical ventilation. Neutropenia and dialysis were rare conditions which was only documented in only 35 case patients (3.55%) and 12 patients (1.21%) respectively. Invasive *Candida* spp. infection complications such as endocarditis or endophalmitis were infrequent and with 17 cases documented for the former complication (2%) and 3 patients for the later.

Variable	Value for all total cases	Value for species			
		C. albicans	*C. parapsilosis*	*C. tropicalis*	*C. glabrata*
Average age (range)	41 (0–96)	46 (0–92)	48 (0–96)	33 (0–89)	52 (0–88)
No. of males	577 (58.64)	273 (56.52)	182 (89.21)	51 (48.11)	62 (46.27)
No. of outpatients	7 (0.71)	3 (0.62)	1 (0.49)	3 (2.83)	0 (0.00)
Median no. of days (range) until candidemia	20 (0–385)	20 (0–114)	19 (0–385)	19 (0–47)	19 (0–115)
No. of cases of underlying diseases					
Cancer	311 (31.61)	127 (26.29)	86 (42.16)	34 (32.07)	26 (19.40)
Hematological malignancy	20 (2.03)	5 (1.04)	6 (2.94)	1 (0.94)	1 (0.75)
Coronary artery disease	82 (8.33)	33 (6.83)	23 (11.27)	5 (4.72)	8 (5.97)
Chronic Obstructive Pulmonary disease (COPD)	71 (7.21)	40 (8.28)	11 (5.39)	5 (4.72)	9 (6.71)
Neurological disease	35 (3.55)	14 (2.80)	12 (5.88)	2 (1.89)	2 (1.49)
Diabetes	120 (12.20)	53 (10.97)	22 (10.78)	8 (7.55)	20 (14.93)
Organ transplantation	45 (4.57)	14 (2.90)	21 (10.29)	2 (1.89)	3 (2.23)
HIV infection	33 (3.35)	18 (3.73)	3 (1.47)	3 (2.83)	3 (2.24)
Parenteral drug abusers	22 (2.23)	10 (2.07)	4 (1.96)	2 (1.89)	1 (0.75)
No. of patients with characteristic					
Previous or actual corticosteroid therapy	180 (18.29)	80 (16.56)	50 (24.50)	13 (12.26)	21 (15.67)
Immunosuppressive therapy and/or neutropenia	265 (26.93)	102 (21.12)	75 (36.76)	28 (26.41)	28 (20.90)
In the ICU at diagnosis	252 (25.61)	120 (24.84)	68 (33.33)	21 (19.81)	25 (18.66)
Mechanical ventilation	265 (26.93)	133 (27.54)	71 (34.80)	15 (14.15)	26 (19.40)
Hemodialysis at diagnosis	12 (1.22)	2 (0.41)	4 (1.96)	1 (0.94)	3 (2.24)
Previous surgery	311 (31.61)	148 (30.64)	82 (40.20)	19 (17.92)	36 (26.87)
Central venous catheter	659 (66.79)	295 (61.07)	187 (91.66)	52 (49.06)	61 (45.52)
Urinary catheter	450 (45.73)	207 (42.86)	112 (54.90)	31 (29.25)	52 (38.81)
Prior antibiotic therapy	747 (75.91)	337 (69.77)	106 (51.96)	60 (56.60)	71 (52.98)
Prior fluconazole use	78 (7.93)	29 (6.00)	10 (4.90)	12 (11.32)	9 (6.71)
Death attributed to candidemia	134 (13.62)	60 (12.42)	20 (9.80)	13 (12.26)	15 (11.19)
Mortality due to other conditions	103 (10.47)	48 (9.94)	36 (17.65)	7 (6.60)	14 (10.45)
Overall mortality	237 (24.10)	108 (22.36)	56 (27.45)	20 (18.87)	29 (21.64)

Table 3. Demographics, clinical characteristics, and mortality for *Candida* spp. BSI episodes identified during prospective sentinel surveillance conducted in Spain from June 2008 to June 2009.

There were no statistically significant differences when the risk mentioned above were analyzed for the pediatric population of patients.

4. Antifungal susceptibility

In vitro susceptibility testing of the 984 BSI isolates of Candida species against amphotericin B, fluconazole, voriconazole, caspofungin and anidulafungin revealed that when globally analyzed *Candida* strains causing BSI are rarely resistant to a wide number of antifungal agents. However, the resistance rates among the different species vary a lot as it can be shown on Table 4.

Species	Antifungal agent	MIC (ug/ml) Range	50%	90%	No. of resistant or SDD isolates
C. albicans (483)	Amphotericin B	0.125–1.0	0.5	1.0	0 (0.00)
	Fluconazole	0.125–64	0.5	2.0	10 (2.07)
	Voriconazole	< 0.03–4	0.03	0.03	5 (1.04)
	Caspofungin	<0.03–4	0.25	2.0	3 (0.62)
	Anidulafungin	<0.03–2	0.03	0.03	0 (0.00)
C. parapsilosis (204)	Amphotericin B	0.25–1.0	1.0	1.0	0 (0.00)
	Fluconazole	0.125–64	0.5	4.0	11 (5.39) [a]
	Voriconazole	0.03–2	0.03	0.125	3 (1.47) [b]
	Caspofungin	0.125–64	1.0	2.0	12 (5.88)
	Anidulafungin	0.03–64	1.0	2.0	7 (3.43)
C. glabrata (134)	Amphotericin B	0.25–1.0	0.5	1.0	0 (0.00)
	Fluconazole	1.0–64	4.0	32	25 (18.67)
	Voriconazole	0.03–4.0	0.125	0.5	3 (2.24)
	Caspofungin	0.03–0.5	0.06	0.125	0 (0.00)
	Anidulafungin	0.06–0.5	0.06	0.125	0 (0.00)
C. tropicalis (106)	Amphotericin B	0.125–1.0	0.5	1.0	0 (0.00)
	Fluconazole	0.25–128	1	2	2 (1.89)
	Voriconazole	0.03–8	0.06	0.125	2 (1.89)
	Caspofungin	0.03–0.5	0.06	0.125	0 (0.00)
	Anidulafungin	0.03–0.5	0.03	0.125	0 (0.00)
C. krusei (21)	Amphotericin B	0.125–2.0	0.25	0.75	0 (0.00)
	Fluconazole	16–128	4.0	8.0	21 (100.00)
	Voriconazole	0.03–4.0	0.25	1.0	2 (9.52)
	Caspofungin	0.125–8	0.125	1.0	1 (4.76)
	Anidulafungin	0.03–8	0.06	0.25	1 (4.76)

[a] All the isolates except one exhibit decreased susceptibility (SDD) to fluconazole. [b] All the isolates are SDD to voriconazole.

Table 4. Antifungal susceptibility test results for selected species of *Candida* isolated during prospective, sentinel surveillance in Spain from June 2008 to June 2009

When we considered the *C. glabrata* isolates obtained during the study only the 81.33% of them were were susceptible to fluconazole and 97.76% were susceptible to voriconazole, but on the contrary, 97.93% and 98.96% of the isolates of *C. albicans* were susceptible to fluconazole and voriconazole respectively. The proportion of isolates that was resistant to the studied azole drugs was comparable with that observed in the other recently published studies. (Messer et al., 2009, Pemán et al., 2011).

The antifungal activities of voriconazole, fluconazole, amphotericin B, caspofungin and anidulafungin against the 984 *Candida spp* isolated during the study period are summarized in Table 4. Among the azole compounds, voriconazole was the most active drug overall with an MIC90 of 0.25 μg/ml. Against *C. albicans, C. parapsilosis* and *C. tropicalis* isolates, voriconazole (MIC90 range 0.03-0.25 μg/ml) was much more active than fluconazole (MIC90, 2-4). Although these differences in the drug activity, both azole compounds showed lower MICs for fluconazole and voriconazole for the species mentioned before when compared to *C. glabrata* and *C. krusei* isolates. Despite this good susceptibility profile, we found five *Candida albicans* isolates with a MIC greater than 4 μg/ml to voriconazole and two *C. krusei* isolates that had a voriconazole MIC of 2 ug/ ml. All these isolates were also resistant to fluconazole.

We found that there was a statistically significant moderate linear correlation between fluconazole and voriconazole MICs (r = 0.574; $P \leq 0.01$). having higher voriconazole MICs those isolates from patients who received fluconazole before the candidemia episode when compared to those without previous exposure to fluconazole (MIC90s of 0.25 μg/ml and 0.06 μg/ml, respectively; $P \leq 0.05$

Table 5 summarize the risk factors we identified during the study with a candidemia episode due to an isolate with decreased susceptibility (SDD or resistant) to fluconazole using univariate statistical techniques.

	No of isolates (%) susceptible to fluconazole	No. of isolates (%) with decreased susceptibility or resistant to fluconazole	P - value
Neoplasia	27 (2.95)	6 (8.70)	≤ 0.01
Neutropenia	37 (4.04)	11(15.94)	≤ 0.01
Prior fluconazole use	27 (2.95)	10 (14.49)	≤ 0.01

[a] Only statistically significant variables are summarized in the table

Table 5. Summary of univariate statistical analysis between fluconazole susceptible isolates vs. resistant or SDD ones

We found that this condition was associated with neoplasia (9% versus 3%; $P \leq 0.01$), current neutropenia (16% versus 4%; $P \leq 0.01$), and prior fluconazole use (14% versus 3%; $P \leq 0.001$). These independent factors identified using the univariate statistical approach, were analyzed more deeply using a repeated measures logistic regression model. We obtained significant results for neoplasia (odds ratio, 2.9; 95% confidence interval, 1.4 to 5.9; $P \leq 0.05$) and prior use of fluconazole (odds ratio, 3.8; 95% confidence interval, 1.7 to 8.2; $P \leq 0.01$). (Table 6).

	Odds ratio	95 percent confidence Limits	P - value
Neoplasia	2.9	1.4 - 5.9	≤ 0.05
Prior fluconazole use	3.8	1.7 - 8.2	≤ 0.01

[a] Only statistically significant variables are summarized in the table.

Table 6. Summary of multivariate statistical analysis of risk factors for candidemia caused by fluconazole susceptible isolates vs. resistant or SDD ones [a]

Caspofungin and anidulafungin resistance was low (16 cases for caspofungin and 8 cases for anidulafungin) (Table 4). Despite this low rate of in vitro resistance to echinocandins of the isolates studied MICs from *C. parapsilosis* and *C. guilliermondi* were higher compared to the MIC obtained from other *Candida spp.* as it has been described in others studies.

5. Antifungal treatment

At the time of diagnosis and inclusion in this study, 122 case patients (12.3%) were receiving a systemic antifungal agent and were considered breakthrough infections (fluconazole, 78 patients, amphotericin B, 31 patients, itraconazole and voriconazole, 3 patient each; and echinocandins, 5 patients). Although the reason for this high rate of breakthrough infections is not clear, it is possible that other factors besides the antifungal resistance have got a role in the explanation of this phenomenon. A deep analysis of these 122 cases showed that either the antifungal therapy duration or the election of the antifungal drug was inadequate. A total of 536 case patients (54.5%) received antifungal therapy, started at a median of 3 days from the *Candida* isolation or onset of candidemia.

6. Mortality

The crude mortality rate was 24.10%, but the mortality rate among children was significantly lower. (see Table 3) As it has been described in different studies published in the medical literature candidemia due to *C. parapsilosis* had a lower mortality rate than the rate due other Candida species (Morgan et al., 2005, Pappas et al., 2004, Pemán et al., 2002), but no statistically significant result when analyzing the death rate of patients infected by a susceptible isolate (54%) or a less-susceptible isolate (SDD or resistant) (64%) among patients who received fluconazole as treatment. ($P \leq 0.44$).

7. Discussion and remarks

This prospective candidemia surveillance study represents one of the largest multicenter studies conducted in Spain and provide one of the most representative data on the epidemiology of candidemia to date. The first remarkable finding of our study was the higher incidence of candidemia than those reported from centers located in the Northern Hemisphere which ranged between 0.28 to 0.96 per 1,000 admissions (Banerjee et al., 1991, Doczi et al., 2002, Marchetti et al., 2002, Pfaller et al., 1998, Pfaller et al., 2004, Richet et al., 2002, Sandven et al., 1998, Tortorano et al., 2002, Tortorano et al., 2004) and including those published before in Spain (0.76 to 0.81 per 1,000 admissions) (Almirante et al., 2005, Alonso-Valle et al., 2003, Pemán et al., 2002, Pemán et al., 2011, San Miguel et al., 2005). Although the reasons for this high rate are not entirely clear, it is possible that this may be related to a combination of multiple factors, including differences in medical care resources, transplantation programs, implementation of infection control measures in hospitals, empirical antifungal therapy and prophylaxis for high-risk patients. Another possibility is that our series may not reflect the current trends, but the data from a prospective study held in Spain and recently published by Peman *et al.* support our data (Pemán et al., 2011, Pfaller & Diekema, 2007) (see Table 7).

Country and period	Total number of isolates	% of total by most representative species				
		C. albicans	*C. parapsilosis*	*C. tropicalis*	*C. glabrata*	*C. krusei*
USA 1992-1993	837	52	21	10	12	4
USA 1993-1995	79	56	15	10	15	-
USA 1995-1997	1593	46	14	12	20	2
USA 1995-1998	934	53	10	12	20	3
USA 1998-2000	935	45	13	12	24	2
USA 2001-2004	2773	51	14	7	22	2
USA 2008-2009	1354	48	17	10	18	2
Canada 1992-94	415	69	10	7	8	1
Latin America 1995-1996	145	37	25	24	4	1
Latin America 2001-2004	1565	50	16	20	7	2
Asia-Pacific 2001-2004	1344	56	16	14	10	2
Taiwan 1994-2000	1095	50	14	21	12	<1
Europe 1992-94	249	49	11	11	10	9
Europe 1997-99	2089	56	13	7	14	2
Europe 2001-2004	2515	60	12	9	10	5
Norway 1991-2003	1415	70	6	7	13	2
Denmark 2003-2004	307	63	4	4	20	3
Spain 2002-2003	351	51	23	10	9	4
Spain 2001-2006	1997	47	19	10	12	5
Spain 2008-2009	984	49	21	13	11	2
Spain 2009-2010	1377	45	29	12	8	2

Table 7. Summary of geographical differences in species distribution in Candida BSI isolates. (Adapted and modified from Pemán et al., 2001 and Pfaller & Diekema, 2007).

Despite this fact, it seems that probably a combination of factors may have affected the overall rates of fungemia cases in Spain. The differences appeared in the average age of our patients when compared to other surveillance series from the United States (Ostrosky-Zeichner et al., 2003, Pappas et al., 2003), are probably due to the high proportion of children in our study, especially in the Spanish hospitals located in the Southern part of the country (32% of children in the Spanish hospitals from the Southern part of the country compared to 9% described in the study from the United States) (data not shown). Therefore, this condition reflects that there are great differences among patients of different geographical locations as it was mentioned in the introduction and the demographical composition and lastly the risk factors, could be very different from one population to another. (Table 7). In fact, the number of cases of invasive candidemia was not homogeneous across the country., the distribution of the clinical isolates obtained during the study period along four different geographical areas in Spain,. (North, Center, East and South). *C. albicans* covers almost half (49.08%) of the global cases, remaining as the most frequently isolated specie, but the rates between the four different areas were not homogenous., for instance, in the Southern part of the country the rate of isolates of C. albicans (39.2%) was similar to the one of *C. parapsilosis* (37.4%).

Some studies have reported a shift in the etiology of candidemia reporting an increase of candidemia cases caused by non-*albicans Candida* species during the last decade (Colombo et al., 2006, Richet et al., 2002, Tortorano et al., 2004) (Table 7). Although C. albicans remain the most frequently isolated specie, reasons for the emergence of non-*albicans* species remain unclear, but some medical conditions may explain increasing incidence of candidemia due to non-*albicans* species. It has been noted in previous reports that infections due to *C. tropicalis* candidemia is associated with neoplasia and neutropenia (Komshian et al., 1989) and those attributable to *C. parapsilosis* are often associated with the presence of intravascular catheters and are not influenced by exposure to fluconazole or other antifungal agents (Clark et al., 2004, Girmenia et al., 1996, Levy et al., 1998, Sandven et al., 1998). The last situation, may us to consider *C. parapsilosis* as an exogenous pathogen and breaches of catheter care and of infection control practice should be investigated and revised within institutions where this species has become a common blood culture isolate.

The increasing incidence some of non-*albicans Candida* species with reduced susceptibility to azoles, such as *C. glabrata,* creates new therapeutic challenges and leads to another important question such as the influence of previous antifungal therapy in the development of non-*albicans* species candidemia. Recent studies, such as those published by Marr *et al.* and Tortorano *et al.* had addressed this question and showed interesting results about the association with previous exposure to azoles and the risk of development of fungemias due to *C. krusei* and / or *C. glabrata* (Marr et al., 2000, Tortorano et al., 2004). In fact, the differences in antifungal susceptibilities among isolates between different regions in Spain was almost entirely attributable to high-level resistance to azoles observed among *C. glabrata* and *C. krusei* isolates (Table 4).

We are not aware of these epidemiological changes mentioned in the paragraph above and our findings from our study are supportive of them. *C. parapsilosis* fungemia account for the large majority of non-*albicans* species (in the same manner that that been described for other European countries) and candidemia due to *C. krusei* is rare in Spain as it has been described in other series (Almirante et al., 2005, Alonso-Valle et al., 2003, Ostrosky-Zeichner et al., 2003, Pemán et al., 2002, Pemán et al., 2011, Tortorano et al., 2004). The explanation for this species distribution in Spain which is more or less similar to other Latin American countries is not clear and perhaps many factors are involved. However, this species distribution has got a great importance in the developing of therapeutic schemes and in the prevention of antifungal resistance.

While most non-albicans *Candida* species are associated with high fluconazole minimum inhibitory concentrations (MIC), *C. parapsilosis* is typically susceptible to most antifungals, although is associated with higher echinocandin MIC that vary between different agents. Moreover, the rate of persistently positive fungemia in patients treated with caspofungin was reported as almost double for *C. parapsilosis* versus other Candida species. Even more, if we consider clinical patients at risk of suffering a candidemia episode, such as immunocompromised patients, where clinical responses are poorer the picture is not good. Summarizing, we are concerned about the use of echinocandins alone based on the identification of non-albicans *Candida* specie. Grouping these agents into one treatment scheme is difficult due to the variability not only in the susceptibility of the isolates, as well as the microbiological responses seen between different echinocandins.

Regarding the susceptibility of the studied isolates, antifungal resistance was an infrequent finding in our study and was restricted to a few isolates, and none of them were resistant to amphotericin B. This condition is similar to the findings published in three recent studies (Almirante et al., 2005, Messer et al., 2009, Pemán et al., 2011). Our proportion of fluconazole-resistant isolates (6.32%) was low, similarly to the rate observed with Spanish (Almirante et al., 2005, Pemán et al., 2011) European (5.2%) and North American isolates (6.6%) (Messer et al., 2009, Richardson & Lass-Flörl et al., 2008) (see Table 7). Mixing the ideas exposed above we can argue that the differences in the activity and susceptibility of the antifungal compounds studied suggest that azole drugs and echinocandins have got a complementary susceptibility profile. While azoles has got excellent in vitro activity to *C. albicans, C. parapsilosis* and *C. tropicalis* bloodstream isolates, echinocandins showed excellent activity against *C. glabrata* and *C. krusei* which are are associated with higher azole MICs. On the contrary, species with high MICs to echinocandins such as *C. parapsilosis* and *C. guilliermondii* showed excellent activity to azole agents. (Table 8).

Specie of *Candida*	Susceptibility to antifungal agent				
	Amphotericin B	Fluconazole	Voriconazole	Caspofungin	Anidulafungin
C. albicans	S	S	S	S	S
C. parapsilosis	S	S	S	S - I	S - I
C. glabrata	S - NS	S - SDD - R	S - NS	S	S
C. tropicalis	S	S	S - NS	S	S
C. krusei	S	R	S	S	S

[a] S, susceptible; NS, non-susceptible (intermediate for CLSI M27-A2 clinical breakpoints); SDD, sensitive dose-dependent; R, resistant.

[b] The clinical breakpoints adopted in this table are those reflected in the CLSI M27-A2 methodology. No new clinical breakpoints or epidemiological cut-offs were used, in order to make the data comparable to the one reflected in our work.

Table 8. Summary of commonly associated in-vitro susceptibility profiles for *Candida* spp. BSI isolates. (Adapted and modified from Richardson & Lass-Flörl, 2008) [a, b]

These ideas are of great importance because previous exposure to fluconazole was a strong and independent factor associated with candidemia caused by fluconazole non-susceptible isolates as it had been reported previously by Marr *et al.* and Lin and colleagues and higher voriconazole MICs tended to be associated with prior exposure to fluconazole. Although these obtained results are statistically significant, they must be taken with some caution because the low resistant proportion of isolates in our study. However, they depict a situation of concern and illustrate the potential problem of cross-resistance between azoles with a direct impact in treatment failure and the outcome of the patient. Moreover, the potential for voriconazole resistant *C. glabrata* to emerge as a threat in people receiving voriconazole therapy and or prophylaxis has been raised in reports of breakthrough infections (Imhof et al., 2004, Pfaller et al., 2004).

Despite these concerning matters exposed above, voriconazole was the azole which exhibited the best in vitro antifungal activity in our study, and only one of six fluconazole-resistant isolates was cross-resistant to voriconazole. The combination of a third generation azole such as voriconazole or posaconazole with an echinocandin could be of benefit for some patients, especially in those with persistent candidemia.

The crude mortality rate observed in our study was similar to that reported in other series (Almirante et al., 2005, Colombo et al., 2006, Gudlaugsson et al., 2003, Pappas et al., 2003, Pfaller et al., 2004). Adults had higher mortality rates than pediatric patients (24.10% to 16%). Similar to other reports, patients with *C. parapsilosis* candidemia had the lowest death rates (Nucci et al., 1998, Pappas et al., 2003).

Summarizing, the epidemiological and susceptible data described along the text, document important differences and similarities in the epidemiology of candidemia in Spain compared to updated reports from other countries. This report shows that candidemia is a source of significant morbidity and mortality with high associated healthcare costs. Although our high rates of candidemia may be related to many factors, reasons for them are not clear and further study is necessary. Determining them may lead to identify potential measures that can help in disease prevention. In addition, our data support that fluconazole non-susceptibility could be associated with prior fluconazole exposure and suggest that such exposure could lead to other new azoles cross-resistance and complicate the clinical outcome of some patients.

8. Acknowledgments

To the Spanish Candidemia Surveillance Group composed in this study, by 40 hospitals distributed in four diferents Areas of Spain, North, Center, East and South.

9. References

[1] Al-Jasser, A. M., and N. A. Elkhizzi. 2004. Distribution of *Candida* species among bloodstream isolates. *Saudi Med. J.* 25:566–569.

[2] Almirante, B., D. Rodriguez, B. J. Park, M. Cuenca-Estrella, A. M. Planes, M. Almela, J. Mensa, F. Sanchez, J. Ayats, M. Gimenez, P. Saballs, S. K. Fridkin, J. Morgan, J. L. Rodriguez-Tudela, D. W. Warnock, and A. Pahissa. 2005. Epidemiology and predictors of mortality in cases of *Candida* bloodstream infection: results from population-based surveillance, Barcelona, Spain, from 2002 to 2003. *J. Clin. Microbiol.* 43:1829–1835.

[3] Alonso-Valle, H., O. Acha, J. D. Garcia-Palomo, C. Farinas-Alvarez, C. Fernandez-Mazarrasa, and M. C. Farinas. 2003. Candidemia in a tertiary care hospital: epidemiology and factors influencing mortality. *Eur. J. Clin. Microbiol. Infect. Dis.* 22:254–257.

[4] Antunes, A. G., A. C. Pasqualotto, M. C. Diaz, P. A. d'Azevedo, and L. C. Severo. 2004. Candidemia in a Brazilian tertiary care hospital: species distribution and antifungal susceptibility patterns. *Rev. Inst. Med. Trop. Sao Paulo* 46:239–241.

[5] Asmundsdottir, L. R., H. Erlendsdottir, and M. Gottfredsson. 2002. Increasing incidence of candidemia: results from a 20-year nationwide study in Iceland. *J. Clin. Microbiol.* 40:3489–3492.

[6] Banerjee, S. N., T. G. Emori, D. H. Culver, R. P. Gaynes, W. R. Jarvis, T. Horan, J. R. Edwards, J. Tolson, T. Henderson, W. J. Martone, et al. 1991. Secular trends in nosocomial primary bloodstream infections in the United States, 1980–1989. *Am. J. Med.* 91:86S–89S.

[7] Berenguer J, M Buck, F Witebsky, *et al.* 1993. Lysis-centrifugation blood cultures in the detection of tissue-proven invasive candidiasis. disseminated versus single-organ infection. *Diagn Microbiol Infect Dis.* 7:103-109.)

[8] Blumberg, H. M., W. R. Jarvis, J. M. Soucie, J. E. Edwards, J. E. Patterson, M. A. Pfaller, M. S. Rangel-Frausto, M. G. Rinaldi, L. Saiman, R. T. Wiblin, R. P. Wenzel, et al. 2001. Risk factors for candidal bloodstream infections in surgical intensive care unit patients: the NEMIS prospective multicenter study. *Clin. Infect. Dis.* 33:177–186.

[9] Clark, T. A., S. A. Slavinski, J. Morgan, T. Lott, B. A. Arthington-Skaggs, M. E. Brandt, R. M. Webb, M. Currier, R. H. Flowers, S. K. Fridkin, and R. A. Hajjeh. 2004. Epidemiologic and molecular characterization of an outbreak of *Candida parapsilosis* bloodstream infections in a community hospital. *J. Clin. Microbiol.* 42:4468–4472.

[10] L. Colombo, M. Nucci, B. J. Park, S. A. Nouér, B. Arthington-Skaggs, D. A. da Matta, D. Warnock, and J. Morgan for the Brazilian Network Candidemia Study. 2006. Epidemiology of candidemia in Brazil: a nationwide sentinel surveillance of candidemia in eleven medical centers *J. Clin. Microbiol.* 44:2816–2823.

[11] Costa, S. F., I. Marinho, E. A. Araujo, A. E. Manrique, E. A. Medeiros, and A. S. Levin. 2000. Nosocomial fungaemia: a 2-year prospective study. *J. Hosp. Infect.* 45:69–72.

[12] Diekema, D. J., S. A. Messer, A. B. Brueggemann, S. L. Coffman, G. V. Doern, L. A. Herwaldt, and M. A. Pfaller. 2002. Epidemiology of candidemia: 3-year results from the emerging infections and the epidemiology of Iowa organisms study. *J. Clin. Microbiol.* 40:1298–1302.

[13] Doczi, I., E. Dosa, E. Hajdu, and E. Nagy. 2002. Aetiology and antifungal susceptibility of yeast bloodstream infections in a Hungarian university hospital between 1996 and 2000. *J. Med. Microbiol.* 51:677–681.

[14] Fraser, V. J., M. Jones, J. Dunkel, S. Storfer, G. Medoff, and W. C. Dunagan. 1992. Candidemia in a tertiary care hospital: epidemiology, risk factors, and predictors of mortality. *Clin. Infect. Dis.* 15:414–421.

[15] Garbino, J., L. Kolarova, P. Rohner, D. Lew, P. Pichna, and D. Pittet. 2002. Secular trends of candidemia over 12 years in adult patients at a tertiary care hospital. *Medicine* (Baltimore) 81:425–433.

[16] Girmenia, C., P. Martino, B. F. De, G. Gentile, M. Boccanera, M. Monaco, G. Antonucci, and A. Cassone. 1996. Rising incidence of *Candida parapsilosis* fungemia in patients with hematologic malignancies: clinical aspects, predisposing factors, and differential pathogenicity of the causative strains. *Clin. Infect. Dis.* 23:506–514.

[17] Gudlaugsson, O., S. Gillespie, K. Lee, B. J. Vande, J. Hu, S. Messer, L. Herwaldt, M. Pfaller, and D. Diekema. 2003. Attributable mortality of nosocomial candidemia, revisited. Clin. Infect. Dis. 37:1172–1177. 19. Hsueh, P. R., L. J. Teng, P. C. Yang, S. W. Ho, and K. T. Luh. 2002. Emergence of nosocomial candidemia at a teaching hospital in Taiwan from 1981 to 2000: increased susceptibility of *Candida* species to fluconazole. *Microb. Drug Resist.* 8:311–319.

[18] Imhof, A., S. A. Balajee, D. N. Fredricks, J. A. Englund, and K. A. Marr. 2004. Breakthrough fungal infections in stem cell transplant recipients receiving voriconazole. *Clin. Infect. Dis.*39:743–746.

[19] Kao, A. S., M. E. Brandt, W. R. Pruitt, L. A. Conn, B. A. Perkins, D. S. Stephens, W. S. Baughman, A. L. Reingold, G. A. Rothrock, M. A. Pfaller, R. W. Pinner, and R. A. Hajjeh. 1999. The epidemiology of candidemia in two United States cities: results of a population-based active surveillance. *Clin. Infect. Dis.* 29:1164–1170.

[20] Komshian, S. V., A. K. Uwaydah, J. D. Sobel, and L. R. Crane. 1989. Fungemia caused by *Candida* species and *Torulopsis glabrata* in the hospitalized patient: frequency, characteristics, and evaluation of factors influencing outcome. *Rev. Infect. Dis.* 11:379–390.

[21] Levy, I., L. G. Rubin, S. Vasishtha, V. Tucci, and S. K. Sood. 1998. Emergence of *Candida parapsilosis* as the predominant species causing candidemia in children. *Clin. Infect. Dis.* 26:1086–1088.

[22] Luzzati, R., G. Amalfitano, L. Lazzarini, F. Soldani, S. Bellino, M. Solbiati, M. C. Danzi, S. Vento, G. Todeschini, C. Vivenza, and E. Concia. 2000. Nosocomial candidemia in non-neutropenic patients at an Italian tertiary care hospital. *Eur. J. Clin. Microbiol. Infect. Dis.* 19:602–607.

[23] Marchetti, O., J. Bille, U. Fluckiger, P. Eggimann, C. Ruef, J. Garbino, T. Calandra, M. P. Glauser, M. G. Tauber, and D. Pittet. 2004. Epidemiology of candidemia in Swiss tertiary care hospitals: secular trends, 1991–2000. Clin. Infect. Dis. 38:311–320.

[24] Marr, K. A., K. Seidel, T. C. White, and R. A. Bowden. 2000. Candidemia in allogeneic blood and marrow transplant recipients: evolution of risk factors after the adoption of prophylactic fluconazole. *J. Infect. Dis.* 181:309–316.

[25] Messer S.A. Moet G.J. Kirvy J. T. and Jones R.N. 2009. Activity of contemporary antifungal agents, including the novel echinocandin anidulafungin, tested against *Candida* spp. *Cryptococcus spp.* and *Aspergillus* spp.: Report from the SENTRY antimicrobial surveillance program (2006 to 2007) *J. Clin. Microbiol.* 47 (6): 1942-1946.

[26] Morgan, J., M. I. Meltzer, B. D. Plikaytis, A. N. Sofair, S. Huie-White, S. Wilcox, L. H. Harrison, E. C. Seaberg, R. A. Hajjeh, and S. M. Teutsch. 2005. Excess mortality, hospital stay, and cost due to candidemia: a case-control study using data from population-based candidemia surveillance. *Infect. Control Hosp. Epidemiol.* 26:540–547.

[27] National Committee for Clinical Laboratory Standards. 2002. Reference method for broth dilution antifungal susceptibility testing of yeasts; approved standard, 2nd ed. Document M27-A2. National Committee For Clinical Laboratory Standards, Wayne, Pa.

[28] Nguyen, M. H., C. J. Clancy, V. L. Yu, Y. C. Yu, A. J. Morris, D. R. Snydman, D. A. Sutton, and M. G. Rinaldi. 1998. Do in vitro susceptibility data predict the microbiologic response to amphotericin B? Results of a prospective study of patients with *Candida* fungemia. *J. Infect. Dis.* 177:425–430.

[29] Nucci, M., A. L. Colombo, F. Silveira, R. Richtmann, R. Salomao, M. L. Branchini, and N. Spector. 1998. Risk factors for death in patients with candidemia. *Infect. Control Hosp. Epidemiol.* 19:846–850.

[30] Ostrosky-Zeichner, L., J. H. Rex, P. G. Pappas, R. J. Hamill, R. A. Larsen, H. W. Horowitz, W. G. Powderly, N. Hyslop, C. A. Kauffman, J. Cleary, J. E. Mangino, and J. Lee. 2003. Antifungal susceptibility survey of 2,000 bloodstream *Candida* isolates in the United States. *Antimicrob. Agents Chemother.* 47:3149-3154.

[31] Pappas, P. G., J. H. Rex, J. Lee, R. J. Hamill, R. A. Larsen, W. Powderly, C. A. Kauffman, N. Hyslop, J. E. Mangino, S. Chapman, H. W. Horowitz, J. E. Edwards, and W. E. Dismukes. 2003. A prospective observational study of candidemia: epidemiology, therapy, and influences on mortality in hospitalized adult and pediatric patients. *Clin. Infect. Dis.* 37:634–643.

[32] Pemán J, Cantón E, Orero A, Viudes A, Frasquet J, Gobernado M. 2002. Epidemiology of candidemia in Spain - Multicenter study. *Rev Iberoam Micol.* 19(1):30-35.

[33] Pemán J, Cantón E, Miñana JJ, Florez JA, Echeverria J, Ortega DN, Alarcón JM, Fontanals D, Sard BG, Moreno BB, Torroba L, Ayats J, Pérez MÁ, Fernández MA, Reus FS, Natal IF, García GR, Ezpeleta G, Martín-Mazuelos E, Iglesias I, Rezusta A, de Ocariz IR, Nieto AG; el Grupo de Estudio FUNGEMYCA. 2011. Changes in the epidemiology of fungaemia and fluconazole susceptibility of blood isolates during the last 10 years in Spain: results from the FUNGEMYCA study]. *Rev Iberoam Micol.* Apr-Jun;28(2):91-9

[34] Pfaller, M. A., R. N. Jones, G. V. Doern, H. S. Sader, R. J. Hollis, and S. A. Messer for the SENTRY Participant Group. 1998. International surveillance of bloodstream infections due to *Candida* species: frequency of occurrence and antifungal susceptibilities of isolates collected in 1997 in the United States, Canada, and South America for the SENTRY Program. *J. Clin. Microbiol.* 36:1886–1889.

[35] Pfaller, M. A., S. A. Messer, L. Boyken, S. Tendolkar, R. J. Hollis, and D. J. Diekema. 2004. Geographic variation in the susceptibilities of invasive isolates of *Candida glabrata* to seven systemically active antifungal agents: a global assessment from the ARTEMIS Antifungal Surveillance Program conducted in 2001 and 2002. *J. Clin. Microbiol.* 42:3142–3146.

[36] Pfaller M. A. and D. J. Diekema. 2007. Epidemiology of invasive candidiasis: a persistent public health problem. *Clin. Microbiol. Rev.* 20: 133 –163.

[37] Richardson M. And C. Lass-Flörl. 2008. Changing epidemiology of systemic fungal infections. *Clin. Microbiol. Infect.* 14 (Suppl. 4): 5–24.

[38] Richet, H., P. Roux, C. C. Des, Y. Esnault, and A. Andremont. 2002. Candidemia in French hospitals: incidence rates and characteristics. *Clin. Microbiol. Infect.* 8:405-412.

[39] Sandven, P., L. Bevanger, A. Digranes, P. Gaustad, H. H. Haukland, and M. Steinbakk. 1998. Constant low rate of fungemia in Norway, 1991 to 1996. The Norwegian Yeast Study Group. *J. Clin. Microbiol.* 36:3455–3459.

[40] San Miguel, L. G., J. Cobo, E. Otheo, A. Sanchez-Sousa, V. Abraira, and S. Moreno. 2005. Secular trends of candidemia in a large tertiary-care hospital from 1988 to 2000: emergence of *Candida parapsilosis. Infect. Control Hosp. Epidemiol.* 26:548–552.

[41] Silva, V., M. C. Diaz, and N. Febre. 2004. Invasive fungal infections in Chile: a multicenter study of fungal prevalence and susceptibility during a 1-year period. *Med. Mycol.* 42:333–339.

[42] Tortorano, A. M., E. Biraghi, A. Astolfi, C. Ossi, M. Tejada, C. Farina, S. Perin, C. Bonaccorso, C. Cavanna, A. Raballo, and A. Grossi. 2002. European Confederation

of Medical Mycology (ECMM) prospective survey of candidaemia: report from one Italian region. *J. Hosp. Infect.* 51:297–304.

[43] Tortorano, A. M., J. Peman, H. Bernhardt, L. Klingspor, C. C. Kibbler, O. Faure, E. Biraghi, E. Canton, K. Zimmermann, S. Seaton, and R. Grillot. 2004. Epidemiology of candidaemia in Europe: results of 28-month European Confederation of Medical Mycology (ECMM) hospital-based surveillance study. *Eur. J. Clin. Microbiol. Infect. Dis.* 23:317–322.

[44] Trick, W. E., S. K. Fridkin, J. R. Edwards, R. A. Hajjeh, and R. P. Gaynes. 2002. Secular trend of hospital-acquired candidemia among intensive care unit patients in the United States during 1989–1999. *Clin. Infect. Dis.* 35: 627–630.

[45] Viudes, A., J. Peman, E. Canton, P. Ubeda, J. L. Lopez-Ribot, and M. Gobernado. 2002. Candidemia at a tertiary-care hospital: epidemiology, treatment, clinical outcome and risk factors for death. *Eur. J. Clin. Microbiol. Infect. Dis.* 21:767–774.

[46] Voss, A., J. A. Kluytmans, J. G. Koeleman, L. Spanjaard, C. M. Vandenbroucke-Grauls, H. A. Verbrugh, M. C. Vos, A. Y. Weersink, J. A. Hoogkamp-Korstanje, and J. F. Meis. 1996. Occurrence of yeast bloodstream infections between 1987 and 1995 in five Dutch university hospitals. *Eur. J. Clin. Microbiol. Infect. Dis.* 15:909–912.

2

Epidemiology of Dermatomycoses in Poland over the Past Decades

Katarzyna Kalinowska
Wroclaw Medical University
Poland

1. Introduction

Dermatophytes are keratinophilic and keratinolytic fungi. They are characterized by high affinity to keratin-containing tissues, what make them responsible for superficial mycoses of skin (*tinea faciei, tinea barbae, tinea corporis, tinea cruris, tinea manuum* or *tinea pedis*), nails (*onychomycosis, tinea unguium*) and hair (*tinea capitis*) (Kalinowska et al., 2009a).

Infections caused by dermatophyte fungi are very serious problem, not only clinical, but also epidemiological and therapeutic. The incidence of skin, hair and nail diseases does not depend on sex, age or social status.

2. Short characteristic of dermatophytes

There are many species of dermatophytes causing mycoses, so it is very important to assay them properly through mycological examination. Correct identification of the pathogen responsible for disease allows choosing a right treatment for patient.

Natural reservoir of dermatophytes is soil and keratin contained in soil is used as main nutrient for these fungi. However, evolutionary progress adapted these microorganisms to a various environments, so they generated ability to metabolize keratin derived not only from soil (Dworacka-Kaszak, 2004).

For that reason dermatophytes, with regard to their habitat, may be divided into antropophilic, zoophilic and geofilic species. For antrophophilic dermatophytes natural reservoir and carrier is human, zoophilic dermatophytes grow on domestic and stock animals and geophilic dermatophytes are found in soils (Adamski & Batura-Gabryel, 2007).

In laboratory practice dermatophyte fungi belonging to three genera (*Trichophyton, Microsporum, Epidermophyton*), are known. *Trichophyton* and *Microsporum* genera are the most numerous and diverse, there are over 40 species belonging to these two taxonomic groups. *Epidermophyton* genus has only one representative – *Epidermophyton floccosum* species.

The genera *Trichophyton* is numerous and diverse, for example, in the Lower Silesia region, in years 2003 - 2007, these fungi were isolated in 92% of all cultures (Jankowska-Konsur et al., 2011).

In Poland, there are only few *Trichophyton* species, which are common, including:

- *Trichophyton rubrum* - antropophilic dermatophyte, distributed worldwide, usually specific to human, but infections in animals also have been reported. It may be the cause of practically all infections of body surface areas (with exception of fungal infections of the scalp). Most commonly it causes onychomycosis and athlete`s foot (*tinea pedis*). It may also cause infections of glabrous skin (*tinea corporis, tinea faciei*), groin (*tinea cruris*), hands (*tinea manuum*) or nails (*tinea ungiuim*). This fungus causes persistent, chronic infections.
- *Trichophyton mentagrophytes* - zoophilic dermatophyte, cosmopolitan fungus, distributed worldwide. It causes infections in animals (cats, dogs, rabbits, guinea pigs, rodents, hedgehogs) as well as in human. Most commonly it causes infections of glabrous skin (*tinea corporis, tinea faciei*) and scalp infections (*tinea capitis*). Lesions often proceed with a large inflammatory reactions.
- *Trichophyton tonsurans* - antropophilic species, usually specific to human, practically cosmopolitan. Most commonly it causes infections of the scalp (*tinea capitis*) and it may also cause infections of glabrous skin (*tinea corporis*), especially in the "shower area" - on neck, shoulder, back, buttocks, and feet, when inoculum is washed off from head on the other parts of the body, while taking shower. Infections usually proceed with mild inflammatory reaction, but cases with severe inflammatory responses also have been reported. This fungus often causes family and school outbreaks. It is also responsible for infections among wrestlers and judo competitors (*tinea corporis gladiatorum*). This dermatophyte is resistant to the adverse impact of external conditions and it is transferred by asymptomatic carriers.
- *Trichophyton interdigitale* - antropophilic species, distributed worldwide. It causes infections of feet (aspecially in the interdigital spaces) and hands (*tinea manuum*), sometimes it can also infect nails (*tinea unguium*).
- *Trichophyton verrucosum* - zoophilic species, the mostly isolated from cattle, it infects people, who work with these animals (farmers). Cosmopolitan fungus, it causes diseases of exposed parts of the body (*tinea corporis*) and face (*tinea faciei*), beard (*tinea barbae*) or head (*tinea capitis*).
- *Trichophyton violaceum* - antropophilic species, mostly it causes infections of the scalp (*tinea capitis*) and glabrous skin (*tinea corporis*), aspecially in the "shower area". It can also cause onychomycosis. It is specific to human, but it also can be pathogenic for animals. It is the cause of family and institutional outbreaks.
- *Trichophyton schoenleinii* - antropophilic species, it causes *favus*. Nowadays is practically unique.

Among *Microsporum* genera, only few species are common in lab-practice:

- *Microsporum canis* - zoophilic species, cosmopolitan, distributed worldwide. It is very contagious aspecially for young cats and dogs. In human it causes infections of the scalp (*tinea capitis*) and beard (*tinea barbae*) or infections of glabrous skin or face (*tinea corporis, tinea faciei*).
- *Microsporum audouinii* - antropophilic species, cosmopolitian, however, the incidence of fungal infections caused by this pathogen in Poland is very small. It causes infections of the scalp (*tinea capitis*), glabrous skin (*tinea corporis*), face (*tinea faciei*), affecting mostly school-age children (boys:girls=4:1), however cases of dermatomycoses in adults,

caused by *Microsporum audouinii* also were described. Although it is human pathogen, it was isolated from fur of guinea pigs and rarely, from dog`s fur.

- *Microsporum gypseum* - geophilic species, ubiquitous, isolated from soils worldwide. Most exposed to infections are people, who cultivate the soil (farmers, gardeners), percentage of males prevails over females. Sometimes infection could be transmitted from animals . In human it causes infections of the scalp (*tinea capitis*) and glabrous skin (*tinea corporis*).
- *Microsporum nanuum* - zoophilic species, isolated also from soil. It causes infections among breeding cattle, mostly in pigs. In human it causes infections of the glabrous skin (*tinea corporis*) and the scalp (*tinea capitis*) proceeding with or without severe inflammation.
- *Microsporum persicolor* - zoophilic species, cosmopolitan. In human it causes infections of the scalp (*tinea capitis*), glabrous skin (*tinea corporis*) and feet (*tinea pedis*). Infections proceed with significant inflammatory reaction.

The genera *Epidermophyton* has only one representative, quite often isolated form lesions:

- *Epidemophyton floccosum* - antropophilic species, cosmopolitan. In human it causes mostly infections of the groin (*tinea cruris*), rarely of glabrous skin (*tinea corporis*), feet (*tinea pedis*) and very rarely of toenais (*onychomycosis*).

2.1 Methods of pathogen transmission – a short description

Dermatophytes are keratinophilic fungi, which parasitize on corneous structures, such as stratum corneum, hair or nails (Kobierzycka et al., 2005). Dermatophyte species are equipped with numerous enzymes, enabling them to survive on the skin and its appendages, because they have a proteolytic, keratinolytic and lipolytic activity. Furthermore the skin environment is conducive to dermatophytes because the corneal layer lacks blood vessels making it difficult to contact with immunologically competent cells and activate the defense mechanisms. On the surface of the epidermis are proteins, carbohydrates and micronutrients (including iron ions), which may provide substrates for the metabolism of fungi and help them to survive. Of great importance may also be some specific anatomic regions of the skin, greatly facilitating the colonization by fungi. Scalp hair can therefore arrest arthrospores spreaded by air. Similarly, spores are arrested in the hyponychium under or in the interdigital spaces, or in the folds of the skin where additionally oclusion helps them to develop (Dworacka-Kaszak, 2004). The spores are particularly resistant to environmental conditions, such as variable temperature and drying (Hryncewicz-Gwozdz et al., 2005; Kobierzycka et al., 2005). It is known that they can survive outside the host organism and colonize the skin and its appendages under favorable conditions, for example, in warm and humid environment, with increased amounts of CO_2, which prevails in the poorly sheered shoes, it can lead to growth of the fungi and invasion of the skin structures.

To narrowly understand epidemiology of dermatomycoses, methods of pathogen transmission, are described below.

The sources of dermatophyte fungi infection are: human, animals and soil.

Infection with antropophilic dermatophytes may happen through direct contact with infected person, moreover spores of dermatophyte fungi can survive on skin and its appendixes without causing the disease (asymptomatic carrier) (Adamski & Batura-Gabryel, 2007).

Infection may occur also through some objects on which infectious material can be found (stratum corneum or hair with spores of fungi). The source of trunk, groin or extremities infections may be clothes, underwear or towels and sponges. Scalp diseases may happen through using the same brushes or combs. Shoes, socks, accessories for feet care or cosmetic pedicure are often the source of infections of feet and toenails.

Nails diseases are often connected with cosmetic manicure, infection may be a result of unsuitable disinfection of nails care accessories in cosmetic salons.

Also some public places could be potential source of antropophilic dermatomycoses - for example swimming-pools, toilets, showers, hotels, schools and similar (Bolinski et al., 2003, Szepietowski & Baran, 2005).

Recently some cases of *tinea corporis gladiatorum* were described in literature. This type of dermatomycosis is common among wrestlers and judo competitors. The source of infection are athletes and wrestling mats (Hryncewicz-Gwozdz et al., 2011).

Similarly with zoophilic species - transmission of pathogen may happen through direct contact with an infected animal or animal being carrier of fungus. Zoophilic dermatophytes can be also transmited from human to human. The source of infection in children and adults are mostly domestic animals - cats, dogs, hamsters, guinea pigs, rabbits or even some birds. Farmers also often suffer from dermatomycoses transmitted from breeding cattle (pigs, cows, sheep, horses, goats) (Adamski Z & Batura-Gabryel H., 2007).

Infection with geophilic dermatophytes usually happens as a result of contact with soil and it is common among people, who cultivate the soil (gardeners, farmers). The disease more often affect males than females. Working without protective gloves and unsuitable hygiene is conductive for transmission of pathogen. In literature were also described cases of transmission of geophilic dermatophytes through some animals (for example monkeys, mouses, leopards, rats, tigers) and insects (flies). Infection through direct contact with ill peoples occurs rather rarely (Kalinowska et al., 2009b)

2.2 Clinical picture of dermatomycosis

Fungi are present both in the natural environment and in the immediate surroundings of man. The host organism reaction to the infection with these pathogens is different and it depends greatly on what kind of dermatophyte causes it.

The main factor favourable to the development of fungal infection is a disorder of right microclimate of the skin, which is often caused by occlusion (poorly sheered clothes, shoes made of synthetic fabric) and microinjuries. Some diseases like diabetes and circulation disorders are of great importance in the development of mycoses (Macura & Pawlik, 1998).

Clinical pictures of superficial mycoses are diverse, types of fungi infections are:

- *Tinea capitis* - infection of the scalp. When it is caused by antropophilic and zoophilic species ringworm of the scalp reveals the presence of foci of alopecia and scaling. The changes develop on erythematous base, but the severity of the inflammation is very diverse and in some individuals may it be a slight erythema. In extreme cases, the changes are soft with the presence of pustules and inflammatory tumors with pus or yellow crusts. This condition is called deep mycosis (kerion) and is the result of an inflammatory response to the presence of the fungus. Apart from very severe forms of deep fungal infection of the scalp, hair loss is usually transient. Even in the worst cases, regrowth occurs at a surprisingly high proportion. Exception is infection with antropophilic *Trichophyton schoenleinii*, which leads to scarring and permanent alopecia foci formation. Lesions very often are accompanied with itching.

- *Tinea corporis* - infection of the trunk and also extremities. Caused by antropophilic, zoophilic and geophilic species. Fungi, after infection of the skin form colonies and grow centrifugally. Lesions caused by antropophilic species form round or oval patches, which are spreading peripherally, and resolving and disappearing in the middle. In the part of the peripheral states moderate inflammation, redness and slight swelling, and even the production of pustules is seen. Lesions caused by zoophilic species characterize with significant inflammation, are well separated from the healthy skin, with exfoliation on the whole surface. Lesions are very often accompanied with itching.
- *Tinea barbae* - infection of the bearded area of men. Mostly it is caused by zoophilic species. Generally, the infection occurs as a follicular inflammation, or as a cutaneous granulomatous lesion, i.e. a chronic inflammatory reaction. It is one of the causes of folliculitis. Lesions are accompanied with itching. This infection is most common in farmers.
- *Tinea faciei* - infection of the glabrous skin of the face. It is caused by antropophilic and zoophilic species. Itchy lesions appearing on the face may be erythematous with exfoliation in the peripheral part or they may proceed with significant inflammation with the exfoliation on the entire surface.
- *Tinea pedis* - infection of feet and the interdigital spaces. Mostly it is caused by antropohilic species. In the interdigital variety, lesion appear in the folds between 3rd and 4th toes. The lateral surfaces of the toes and the bottom of folds are covered with layers and scales of keratinized epidermis. In the depth of the fold may appear cracks of the skin. Lesions may proceed on the dorsal and the basal surface of toes. There is a slight redness and exfoliation of the skin, and sometimes tiny vesicles and pustules may appear. The course is usually chronic, but it may be subject to intensify. On the plantar surface of feet occur eruptions similar to eczema. There are itchy follicles of various sizes. The course is chronic and recurrent, sometimes severe, however,complicated by purulent secondary infection and secondary prone to allergization.
- *Tinea manuum* - fungal infections of hands, it is caused by antropophilic species. Fungal infection of hands is almost always secondary to athlete's foot. Very rare primary form may develop in the case of occupational exposure to dermatophytes. Dermatophyte infections of hands can take several different clinical forms. The most commonly occurring is hiperkeratotic form, which is characterized by excessive keratosis of hands skin, with the presence of small and very adherent scales on erythematous base. Infectious process is typically subject to the fingertips. Also often coexists nail fungal infection. Less common is intertrigous form.
- *Tinea cruris* - dermatophyte infection of the groin, caused mostly by antropophilic species. In many patients the development of groin ringworm occurs through auto-infection from

feet. It is revealed by the appearance of a typical erythematous lesions associated with exfoliation and itching, which spread on the upper surface of the thighs and crotch.

- *Tinea unguium, Onychomycosis* – dermatophyte infection of the nail plates. Mostly caused by antropophilic and very rarely by geophilic species. Changes within nail plates begin on free edge of nail and can cause excessive callus and fragility, appearance of grooves and fractures on surface of nail, the most often nail plates are turning yellow. Infected, untreated nails undergo gradually diminishing. Toenails are more often infected than fingernails. Fungal infection of toenails is often a result of athlete`s foot.

2.3 Treatment of dermatomycosis

There are many antifungal drugs, allowing for treatment dermatomycoses effectively.

These drugs can be divided to several groups :

- Antifungal antiseptics:

1. Iodine compounds
2. Phenol derrivates
3. Sulphur and its derrivates
4. Alcohol
5. Inorganic acids
6. Organic acids and their derrivates
7. Derrivates of unsaturated fatty acids
8. Aniline dyes
9. Heavy metals compounds
10. Quaternary ammonium hydroxides
11. Quinoline derrivates
12. Benzimidazole derrivates

- Antifungal antibiotics:

1. Polyene antibiotics (Natamycin)
2. Non-polyene antibiotcs (Gryzeofulvin)

- Antifungal chemioterapeutics :

1. Fluorpirimidine derrivates - flucytosine
2. Imidazole derrivates:

a. Azole drugs of the 1st generation - Chlormidazole, Clotrimazole, Miconazole, Econazole, Izoconazole, Tioconazole, Bifonazole
b. Azole drugs of the 2nd generation - Ketoconazole
c. Azole drugs of the 3rd generation – Itraconazole, Fluconazole, Voriconazole, Posaconazole

3. Allyloamin derrivates - Naftifine, Terbinafine
4. Morpholine derrivates - Amorpholine
5. Pyridone derrivates - Cyclopirox

The mechanism of action of antifungal drugs is based on disruption of a fungal cell membrane or inhibition or disruption of DNA or RNA synthesis or inhibition of egrosterole synthesis in fungal cells.

Antifungal therapy should be selected to the type of dermatomycosis, some of them can be treated topically, others require systemic treatment. Sometimes, when fungal infection is difficult to treat, both of these therapies should be involved.

Topical antifungal therapy is often the only procedure in the superficial mycoses of skin, it is decisive for the effectiveness of therapy. In cases of extensive and chronic superficial fungal infections of the scalp and nails, topical treatment is usually an essential element of combined therapy, shortening its duration and improves the treatment results.

The main indications for oral antifungal agents include the following infections :

- Fungal infections of nails and scalp
- Fungal infections involving large areas of skin
- Fungal infections in patients with immune disorders
- In a situation where there is a poor penetration of topical drug to the foci of fungal infection
- Persistent focus of fungal infection

To effectively treat fungal infections following conditions should be also applied:

- The correct mycological diagnosis before starting treatment.
- Removal of the factors predisposing to the development of fungal infection.
- Appropriate selection of drug.
- Knowledge of the principles of conducting antifungal treatment.
- Good cooperation with the patient.
- Control after treatment (clinical and mycological).

After complete cure of fungal infection, the physician should inform the patient about the the principles of prevention. This is especially important for onychomycosis, because these infections are often recurrent and chronic. For this purpose, patient should frequently disinfect shoes, wear cotton socks and avoid places with high humidity such as saunas, steam baths or swimming pools (Adamski & Batura-Gabryel, 2007).

3. Epidemiology of dermatomycoses in Poland over the past decades

Within the past decades changes in percentage of fungal infections and spectrum of dermatophytes were observed - in given geographical regions appear new species, replacing the existing ones. Migration of population, industrialization, economic and cultural development, ageing of society, increased percentage of diseases like diabetes, circulation disorders, antibiotic therapy or taking of immunosuppressive medicines - these are the factors that are conductive to this phenomenon. There is a close relation between mycological biota isolated from skin and its appendages and changing spectrum of dematophyte fungi in environment (Wronski & Nowicki, 2005).

3.1 Geographical distribution of dermatophytes in Poland

Studies on epidemiology of dermatomycoses in different parts of the world show how large changes can occur in the fungal biota in just a few decades. This phenomenon concerns also Poland and it is affected by changing environmental factors, including the formation of ever larger urban agglomerations, permanently changing profiles of the economy, and also clearly present in the last 15 - 20 years the changes in climatic conditions (Kobierzycka et al., 2005; Macura & Pawlik, 1998; Szepietowski & Baran, 2005). Of great importance is also easy to move to distant climatic - geographical regions - both tourist travel and mass migration for economic reasons. Thereby, various species of fungi appear far beyond the borders of the endemic areas.

The accumulated epidemiological data indicate how much the fungal biota of the given area, including Poland, changes over time. In the first half of the twentieth century in Central and Western Europe dominated zoophilic dermatophyte *Trichophyton mentagrophytes*, and today the predominant species is *Trichophyton rubrum*, antropophilic dermatophyte originating from Asia (Bajcar & Ratka, 2002; Glinski et al., 2002, Szepietowski et al., 2001). Currently it is the most common etiological agent of fungal infections of toenails in Poland.

The increasing dominance of infections caused by *Trichophyton rubrum* appears to be a negative phenomenon, because these types of diseases are particularly chronic and often recurrent. As fungal infections of the skin and its appendages in different regions of the world are caused by different species of fungi, mycological biota present in the skin lesions is associated with changes in the natural environment and man's artificial environment. It is known that *Trichophyton rubrum* came to Poland during the mass migration after World War II (Macura&Pawlik, 1998). This species was rare then, but over the years it has achieved a dominant position, while causing a permanent reduction in the participation of other dermatophyte infections of the skin and its appendages. Similarly, the major change relates to the presence on Polish territory The fungus *Trichophyton schoenleinii*. Today infections caused by this species are not found in Poland, but they occurred very often throughout the country in the first half of the twentieth century. Between 50\`s and 60\`s it caused only 5.7% of fungal infections, and in the late 90\`s its isolation has already belonged to the casuistic rarity (Macura & Pawlik, 1998; Szepietowski & Baran, 2005). Increasing number of infections caused by other antropophilic dermatophyte was observed instead. Although *Epidermophyton floccosum* was only 0.7% of all isolated dermatophytes in the 70\`s, then after 20 years the percentage of fungal infections increased 3-fold, up to 2.23%. Moreover, in place of *Microsporum gypseum*, which was only sporadically isolated in the 70\`s of the twentieth century, occured an unprecedented then species *Microsporum canis*, taking the 3rd position among the dermatophytes (2.64%) (Macura&Pawlik, 1998).

Mass migrations are particularly important and confirmed by epidemiological importance. It contributes to a large extent with spreading of fungal pathogens, especially antropophilic dermatophytes. The example is the African species (*Trichophyton soudanense*), and in the recent decades continuously isolated in Europe from immigrants coming from endemic areas. Similarly, in the U.S. athlete's foot cases caused by *Trichophyton violaceum* in immigrant from Asia, where this fungus is found endemic, were reported (Kobierzycka et al., 2005).

Interestingly, some species of dermatophytes found throughout the world, such as *Microsporum audouinii* and *Trichophyton schoenleinii*, are now very rare in the U.S. and Western Europe, although they are common in the other areas, particularly in Africa (Kobierzycka et al, 2005). Epidemiological data indicate that the changes that constantly occur in the distribution of pathogenic fungal biota are dependent on many factors. In addition to the progressive migration and climate change, social and economic conditions that affect skin exposure to fungal pathogens, and therapeutic methods are also important Szepietowski & Baran, 2005). These factors significantly affect the changes in the proportion of different species of fungi at the time in a given area. Extremely rare occurrence of *tinea capitis* caused by *Trichophyton schoenleinii* in Poland now is mainly associated with progressive, improved sanitation in the second half of the twentieth century (Szepietowski & Baran, 2005).

Given the fact that people are constantly exposed to the possibility of contact with dermatophytes, since infectious material is commonly present in the environment, in the case of infection with widespread antropophilic species it is difficult to identify the source and route of infection. Conversely, if the fungal infection is caused by zoophilic dermatophyte with a relatively narrow specificity of the species (*Microsporum canis*, *Trichophyton verrucosum*), and the number of actual cases is not large, the epidemiological investigation may allow to trace the spread of infection and determine its source (Kobierzycka et al., 2005).

Many years of studies of mycological biota indicate that one of its characteristics are constant changes in time, related to the presence of particular species of fungi in the natural environment and their involvement in causing infections of the skin and its appendages in human. Changing mycological biota varies in different geographical regions. Moreover, it was found that the clinical forms of fungal infections in different parts of the world are caused by different species of fungi (Chong & Sinclair, 2000; Cribier & Paul, 2001; Gupta, 2001). Tracing this variability is essential for epidemiological research, as it allows to prove the existence of variation ranges of the different species of dermatophytes. It also has no less important from the standpoint of public health, makes it possible to forecast the development of fungal infections in the population. Although Poland is a relatively small territory, epidemiological studies conducted in different parts of the country consistently show the changes in the fungal biota during the last 50 years.

Baran and Szepietowski analyzed results of mycological examinations from years 1988 - 1992, conducted across the country, updating epidemiological map of Poland (Baran & Szepietowski, 1994). These researchers have demonstrated a definite advantage in the incidence of anthropophilic dermatophytes (64.3% of all dermatophytes) over zoophilic dermatophytes (35%). In addition, they found that infections with geophilic dermatophytes occured occasionally (0.7% of all isolated pathogens) (Figure 1).

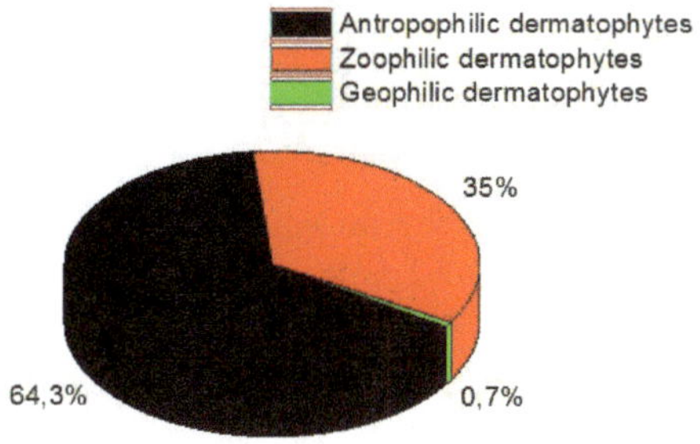

Fig. 1. Dermatophytes in Poland in years 1988-1992.

Anthropophilic dermatophytes dominance was observed in almost all regions of the country, but particularly clearly in the centraleastern region (75.9%), midwestern region (75.5%), southwestern region (72.1%) and southeastern region (70.4%). Only in the northern region of the country, this advantage was small, anthropophilic fungi accounted for only 54.6% of the total number of dermatophytes (Szepietowski & Baran, 2005; Baran & Szepietowski, 1994).

Quite different results were obtained in the province of Bialystok. Only in this region anthropophilic dermatophytes formed a minority, accounting for just 45.1% of all dermatophytes isolated in the area. It also appeared that the zoophilic fungi were the most common dermatophytes (54.9%) in Bialystok province (northeastern Poland) (Szepietowski & Baran, 2005; Baran & Szepietowski, 1994). Authors found a clear upward trend in a southerly direction for the anthropophilic dermatophytes, closely associated with the occurrence of an inverse trend for zoophilic fungi (Szepietowski & Baran, 2005). It turned out that zoophilic dermatophytes are the most commonly reported in the northern region (45.4%) and least often in the middleeastern region (24.1%). Baran and Szepietowski thus agreed that the distribution of zoophilic dermatophytes is the reverse of the map of anthropophilic dermatophytes distribution (Szepietowski & Baran, 2005; Baran & Szepietowski, 1994).

Among the anthropophilic fungi *Trichophyton rubrum* was isolated most frequently, it accounted for 45.5% off all dermatophytes and for anthropophilic dermatophytes - 70.8%. This species occurred most frequently in the southwestern region (59.1% of all dermatophytes), midwestern region (55.8%) and southeastern region (53.4%). Least often it was isolated in the northern region (7.7% of all dermatophytes ascertained in this area). The second in the order, *Trichophyton interdigitale* usually occurred in the northern region (34.0% of all dermatophytes), slightly less often (24.5%) in the central-eastern parts of the country, but only occasionally - in the West (0.6%). *Epidermophyton floccosum* was found the most frequently in the northeastern region (19.5%) and the midwestern region (15.6%), with a clear decrease in the incidence in the southern direction. Other species of anthropophilic dermatophytes were very rare, they were isolated only sporadically. In the group of zoophilic fungi *Trichophyton mentagrophytes* was mostly isolated. It accounted for 22.4% of all dermatophytes and among zoophilic dermatophytes it accounted for 64.4%, and most occurred in the northeastern region (31.5% of all dermatophytes), and the least in the region of central-western and south-western regions. Isolated somewhat less *Microsporum canis* constituted 9.7% of all dermatophytes and 27.6% of zoophilic dermatophytes. This fungus was typically found mostly in the northern region (21.5% of dermatophytes in this area), in the central region (12.1%) and least often in the centraleastern region and northeastern regions (3.8 % and 0.5%, respectively) (Baran & Szepietowski, 1994).

Among the geophilic fungi, *Microsporum gypseum* was isolated most often. It represented only 0.6% of all dermatophytes and among geophilic dermatophytes - 82.8%, and most frequntly occurred in the central region (Szepietowski & Baran, 2005; Baran & Szepietowski, 1994).

The authors analyzed the results of mycological examinations from the years 1988-1992 conducted across the country. The most often isolated fungus was antropophilic *Trichophyton rubrum*. Only in the northeastern region, in the province of Bialystok *Trichophyton mentagrophytes* was the most frequently observed species (40.7% of all dermatophytes in the province). In the northern part of the Poland dominated *Trichophyton interdigitale* (34% of all dermatophytes), although in the Gdansk region dominated infections caused by *Microsporum canis* (30.5% of isolated dermatophytes) (Baran & Szepietowski, 1994).

The results of this analysis showed how great epidemiological changes took place in relation to the occurrence of fungal pathogens, at a relatively small area of Poland in about 30 years. In the earlier years (1952-1967) a distinct advantage of zoophilic dermatopytes, representing 69.6% of the total dermatophytes over antropophilic (30.3%) and geophilic dermatophytes (0.1%) was observed (Figure 2). At that time, the dominance of zoophilic fungi did not concern only the region of Bialystok, where antropophilic dermatophytes accounted for 58.2% (Wronski & Nowicki, 2000).

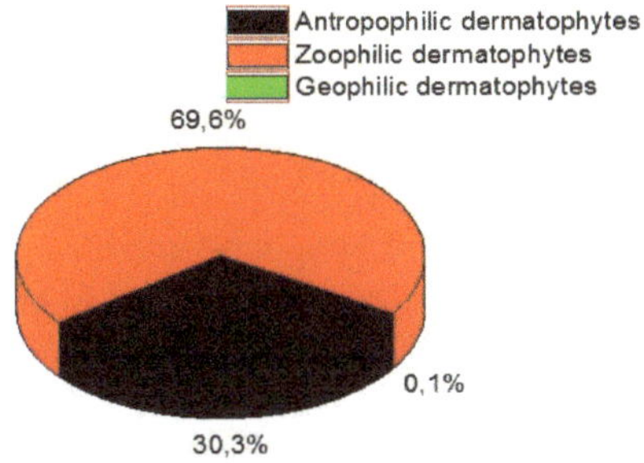

Fig. 2. Dermatophytes in Poland in years 1952-1967.

In the following years (1974-1979) more pronounced changes were observed in Poland, and the incidence of infections due to zoophilic and antropophilic dermatophytes became similar and amounted to 50.9% and 48.1%, respectively (Lange et al., 2002). Geophilic dermatophytes constituted then only 1% (Hryncewicz-Gwozdz et al, 2005).

In the region of Olsztyn (northeastern Poland) incidence of zoophilic dermatophytes decreased from 51.7% in 1978-1981 to 48.8% in 1982-1986 (Nowicki & Bykowska, 2006).

Increased frequency of isolation of anthropophilic fungi in relation to the zoophilic species, is confirmed by other studies - Ratka (1977-1988) and Baran *et al* in Lower Silesia (southwestern Poland) region (1977-1991) (Baran et al, 1993; Ratka, 1990). Over the years steadily increased the frequency of isolation of anthropophilic fungi among the dermatophytes. Previous studies showed that more than 40 years ago, most often isolated fungus in Poland was zoophilic *Trichophyton mentagrophytes* and Baran and Szepietowski showed that nowadays the most common species in Poland is *Trichophyton rubrum* (Baran & Szepietowski, 1994; Wronski & Nowicki, 2005) .

In the years 1987-1996 Kaszuba *et al*, studied fungal infections of the skin and its appendages in the Lodz region (Central Poland), they found that in the 51.7% of cases dermatophytes were the etiologic agent, including genera: *Trichophyton* (75.39%), *Microsporum* (15.35%) and *Epidermophyton* (9.35%). Compared with studies from the years 1982-1986 the authors pointed out an increase in isolation of dermatophyte fungi in the Lodz region. The main etiological agent was *Trichophyton rubrum* (34.15%), the second most common pathogen was *Trichophyton mentagrophytes* (33.19%), and further were *Microsporum canis* and *Epidermophyton floccosum*. An interesting observation of the authors was significant change in the isolation frequency of *Trichophyton mentagrophytes* and *Trichophyton rubrum* species. It has been found a decrease of the incidence of *Trichophyton mentagrophytes* from over 50% to 33%, while the number of isolation of *Trichophyton rubrum* has increased from 25% to 34% which places this species in the first place among diagnosed dermatophytes (Kaszuba et al., 1997).

Between 1995-1999 survey of fungal infections in the Wroclaw (Lower Silesia) region conducted Sikora *et al* (Sikora et al., 2000). A large variety of mycological biota was found. Among the dermatophytes, most often because 62.7% of infections concerned *Trichophyton mentagrophytes*, *Trichophyton rubrum* was isolated less frequently (27.8%), *Epidermophyton floccosum* (6.2%) and least often *Microsporum canis* (3%). An important observation was a significant decrease in the number of infections caused by *Trichophyton rubrum* (32.9%) and *Epidermophyton floccosum* (25.6%). Moreover, the frequency of isolation of *Trichophyton mentagrophytes* grew by 61.5%. In the case of *Microsporum canis* infections with this species increased to 1997, with subsequent later decrease of the number of infections (Sikora et al., 2000).

Between years 1996-2000 in region of Bydgoszcz (Central Poland) antropophilic *Trichophyton rubrum* was isolated in 41.6% of cases, followed by antropophilic *Trichophyton interdigitale* (26.9%). Zoophilic *Microsporum canis* was isolated in 8.2% of cases (Mrotek et al., 2001).

In the years 1996-2001 further studies concerned analysis of mycological biota and assessment of the incidence of fungal infections in patients from the urban environment of Bialystok. Anthropophilic dermatophytes were found in 40.1% of all isolates and among them most often were: *Trichophyton rubrum*, *Trichophyton interdigitale*, and *Epidermophyton floccosum*. Zoophilic dermatophytes represented 34.4% of fungi and most often occurred *Trichophyton mentagrophytes*. The results of studies conducted in region of Bialystok indicated the anthropophilic dermatophytes as the main etiological agents of fungal infections of the skin and its appendages (Bolinski et al., 2003).

Multiannual mycological research (1984-2001) were conducted in the Subcarpathian region (southeastern Poland) by Bajcar and Ratka. They compared in terms of epidemiology two periods: the years 1984-1993 and 1994-2001. Among isolated dermatophytes prevailed *Trichophyton rubrum* (68.9% of all infections), and *Trichophyton interdigitale* was found in 11.3% of cases, *Epidermophyton floccosum* in 9.1% of cases, and *Trichophyton tonsurans* in 6.2% of cases. Zoophilic fungi were isolated rarely, in 4.1% of cases *Trichophyton mentagrophytes* was isolated. Comparing the results of research conducted in the years 1994-2001 with data obtained in the previous decade, Bajcar and Ratka observed in the Subcarpathian region continuing dominance of antropophilic fungi infections. Among the antropophilic dermatophytes was observed a decrease in the number of infections caused by *Trichophyton rubrum* (9.5%) and an increased participation of *Trichophyton interdigitale* (9.4%). An important observation of the authors was the emergence in the region of Subcarpathian an unprecedented *Trichophyton violaceum* species (0.4% of isolates) - species frequent in Eastern Europe. Comparing the two periods also a slight increase of fungal infections with zoophilic fungi was observed: *Trichophyton mentagrophytes* (from 4.1% to 5.5%) and *Trichophyton verrucosum* (from 0.2% to 1.1%) (Bajcar & Ratka, 2002).

In the region of Gdansk Szarmach and Nowicki in years 1994-1998 found large share of dermatophytes as etiological agents of onychomycosis. They accounted for 44.8% of all fungal pathogens and most often isolated species were: *Trichophyton rubrum* and *Trichophyton interdigitale* (Szarmach & Nowicki, 2001).

Further studies conducted in Gdansk (midsouthern region of Poland) in years 2003-2005 showed an increase in the number of infections and variability of pathogenic fungi species. Among dermatophytes *Trichophyton rubrum* and *Trichophyton mentagrophytes* were recognized the most often (43.9% and 35.6%, respectively). These fungi were isolated mainly from toenails. *Microsporum canis* was isolated from 8.4% of patients, mostly from children it caused infections of the scalp (65.7%) and glabrous skin (34.3%) (Nowicki & Bykowska, 2006). Moreover, this dermatophyte is the most common fungal pathogen among children in Gdansk region since 1984 (Wilkowska & Nowicki, 1991).

Kalinowska *et al* studied dermatomycoses in Lower Silesia in years 2004 - 2008. The author found, that pathogen isolated most fequently (59.27%) was antropophilic *Trichophyton rubrum*, sencond most frequently isolated fungus was *Trichophyton mentagrophytes* (22.09%). Interestingly, the incidence of dermatomycoses caused by *Trichophyton tonsurans* increased, and this dermatophyte was placed on the third position (10.45%), followed by *Microsporum canis* (4.74%) (Kalinowska et al., 2010).

Previous mycological research carried out in different regions of Poland indicate the need for constant observation and epidemiological analyses, to monitor ongoing changes of the fungal biota and its contribution to infections in human.

International Studies (Achilles project) conducted in 1989-1999 showed that Poland takes 4th place after Russia, Hungary and the Czech Republic in the incidence of fungal infections in European countries (Glinski et al, 2002).

Among the 40,000 surveyed Poles 42% of them were diagnosed with athlete's foot and 21% with onychomycosis. The results of these studies additonally support the view that the epidemiological data of fungal infections must be constantly updated to confirmed variations of fungal biota in the natural environment.

From the 50`s of the past centrury, mycoses caused by zoophilic species represented up to almost 70% of diagnosed mycoses, whereas infections caused by antropophilic dermatophytes represented 30% and infections caused by geophilic dermatophytes represented 0.1% of all dermatomycoses. This situation has changed entirely in next decades, so different data are shown in literature from 1980s and 1990s - the most common were antropophilic dermatophytes (64.3%), less common zoophilic dermatophytes (35.0%) and infections caused by geophilic dermatophytes represented 0.7%. Among antropophilic dermatophytes, *Trichophyton rubrum* is in the lead over past fifty years, this species is commonly responsible for onychomycosis. Among zoophilic dermatophytes, most frequently *Trichophyton mentagrophytes* was isolated. Among geophilic dermatophytes *Microsporum gypseum* was isolated most frequently.

Nowadays, depending on geographical region of Poland, antropophilic species represent about 45 - 75 % of all dermatophytes and zoophilic species represent about 30 - 55%.

3.2 Epidemiology of different types of dermatomycoses in Poland

Fungal infections are now a major epidemiological and social problem worldwide. According to various data relating to different geographical regions, they concern from 10 to 40% ofthe world's population (Bolinski et al., 2003; Foster et al., 2004; Kaszuba et al., 1997; Szepietowski & Baran, 2005). Research conducted among people living in moderate climate zones showed chronic fungal infections among 10-20% of the population (Bolinski et al., 2003; Glinski et al., 2002). Fungi pathogenic for human usually cause infections of the skin and its appendages, although in recent years also increasing recognition of fungal infections of internal organs is seen.

Among the more than 200 000 species of fungi about 200 are pathogenic to human (Szepietowski & Baran, 2005). Their high morphological diversity allows them to survive in different ecosystems. Polymorphism of fungi is also a result of their diverse needs for growth substances in certain ecological niches, because they have a high potential to adapt to the changing resources of their environment (Dworacka-Kaszak, 2004). Among potential fungal skin pathogens are fungi not only highly adapted for parasite on the skin - dermatophytes, but also yeasts and molds.

Observed in recent decades, the increasing incidence of fungal infections of the skin is mainly associated with the constant presence, and even an increase in risk factors for fungal infections. It was established a number of factors predisposing to the development of fungal infections, some of which relate to the host, and other to biological characteristics of the fungal pathogens. One of the main factors is prolongation of the average life span, age proved to be a physiological risk factor for fungal infection. Particularly predisposed group are not only people over 65 years, but also premature newborns and infants. It was found that the presence of multifocal skin infections increases with age and is 2-fold more frequent in men than in women (Kobierzycka et al., 2005).

One of the most important factors influencing the increasing number of fungal infections is the progress in medical science, it now allows the survival of patients with an impaired immune response in the course of chronic, severe illnesses such as cancer, metabolic and endocrine diseases, renal failure, HIV infection and other (Hryncewicz, Gwozdz et al., 2006; Miroszewska-Sobanska & Adamski, 2000). This is related to the development of intensive medical care, dialysis, parenteral nutrition and artificial ventilation, conducting invasive diagnostics, catheterization of vascular and body cavities, and also with the use of modern cardiac transplantation techniques (Glisnki et al., 2002). Very important is also antibiotic therapy, treatment with cytostatics, immunosuppressants and corticosteroids (Krajewska-Kulak et al., 2000).

Superficial mycoses of skin and its appendages are diagnosed in Poland very often. Among the clinical forms of mycoses of skin and its appendages special place because of the prevalence takes athlete's foot and onychomycosis. Athlete's foot occurs mostly in adults, rarely in children and often is acquired early in adolescence.

For example, studies of Kalinowska *et al* on lowersilesian population in years 2004-2008 indicated, that *tinea pedis* and onychomycosis were very often in adults, whereas in children and adolescents *tinea capitis* and *tinea corporis* were predominated (Kalinowska et al., 2010). It is believed that in developed countries athlete`s foot may affect up to 10% of the total population. In recent years, it was found that for most cases of athlete's foot are responsible three anthropophilic species of dermatophytes: *Trichophyton rubrum, Trichophyton interdigitale* and *Epidermophyton floccosum* (Kobierzycka et al., 2005).

Studies of Szepietowski *et al* indicate that the athlete's foot was 28% of all fungal infections of skin and nails in Poland and it is the second most common after onychomycosis. Other authors estimate the incidence of fungal infection rates similar of 25-30% in the general population, although this is difficult to determine it because in the special risk groups (athletes, miners), it can grow up to 60-70%. In studies of Szepietowski *et al* most common type of *tinea pedis* was a athlete's foot (45.5%), and the most common pathogens causing it were dermatophytes, which were isolated in 88.8% of all patients with fungal infections. Among the most commonly cultured dermatophytes were *Trichophyton rubrum* (51%), followed by *Trichophyton mentagrophytes* (33.1%) (Szepietowski et al., 2001).

The authors found that athlete's foot in 75.2% of patients occurred together with the other forms of fungal infection of the skin, the most common was onychomycosis found in 69.2% of patients. Described in the literature the simultaneous occurrence of fungal infection of the both feet with one hand forming the so-called two feet and one hand syndrome and was rarely observed, because only in 2.5% of patients (Szepietowski et al., 2001). It is believed that the probability of developing athlete's foot is lower in women than in men. The differences are likely to result from increased exposure to pathogenic fungi associated with wearing heavy occlusive footwear by men (Kobierzynska et al., 2005).

Onychomycosis is often concomitant with athlete`s foot, it is developed by the occurrence of the same favorable environmental conditions for fungi (Elewski, 2000a; Hryncewicz-Gwozdz et al., 2005; Wronski & Nowicki, 2005). Infections concerns mostly the elderly, after 65 years. Its occurence is much rarer in children, it is associated with rapid growth of the nails in young people which hinders the development of infection because the fungus is removed together with the growing plate (Hryncewicz-Gwozdz et al., 2006; Lange & Bykowska, 2004). Epidemiological data from recent years show significant dominance of dermatophyte fungi as a etiological agents of onychomycosis. It is assumed that currently about 80% of fungal infections of nails are caused by *Trichophyton rubrum* (Wronski & Nowicki, 2000).

Fungal infection of hands is most common as a secondary infection in patients with athlete`s foot. It can then concern the dominant hand and form the aforementioned two feet and one hand sydrome (Szepietowski et al., 2001). In most cases the etiological factors for mycosis of hands are anthropophilic species of dermatophytes that also cause athlete's foot also: *Trichophyton rubrum*, rarely *Epidermophyton floccosum* and *Trichophyton interdigitale*. Much less fequently hand`s skin can be infected by antropohilic species *Trichophyton violaceum* and some zoophilic species such as *Trichophyton mentagrophytes* (Kobierzycka et al., 2005; Hryncewicz-Gwozdz et al., 2005) .

The development of fungal infection of the hands may facilitate various factors causing maceration of the skin, such as wearing rings, watches, anatomical deformities, and environmental factors associated with the professional activities (Kobierzycka et al., 2005).

Species of dermatophytes that cause athlete's foot can also cause fungal infection of the groin. The most common pathogen is *Trichophyton rubrum*, while *Trichophyton interdigitale* and *Epidermophyton floccosum* more rarely cause infections of this area. This infection is a common disease, occurring more often in men than in women, but it is rarely observed in children. *Tinea cruris* is a very widespread in the tropics, particularly among immigrants from countries with temperate climates, especially when factors that makes them predisposed to the formation of intertrigos and development of fungal infections are accumulated (Kobierzycka et al., 2005).

Most dermatophytes can infect hair, the exceptions are, however, some species such as *Epidermophyton floccosum*, *Trichophyton rubrum*, *Trichophyton interdigitale*. Conversely, some dermatophytes (*Microsporum audouinii*, *Trichophyton schoenleinii*, *Trichophyton violaceum*) have a strong affinity for hair structures. It was found that all the dermatophytes, which cause fungal infections of the scalp can also infect glabrous skin (Kobierzycka et al., 2005). Pathogens that cause *tinea capitis* differs between countries and geographic regions. In recent years, it has been observed in most European countries, an increase in the frequency of infections caused by *Microsporum canis*, whereas in the U.S. urban environments - a larger share *Trichophyton tonsurans* was seen (Elewski, 2000b). Mycosis of the scalp concerns mainly children. Peak incidence falls on 4 – 6 years of age, and the infection is spreading especially in boys. Higher incidence of fungal infections in children is associated with the difference of biological characteristics of the skin, including the different composition of sebum in children and adults (Szepietowski & Baran, 2005).

In a study of Lange *et al*, of the pediatric population in the region of Gdansk (midsouthern Poland), fungal infections of skin were usually caused by dermatophytes, which accounted for 60% of all infections. The highest incidence of skin fungal infections was observed in children aged 4-7 years. In this age group, the lesions caused by *Microsporum canis* affected the scalp. In slightly older children, aged 8-12 years, the number of infections of the scalp decreased rapidly, and over 13 years of age lesions in this location rarely have been observed. Most common form of fungal infection, that was seen in the pediatric population studies, was fungal infection of the glabrous skin (30%), mostly caused by *Microsporum canis*, rarely by *Trichophyton mentagrophytes* and by *Trichophyton rubrum*, occurring most often in children aged 8 - 15 years. It is interesting that in children above 12 years of age athlete's foot was also observed (11%), in most cases caused by *Trichophyton rubrum* and *Trichophyton mentagrophytes*, and also fungal infections of the toenails (8%) caused by *Trichophyton rubrum* were seen (Lange et al., 2002). Similar results were obtained in the studies of pediatric patients in the region of Poznan (Central-West Poland) (Zaba & Danczak-Pazdrowska, 2001).

Many authors underline the rarity of these forms of mycoses in children before puberty, in contrast to the fungal infections of glabrous skin and scalp, considered to be typical for the childhood. Accepted view is that the athlete's foot and onychomycosis are very common skin and nails diseases in adults, and their incidence increases with age. However, epidemiological studies on the population of children of different ages and in different regions of the world indicate that the athlete's foot may relate to 2.2-8.2% of the pediatric population (Lange & Bykowska, 2004) In addition, there are also cases of athlete's foot in pediatric patients like *tinea incognito*, proceeding without symptoms or mistakenly acknowledged as bacterial lesions or allergic changes and treated with antibiotics or topical cortycosteroids (O`Grady & Sahn, 1999).

Studies of Lange and Bykowska on recognition of fungal infections in pediatric patients in years 1993-2002 showed an increase in the prevalence rates of onychomycosis in children (Lange & Bykowska, 2004). In the literature, individual national studies of mycoses of the feet and toenails in children and adolescents refers to the area of Wroclaw (Lower Silesia, southwestern Poland), where there has been considerable percentage of fungal infection of the feet and toenails in children under 15 years of age (16.3% and 21%, respectively) (Szepietowski, 1997).

Also, Zaba and Danczak-Pazdrowska examining children and adolescents to 18 years of age, living in the area of Greater Poland, found fungal infections of toenails in 34.5% patients and mycoses of hands and feet in 26.1% of cases (Zaba & Danczak-Pazdrowska, 2001). It seems that a particular risk factor in children is a participation in sport activities. It turned out that in this group superficial mycosis of the feet occurs several times more often than in children not involved in sport, which is related to use of occlusive footwear, as well as frequent, repetitive injuries of fingers and toenails. Thus, the results of the Polish authors suggest that fungal infection of the feet and toenails in children and adolescents currently are not that uncommon. Moreover, as in adults, athlete's foot in children can coexist with other clinical forms of fungal infection, especially fungal infection of the toenails (Lange & Bykowska, 2004).

The analysis of few described so far cases in the world of dermatomycosis in newborns showed that it could even occur on the second day of life and can be caused both by anthropophilic dermatophytes (*Trichophyton rubrum*) and as well as zoophilic dermatophytes (*Microsporum canis*). The source of infection in case of antropophilic dermatophytes was immediate family and in case of zoophilic dermatophytes - pets, especially cats. Descriptions analyzed by Szepietowski of dermatomycosis in newborns come mostly from India and Japan, which is probably related both to climatic conditions, as well as significantly to local practices for baby care (Szepietowski, 1997).

4. Conclusion

Fungal infections are a serious problem - not only clinical, but also therapeutic and social. Fungi are widespread in the environment of human life, are ubiquitous, so the disorders caused by them could be classified as a lifestyle diseases, affecting people independtly of age, sex, race or social status. Fortunately, our knowledge about these parasites of the skin and its appendages is growing, new therapies and new methods of treatment of fungal diseases are developed, which allows us to effective protection against these pathogens.

5. References

Adamski, Z. & Batura - Gabryel, H. (2007). *Medical mycology for physicians and students, 2nd edition.* Scientific Publishing of Poznan Medical University, Poznan, Poland, ISBN 978-83-60187-76-0

Bajcar, S & Ratka P. (2002). Epidemiology of dermatophyte infections among inhabitans of Subcarpathian region in years 1984-2001. *Mikologia Lekarska,* Vol. 9, No. 2 (June), pp. 101-104, ISSN 1232-986X

Baran, E. & Szepietowski J. (1994). Geographical distribution of dermatophytes isolated from skin lesions in Poland. *Mikologia Lekarska,* Vol. 1, No. 1 (March), pp. 11-18, ISSN 1232- 986X

Baran, E. et al. (1993). Fungal infections in Lower Silesia region in years 1974-1988. *Przeglad Dermatologiczny,* Vol. 80, pp. 49-58, ISSN 0033-2526

Bolinski, J. et al. (2003). Epidemiology of infections of skin and its appendages in material of Dermatology Clinic in Bialystok. *Mikologia Lekarska,* Vol. 10, No. 2 (June), pp. 119-127, ISSN 1232-986X

Chong, A. & Sinclair, R. (2000). Diagnosing superficial mycoses. *American Journal of Clinical Dermatology*, Vol. 1, No. 2 (March-April), pp. 125-131, ISSN 1175-0561

Criber, B. & Paul, C. (2001). Long-term efficacy of antifungals in toenail onychomycosis: a critival review. *British Journal of Dermatology*, Vol. 145, No. 3, pp. 446-452, ISSN 1365- 2133

Dworacka-Kaszak, B. (2004). Dermatophytes. Keratophilic fungi and their role in environment. *Mikologia Lekarska*, Vol. 11, No. 4 (December), pp. 317-322, ISSN 1232-986X

Elewski, B. (2000a). Onychomycosis. Treatment, quality of life and economic issues. *American Journal of Clinical Dermatology*, Vol. 1, No. 1 (January-February), pp. 19-26, ISSN 1175-0561

Elewski, B. (2000b). Tinea capitis: a current perspective. *Journal of the American Academy of Dermatology*, Vol. 42, No. 1 (January), pp. 1-20, ISSN 1175-0561

Foster, K., Ghannoum, M. & Elewski, B. (2004). Epidemiologic surveillance of cutaneous fungal infections in the United States from 1999-2001. *Journal of the American Academy of Dermatology*,Vol. 50, No. 5 (May), pp. 748-752, ISSN 1097-6787

Glinski, W. et al., (2002). Consensus concerning treatment of superficial fungal infections. *Przeglad Dermatologiczny*, Vol. 89, pp. 85-92, ISSN 0033-2526

Gupta, A. (2001). Cyclopirox: an overview. *International Journal of Dermatology*, Vol. 40, No. 5 (May), pp. 305-310, ISSN 1365-4632

Hryncewicz-Gwozdz, A., Plomer-Niezgoda, E & Maj, J. (2005). Mycoses of feet, hands and nails - epidemiology, symptoms, treatment. *Mikologia Lekarska*, Vol. 12, No. 1 (March), pp. 57-62, ISSN 1232-986X

Hryncewicz-Gwozdz, A. et al. (2011). *Tinea Capitis* and *Tinea Corporis* with a Severe Inflammatory Response due to *Trichophyton tonsurans*. *Acta Dermato-Venereologica*, Epub ahead of print, ISSN 0001-5555

Hryncewicz-Gwozdz, A. et al. (2006). Mycosis of nails - current clinical and epidemiological aspects in Poland. *Mikologia Lekarska*, Vol. 13, No. 2 (June), pp. 137-142, ISSN 1232-986X

Jankowska-Konsur, A. et al. (2011). A 5-year survey of dermatomycoses in southwest Poland, years 2003–2007. *Mycoses*, Vol. 54, No. 2 (March), pp. 162-167, ISSN 1439-0507

Kalinowska, K., Hryncewicz-Gwozdz A. & Plomer-Niezgoda E., (2009a). Differential of *Trichophyton* species. *Mikologia Lekarska*, Vol. 16, No. 3 (September), pp. 171-177, ISSN 1232-986X

Kalinowska K, Hryncewicz-Gwozdz A. & Plomer-Niezgoda E. (2009b). Dermatomycoses due to *Microsporum audouinii* and *Microsporum gypseum*. *Mikologia Lekarska*, Vol. 16, No. 3 (September), pp. 179-183, ISSN 1232-986X

Kalinowska, K. et al. (2010). Epidemiology of dermatophytoses in Lower Silesia in years 2004-2008. *Mikologia Lekarska*, Vol. 17, No. 3 (September), pp. 165-168, ISSN 1232-986X

Kaszuba, A. et al. (1997). Dermatophytes in infections of skin and its appendages in people I n Lodz region. *Mikologia Lekarska*, Vol. 4, No. 4 (December), pp. 211-216, ISSN 1232-986X

Kobierzycka, M. et al. (2005). Epidemiology and diagnostic of the most common mycoses of glabrous and hairy skin. *Terapia*, Vol. 13, No. 1, pp. 53-58, ISSN 1230-3917

Krajewska-Kulak, E., et al. (2000). Nosocomial fungal infections-an increasing problem. *Mikologia Lekarska*, Vol. 7, No. 3, (September) pp. 159-163, ISSN 1232-986X

Lange, M. et al. (2002). Mycotic infections of skin and and mucous membranes in children in the district of Gdansk between 1999-2001. *Mikologia Lekarska*, Vol. 9, No. 2 (June), pp. 75-81, ISSN 1232-986X

Lange, M. & Bykowska, B. (2004). Tinea pedis and toenail onychomycosis in children and adolescents - clinical types and pathogens. *Mikologia Lekarska*, Vol. 11, No. 1 (March), pp. 63-69, ISSN 1232-986X

Macura, A. & Pawlik, B. (1998). Analysis of mycological flora causing superficial fungal infections in the last decade. *Mikologia Lekarska*, Vol. 5, No. 1, pp. 51-61, ISSN 1232-986X

Miroszewska-Sobanska, T., Adamski, Z. (2000). Prophylaxis of fungal infections. *Postepy Dermatologii i Alergologii*, Vol. 18, No. 3, pp. 181-188, ISSN 1642-395X

Mrotek, M. et al. (2001). Pathogenic fungi in the material of Mycological Laboratory of the Dermatology Clinic in Bydgoszcz in the period January 1996-August 2000. *Mikologia Lekarska*, Vol. 8, No. 3 (September), pp. 153-157, ISSN 1232-986X

Nowicki, R. & Bykowska, B. (2006). Dermatomycoses among inhabitants of the Pomeranian province in the years 2003-2005. *Mikologia Lekarska*, Vol. 13, No. 2 (June), pp. 119-122, ISSN 1232-986X

O`Grady, T. & Sahn E. (1999). Investigation of asymptomatic *tinea pedis* in children. *Journal of the American Academy of Dermatology*, Vol. 24, No. 4, pp. 660-661, ISSN 1097-6787

Ratka, P. (1990). Epidemiology of fungal infections in Poland in years 1977-1988. *Postepy Dermatologii i Alerologii*, Vol. 7, pp. 207-213, ISSN ISSN 1642-395X

Sikora, M. et al. (2000). Analysis of fungal skin and skin appendages infections in the region of Wroclaw in the years 1995-1999. *Mikologia Lekarska*, Vol. 7, No. 3 (September), pp. 145-151, ISSN 1232-986X

Szarmach, A. & Nowicki, R. (2001). Mycosis of nails due to dermatophytes in the material of Dermatology Clinic of Gdansk Medical University in the years 1994 - February 1998 -mycological, morphological and clinical aspect. *Mikologia Lekarska* Vol. 8, No. 2 (June), pp. 55-62, ISSN 1232-986X

Szepietowski, J. & Baran, E. (2005). Epidemiology of mycoses. In: Outline of mycology of nurses. E. Krajewska-Kulak (Ed.), 31-35, Czelej Publishing, Lublin, Poland, ISBN 83- 89309-54-8

Szepietowski, J., Baran, E. & Wild, E. (2001). Mycosis of feet - clinical types and pathogens. *Przeglad Dermatologiczny*, Vol. 886, pp. 497-502, ISSN 0033-2526

Szepietowski, J. (1997). Mycosis of skin in newborns. *Mikologia Lekarska*, Vol. 4, No. 1 (March), pp. 41-45, ISSN 1232-986X

Wilkowska, A. & Nowicki, R. (1991). Microsporiasis in patients treated in Dermatology Clinic of Gdansk Medical University. *Przeglad Dermatologiczny*, Vol. 78, pp. 38-42, ISSN 0033-2526

Wronski A. & Nowicki, R. (2000). Etiology of superficial fungal infection in contemporary mycological diagnostic methods. *Mikologia Lekarska*, Vol. 12, No. 3 (September), pp. 197-202, ISSN 1232-986X

Zaba, R. & Danczak-Pazdrowska, A. (2001). Analysis of mycoses in children - patients of City Hospital in Poznan in the years 1996-2000. *Mikologia Lekarska*, Vol. 8, No. 2 (June), pp. 106-109, ISSN 1232-986X

3

Microsatellite Typing of Catheter-Associated *Candida albicans* Strains

Astrid Helga Paulitsch-Fuchs[1,2], Bettina Heiling[1], Birgit Willinger[3] and Walter Buzina[1]
[1]*Institute of Hygiene, Microbiology and Environmental Medicine Medical University of Graz, Graz*
[2]*Wetsus Centre of Excellence for Sustainable Water Technology, Leeuwarden*
[3]*Division of Hygiene and Medical Microbiology, Medical University of Vienna, Vienna*
[1,3]*Austria*
[2]*The Netherlands*

1. Introduction

Candida albicans is the most common pathogenic fungus and occurs frequently in the digestive tract (Bernhardt, 1998; Doskey, 2004). Vaginal candidiasis (Mohanty et al. 2007; Paulitsch et al., 2006; Sobel, 2007) is also a wide spread problem. This species can become invasive, causing infections on many different sites in patients with severe underlying diseases (Marol & Yükesoy, 2008; Odds et al., 2007).

Catheter or shunt related infections caused by *C. albicans* (Pierce 2005) were reported e.g. by Sánchez-Portocarrero et al. (1994), David et al. (2005) and Tumbarello et al. (2007).

The classical picture of yeast cells as unicellular life forms is based on the pure-culture model of growth. In their natural habitat microorganisms including yeasts are mostly organized in biofilm ecosystems which are often ´multicultural´, made not only of yeasts but also of bacteria (El-Aziz et al., 2004; López-Ribot, 2005; Ramage et al., 2005; Nobile et al., 2006). The possibility to adhere to a surface is a very important factor for the development of fungal (Hogan, 2006; Verstrepen & Klis, 2006) and bacterial biofilms (Dolan, 2001).

Microsatellites, which are also known as short tandem repeats, are repeated nucleotide sequences with a length from 2 up to 7 base pairs. These polymorphic DNA loci are variable within a population and in this way multiple alleles are created for a single microsatellite locus. These different multilocus genotypes are used to distinguish strains within a single species (Applied Biosystems [AB], 2005). Microsatellite markers provide the possibility to discriminate strains of the same species and to trace their epidemiological pathways (Botterel et al., 2001; Sampaio et al., 2005).

For this study, pairs for three loci (CDC3, EF3, and HIS3) on three different chromosomes developed by Botterel et al. (2001) were used to compare the *C. albicans* strains which were found to produce a biofilm, with those strains which did not produce a biofilm on the investigated catheter material. The differentiation of biofilm and non-biofilm forming strains was based on scanning electron microscopical findings (Paulitsch et al., 2009). Different primer pairs and also different combinations of primer pairs for the subtyping of *C. albicans* were reported elsewhere, see e.g. the works of Sampaio et al. (2005) or Fan et al. (2007).

For each marker and for a given isolate one or two bands were observed, and each observed band was assigned to an allele. Because *C. albicans* is diploid each strain can be characterized by six alleles with the method used.

The discriminatory power (DP) is a numerical index to describe the probability that two unrelated samples of a test group are placed in two different typing groups. The DP of EF3 is 0.86, the DP of CDC3 is 0.77, and the DP of HIS3 is 0.91 (Botterel et al., 2001). The combined DP of all three markers was 0.97. In order to get reliable results, this index has to be greater than 0.90 (Botterel et al., 2001).

2. Microsatellite typing

2.1 Material and methods

The 123 *C. albicans* (64 [52%] of them biofilm positive) strains for this study were collected during a study in biofilm forming abilities of yeast on indwelling devices (Paulitsch et al., 2009). The strains were stored at -70°C until examination.

Strains were subcultured on Sabouraud agar plates for 24 h at 35°C. For DNA extraction the PrepManTM Ultra Kit (Applied Biosystems [AB], Foster City, California) was used. For the microsatellite typing three different primer pairs were used (Botterel et al., 2001). The unmarked primers were HIS3R, CDC3R, and EF3 (Invitrogen, Lofer, Austria). The fluorescence labeling of the primers HIS3 (NEDTM, yellow), CDC3 (VICTM, green), and EF3R (6-FAMTM, blue) (all AB) was fitted to the DyeSet DS-33 (AB) which is recommended for 5-dye custom primer analyses. PCR was performed using the 96 well GeneAmp PCR System 9700 or the 96 well 2700 Thermal Cycler (both AB). PCR reactions were carried out as singleplex reactions for each primer pair. The samples were initially incubated for 2 minutes at 94°C to activate the Taq Polymerase (Eppendorf, Hamburg, Germany) and to denature the DNA. After thermal cycling (30 cycles; 94°C for 45 s, 48°C for 45 s, 68°C for 90 s) samples were kept at 68°C for another 5 minutes to complete partial polymerization.

Sample preparation for the injection in the 3100 Automatic Sequencer (AB) was done following the instructions. For analysis 1 µL of PCR product, 0.3 µL of size standard (GeneScanTM 500-LIZ®, AB) and 10 µL Hi-DiTM Formamide (AB) were mixed and transferred into a 96 well plate. The samples were denatured for 4 minutes at 94°C in a thermal cycler and immediately placed on ice. In every run three samples were used as internal control. The plate was transferred in the sequencer and processed using the Foundation Data Collection 3.0 software of the sequencer.

Data analysis was done with the GeneMapper® v3.7 software. Therefore it was necessary to set up the microsatellite analyses following the instructions of the manual (AB, 2005). The peaks were automatically detected (Auto Binning) with the created bin set, low quality data were checked manually and corrected. The results were exported in a Microsoft Excel sheet for documentation.

2.2 Results

Typing of 123 *C. albicans* strains was done with the above mentioned three primer pairs. Only from strain number 85 (sample W60) no data from the EF3 locus was producible. Although the DNA was isolated a second time and several PCR reactions were done for this locus, no peaks could be generated. In table 1 detailed information of all three loci for each strain is listed.

		CDC3/CDC3R		EF3/EF3R		HIS3/HIS3R	
	sample	allele 1	allele 2	allele 1	allele 2	allele 1	allele 2
1	*K7*	117	129	130	139	154	154
2	K10	125	125	133	133	174	186
3	*K11*	117	129	130	139	154	154
4	*K13*	125	125	126	133	166	182
5	K14	117	129	130	139	154	154
6	K15	125	125	123	123	174	182
7	*K16*	125	125	126	126	174	182
8	*K17*	117	129	130	139	154	154
9	K18	117	129	129	139	154	154
10	*K19*	117	125	120	129	162	218
11	*K21*	117	117	120	126	162	186
12	*K22*	117	125	120	129	162	162
13	K23	125	125	126	126	214	234
14	*K24*	117	125	120	129	162	214
15	*K25*	121	129	130	139	154	154
16	K26	117	129	130	139	154	154
17	*K27*	117	117	123	129	150	162
18	*K28*	125	129	123	123	154	166
19	*K29*	117	129	130	139	154	154
20	K30	117	117	130	139	154	154
21	K31	117	125	120	129	162	202
22	K32	117	121	126	129	162	182
23	*K35*	117	125	120	129	162	214
24	K36	117	125	120	129	162	166
25	K37	113	117	123	130	150	162
26	K38	121	125	123	137	154	166
27	*K39*	117	117	123	129	174	178
28	K40	125	125	123	137	158	158
29	K41	121	129	129	139	154	154
30	*K45*	125	125	123	137	154	166
31	K49	117	125	120	129	162	198
32	*K50*	117	125	120	129	162	198
33	K51	117	129	129	139	154	154
34	K53	117	129	129	139	146	154
35	K54	121	125	123	137	154	166

	sample	CDC3/CDC3R allele 1	CDC3/CDC3R allele 2	EF3/EF3R allele 1	EF3/EF3R allele 2	HIS3/HIS3R allele 1	HIS3/HIS3R allele 2
36	K57	117	117	126	137	154	182
37	*K58*	117	117	129	133	150	170
38	*K59*	117	129	129	137	154	154
39	K60	117	129	130	139	154	154
40	K62	121	125	123	137	154	166
41	K63	117	129	129	139	143	154
42	K64	117	125	120	129	166	230
43	K65	111	117	123	130	154	198
44	K66	125	125	123	133	166	182
45	*K67*	117	117	130	139	154	158
46	*K68*	117	125	120	120	162	198
47	*K69*	117	129	130	139	154	158
48	K71	121	125	123	123	166	166
49	W2	113	117	123	129	150	162
50	W3	117	125	129	129	162	162
51	*W4*	117	117	126	139	154	186
52	*W5*	117	125	120	129	162	198
53	*W6*	117	129	130	139	154	154
54	*W8*	117	125	120	129	162	162
55	*W9*	117	125	120	120	162	206
56	W11	117	125	120	120	154	162
57	W13	117	121	129	129	150	150
58	W14	117	125	126	126	162	162
59	W15	125	125	126	133	166	182
60	W16	125	125	123	133	166	182
61	*W17*	117	125	129	133	186	206
62	W18	117	125	126	126	178	178
63	W19	117	125	120	129	162	198
64	*W20*	117	125	129	129	190	202
65	W21	125	125	126	126	186	222
66	*W22*	125	125	123	139	166	166
67	W25	117	125	120	129	206	210
68	*W26*	117	117	126	139	142	154
69	*W27*	109	117	129	139	154	154
70	W34	117	117	126	139	154	158
71	*W37*	117	125	126	126	162	186
72	*W38*	113	117	123	129	150	162
73	W39	117	125	126	126	162	186
74	W44	117	129	130	139	154	154
75	*W45*	117	129	130	139	154	154
76	W47	109	117	126	131	154	154
77	W48	117	125	130	133	154	162

		CDC3/CDC3R		EF3/EF3R		HIS3/HIS3R	
	sample	allele 1	allele 2	allele 1	allele 2	allele 1	allele 2
78	W51	117	125	126	133	166	166
79	*W52*	117	125	120	129	162	194
80	W53	125	129	130	139	166	166
81	W54	125	125	126	133	182	194
82	*W55*	117	125	120	120	162	214
83	*W56*	113	117	123	129	150	162
84	*W58*	121	129	139	139	154	154
85	*W60*	117	125			162	210
86	*W61*	117	129	130	141	154	154
87	W62	117	121	126	126	162	190
88	*W63*	125	125	133	133	194	198
89	*W64*	117	129	129	139	154	154
90	*W65*	109	117	126	137	154	214
91	*W67*	117	125	120	129	170	206
92	*W68*	121	121	120	129	162	202
93	*W69*	117	125	129	139	162	202
94	W70	117	129	129	139	154	154
95	W71	113	117	126	139	150	162
96	*W73*	117	117	126	137	154	186
97	*W74*	117	125	120	129	166	226
98	*W75*	109	117	126	129	162	186
99	*W76*	117	117	126	139	154	182
100	*W77*	117	129	130	130	154	186
101	*W78*	117	129	129	129	154	162
102	W79	121	129	130	141	154	154
103	W80	117	129	120	129	194	206
104	W82	117	117	123	129	150	150
105	*W83*	117	125	120	120	162	198
106	*W84*	113	117	129	129	162	162
107	*W85*	117	125	120	129	162	206
108	*W87*	117	117	120	129	162	178
109	*W91*	117	129	129	139	142	142
110	W92	117	125	123	133	166	186
111	W94	117	129	129	139	154	154
112	W96	113	117	129	129	150	150
113	W97	117	117	123	130	178	182
114	*W98*	121	129	130	139	154	154
115	*W101*	117	117	126	137	154	154
116	W102	125	125	123	133	166	182
117	W103	125	125	126	133	182	186
118	*W104*	117	129	130	139	154	154
119	*W106*	121	125	123	137	158	166

		CDC3/CDC3R		EF3/EF3R		HIS3/HIS3R	
	sample	**allele 1**	**allele 2**	**allele 1**	**allele 2**	**allele 1**	**allele 2**
120	W107	117	129	129	139	154	158
121	W108	117	129	123	133	162	202
122	*W110*	121	125	123	137	154	166
123	*W113*	117	125	129	133	178	178

(samples in italic letters: biofilm positive)

Table 1. Microsatellite data for 123 *C. albicans* strains.

A comparison of the results did not reveal information of typical microsatellite models for *C. albicans* strains which produced biofilms in this study. Only 41 of the investigated strains showed a similarity with one or up to six other strains (Table 2).

CDC3/CDC3R		EF3/EF3R		HIS3/HIS3R		n		
allele 1	**allele 2**	**allele 1**	**allele 2**	**allele 1**	**allele 2**	**+**	**-**	**total**
113	117	123	129	150	162	2		2
117	129	129	139	154	154	1	4	5
117	129	130	139	154	154	7	4	11
121	129	130	139	154	154	2		2
121	125	123	137	154	166	1	3	4
117	125	120	129	162	162	2		2
117	125	126	126	162	186	1	1	2
117	125	120	120	162	198	2		2
117	125	120	129	162	198	2	2	4
117	125	120	129	162	214	2		2
125	125	123	133	166	182		3	3
125	125	126	133	166	182	1	1	2
						23	18	41

(+: biofilm positive; -: biofilm negative)

Table 2. Microsatellite models.

The most convergent data were generated with the CDC3 primer pair, only 12 different allele pairs were; found, with the EF3 primer pair 25 different pairs were located, and HIS3 primers provided 50 different pairs of alleles.

From six patients two strains were available, each of them originated from different samples and showed *C. albicans* infections in routine diagnostics. Both samples from one patient were biofilm positive, from another patient both samples were negative. The microsatellite data of these catheters are listed in table 3. When only HIS3 and CDC3 alleles were compared, five out of the six patients showed the same strain two times, when they were also compared with EF3 primer alleles, only one patient had the same strain two times.

The comparison of the genotyping of biofilm forming *C. albicans* strains (e.g. see figure 1) with non-biofilm forming *C. albicans* species shows also a consistent distribution of genotypes.

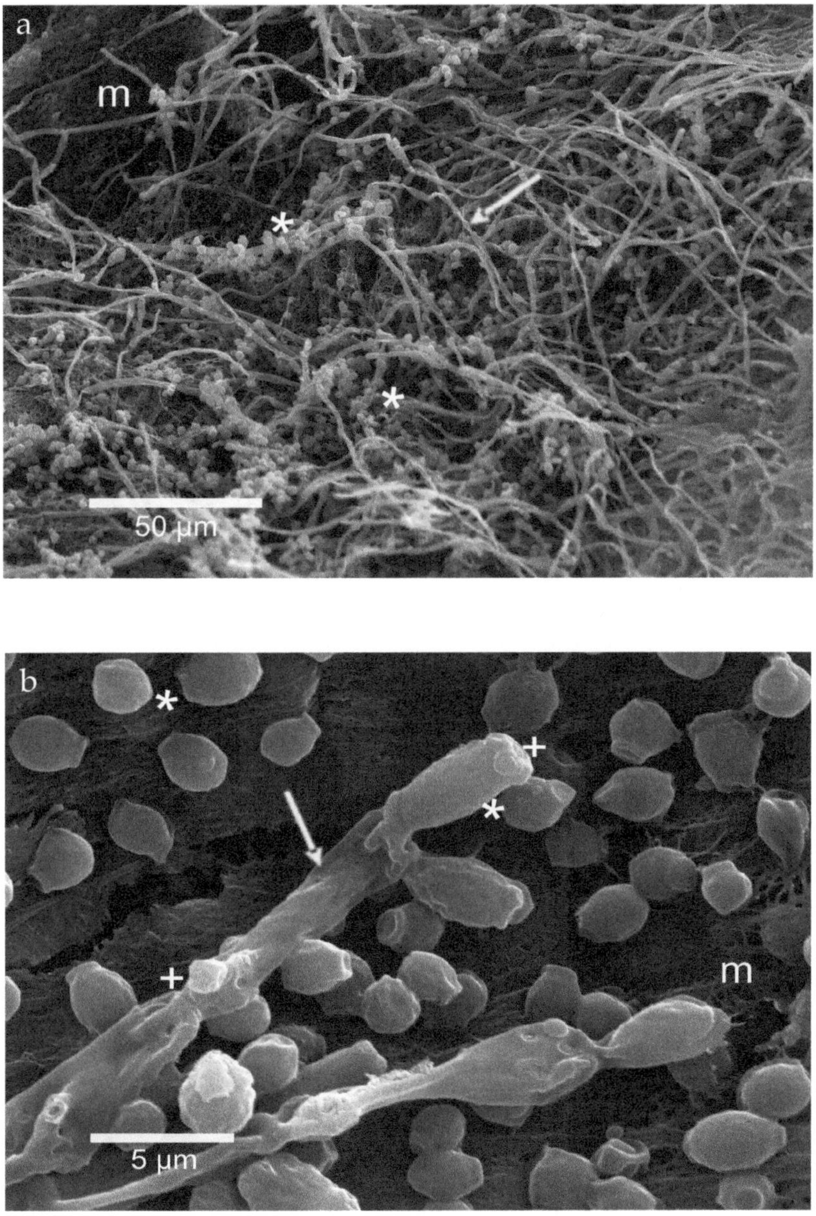

Fig. 1. (a) Biofilm of *C. albicans* (W65) in catheter lumen. (b) Biofilm detail of *C. albicans* (W91). *: yeast cells; +: bud scars; m: matrix material; arrow: hyphae. SEM micrographs were taken with a Philips XL30 ESEM scanning electron microscope using the high vacuum mode (emission electrons detection, acceleration voltage 20 kV, operating distance 10 mm).

			CDC3/CDC3R		EF3/EF3R		HIS3/HIS3R	
Patient	sample	biofilm	allele 1	allele 2	allele 1	allele 2	allele 1	allele 2
1	K15	-	125		126	133	166	182
	K16	+	125		123	133	166	182
2	K17	+	117	129	130	139	154	
	K18	-	117	129	129	139	154	
3	K49	-	117	125	120	129	162	198
	K50	+	117	125	120	129	162	198
4	K59	+	117	129	129	137	154	
	K60	-	117	129	130	139	154	
5	K67	+	117		130	139	154	158
	K69	+	117	129	130	139	154	158
6	W15	-	125		126	133	166	182
	W16	-	125		123	133	166	182

(+: biofilm positive; -: biofilm negative)

Table 3. Microsatellite models of 12 strains from six patients (two strains each).

3. Discussion

The catheters which were investigated in this study originated from many different stations of mainly two hospitals. The analyses of the genotypes of 123 *C. albicans* strains collected from these samples give many interesting points to think about. The comparison of the CDC3, EF3, and HIS3 genotyping results from the two hospitals (data not shown) did not provide suitable data for distinguishing the epidemiological distribution of *C. albicans*. The contribution of the genotypes was consistent within the University Hospital of Graz compared with the AKH Vienna hospital. This was also true for the aggregation of the data, no significantly dominant genotype was detected, only a group of 11 (8.9%) strains (Table 2) was found to be the most frequent genotype with the multilocus genotype characterised by CDC3: 117-129, EF3: 130-139, and HIS3 154-154. All other groups within this study consist of at most 5 strains. These results are comparable to those of Eloy et al. (2006) who studied the genotypes of *C. albicans* in two different hospitals using the CDC3, EF3, and HIS3 typing system. An overall number of 67 isolates were tested and 50 different genotypes were found. Eight patients shared the same genotype in one hospital; the same genotype was also present in 3 strains in the second hospital. Botterel et al. (2001) tested 100 isolates for their microsatellite profile. They detected 5, 12, and 18 alleles in the CDC3, EF3, and HIS3 system, respectively. The different associations of this alleles led to 10 CDC3, 22 EF3, and 25 HIS3 allele associations within this system. A group of 17 isolates was found to share the genotype.

This genotype was the same as reported by Eloy et al. (2006) in the group of 11 genotype identical strains. Both authors reported the multilocus genotype characterised by CDC3: 117-125, EF3: 126-135, and HIS3 162-162 for their most common strains.

Totally different data were provided from Shi et al. (2007) who collected isolates by female and male patients with genital infection, rectal and oral samples. The authors reported 54.9% of the strains investigated to show the same multilocus genotype, these results were clearly different from all other studies.

The CDC3 locus showed 12 different allele pairs, the EF3 locus 25 allele pairs, and the HIS3 locus 50 allele pairs. This is convergent with the data within the three loci and leads to 94 multilocus genotypes. When compared with the results of Botterel et al. (2001) who reported 65 different multilocus genotypes with different allele associations of 10 for CDC3, 22 for EF3, and 25 for HIS3, it is obvious that the HIS3 locus was clearly more divergent within the current study. However, it remains unclear whether this variation is typical for *C. albicans* strains collected from BSI, or if the discriminatory power (DP) of the HIS3 locus (0.91) is not strong enough. The calculated overall DP for the CDC3, EF3, and HIS3 multilocus genotyping was 0.97. It is worth noting that the DP of HIS3 alone was the highest of the three loci (CDC3: 0.77, EF3: 0.86) (Botterel et al., 2001). Nevertheless, a comparison of the typing information without the HIS3 locus showed that the groups of strains sharing the same genotype do not increase significantly (data not shown).

The comparison of the genotyping of biofilm forming *C. albicans* strains with non-biofilm forming *C. albicans* species shows also a consistent distribution of genotypes. There is no literature to compare these specific results with, but as aforementioned, a consistent contribution of genotype data collected with the CDC3, EF3, and HIS3 multilocus genotyping system seems to be normal for *C. albicans* strains.

The collected information about strains from the same patients are worth a closer look: Only one patient out of six showed 2 strains sharing the multilocus genotype. Using the same typing system, Beretta et al. (2006) investigated 14 isolates of eight patients and reported 4 strains with the same genotype for one patient out of three. Another patient had 2 of 3 strains sharing the genotypes (Beretta et al., 2006). When only HIS3 and CDC3 alleles were compared, five out of the six patients in the current study show the same strain twice. Because of these findings, the typing was done without EF3 locus information, and as it is mentioned above for the typing without HIS3 allele information, no significant increase in the numbers of strains sharing the same multilocus genotype could be seen (data not shown).

Recapitulating the multilocus genotyping with the CDC3, EF3, and HIS3 system during this study, the data presented here is in good agreement with the authors mentioned above.

4. Conclusion

The multilocus genotyping with the CDC3, EF3, and HIS3 system during this study did work well and provided data comparable to former studies. Therefore it is strongly indicated that the genotyping of *C. albicans* strains should be continued in future studies. Aditionally the results give possible evidence that genotypes do not matter in the connection to biofilm forming abilities, so that potentially all *C. albicans* strains are able to form such ecosystems. In that case, studies like the recent one can only give evidence of epidemiological behavior of the species investigated.

Another set of microsatellite markers is likely to give more information about those strains which are able to form biofilms on indwelling devices or about the epidemiological behavior of clinically important strains.

5. Acknowledgment

This work was partly funded by the Hygiene Fund of the Medical University of Graz. This work was performed in the TTIW-cooperation framework of Wetsus, centre of excellence for sustainable water technology (www.wetsus.nl). Wetsus is funded by the Dutch Ministry of Economic Affairs. The authors like to thank the participants of the research theme "DNA based detection technologies" for the fruitful discussions and their financial support.

6. References

Applied Biosystems. 2005. *GeneMapper® Software Version 4.0 Microsatellite Analysis Getting Started Guide*. Applied Biosystems, Foster City, California.

Beretta, S.; Fulgencio, J.P.; Enache-Angoulvant, A.; Bernard, C.; El Metaoua, S., Ancelle, T.; Denis, M. & Hennequin, C. (2006). Application of microsatellite typing for the investigation of a cluster of cases of Candida albicans candidaemia. *Clinical Microbiology and Infection*, Vol.12, No.7, pp. 674-676, ISSN 1198-743X

Bernhardt, H. (1998). Fungi in the intestine - normal flora or pathogens? *Zeitschrift für ärztliche Fortbildung und Qualitätssicherung*, Vol.92, No.3, pp. 154-156

Botterel, F.; Desterke, C.; Costa, C. & Bretagne, S. (2001). Analysis of microsatellite markers of Candida albicans used for rapid typing. *Journal of Clinical Microbiology*, Vol.39, No.11, pp. 4076-4081, ISSN 0095-1137

David, A.; Risitano, D.C.; Mazzeo, G.; Sinardi, L.; Venuti, F.S. & Sinardi, A.U. (2005). Central venous catheters and infections. *Minerva Anestesiologica*, Vol.71, No.9, pp. 561-564, ISSN 0375-9393

Donlan, R.M. (2001). Biofilm formation: a clinically relevant microbiological process. *Clinical Infectious Diseases*, Vol.33, No.8, pp. 1387-1392, ISSN 1058-4838

Donskey C.J. (2004). The role of the intestinal tract as a reservoir and source for transmission of nosocomial pathogens *Clinical Infectious Diseases*, Vol.39, No.2, pp. 219-226, ISSN 1058-4838

El-Azizi, M.A.; Starks, S.E & Khardori, N. (2004). Interactions of Candida albicans with other Candida spp. and bacteria in the biofilms. *Journal of Applied Microbiology*, Vol.96, No.5, pp. 1067-1073, ISSN 1365-2672

Eloy, O.; Marque, S.; Botterel, F.; Stephan, F.; Costa, J.M.; Lasserre, V. & Bretagne, S. (2006). Uniform distribution of three Candida albicans microsatellite markers in two French ICU populations supports a lack of nosocomial cross-contamination. *BMC Infectious Diseases*, Vol.13, No.6, pp. 162, ISSN 1471-2334

Fan, S.R.; Liao, Q.P.; Li, J.; Liu, X.P.; Liu, Z.H. & Bai, F.Y. (2007). Genotype distribution of Candida albicans strains associated with different conditions of vulvovaginal candidiasis, as revealed by microsatellite typing. *Sexually Transmitted Infections*, Vol.84, No.2, pp. 103-106, ISSN 1472-3263

Hogan, D.A. (2006). Talking to themselves: autoregulation and quorum sensing in fungi. *Eukaryotic Cell*, Vol.5, No.4, pp. 613-619, ISSN 1535-9778

López-Ribot, J.L. (2005). Candida albicans biofilms: more than filamentation. *Current Biology*, Vol.15, No.12, pp. 453-455, ISSN 0960-9822

Marol, S. & Yücesoy, M. (2008). Molecular epidemiology of Candida species isolated from clinical specimens of intensive care unit patients. *Mycoses*, Vol.51, No.1, pp. 40-49, ISSN 0933-7407

Mohanty S, Xess I, Hasan F, Kapil A, Mittal S, Tolosa JE. 2007. Prevalence & susceptibility to fluconazole of Candida species causing vulvovaginitis. *The Indian Journal of Medical Research*, Vol.126, No.3, pp. 216-219, ISSN 0971-5916

Nobile, C.J.; Andes, D.R.; Nett, J.E.; Smith, F.J.; Yue, F.; Phan, Q.T.; Edwards, J.E.; Filler, S.G. & Mitchell, A.P. (2006). Critical role of Bcr1-dependent adhesins in C. albicans biofilm formation in vitro and in vivo. *PLoS Pathogens*, Vol.2, No.7, pp. e63, ISSN 1553-7366

Odds, F.C.; Hanson, M.F.; Davidson, A.D.; Jacobsen, M.D.; Wright, P.; Whyte, J.A.; Gow, N.A. & Jones, B.L. (2007). One year prospective survey of Candida bloodstream infections in Scotland. *Journal of Medical Microbiology*, Vol.56, No. 8, pp. 1066-1075, ISSN 0022-2615

Paulitsch, A.; Weger, W.; Ginter-Hanselmayer, G.; Marth, E. & Buzina, W. (2006). A 5-year (2000-2004) epidemiological survey of Candida and non-Candida yeast species causing vulvovaginal candidiasis in Graz, Austria. *Mycoses*, Vol.49, No.6, pp. 471-475, ISSN 0933-7407

Paulitsch, A.H.; Willinger, B.; Zsalatz, B.; Stabentheiner, E.; Marth, E. & Buzina, W. (2009). In-vivo Candida biofilms in scanning electron microscopy. *Medical Mycology*, Vol.47, No.7, pp. 690-696, ISSN 1369-3786

Pierce, G.E. (2005). Pseudomonas aeruginosa, Candida albicans, and device-related nosocomial infections: implications, trends, and potential approaches for control. *Journal of Industrial Microbiology & Biotechnology*, Vol.32, No.7, pp. 309-318, ISSN 1367-5435

Ramage, G.; Saville, S.P.; Thomas, D.P. & López-Ribot, J.L. (2005). Candida biofilms: an update. *Eukaryotic Cell*, Vol.4, No.4, pp. 633-638, ISSN 1535-9778

Sampaio, P.; Gusmão, L.; Correia, A.; Alves, C.; Rodrigues, A.G.; Pina-Vaz, C.; Amorim, A. & Pais, C. (2005). New microsatellite multiplex PCR for Candida albicans strain typing reveals microevolutionary changes. *Journal of Clinical Microbiology*, Vol.43, No.8, pp. 3869-3876, ISSN 0095-1137

Sánchez-Portocarrero, J.; Martín-Rabadán, P.; Saldaña, C.J. & Pérez-Cecilia, E. (1994). Candida cerebrospinal fluid shunt infection. Report of two new cases and review of the literature. *Diagnostic Microbiology and Infectious Disease*, Vol.20, No.1, pp. 33-40, ISSN 0732-8893

Shi, W.M.; Mei, X.Y.; Gao, F.; Huo, K.K.; Shen, L.L.; Qin, H.H.; Wu, Z.W. & Zheng, J. (2007). Analysis of genital Candida albicans infection by rapid microsatellite markers genotyping. *Chinese Medical Journal*, Vol.120, No.11, pp. 975-980, ISSN 0366-6999

Sobel, J.D. (2007). Vulvovaginal candidosis. *Lancet*, Vol.369, No.9577, pp. 1961-1971. ISSN 0140-6736

Tumbarello, M.; Posteraro, B.; Trecarichi, E.M.; Fiori, B.; Rossi, M.; Porta, R.; de Gaetano Donati, K.; La Sorda, M.; Spanu, T.; Fadda, G.; Cauda, R. & Sanguinetti, M. (2007). Biofilm production by Candida species and inadequate antifungal therapy as predictors of mortality for patients with candidemia. *Journal of Clinical Microbiology*, Vol.45, No.6, pp. 1843-1850, ISSN 0095-1137

Verstrepen, K.J. & Klis, F.M. (2006). Flocculation, adhesion and biofilm formation in yeasts. Molecular Microbiology, Vol.60, No.1, pp. 5-15

Section 2

Epidemiology Molecular of Methicillin-Resistant *Staphylococcus aureus* (MRSA) Isolated from Humans and Animals

4

MRSA Epidemiology in Animals

Patrícia Yoshida Faccioli-Martins and
Maria de Lourdes Ribeiro de Souza da Cunha
UNESP- Univ. Estadual Paulista, Biosciences Institute, Botucatu, SP
Brazil

1. Introduction

Until the 1990s, methicillin-resistant *Staphylococcus aureus* (MRSA) was traditionally considered a pathogen causing nosocomial infections, being the so-called HA-MRSA (healthcare-associated methicillin-resistant *Staphylococcus aureus*). However, over time, cases of MRSA-positive individuals were observed who never had contact with hospital services, and strains from these individuals were identified and named CA-MRSA (community-associated methicillin-resistant *Staphylococcus aureus*). In 2003 in the Netherlands, a new MRSA strain arose in patients that could not be typed through PFGE (pulsed field gel electrophoresis) with *Sma*I, with resistance to digestion by this enzyme (Bens et al., 2006), being called since then NT-MRSA (non typeable methicillin-resistant *Staphylococcus aureus*). Investigations of this NT-MRSA intensified, and it was observed that these patients carrying this strain had previous contact with pigs and the geographic distribution of cases showed clusters near pig farms (van Loo et al., 2007). With more advanced studies, it was possible to determine strains strictly related to animals, such as those found in pigs, which were named LA-MRSA (livestock-associated methicillin-resistant *Staphylococcus aureus*) in 2010 (Vanderhaeghen et al., 2010).

The resistance to methicillin in staphylococci is mediated by the *mecA* gene that encodes a modified penicillin-binding protein (PBP), the PBP2a or 2′, which shows reduced affinity to the resistant penicillins to penicillinase, such as methicillin and oxacillin and for all other beta-lactam antibiotics (van Duijkeren et al., 2004). Due to the need for better characterizing these isolates, they have been classified in a more detailed manner, beginning with the SCC*mec* types and patterns identified by PFGE, and are currently based on sequence type and *spa* typing. With the use of techniques such as MLST (multi locus sequence typing) and *spa* typing, characteristic clones from animals have been observed, and it is suspected that some have tropism by determined host species. An example of this is ST398, which in addition to being strictly linked to pigs, has carried novel types of SCC*mec*. Li et al. (2011) analyzed the *SCCmec* element structure carried by 31 CC398 MRSA strains isolated from participants of a conference. The strains were classified into novel types, IX and X, type V (5C2&5) subtype c and type IVa, all carriers of genes conferring resistance to metals. The SCC*mec* structures from CC398 strains were distinct from those usually found in humans, complementing evidence that humans are not the original host for CC398. With the absence of a complete evaluation of risk factors for carrying this strain as much in animals as in humans, Graveland et al. (2010) carried out the first study that showed direct association between animal and human carriage of ST398. This association, in addition to the association between MRSA and the antimicrobial use in calves, highlights the need for prudent use of antibiotics in farm animals.

One clone of special interest in ruminants is the CC133. The great majority of isolates from small ruminants is represented by this clonal complex of *S. aureus*, but its evolutionary origin and molecular basis for its host tropism remain unknown. Guinane et al. (2010), attempting to determine whether the CC133 developed as result of a transmission from human host to ruminant followed by an adaptative diversification of the genome, carried out a comparative sequencing of the complete genome. Several novel mobile genetic elements were observed in the CC133 isolates encoding virulence proteins with attenuated or enhanced activity and they were widely distributed, suggesting a key role in their host-specific interaction. These data provide broad and new insights into the origin and basis molecular of *S. aureus* ruminant host specificity. The MRSA evolution and epidemiology in animals are discussed in this chapter.

2. History of MRSA in animals

The first report of MRSA in animals was in milk from Belgium cows with mastitis (Morgan, 2008). Until 2000, MRSA had been isolated sporadically from animals, in particular cows, small companion animals, and horses. With exception of some equine isolates, the nature of these cases suggested a human origin and no epidemics have been reported. In this respect, until the end of 20th century, both the scientific community and policy makers were convinced that animal husbandry was of little relevance for MRSA causing diseases in humans, but was particularly a problem based on antimicrobial use in human medicine. The situation has changed with a growing number of reports of MRSA in livestock, especially pigs and veal calves. MRSA has also been reported in companion animals and horses, as well as transmission between humans and animals (Catry et al., 2010). Calling attention to this dramatic increase of MRSA in animals, van Duijkeren et al. (2010) at the Veterinary Microbiological Diagnostic Center, in the Netherlands, reported 0% MRSA in isolates from equine clinical samples in 2002 and then 37% in 2008.

3. The importance of the different animal species

Various species have been identified as host and carriers of MRSA in different countries and settings, including dogs, cats, sheep, chickens, horses, pigs, rabbits, seals, psittacine birds, and one turtle, bat, guinea pig and chinchilla (Morgan, 2008). With differences between strains isolated from pets, wild animals and cattle, it is important to evaluate each species individually, because they present peculiar characteristics, including the series of resistance genes. Thus, the concern for MRSA types in animals has grown considering their role as a potential reservoir or vector for human infection by MRSA in the community. However the data available on MRSA transmission between humans and companion animals are limited, and further epidemiological studies are needed on this transmission and its impact on public health (Loeffler & Lloyd, 2010).

3.1 Companion animals

Pets have been shown to act as reservoirs of bacteria resistant to antimicrobials, and MRSA transmission between humans and animals has been described. For strains of MRSA with a low specificity to the host, the transference is likely to occur in both directions between humans and pets living at the same household (Nienhoff et al., 2009). The infections by MRSA in companion animals are predominantly of skin and soft tissues, especially during post-surgical (Morgan, 2008).

Nienhoff et al. (2009) reported two cases of transmission of MRSA strains between humans and dogs. Three positive dogs to MRSA were identified in a survey carried out in 803 dogs and 117 cats admitted to the Small Animal Clinic of the University of Veterinary Medicine Hannover, Germany. The first case was a 6-month-old female admitted to the clinic for teeth extraction. The owner, MRSA-positive, was a specialist veterinarian in swine diseases, working in pig barns 4-5 days per week and having access to MRSA ST398-positive farms. The dog and owner strains were identical through molecular typing, belonging to ST398 and *spa* type t034. The second case was an 11-year-old male admitted to the clinic because of a cardiac problem. The likely origin of the strain was the mother-in-law of the dog's owner, who is diabetic, having received nursing care at home and presenting an infected wound on the foot and an ulcer in the right eye. The MRSA isolates found in these lesions and in the dog belonged to ST225, which is frequently found in humans.

3.2 Cattle

Cows with mastitis have been the most likely to harbor MRSA, and they may be related to horizontal transfer via wet hands of colonized or infected dairy farm workers, and selection by the use of antibiotics to treat mastitis (Morgan, 2008). The first known case of MRSA transmission between cows and a person was reported by Juhász-Kaszanyitzky et al. (2007). MRSA strains isolated from cows with subclinical mastitis were phenotypically and genotypically indistinguishable from the strain from the person who worked with these animals. These strains were determined as ST1, *spa* type t127, SCC*mec*IVa. The authors considered these strains epidemiologically related, indicating transmission from cow to human or from human to cow.

Feβler et al. (2010) studied 25 MRSA ST398 isolates from cases of bovine clinical mastitis and two isolates from farm workers originating from 17 dairy farms in Germany, evaluating the genetic relatedness, antimicrobial resistance and virulence properties. Nine major ApaI PFGE patterns were found, three *spa types* (t011, t034 and t2576) and two types of SCC*mec* (IV and V) were identified. As described previously for ST398 from pigs, isolates from this sequence type originating in cases of bovine mastitis have also shown a high degree of variability when the ApaI PFGE profile and other genotypic and phenotypic characteristics were compared. A uniform pattern of virulence genes appeared to be conserved between ST398 isolated from both animal species.

Türkyılmaz et al. (2010) detected 14 of 16 strains from bovine milk of the lineage MRSA ST-239-III in which one was related to hospital-associated clones, and two strains were ST8/IV, which correspond to USA300, which causes severe community-acquired infections. The presence of MRSA ST239-III lineage can indicate a transmission from humans to animals, and the presence of ST8-IV can show emergence of strains from the community in the Aydin region in Turkey. This study underscores the necessity to take measures to avoid MRSA transmission between humans and animals.

3.3 Horses

In horses, MRSA have been reported in infections of skin and soft tissues, bacteraemia, septic arthritis, osteomyelitis, implant-related infections, metritis, omphalitis, catheter-related infections and pneumonia. The first MRSA outbreak in horses was observed in 1993, with 11 infected horses in the post-surgical in a veterinary teaching hospital in Michigan. Subsequent outbreaks have occurred on Japan, Austria, the UK, Ireland, Canada, and other areas of the USA (Morgan, 2008).

In 2009, Loeffler et al. reported the first isolation of MRSA ST398 *spa* type t011 in animals from the UK. They were two horses in southeastern England, with isolates with identical phenotypic and genotypic characteristics as reported in horses in Belgium, Austria and Germany, which also carried the SCC*mec* type IVa. They vary from those commonly found in pigs (*spa* type t108, t034 or t571) and frequently carry SCC*mec* V, possibly indicating host-specific variation within this lineage or independent evolution. One interesting fact is that isolates from pigs and horses commonly show resistance to tetracycline and/or gentamicin, both agents frequently used in pigs and horses, respectively. These findings demonstrate the introduction of ST398 in England and provide more evidence of successful dissemination of this zoonotic pathogen in the animal reservoir. The authors recommended vigilance for MRSA ST398 in both animals and humans.

Outbreaks of MRSA were observed in horses and horse personnel in the Netherlands in the period of 2006-2008. The isolates belonged to ST8, *spa* type t064, and to ST398, *spa* types t011 and t2123, predominantly. During the outbreak of post-surgical infections by MRSA in horses in a veterinary teaching hospital, isolates from *spa* type t2123 were isolated from 7 horses, and 4 of 61 personnel indicating a zoonotic transmission; after intervention, the outbreak stopped. In another outbreak that occurred in 2008, 17 horses with MRSA were detected, with 12 *spa* type t011, 4 *spa* type t2123 and 1 *spa* type t064. From 170 personnel, 16 were positive for MRSA, with 11 *spa* type t011 and 5 *spa* type t2123. From 106 personnel who maintained close contact with horses, 15 were MRSA-positive compared with 1 MRSA-positive of 64 personnel who had no close contact with the animals. Furthermore, screening carried out on the horses on admission showed that 9.3% were MRSA-positive, predominantly *spa*-type t011. Weekly cross-sectional sampling from all horses hospitalized for 5 weeks demonstrated that 42% were MRSA-positive at least once, again predominantly with *spa* type t011, which suggests that a nosocomial transmission appeared. The research of environmental samples from veterinary hospital revealed the presence of 53% of MRSA, including samples from students and staff member rooms, all *spa* type t011, indicating that humans contribute to the microorganism dissemination. The samples cultured employing pre-enrichment with high-salt concentration presented better results than the method without pre-enrichment. These results demonstrate that the nosocomial transmission in equine clinics occurs and suggest that personnel play a role in the transmission (van Duijkeren et al., 2010).

3.4 Poultry

The first reports of MRSA in chicken meat occurred in Korea in 2003 (Lee, 2003) and Japan in 2005 (Kitai et al., 2005), but it was not determined as livestock-associated, raising the hypothesis of meat contamination with human strains through handlers.

LA-MRSA was reported primarily in health poultry in 2008 in Belgium, with ten recent isolates classified as ST398 *spa* types t011 and t567. In this study, strains isolated in 1970s and strains isolated recently in 2006 were evaluated. It was observed that from 12 antimicrobial agents tested, eight presented percentage of resistance significantly higher in the recent isolates (Nemati et al., 2008).

Persoons et al. (2009) evaluated samples from 50 laying hens and 75 broiler chickens in Belgium. MRSA was found in 8 broiler chickens from 2 of 14 farms sampled, belonging to ST398 *spa* type t1456. According to the author, it still remains unclear as to whether this strain is associated with poultry.

3.5 Pigs

Mounting evidence suggests that livestock, particularly pigs, can represent an important reservoir of CA-MRSA (community-associated - CA) strains that can colonize and infect humans in close contact with them. ST398 is the most commonly reported MRSA sequence type among large livestock in Europe. These strains frequently carry genes encoding for non-beta-lactam antimicrobial resistance, including a plasmid-borne gene with resistance to trimetoprim, *dfrK*, identified in an isolate from a pig from Germany. Furthermore, these isolates are referred to often as nontypeable by PFGE because their genome is not digested by SmaI enzymes, several common *spa* types have been associated with them, carrying SCC*mec* types IV and V and they typically lack PVL genes (David & Daum, 2010).

In 2008, with the aim of evaluating whether other professionals in contact with pigs, in addition to farmers and veterinarians, have a higher risk of carrying MRSA than the population in general, a study was carried out with 272 participants of a conference on swine health in Denmark. In total, 34 (12.5%) participants from 9 countries carried MRSA, being that 31 isolates were not typeable by PFGE with *Sma*I. They belonged to ST398, *spa* types t011, t034, t108, t571, t567 and t899. The MRSA transmission from pigs to staff demonstrated to be an international problem, creating a new reservoir for a strain that was still considered CA-MRSA (Wulf et al., 2008).

Horgan et al. (2010) evaluated the prevalence of MRSA in the swine population in Ireland. A total of 440 pigs were evaluated from 41 geographically distributed farms and 100 individuals involved in the pig industry. No MRSA isolate was recovered from pigs but two humans tested were identified as MRSA carriers. These individuals were working in the wider pig industry. These isolates belonged to ST22 and ST1307, indicating that during the period of study the porcine colonization by MRSA, in particular the animal-related strain ST398, was not common in Ireland.

Wagenaar et al. (2009) published the first report of MRSA on pig farms in China, and it was the first time that MRSA ST9 in 4 pig farms and one *single locus variant* of MLST ST9 (ST1376) were detected in a pig farm. This study shows that LA-MRSA is not restricted to the clonal lineage ST398 found in Europe and North America in commercial pigs, but that other MRSA lineages are able to spread in the livestock in the same manner, also confirming that livestock can act as a reservoir of MRSA.

Despite that LA-MRSA appears be the predominant MRSA strain in pigs, some studies mention the detection of non-LA-MRSA strains in these animals, possibly by transmission of human strains to the animals. In Singapore, ST22-MRSA-IV was isolated from pigs and this strain was previously found increasingly important in the hospital population there. Notably the ST22-MRSA-IV is also a major hospital clone, as is the UK-EMRSA-15 found in the UK, with both strains indicating a contamination of human origin. In Canada, 14% of MRSA isolated from pigs appeared to belong to the human epidemic clone CMRSA-2 (Canadian epidemic MRSA-2, known as USA100), while 74.4% of isolates were LA-MRSA. The remaining strains belonged to rare clones, not related to LA-MRSA or CMRSA-2. Most reports on LA-MRSA in pigs originate from the Netherlands. In Europe, LA-MRSA has also been found in pigs in Germany, Denmark and Belgium, and beyond Europe, in Canada, Singapore and the USA (Vanderhaeghen et al., 2010).

3.6 Products of animal origin

Besides the importance of living animals as a source of MRSA, animal origin products also play a role in disseminating these strains to the humans. Lozano et al. (2009) detected MRSA ST398 in food samples in Spain. A total of 318 samples of raw food were evaluated from food-producing animals (148 from chicken, 55 from pork, 46 from veal, 19 from lamb, 10 from turkey, 8 from rabbit and 12 minced-meat samples) and of wild animals (8 *game birds*, 4 wild boar, 4 deer and 4 hare samples). MRSA was detected in 5 of 318 (1.6%) food samples (pork, chicken, rabbit, veal and wild boar). The two strains from pork and veal corresponded to ST398-SCC*mec*V clone (*spa* types t011 and t1197, respectively), the two strains from chicken and rabbit were typed as ST125-SCC*mec*IVa-t067, and the strain from one wild boar was ST217-SCC*mec*IVa-t032, with all the MRSA being PVL negative. The characteristics of these strains suggest that they can be of both animal and human origin, and although the presence of MRSA in food is low, it must be monitored, because it can contribute to its dissemination.

Recently, Weese et al. (2011) evaluated the presence of MRSA in feedlot cattle, close to the time of slaughter, in nasal and rectal fecal samples. It was not possible to detect MRSA in these animals, in contrast to recent studies on retail beef (Weese et al., 2010), demonstrating the need for more studies of livestock, as well as farms, processing and retail environments to elucidate the epidemiology of contamination with MRSA in meat.

4. MRSA as zoonosis or humanosis

Several studies have been done to determine the degree to which MRSA plays a role in zoonosis or humanosis. It has been observed that usually the strains originating from companion animals are originally human strains, and that the infection with this MRSA type is considered humanosis. On the other hand, the strains orginating from livestock (livestock-associated - LA) are often divergent from human strains and the infection with this type of LA-MRSA could be considered zoonosis, and in this case MRSA would be an emergent zoonotic agent. Within this context, veterinarians, cattle farmers and pet owners are considered risk groups for acquiring MRSA (Morgan, 2008).

In 2011, a case of empyema was reported in a 79-year-old man in Spain with isolation of MRSA ST398 in purulent exudates from the thorax and trachea and nasal swabs. The ineffective initial therapy with levofloxacin was modified to intravenous linezolid, but the clinical situation of the patient rapidly deteriorated, and he died of multiorgan failure. The three MRSA strains were typed as ST398, *spa*-type t011, SCC*mec* V and *agr*I and presented the same phenotypic resistance, including β-lactam, tetracycline, clindamycin (but not erythromycin), ciprofloxacin and levofloxacin. It is important to point out that the patient lived with his wife and two sons near a pig farm. Both sons worked on the farm. The patient, but not his wife, sporadically helped on the farm. Nasal samples from three family members indicated MRSA carriage in one son. The characteristics of this isolate were identical to the isolate from the patient. Furthermore, nasal swabs of 18 pigs from the farm were randomly collected, and MRSA isolates were detected in 9 (50%) pigs. One MRSA isolated in each animal was minutely characterized. Eight isolates were typed as ST 398/t011/SCC*mec* V/*agr*I and one remaining isolate as ST398/t1451/SCC*mec* V/*agr*I. All MRSA isolated from the animals had the same phenotypic and genotypic resistance comparing MRSA isolated from the patient and son. These findings indicate potential pig-human zoonosis transmission of MRSA ST398 and that this clone can be associated with severe respiratory pathology in immunocompromised patients, and this microorganism can also be resistant to other first-line antimicrobial agents, such as fluoroquinolones, used to treat these infections. Furthermore, the unusual clindamycin-resistance/erythromycin-susceptibility phenotype can be a key marker (in addition to tetracycline resistance) of the possible presence of livestock-associated MRSA (Lozano et al., 2011).

As seen in the reports, animal reservoirs for MRSA are becoming recognized worldwide with increasing awareness of MRSA ST398 colonizing pig and veal farmers, and attending veterinarians, at high rates. In The Netherlands, these groups are now considered high risk, and if admitted to a hospital, they are immediately conducted to isolation, screening for MRSA and decolonization (Loeffler et al., 2009).

MRSA isolates originating from animals have been shown to hold important genes of resistance which could be transferred to less pathogenic human strains, but well adapted, in a nasal co-colonization and resulting in new human lineages, for example (Springer et al., 2009). The gene *czrC,* which confers resistance to cadmium and zinc, was determined in isolates of MRSA CC398 of SCC*mec* type V originating from 23 (74%) pigs and 24 (48%) humans from Denmark. It is suggested that resistance to heavy metals can play a role in coselection of MRSA, because it was strongly related to the clone CC398 (Cavaco et al., 2010).

In lineages MRSA ST398 and MSSA ST9 isolated from pigs in Germany, the major reservoir of these lineages, the gene *cfr* was found, a gene of multi-resistance to the drugs phenicol/lincosamine/oxazolidinone/pleuromutilin/streptogramin A. The risk of its transference to humans with exposure to pig farms is of concern since these lineages can colonize and cause infections in humans (Kehrenberg et al., 2009).

Genes encoding virulence factors can also be carried by animal strains. An example is the PVL gene, encoding an important virulence factor related to MRSA, rarely reported in animals, but can be found in companion animals. PVL-positive CA-MRSA has been reported in cats, dogs, rabbits, birds, bats, turtles, pigs and cattle. The strains associated with pigs that have been rapidly disseminating are currently PVL-negative (Morgan, 2008).

As for animal origin food, meats of several animal species have been evaluated for detection of MRSA. The contamination has been reported in meats of turkey, chicken, veal, pork, beef and lamb. The majority of the isolates were non typeable MRSA. Considering the low number of non typeable MRSA in patients, the role of food products in disseminating MRSA seems to have been overlooked (Morgan, 2008).

5. MRSA detection in animals

Animal studies of MRSA are limited by certain research bottlenecks compared to human studies, including a lack of standardization regarding culture methodology, susceptibility testing, definition of genetic profile and sampling methods, which ultimately renders comparison difficult. A mass animal screening is logistically difficult, expensive, and impractical in many situations. Moreover, physical challenges exist: for example, carrying out a nasal swab in cats is only possible with appropriate animal restraints (Morgan, 2008).

Despite these drawbacks, several studies have been carried out, as more detailed studies of epidemiological aspects of animal MRSA are indispensable, primarily in food-producing animals of particular concern. These animals are not only reported as the primary source of a recently emergent new type of MRSA, LA-MRSA, but studies also suggest that they are involved in transmission of other strains of MRSA between animals and humans (Vanderhaeghen et al., 2010). MRSA screening must be performed in all diagnostic laboratories, even if done through disk diffusion with oxacillin, which is better than methicillin related to the resistance to degradation and the detection of heteroresistant strains (Weese et al., 2004).

MRSA detection in animals has been performed, generally, with isolation from samples from nasal and oral mucosae and perineum in small animals (Loeffler et al., 2005; Nienhoff et al., 2009), samples from milk in cows (Kwon et al., 2005), samples from nasal, oral and/or perineal swab, in pigs and horses (Baptiste et al., 2005; Voss et al., 2005; Huijsdens et al., 2006), samples from nose and cloacae in poultries (Nemati et al., 2008) and samples from meats (Lozano et al., 2009).

The samples were pre-enriched in different selective mediums with the aim of increasing the sensitivity of the culture technique. Lozano et al. (2009), to detect MRSA in meat, pre-enriched the samples in BHI broth (brain heart infusion) containing 6.5% of sodium chloride at 35°C for 24 h. An aliquot of each growth was seeded on ORSAB plates (oxacillin resistance screening agar base) with oxacillin (2mg/L) and incubated at 35°C for 36 h. Van Duijkeren et al. (2010) compared two methods of culture technique; the first was Müeller Hinton Broth containing 6.5% sodium chloride, which after overnight incubation at 37°C, was transferred to phenol red mannitol broth with 5μg/ml of ceftizoxime and 75μg/ml of aztreonam and after overnight incubation at 37°C was plated onto sheep blood agar and brilliance MRSA agar. In the second method, Tryptone Soy Broth was used containing 4% sodium chloride, 1% mannitol, 16μg/ml of phenol red, 50μg/ml of aztreonam and 5μg/ml ceftizoxime, plating onto sheep blood agar and MRSA brilliance agar after 48 hours of incubation at 37°C. The first method, with the pre-enrichment containing higher salt concentration, presented better results. Weese et al. (2011) used as pre-enrichment a broth containing tryptone, sodium chloride, mannitol, yeast extract and incubated at 35°C for 24 h to evaluate MRSA presence in feedlot cattle, as well the nose samples as feces. An aliquot of the growth was inoculated onto MRSA Chromogenic agar and incubated at 35°C for 48 hours.

Many methodologies have been employed to identify and characterize strains, ranging from phenotypic to genotypic. Both present advantages and disadvantages and must be performed in accordance with the need of the study and the material and personnel available in each laboratory. Relative speed and the reliability are the desirable characteristics in both methods, because the choice of treatment and infection control measures are determined by the results of such testing (Kaya et al., 2009). Phenotypic methods at first are more accessible and nearly always cheaper; however they depend on the characteristic expression and visualization that cannot occur or be reduced, as for example, by environmental influences and/or regulatory genes (Berger-Bächi, 2002; Mohanasoundaram & Lalitha, 2008).

Methicillin-resistant *S. aureus* can be identified through different genotypic methods, such as species-specific primers for detection of DNA fragment of *S. aureus*-specific (van Duijkeren et al., 2010, as cited in Martineau et al., 1998) and with gene *mecA* (Murakami et al., 1991) by PCR (polymerase chain reaction), or the detection of DNA fragment of *S. aureus*-specific and gene *mecA* by multiplex PCR (Huijsdens et al., 2006), for example.

To determine the MRSA clones involved, in the beginning of 1990s the pulsed-field gel electrophoresis (PFGE) of genomic SmaI macrorestriction fragments were introduced and still represents the gold standard with respect to discriminatory power. The clonal groups determined by cluster analysis through PFGE are largely congruent with those defined by MLST. However, with the presence of some lineages of special interest (for example ST398) that are non typeable by the standard restriction enzyme SmaI, other methods have been used (Cuny et al., 2010).

As observed in the majority of studies discussed in this chapter, from genotypic methods for classification of predominant strains and determination of evolutionary pathways, MLST and *spa* typing have been the most widely employed: the first because it is an unambiguous discriminatory method for studying MRSA epidemiology and evolution, with results that can be truly portable between laboratories (Enright, 2003) and the second method to indicate genetic microvariation permitting investigation of outbreaks or accomplishment of phylogenetic analysis (Koreen et al., 2004). MLST characterize bacteria isolates unambiguously using the sequences of internal fragments of seven "housekeeping" genes, being a discriminatory method which permits that related strains recovered from different countries be quickly identified (Enright et al., 2002). The *spa* type identified by DNA sequence analysis of the X region of the protein A gene (*spa*) is less expensive, time-consuming, and error prone than multilocus techniques, such as MLST (Shopsin et al., 1999; Koreen et al., 2004).

The classification by MLST permits that the genomes of strains deposited in the GenBank database to be compared to establish their evolution and characteristic features. Comparing the genome of CA-MRSA and HA-MRSA from the same clonal lineage as well as their most probable MSSA ancestor, about 78% of the genes are conserved, and the remaining 22% comprise an "accessory genome" including genomic islands, pathogenicity islands, prophages, integrated plasmids, and transposons. However, comparing the *S. aureus* genome from cattle mastitis (ST151) with human *S. aureus*, it has been demonstrated that this bovine clone probably evolved from a common ancestor by acquiring foreign DNA. Subsequent microarray studies on recent epidemic strains of bovine origin (such as ST97) also revealed the presence of mobile genetic elements absent from *S. aureus* of human origin. Even with these impressive insights into the evolution of *S. aureus*, research has not yet provided many clues on the adaptation of the pathogen to the host, since only limited data are available (Cuny et al., 2010). In this respect, further research is needed to address these gaps, as well as to better understand the evolution of these strains in humans and animals.

6. MRSA prevention and control in animals

All studies on animal MRSA have helped establish critical measures for its control. Numerous reports on MRSA control in humans have been published and many of the principles may also be applied to control in animals. However, caution is necessary for extrapolating these human guidelines to animals, as disease epidemiology can differ significantly (Leonard & Markey, 2008).

It has been observed that exposure to antimicrobials is a risk factor for the acquisition and dissemination of MRSA in humans and also most probably in animals. In this respect, strategies for prevention and management of MRSA in animals should be, as much as possible, related to the use of antimicrobials. If the antimicrobial treatment is necessary in individual cases for the sake of animal welfare, the risk of the emergence of wider resistance in MRSA strains colonizing animals needs to be managed, especially considering zoonotic aspects. Options to manage this risk include the non-use of antimicrobials except as a last resort strategy, decolonization in humans, isolation of animals during treatment, and monitoring the effects of treatment in strain resistance through selective culture and susceptibility tests (CATRY et al., 2010).

6.1 General preventive and control measures

Good hygiene is an important general preventive and control measure, both in homes and human and animal healthcare environments, because environmental contamination with MRSA acts as a reservoir for infection. Known MRSA-positive animals should be nursed apart from other animals, with strict washing of the hands, gloves and gowns if in close contact. Recording the history of contact with human or animal MRSA, as well as an early culture of a wound non-responsive to first-line therapy allows for earlier recognition of MRSA and its appropriate management. Furthermore, when faced with repeated and inexplicable failure of human decolonization, clinicians can investigate nearby exposure to animals and birds that could be the reservoirs (Morgan, 2008).

Below, are some precolonized specific measures cited from (Catry et al., 2010).

6.1.1 Specific measures for livestock animals

- Reduction of antimicrobial selective pressure in livestock by avoiding routine mass medication
- Prevention of transmission of MRSA between and within the farms with sanitary measures of control between herds and during transportation
- Identification and isolation of animals to minimize the risk for zoonotic infection
- Use of contact precautions such as protective outerwear, overalls, aprons or coats and boots or overshoes that are not worn elsewhere
- Protective outerwear and all the items handled during the treatment of MRSA-positive animals should be considered potentially contaminated
- Hands can be hygienically cleaned with alcohol gel pouches, which are essential but need to be used correctly

- Proper cleaning and disinfection of contaminated environments, including transport vehicles. Special attention should be paid to dust in stables
- Animal owners should be informed about the risks and necessary precautions.

6.1.1.1 Reducing carriers on MRSA-positive livestock farms

Control and/or treatment of colonized and infected animals with or without antimicrobials is necessary for the reduction of carriers.

Th1e affected animals need to be immediately separated from healthy animals. In extreme cases culling of infected animals is a further option. Milk of animals with mastitis by MRSA must be destroyed, and in some cases the infected quarter must be prematurely dried-off.

If the antimicrobial treatment is chosen, it is necessary to evaluate its risk-benefit compared with other alternatives. The choice of antimicrobials should always be based on a susceptibility test, and all precautions should be taken that the drug reaches the infected site with appropriate concentrations.

6.1.2 Specific measures for horses

The options of control for colonized horses, as well as livestock animals, include the non-antimicrobial management and the antimicrobial treatment of colonized or infected horses. In a Canadian study, two farms with horses colonized by MRSA drastically reduced the number of affected animals with active screening and strict implementation of control protocols of infection, without the use of antimicrobial therapy. Antimicrobial treatment must be applied only if the colonization is persistent or in cases in which control measures are impossible.

Preventive measures for the infected animals are the same for the previously mentioned livestock animals. In equine hospitals, MRSA management for veterinary practices, guidelines stipulated by the British Small Animal Veterinary Association (BSAVA), for example, can also be applicable. In the confirmed or suspected cases of infection by MRSA, horses must be isolated and treated as if disseminating a nosocomial and zoonotic agent. It is necessary to take precautions with staff hygiene as well, using protective barriers, such as gloves, aprons, and boots. Moreover, the entire animal must be evaluated before being admitted to the hospital to ensure prevention of MRSA dissemination.

6.1.3 Specific measures for companion animals

In colonized animals, it not recommended to decolonize animals having mucosae colonization with MRSA. And it is observed that apparently some pets eliminate the carriage of MRSA spontaneously if the re-colonization is prevented. Antimicrobial therapy is only indicated in exceptionally persistent cases or when control measures are impossible., If the infection is local in infected animals, meticulous management of the wound can avoid the necessity of antimicrobial use. The risk of resistance development, the susceptibility profile of the isolate, the severity of the infection and the presence of systemic disease (fever, leukocytosis), and the patient's underlying disease or any comorbidity must be taken into account when choosing the antimicrobial treatment. In deciding to treat or eventually euthanize, veterinarians must consider the national veterinary guidelines available.

Preventive measures include the strict control practices of the infection in homes, particularly frequent hand washing hygiene, avoiding high-risk contact to minimize the chance of becoming colonized and isolating the animal and other pets. Gloves, masks and eye protection must be used to attend patients, as well as planning surgeries to avoid risk for infection, removing permanent urinary catheters as soon as possible and preventing complications from intravenosous and urinary catheters with appropriate asepsis.

7. Conclusion

This paper summarizes a wide range of information and findings from the literature on MRSA in animals and humans in contact with them. Notwithstanding, there is enormous potential for new research aiming to conclusively address certain unknown questions such as, at which point does an infection play the role of a zoonosis or humanosis? This question has yet to be answered because several animal species are involved, with distinct characteristics of transmission and isolated clones, raising appropriate concern for MRSA in animals.

Steadfast vigilance of MRSA in samples of animal origin in laboratory diagnoses is essential for: consistent and thorough monitoring of the evolution and dissemination of these strains; elucidating characteristics that determine a predilection for a determined host; determing transmission routes; identifying resistance and virulence genes received by these new lineages; and distinguishing molecular markers that allow for discriminating between CA-MRSA, HA-MRSA and LA-MRSA.

Appropriate and effective measures of control and prevention must be better determined and applied to each situation and country, according to previously reported guidelines, aiming to minimize risks to humans, since these strains have housed new virulence and resistance genes which can be transferred to human strains. Veterinarians play an important role in public health, in controlling this pathogen through measures appropriately applied in veterinary medicine, namely, the rational use of antimicrobials and appropriate management of infected animals, together with other health professionals, for prevention of MRSA dissemination.

8. Acknowledgement

The support by FAPESP is gratefully acknowledged.

9. References

Baptiste, K.E.; Williams, K.; Williams, N.J.; Wattret, A.; Clegg, P.D.; Dawson, S.; Corkill, J.E.; O'Neill, T. & Hart, C.A. (2005). Methicillin-resistant staphylococci in companion animals. *Emerging Infectious Diseases*, Vol.11, No.12, pp.1942-1944, ISSN 1080-6059

Bens, C.C.P.M.; Voss, A. & Klaassen, C.H.W. (2006). Presence of a novel DNA methylation enzyme in methicillin-resistant *Staphylococcus aureus* isolates associated with pig farming leads to uninterpretable results in standard pulsed-field gel electrophoresis analysis. *Journal of Clinical Microbiology*, Vol.44, No.5, pp.1875-1876, ISSN 1098-660X

Berger-Bächi, B. (2002). Resistance mechanisms of gram-positive bacteria. *International Journal of Medical Microbiology*, Vol.292, No.1, pp.27-35, ISSN 1438-4221

Catry, B.; van Duijkeren, E.; Pomba, M.C.; Greko, C.; Moreno, M.A.; Pyörala, S.; Ruzauskas, M.; Sanders, P.; Threlfall, E.J.; Ungemach, F.; Törneke, K.; Muñoz-Madero, C. & Torren-Edo, J. (2010). Reflection paper on MRSA in food-producing and companion animals: epidemiology and control options for human and animal health. *Epidemiology and Infection*, Vol.138, No.5, pp.626-644, ISSN 0950-2688

Cavaco, L.M.; Hasman, H.; Stegger, M.; Andersen, P.S.; Skov, R.; Fluit, A.C.; Ito, T. & Aarestrup, F.M. (2010). Cloning and occurrence of *crzC*, a gene conferring cadmium and zinc resistance in methicillin-resistant *Staphylococcus aureus* CC398 isolates. *Antimicrobial Agents and Chemotherapy*, Vol.54, No.9, pp.3605-3608, ISSN 0066-4804

Cuny, C.; Friedrich, A.; Kozytska, S.; Layer, F.; Nübel, U.; Ohlsen, K.; Strommenger, B.; Walther, B.; Wieler, L. & Witte, W. (2010). Emergence of methicillin-resistant *Staphylococcus aureus* (MRSA) in different animal species. *International Journal of Medical Microbiology*, Vol.300, No.2-3, pp.109-117, ISSN 1438-4221

David, M.Z. & Daum, R.S. (2010). Community-associated methicillin-resistant *Staphylococcus aureus*: epidemiology and clinical consequences of an emerging epidemic. *Clinical Microbiology Reviews*, Vol.23, No.3, pp.616-687, ISSN 0893-8512

Enright, M.C.; Robinson, D.A.; Randle, G.; Feil, E.J.; Grundmann, H. & Spratt, B.G. (2002). The evolutionary history of methicillin-resistant *Staphylococcus aureus*. *PNAS*, Vol.99, No.11, pp.7687-7692, ISSN 1091-6490

Enright, M.C. (2003). The evolution of a resistant pathogen - the case of MRSA. *Current Opinion in Pharmacology*, Vol.3, No.5, pp.474-479, ISSN 1471-4892

Feβler, A.; Scott, C.; Kadlec, K.; Ehricht, R.; Monecke, S. & Schwarz, S. (2010). Characterization of methicillin-resistant *Staphylococcus aureus* ST398 from cases of bovine mastitis. *Journal of Antimicrobial Chemotherapy*, Vol.65, No.4, pp.619-625, ISSN 0305-7453

Graveland, H.; Wagenaar, J.A.; Heesterbeek, H.; Mevius, D.; Van Duijkeren, E. & Heederik, D. (2010). Methicillin resistant *Staphylococcus aureus* ST398 in veal calf farming: human MRSA carriage related with animal antimicrobial usage and farm hygiene. *Plos One*, Vol.5, No.6, e10990, pp.1-5, ISSN 1932-6203

Guinane, C.M.; Zakour, N.L.B.; Tormo-Mas, M.A.; Weinert, L.A.; Lowder, B.V.; Cartwright, R.A.; Smyth, D.S.; Smyth, C.J.; Lindsay, J.A.; Gould, K.A.; Witney, A.; Hinds, J.; Boolback, J.P.; Rambaut, A.; Penadés, J.R. & Fitzgerald, J.R. (2010). Evolutionary genomics of *Staphylococcus aureus* reveals insights into the origin and molecular basis of ruminant host adaptation. *Genome Biology and Evolution*, v.2, pp.454-466, ISSN 1759-6653

Horgan, M.; Abbott, Y.; Lawlor, P.G.; Rossney, A.; Coffey, A.; Fitzgerald, G.F.; Mcauliffe, O. & Ross, R.P. (2010). A study of the prevalence of methicillin-resistant *Staphylococcus aureus* in pigs and in personnel involved in the pig industry in Ireland. *The Veterinary Journal, in press*, ISSN 1090-0233

Huijsdens, X.W.; van Dijke, B.J.; Spalburg, E.; van Santen-Verheuvel, M.G.; Heck, M.E.O.C.; Pluister, G.N.; Voss, A.; Wannet, W.J.B. & de Neeling, A.J. (2006). Community-acquired MRSA and pig-farming. *Annals of Clinical Microbiology and Antimicrobials*, Vol.5, No.26, ISSN 1476-0711

Hunter, P.A.; Dawson, S.; French, G.L.; Goossens, H.; Hawkey, P.M.; Kuijper, E.J.; Nathwani, D.; Taylor, D.J.; Teale, C.J.; Warren, R.E.; Wilcox, M.H.; Woodford, N.; Wulf, M.W. & Piddock, L.J.V. (2010). Antimicrobial-resistant pathogens in animals and man: prescribing, practices and policies. *Journal of Antimicrobial Chemotherapy*, Vol.65, suppl.1, pp.i3-i17, ISSN 0305-7453

Juhász-Kaszanyitzky, E.; Jánosi, S.; Somogyi, P.; Dán, A.; Bloois, L.G.; van Duijkeren, E. & Wagenaar, J.A. (2007). MRSA transmission between cows and humans. *Emerging Infectious Diseases*, Vol.13, No.4, pp.630-632, ISSN 1080-6059

Kaya, E.G.; Karakoç, E.; Yağci, S. & Yücel, M. (2009). Evaluation of phenotypic and genotypic methods for detection of methicillin resistance in *Staphylococcus aureus*. *African Journal of Microbiology Research*, Vol.3, No.12, pp.925-929, ISSN 1996-0808

Kehrenberg, C.; Cuny, C.; Strommenger, B.; Schwartz, S. & Witte, W. (2009). Methicillin-resistant and -susceptible *Staphylococcus aureus* strains of clonal lineages ST398 and ST9 from swine carry the multidrug resistance gene *cfr*. *Antimicrobial Agents and Chemotherapy*, Vol.53, No.2, pp.779-781, ISSN 0066-4804

Kitai, S.; Shimizu, A.; Kawano, J.; Sato, E.; Nakano, C.; Uji & T. Kitagawa, H. (2005). Characterization of methicillin-resistant *Staphylococcus aureus* isolated from retail raw chicken meat in Japan. *The Journal of Veterinary Medical Science*, Vol.67, No.1, pp.107-110, ISSN 1347-7439

Koreen, L.; Ramaswamy, S.V.; Graviss, E.A.; Naidich, S.; Musser, J.M. & Kreiswirth, B.N. (2004). *spa* Typing method for discriminating among *Staphylococcus aureus* isolates: implications for use of a single marker to detect genetic micro- and macrovariation. *Journal of Clinical Microbiology*, Vol.42, No.2, pp.792-799, ISSN 1098-660X

Kwon, H.H.; Park, K.T.; Moon, J.S.; Jung, W.K.; Kim, S.H.; Kim, J.M.; Hong, S.K.; Koo, H.C.; Joo, Y.S. & Park, Y.H. (2005). Staphylococcal cassette chromosome *mec* (SCC*mec*) characterization and molecular analysis for methicillin-resistant *Staphylococcus aureus* and novel SCC*mec* subtype IVg isolated from bovine milk in Korea. *Journal of Antimicrobial Chemotherapy*, Vol.56, No.4, pp.624-632, ISSN 0305-7453

Lee, J.H. (2003). Methicillin (Oxacillin)-resistant *Staphylococcus aureus* strains isolated from major food animals and their potential transmission to humans. *Applied and Environmental Microbiology*, Vol.69, No.11, pp.6489-6494, ISSN 0099-2240

Leonard, F.C. & Markey, B.K. (2008). Methicillin-resistant *Staphylococcus aureus* in animals: a review. *The Veterinary Journal*, Vol.175, No.1, pp.27036, ISSN 1090-0233

Li, S.; Skov, R.L.; Han, X.; Larsen, A.R.; Larsen, J.; Sørum, M.; Wulf, M.; Voss, A.; Hiramatsu, K. & Ito, T. (2011). Novel types of staphylococcal cassette chromosome *mec* elements identified in CC398 methicillin resistant *Staphylococcus aureus* strains. *Antimicrobial Agents and Chemotherapy*, Vol.55, No.2, pp.3046-3050, ISSN 0066-4804

Loeffler, A.; Boag, A.K.; Sung, J.; Lindsay, J.A.; Guardabassi, L.; Dalsgaard, A.; Smith, H.; Stevens, K.B. & Lloyd, D.H. (2005). Prevalence of methicillin-resistant *Staphylococcus aureus* among staff and pets in a small animal referral hospital in the UK. *Journal of Antimicrobial Chemotherapy*, Vol.56, No.4, pp.692-697, ISSN 0305-7453

Loeffler, A.; Kearns, A.M.; Ellington, M.J.; Smith, L.J.; Unt, V.E.; Lindsay, J.A.; Pfeiffer, D.U. & Lloyd, D.H. (2009). First isolation of MRSA ST398 from UK animals: a new challenge for infection control teams? *Journal of Hospital Infection*, Vol.72, No.3, pp.269-271, ISSN 0195-6701

Loeffler, A. & Lloyd, D.H. (2010). Companion animals: a reservoir for methicillin-resistant *Staphylococcus aureus* in the community? *Epidemiology and Infection*, Vol.138, No.5, pp.595-605, ISSN 0950-2688

Lozano, C.; López, M.; Gómez-Sanz, E.; Ruiz-Larrea, F.; Torres, C. & Zarazaga, M. (2009). Detection of methicillin-resistant *Staphylococcus aureus* ST398 in food samples of animal origin in Spain. *Journal of Antimicrobial Chemotherapy*, Vol.64, No.6, pp.1325-1346, ISSN 0305-7453

Lozano, C.; Aspiroz, C.; Ezpeleta, A.I.; Gómez-Sanz, E.; Zarazaga, M. & Torres, C. E. (2011). Empyema caused by MRSA ST398 with atypical resistance profile, Spain. *Emerging Infectious Diseases*, Vol.17, No.1, ISSN 1080-6059

Mohanasoundaram, K.M. & Lalitha, M.K. (2008). Comparison of phenotypic versus genotypic methods in the detection of methicillin resistance in *Staphylococcus aureus*. *Indian Journal of Medical Research*, Vol.127, No.1, pp.78-84, ISSN 0971-5916

Morgan, M. (2008). Methicillin-resistant *Staphylococcus aureus* and animals: zoonosis or humanosis? *Journal of Antimicrobial Chemotherapy*, Vol.62, No.6, pp.1181-1187, ISSN 0305-7453

Murakami, K.; Minamide, W.; Wada, K.; Nakamura, E.; Teraoka, H. & Watanabe, S. (1991). Identification of methicillin-resistant strains of staphylococci by polymerase chain reaction. *Journal of Clinical Microbiology*, Vol.29, No.10, pp.2240-2244, ISSN 1098-660X

Nemati, M.; Hermans, K.; Lipinska, U.; Denis, O.; Deplano, A.; Struelens, M.; Devriese, L.A.; Pasmans, F. & Haesebrouck, F. (2008). Antimicrobial resistance of old and recent *Staphylococcus aureus* isolates from poultry: first detection of livestock-associated methicillin-resistant strain ST398. *Antimicrobial Agents and Chemotherapy*, Vol.52, No.10, pp.3817-3819, ISSN 0066-4804

Nienhoff, U.; Kadlec, K.; Chaberny, I.F.; Verspohl, J.; Gerlach, G.F.; Schwarz, S.; Simon, D. & Nolte, I. (2009). Transmission of methicillin-resistant *Staphylococcus aureus* strains between humans and dogs: two case reports. *Journal of Antimicrobial Chemotherapy*, Vol.64, No.3, pp.660-662, ISSN 0305-7453

Persoons, D.; van Hoorebeke, S.; Hermans, K.; Butaye, P.; Kruif, A.; Haesebrouck, F. & Dewulf, J. (2009). Methicillin-resistant *Staphylococcus aureus* in poultry. *Emerging Infectious Diseases*, Vol.15, No.3, pp.452-453, ISSN 1080-6059

Springer, B.; Orendi, U.; Much, P.; Höger, G.; Ruppitsch, W.; Krziwanek, K.; Metz-Gercek, S. & Mittermayer, H. (2009). Methicillin-resistant *Staphylococcus aureus*: a new zoonotic agent? *Wiener klinische Wochenschrift*, Vol.121, No.3-4, pp.86–90, ISSN 0043-5325

Türkyılmaz, S.; Tekbıyık, S.; Oryasin, E. & Bozdogan, B. (2010). Molecular epidemiology and antimicrobial resistance mechanisms of methicillin-resistant *Staphylococcus aureus* isolated from bovine milk. *Zoonoses and Public Health*, Vol.57, No.3, pp.197-203, ISSN 1863-1959

Van Duijkeren, E.; Box, A.T.A.; Heck, M.E.O.C.; Wannet, W.J.B. & Fluit, A.C. (2004). Methicillin-resistant staphylococci isolated from animals. *Veterinary Microbiology*, Vol.103, No.1-2, pp.91-97, ISSN 0378-1135

Van Duijkeren, E.; Moleman, M.; Sloet van Oldruittenborgh-Oosterbaan, M.M.S.; Multem, J.; Troelstra, A.; Fluit, A.C.; van Wamel, W.J.B.; Howers, D.J.; de Neeling, A.J. & Wagenaar, J.A. (2010). Methicillin-resistant *Staphylococcus aureus* in horses and horse personnel: an investigation of several outbreaks. *Veterinary Microbiology*, Vol.141, No.1-2, pp.96-102, ISSN 0378-1135

Van Loo, I.; Huijsdens, X.; Tiemersma, E.; De Neeling, A.; van de Sande-Bruinsma, N.; Beaujean, D.; Voss, A. & Kluytmans, J. (2007). Emergence of methicillin-resistant *Staphylococcus aureus* of animal origin in humans. *Emerging Infectious Diseases*, Vol.13, No.12, pp.1834-1839, ISSN 1080-6059

Vanderhaeghen, W.; Hermans, K.; Haesebrouck & F., Butaye, P. (2010). Methicillin-resistant *Staphylococcus aureus* (MRSA) in food production animals. *Epidemiology and Infection*, Vol.138, No.5, pp.606-625, ISSN 0950-2688

Voss, A.; Loeffen, F.; Bakker, J.; Klaassen, C. & Wulf, M. (2005). Methicillin-resistant *Staphylococcus aureus* in pig farming. *Emerging Infectious Diseases*, Vol.11, No.12, pp.1965-1966, ISSN 1080-6059

Wagenaar, J.A.; Yue, H.; Pritchard, J.; Broekhuizen-Stins, M.; Huijsdens, X.; Mevius, D.J.; Bosch, T. & van Duijkeren, E. (2009).Unexpected sequence types in livestock associated methicillin-resistant *Staphylococcus aureus* (MRSA): MRSA ST9 and a single locus variant of ST9 in pig farming in China. *Veterinary Microbiology*, Vol.139, No.3-4, pp.405-409, ISSN 0378-1135

Weese, J.S. (2004). Methicillin-resistant *Staphylococcus aureus* in horses and horse personnel. *The Veterinary Clinics of North America. Equine Practice*, Vol.20, No.3, pp.601-613, ISSN 0749-0739

Weese, J.S.; Avery, B.P. & Reid-Smith, R. J. (2010). Detection and quantification of methicillin-resistant *Staphylococcus aureus* (MRSA) clones in retail meat products. *Letters in Applied Microbiology*, Vol.51, No.3 ,pp.338–342, ISSN 0266-8254

Weese, J.S.; Hannon, S.J.; Booker, C.W.; Gow, S.; Avery, B.P. & Reid-Smith, R.J. (2011). The prevalence of methicillin-resistant *Staphylococcus aureus* colonization in feedlot cattle. *Zoonoses and Public Health, in press*, ISSN 1863-1959

Wulf, M.W.H.; Sørum, M.; van Nes, A.; Skov, R.; Melchers, W.J.G.; Klaassen, C.H.W. & Voss, A. (2008). Prevalence of methicillin-resistant *Staphylococcus aureus* among veterinarians: an international study. *Clinical Microbiology and Infection*, Vol.14, No.1, pp.29-34, ISSN 1198-743X

5

CA-MRSA: Epidemiology of a Pathogen of a Great Concern

Mariana Fávero Bonesso, Adilson de Oliveira and
Maria de Lourdes Ribeiro de Souza da Cunha
UNESP- Univ. Estadual Paulista, Department of Microbiology and Immunology
Biosciency Institute, Botucatu-SP
Brazil

1. Introduction

The emergence of community-acquired methicillin resistant *Staphylococcus aureus* (CA-MRSA) strains in individuals without traditional risk factors, has caused a drastic change in MRSA epidemiology since community acquired infections are etiologically caused by MSSA (methicillin sensitive *S. aureus*). Initially the most affected social groups were soldiers, men who have sex with men, prisoners, illicit injection drug users, and athletes; people with compromised skin and mucosa, poor hygiene habits and postpartum mastitis; Native Americans of the United States, and children due to their close contact with contaminated nasal secretions.

This change in epidemiology lead to molecular studies aimed at determining pathogenicity, virulence, resistance to different antimicrobial classes and the behavior of these strains against selective pressure of the human immunological system. Associating risk factors with the molecular studies gave rise to Molecular Epidemiology.

Humans are the main source of *Staphylococcus* spp., which can be found in the skin, throat, intestine and nose without causing damage to the host. In hospitals, the asymptomatic host can disseminate *S. aureus* to immunocompromised patients. Since they are ubiquitous, these bacteria can cause several types of infections such as: necrotizing pneumonia, skin and soft tissue infections, bacteremia, as well as food poisoning through enterotoxin production.

Individuals affected by CA-MRSA strains can develop from mild to metastatic and lethal infections, which are directly related to the synthesis of certain toxins, antimicrobial resistance and individual health conditions. One of the most discussed virulence factors is PVL (Panton-Valentine Leukocidine). Since its first association with skin and soft tissue infections, PVL is now believed to contribute to the elevated virulence potential attributed to CA-MRSA.

Methicillin resistance is conferred by *mecA* gene inserted in a mobile genomic island, the Staphylococcal cassette chromosomal (SCC*mec*). Some different SCC*mec* regions are responsible for mobility and regulation, and others for resistance to several antimicrobial classes. According to the presence, lack or genomic variations in these regions, the cassettes can be classified in a range from type I to XI largely used to discriminate hospital and community types.

Community strains are usually more sensitive to other antimicrobial classes compared to multiresistant health care associated strains. In fact, CA-MRSA can be resistant to other antimicrobials besides beta-lactams, thus decreasing the options of drug choices. Another subject of concern is resistance to the drug of choice for treating MRSA, vancomycin. There are few antimicrobials to control the infections caused by MRSA and vancomycin is one of them. Reports of resistance and low level of sensitivity to this drug in health care environments have been reported worldwide.

All of the issues mentioned above, underscore the importance of further research on the behavior of CA-MRSA at the epidemiological and molecular levels enabling establishment and application of preventive measures and treatment in view of infections. The present chapter will outline the main features of CA-MRSA and epidemiological principles involved in the outcome briefly described above.

2. Resistance evolution background

Staphylococcus spp. are gram-positive cocci, catalase positive, belonging to the family Staphylococcaceae and the genus *Staphylococcus,* which currently comprises 45 species (Euzéby, 2011), from which 17 species can be isolated from samples from humans. *Staphylococcus aureus* is the most important species and can be found in both healthy and immunocompromised individuals (Santos et al., 2007).

The *Staphylococcus* genus is classified according to the synthesis of the enzyme coagulase, and those that synthesize are classified as coagulase-positive, represented by the species *Staphylococcus aureus, S. intermedius, S. hyicus, S. schleiferi* subspecie *coagulans, S. delphine* and *S. lutrae,* and in the absence of the synthesis, are represented by other coagulase-negative species (Baba et al., 2002). Both groups can cause infections in humans and, among them, the main species are: *S. aureus, S. epidermidis, S. saprophyticus, S. haemolyticus, S. hominis, S. warneri, S. capitis, S. saccarolyticus, S. lugdunensis, S. cohnii, S. xylosus, S. simulans, S. auricularis, S. caprae* and *S. schleiferi* (Layer et al., 2006).

Humans are the main reservoir of *Staphylococcus aureus,* which can colonize the skin, throat, intestine and nasal passages without causing damage to the host. Asymptomatic carriers in hospitals can spread *S. aureus* increasing risk to immunocompromised patients (Santos et al., 2007). This ubiquity favors the installation of various types of infections such as necrotizing pneumonia, skin and soft tissue infections, food poisoning bacteremia through the synthesis of enterotoxin (Santos et al., 2007; Cunha et al., 2006; Jarraud et al., 2002; Gandhinagar & Silva, 2004).

In 1940, staphylococcal infections were treated with penicillin; however, only two years after its introduction, nosocomial penicillinase producing strains grew resistant to penicillin by the inactivation of the penicillin molecules (Mimica & Mendes, 2007). Shortly thereafter, the same occurred with the strains of community origin necessitating the use of alternative antibiotics to treat infections caused by *S. aureus* (Ricardo, 2004).

In the late 1950s, in Europe, resistant nosocomial and community *Staphylococcus* spp. had penicillin resistance rates of 90% and 70%, respectively (Ricardo, 2004). This finding led to a search for alternatives, and in 1959, adding the acid 6-aminopenicilanic in the penicillin molecule allowed for protecting the precursor of penicillin beta-lactam ring. This semi-synthetic penicillin (Named methicillin (and the analog oxacillin, used in Brazil) proved to be resistant to the action of beta-lactamase. However, both were effective for a short period of time, and in 1961, strains resistant to semisynthetic penicillins emerged. These emerging new strains were named MRSA (Methicillin-Resistant *Staphylococcus aureus*), so far unique to hospital settings (Ricardo, 2004; Salgado et al., 2003).

In the 1980s the first reports emerged of infections caused by *S. aureus* in patients without risk factors for acquisition of nosocomial MRSA (HA-MRSA), resulting in the designation of CA-MRSA (Community-Acquired Methicillin-Resistant *S. aureus*) in the 1990s when reports of CA-MRSA increased (Ricardo, 2004). The community-acquired infections are usually distinct from hospitals in terms of susceptibility and the carriage of the gene that codifies for the synthesis of Panton-Valentine Leukocidin (PVL) responsible for tissue invasion preceding the skin infections (Klevens et al., 2007).

According to criteria, it is considered that individuals affected by CA-MRSA should not report previous MRSA infections; the patient must have a positive culture for MRSA within 48 hours after hospital admission, and must not be hospitalized in the last 12 months, or admitted to nursing homes or homecare, and did not report undergoing dialysis, surgery, catheters or any prior or invasive treatment at the time of MRSA isolation (Salgado et al. 2003).

The transmission of the bacteria occurs through direct contact of susceptible individuals with asymptomatic carriers. There are frequent reports of the spread of CA-MRSA among men who have sex with men, soldiers, athletes, intravenous illicit drug users, prisoners, people with compromised skin and mucous membranes, poor hygiene, postpartum mastitis (Reddy et al., 2007), Native Americans from the U.S. (Klevens et al., 2007; Stemper et al., 2006) and among children due to the contact with contaminated nasal discharge (Klevens et al., 2007).

The transmission of MRSA among family members was reported in a study with 10 families. Strains with PFGE ST8 (USA 300), ST59 (USA 1000), and ST80 PVL-positive were found in this investigation (Huijsdens et al., 2006). Lung infections caused by these strains can be serious because the symptoms are similar to pneumonia in children; therefore, it is important to consider infection by MRSA especially if there were previous reported. (Huijsdens et al., 2006).

Among pathogens that can cause pulmonary infections, CA-MRSA is associated with pneumonia and is frequently associated with pulmonary viral coinfection. Studies indicate that CA-MRSA agents are commonly found in pneumonia during the influenza season, and about 85% of *S. aureus* strains isolated contained the PVL gene. In three cases of severe necrotizing pneumonia, strategies were carried out to prevent the synthesis of Leukocidin, including the administration of antibiotics such as rifampicin, linezolid and clindamycin, and/or applying intravenous immunoglobulin to block the lytic effect of PVL under polymorphonuclear cells (Rouzic et al., 2010). During the influenza season of 2006 and 2007, there were 51 reported cases of pneumonia in health centers caused by *S. aureus*, and 79% were MRSA. Most cases of pneumonia due to MRSA occurred during or after viral infection (Kallen et al., 2008).

The treatment of MRSA infections is variable. Within a hospital environment, there are several options such as linezolid, daptomycin, quinupristin/dalfopristin, but vancomycin is one of the most commonly used to treat several types of infections, but the emergence of strains resistant to this antimicrobial agent limits its use. Historically the emergence of vancomycin resistance occurred primarily in isolates of *Enterococcus* spp. in 1986 and reported only in 1988 in a European hospital. In 1989, in the United States, Vancomycin-Resistant Enterococci (VRE) were detected in clinical isolates and in 1993 accounted for 7.9% of the enterococci samples in nosocomial environments reported by the CDC. The most important reservoir is the gastrointestinal tract and transmission occurs mainly through contact with healthcare workers, and indirectly by contaminated hands in contact with the hospital objects where at least one of the patients had diarrhea (Mayall, 2002).

Vancomycin resistance in VRE is due to the presence of *van* genes (A to G) that encode for the synthesis of peptidoglycan by an alternative pathway that produces precursors ending in D-Ala-D-Lac or D-Ala-D-Ser instead of D-Ala-D-Ala. In *S. aureus,* however the main mechanism involved in vancomycin resistance relies on a thickened cell wall, production of abundant extracellular material that remains not well characterized and it ends up compromising the ability of division. These characteristics result in the synthesis of an altered peptidoglycan with an increased number of terminal D-Ala-Ala-D capable of binding free vancomycin in the outer cell wall, thus leading to a lower availability of the antimicrobial target molecule in the intracellular region. Strains of *S. aureus* with intermediate resistance to vancomycin (VISA) may contain 2 to 4 times more layers of D-Ala-D-Ala than susceptible strains, being capable of binding to three to six times more vancomycin molecules. Some chromosomal changes are necessary to maintain this resistance , and in addition require a larger amount of precursors than normal strains, thus compromising their fitness in an environment free of this antimicrobial. This may explain the reason for the loss of the vancomycin resistance of VISA strains when they are in environments without antibiotics, giving rise to heteroresistant strains called hetero-VISA (Van Bambeke et al., 2004).

3. MRSA colonization and decolonization

Studies on colonization intend to elucidate the mechanism by which certain individuals are persistently or intermittently colonized while others are non-carriers. MRSA colonization is an important predisposing factor, since colonized individuals are at increased risk of acquiring infections (van Belkun et al., 2009). Colonization is well studied in inpatients due to the risk of dissemination and the fact that it can facilitate severe infections.

Nasal colonization is the main form, and colonization can occur in other extra-nasal sites as in the skin, pharynx and perineum, but some sites are considered unusual such as the vagina, axilla and gastrointestinal tract. Studies may help to define carriers as in most cross-sectional studies only a culture classifies individuals as carriers or not, while longitudinal studies usually classify three categories of carriers: intermittent, persistent or non-carriers. Often cultures are harvested in three different time periods to define the carriers (Werthein et al., 2005). A study concluded that a "culture rule" which combines qualitative and quantitative results of two nasal cultures with an interval of one week could accurately classify nasal carriage (Nouwen et al., 2004).

Persistent carriers are usually colonized by a single strain of *S. aureus* over a long period of time, whereas intermittent carriers may carry different strains over time (Werthein et al., 2005). MRSA colonization in individuals in the community remains a low burden as demonstrated in a study of high school boys where no individuals were found colonized with MRSA. The fact that there were no carriers among this population may be a reflection of improvement in hygiene practices among these individuals due to previous reports of outbreaks in team sports (Lear et al., 2011). Although they did not found MRSA in the population, other studies have found colonization rates in individuals in the community ranging from 0.8 to 3% (Keuhnert et al., 2006; Salgado et al., 2003; Ellis et al., 2004).

MRSA colonization in a hospital environment is a matter of utmost importance since it is characterized as a predisposing factor to infection. Nasal decolonization is usually performed with the application of mupirocin and is useful for reducing symptoms and its spread in hospital environments. However, the practice of decolonization with antimicrobials remains controversial because of the risk of acquiring drug resistance, which limits its use. Despite this risk, it is advised to perform decolonization in healthcare settings because of the risk of developing infections especially in individuals who are under invasive treatments and are immunocompromised (Coates et al., 2009).

But how should we manage individuals living in the community who are characterized as persistent carriers of CA-MRSA, but show no clinical manifestations and are healthy? This is a controversial subject because a previous study showed that individuals might be co-colonized with MSSA and MRSA, where the strains of MSSA have better fitness than MRSA, most likely due to the additional mechanism of resistance, which requires a cost in the feasibility and competitiveness of these strains. Thus, when decolonization is performed with mupirocin, both are eliminated and there will be competition, thus increasing the chances of colonization by resistant strains if both were competing for the same ecological niche (Dall'Antonia et al., 2005). Studies are needed to evaluate the cost-effectiveness of nasal colonization among residents in the community as a predisposition to infections, but there are chances of acquisition of resistant strains.

The nasal vestibule is composed of highly keratinized cells including apocrine and sebaceous glands and hair follicles. These factors are poorly studied compared to the mucosa and its linkage to mucins. Some of the pathogen virulence factors contribute to successful colonization; for example, the clumping factor B is highly associated with nasal colonization (Wertheim et al., 2007). Studies have reported the binding of *S. aureus* surface protein G (SasG) to a ligand in nasal epithelial cells. Other factors such as: Teichoic acid and cell wall components recognizing microbial surface adhesive matrix molecules (MSCRAMMS) responsible for the adherence protein in fibronectin, fibrinogen and collagen, may play an important role in colonization (Wertheim et al., 2005).

4. Case reports

Case reports of CA-MRSA emerged worldwide revealing the severity, spread, which has helped to chart the epidemiologic distribution in the various communities and provide a better understanding of the behavior of virulence and resistance profile of these strains involved. Such isolates are associated with diseases of skin and soft tissue (Ribeiro et al., 2005). The infections develop from the skin surface where they penetrate to deeper layers, disrupting natural barriers (Santos et al., 2007). The characteristics of the infection have to be similar to those caused by MSSA (methicillin-sensitive *S. aureus*) (Baba et al., 2002).

Outbreaks of infections caused by CA-MRSA are increasing worldwide among all age groups. Several countries reported their presence as an emerging pathogen, including the United States, Australia, New Zealand, Samoa, several EU countries (Ribeiro et al., 2005) and South America (Brazil, Uruguay and Colombia) (Alvarez et al., 2006). In Brazil there are several case reports confirming the presence of this pathogen in the community involving cases of furunculosis (Razera et al., 2009), metastatic infections with major complications (Strong et al., 2008) and pneumonia (d'Azevedo et al. 2009; Gelatti et al., 2009).

There is transmission of CA-MRSA between humans and animals, and these strains may carry genes codifying for Panton-Valentine Leukocidin (PVL) (Rutland et al., 2009; Van Duijkeren et al., 2005). A diabetic patient first diagnosed with cellulitis in the bicep region in December 2007 was positive for *S. aureus* in February 2008 from ankle biopsies and of nasal swab cultures; both isolates had the same profile of resistance to trimethoprim/ sulfamethoxazole, clindamycin, erythromycin, tetracycline and ciprofloxacin, and were, therefore, treated both times with vancomycin . In February 2008, his eight-year-old female Labrador dog had widespread cellulitis in the neck, which did not respond to treatment with cephalexin. Tissue, blood, and secretion cultures were carried out identifying the same MRSA resistance profile as the dog's owner. Typing performed by pulsed-field isolates of the man and animal was inconsistent with the USA epidemic clones. A *spa* typing (staphylococcal protein A) was performed and identified as *spa*3, the samples were negative for the presence of PVL. Due to the resistance profile of isolates of the patient and his close relationship with the hospital, it is likely that the source of these isolates was the hospital. This study demonstrated that humans could be a source of multiresistant pathogenic microorganisms for their animals (Rutland et al., 2009).

A case study revealed that a woman with successive complications with MRSA transmitted the strain to her relatives as well as her dog. Samples collected from the nose and throat of other asymptomatic relatives were positive for MRSA. Everyone was treated with rifampicin and ciprofloxacin. After six months of treatment, no new samples were recovered in the tests for detection of CA-MRSA among the family members and the dog (Van Duijkeren et al., 2005).

CA-MRSA pneumonia can be hotbeds for metastatic infections leading to vital organ failure. In Sao Paulo, a previously healthy of 17-year-old patient was admitted to the hospital with upper respiratory infection that progressed with worsening of bronchopneumonia, septic shock and respiratory failure in just three days. The course of the infection followed with pulmonary cavitations, empyema and bronchopleural fistula requiring pleural drainage and tracheostomy. On the 16th day of hospitalization, the patient required total colectomy with ileostomy for ischemic colitis. In less than 48 hours, the patient had two blood cultures positive for Gram-positive cocci. Laboratory tests revealed MRSA with resistance to erythromycin and cefoxitin, with MIC for oxacillin of 3μg/ml and vancomycin sensitive (2μg/mL) and teicoplamin (2mg/mL). The strain was sensitive to trimethoprim/ sulfamethoxazole and clindamycin. PCR analysis confirmed the presence of the *mecA* gene, SCC*mec* type IVa in the presence of genes for γ hemolysin, enterotoxin A (*sea*) and was negative for PVL. The treatment was maintained with teicoplamin for 36 days, and from day 7 with meropenem for 14 days, showing progressive improvement and was discharged after 72 days from the hospital. No family member was colonized by CA-MRSA (d'Azevedo et al., 2009).

The presence of CA-MRSA infections involved in high morbidity has been reported. After infection of traumatic injury, a 27-year-old patient, healthy and without history of hospitalization in the previous 12 months, was admitted to the University Hospital Clementino Fraga Filho (Rio de Janeiro, RJ - Brazil) and treated with ceftriaxone and vancomycin. The examination by transtoraxic echocardiography revealed a commitment of the anterior mitral valve and multiple blood cultures positive for MRSA, and molecular analysis detected the PVL toxin and the presence of cassette type IV. The vancomycin MIC performed by E-test was 2μg/mL. Removal of the spleen due to an abscess was carried out, and the patient had a syncope and cerebral mycotic aneurysm. The patient was discharged after 3 months of the treatment (Strong et al., 2008).

Pneumonia and sepsis caused by a localized source of infection caused by CA-MRSA occurred in one patient in Porto Alegre, Brazil, treated at the Pediatric Emergency Room diagnosed with cellulitis and pneumonia. The X-ray of the lesion revealed bone involvement, liver and aneurysm of the pulmonary vessel. Blood culture revealed the presence of *S. aureus* resistant only to oxacillin and cefoxitin. Testing by PCR revealed the presence of *mecA*, the PVL and the cassette type IVc. The clonal profile analyzed by PFGE found that the strain was similar to clone OSPC. The patient remained hospitalized for 50 days and was discharged after treatment with clindamycin and gentamicin (Gelatti et al., 2009).

Reinert et al. (2008), analyzed a culture collection grown between 1995 and 1999 and characterized them by PFGE (electrophoresis in pulsed-field gel). The results showed that the predominant profile (80%) corresponded to the Brazilian Epidemic Clone (BEC). Three of the 50 selected samples, harbored the cassette type IVc, and MLST (Multi Locus Sequence Typing) differed from each other: ST3, ST5 and ST88. These data showed that the presence of CA-MRSA in Brazil is longstanding and well established and must have passed unnoticed in clinical laboratories. It is necessary to detect and monitor these strains in the community and in hospitals for a better understanding of its epidemiology, as well as to inform public health strategies to control its spread (Reinert et al., 2008).

Risk factors for acquisition of CA-MRSA should be evaluated due to widespread character. In areas of close proximity among individuals, there is a greater risk of infection by *S. aureus*. Studies with people who maintain close contacts show that poor hygiene is an important factor in the acquisition of *Staphylococcus aureus*. In addition, younger individuals and the obese are more prone to colonization by MRSA. The objects of common use (soap and towels) and the environment are related to containing outbreaks of infections with this pathogen (Turabelidze et al., 2006).

Antimicrobial agents have different levels of concentration in certain sites of infection and, therefore, can reach subinhibitory levels during the treatment. Studies indicate that these levels may contribute to an increased expression of fibronectin binding proteins in samples having mutant genes for DNA gyrase and topoisomerase IV (*grlA* and *gyrA*, respectively) in MRSA strains. Bisognano et al. (1997) noted that the mutation sites that confer resistance to fluoroquinolones in subinhibitory concentrations of ciprofloxacin somehow increased the

FNB expression of genes that encode the fibronectin binding protein, but the mechanisms have not yet been defined. This may explain why patients who had prior use of ciprofloxacin have a higher likelihood of MRSA colonization.

The colonization by CA-MRSA in adults and children differs in the profiles of resistance to beta-lactam antibiotics, in which it is more typical that multi-sensitive strains colonize and affect children. This is mainly due to different environments they attend and hygienic practices follow. In addition, the antibiotics used in children may differ from those administered to adults, thus providing a different selective pressure in the community. Among adults CA-MRSA strains are more frequently resistant to gentamicin, tetracycline, ciprofloxacin, clindamycin and erythromycin than those observed in isolates from children (David et al., 2006).

One study evaluated *S. aureus* strains isolated from blood cultures as the type of SCC*mec*, the presence of PVL and analyzed the clonal profile by PFGE. In this study, they mainly included cases of HA-MRSA defined by the following isolation criterion for MRSA: must be isolated for 48 hours after hospital admission, previous isolation of MRSA colonized or infected patient during hospitalization or surgical procedures in the 12 months preceding the isolation, patients who underwent installation of a catheter or invasive devices. Of all the samples analyzed, 65% had the cassette type IV and that PVL was present in 92% of these samples. The clonal profile of 92% of samples with SCC*mec* type IV was USA300-ST8 (Gonzalez et al., 2006). The isolation of *S. aureus* resistant to methicillin with the cassette type IV suggests that these strains, particularly the USA300, presents an adaptation that expands beyond the community environment which may cause a change in the epidemiology of CA-MRSA.

5. Genetic characteristics of CA-MRSA

As a result of these observations genetic studies began focusing on molecular mechanisms responsible for the resistance to antibiotics and identification of MRSA strains. These strains had acquired and integrated into their genome harboring resistance genes, called Staphylococcal cassette chromosome *mec* (SCC*mec*). SCC*mec* present the gene responsible for methicillin and other beta-lactamic antibiotic resistance (*mecA*), and can carry genes that determine resistance to other classes of antibiotics. Strains related to community-acquired infections contain the smaller and lighter mobile element, the types and subtypes of SCC*mec* IV or V (21 to 25 kb) (Zhang et al., 2005).

Strains of HA-MRSA carry heavier mobile elements (SCC*mec* I to III) because they have genes that encode for resistance to several antimicrobial classes (Okuma et al., 2002). The mobile element SCC*mec* is characterized by the presence of essential genetic elements: the *mec* complex (classes A to E), the ccr complex (Hanssen & Sollid, 2007), junkyard regions (J) (Zhang et al., 2009) and end 3' is connected to the open reading frame (*ORF*), *orfX*. The SCC*mec* is integrated into the chromosome of *Staphylococcus* called attBscc a specific site located downstream of *orfX* (Zhang et al., 2008). There are several types of SCC*mec* (I to XI) (IWG-SCCmec, 2011) in addition to subtypes IIA to E and the IVg to IVa (Hanssen & Sollid, 2007). The *ccr* complex has five different allotypes for the *ccr*A and the *ccr*B: *ccr*A1 to *ccr*A5, the *ccr*B1 to *ccr*B4 and *ccr*B6 and *ccr*C1 (IWG-SCC*mec*, 2011). The allotypes of the SCC*mec* complexes are characterized by the presence of certain *ccr* genes (Ito et al., 2004). The *ccr*A and *ccr*B genes encode for recombinases of the family "invertase/resolvases." These enzymes mediate the integration within and outside of the SCC*mec* thus giving mobility to the chromosome cassette (Zhang et al., 2005).

The J regions encode several pseudogenes apparently with functions related to the bacterial metabolism (Zhang et al., 2005), and also contain genes for resistance mediated by plasmids or transposons to non beta-lactam antibiotics and heavy metals (Zhang et al., 2009). They are divided into three segments: J1, which is the region between the *ccr* complex the right chromosomal junction and the *ccr* gene complex; J2, between the *ccr* and *mec* regions, and J3 which is located between *orfX* and *mec*. Variations in the J regions within the same *mec*-ccr gene complex are used for defining SCC*mec* subtypes.

The SCC*mec* can be found in several species of *Staphylococcus* spp., such as *S. aureus, S. epidermidis, S. haemolyticus, S. hominis* and *S. warneri* (Hanssen & Sollid, 2007). The origin of SCC*mec* is unknown, and there have been no reports that any other genus than *Staphylococcus* carries the Staphylococal cassette chromosome. The presence of SCC*mec* type IV in *S. epidermidis* in healthy people suggests that this can be responsible for the conversion of CA-MSSA for CA-MRSA (Hanssen et al., 2004) where the transmission of the mobile element occurs mainly by transduction mediated by bacteriophages (Ito et al., 1999).

The *mecA* gene codifies a penicillin binding protein PBP 2 'or 2A (Menegoto & Picoli, 2007) present on the outer surface of the cytoplasmic membrane (Ricardo, 2004). In susceptible strains, conventional PBPs have a high affinity with the beta-lactam antibiotics which prevents the proper formation of cell walls. However, the second PBP has low affinity to this class of antimicrobials, which explains resistance to antimicrobials of the group of methicillin (Menegoto & Picoli, 2007; Ito et al., 2001).

The *mecA* gene is regulated by two genes *mecI* and *mecR1* that have similar functions of the *blaR1* and *blaI* mechanism that regulates the production of beta-lactamase (Chambers, 1997). The *mecA* gene is regulated by a repressor *mecI*, a signal transducer and trans-membrane sensitive to the beta-lactam *mecRI*; both are divergently transcribed. In the absence of beta-lactam antimicrobial, *mecI* represses the expression of *mecA* and *mecRI-mecI*. However in the presence of beta-lactam antibiotics, the *mecI* is cleaved autocatalytically, and a metalloprotease domain, located in the cytoplasmic portion *mecRI*, becomes active. What allows the *mecA* gene transcription and subsequent synthesis of PBP2a is the cleavage of the *mecI* by the metalloprotease and its connection on the operative region of the *mecA* gene (Berger-Bachi & Rohrer, 2002). The presence of insertion sequences IS431 and IS1272 results in the induction of the *mecA* gene (Katayama et al., 2001).

Other resistance mechanisms have been identified in strains that lack the *mecA* gene, for example, the overproduction of beta-lactamase responsible for the inactivation of oxacillin or modified resistance (MOD-SA) mediated by different types of PBPs with changed affinities to this antibiotic. Strains with this profile are called borderline resistant (Wey et al., 1990).

CA-MRSA can express resistance inducible clindamycin resistance, an option for treating both MSSA and MRSA in particular in cases of toxic shock syndrome. In MLSBi positive strains (macrolide-lincosamides-streptogramin B resistance), an inducer promotes methylase production expressed by the gene *emr* and leading to the subsequent methylation of the 23S ribosome unit causing an expression of the resistance to lincosamides (e.g. clindamycin). Phenotypically the strains are resistant to erythromycin and clindamycin sensitive, but when the disk of erythromycin is set at 15mm from the clindamycin disk, the clindamycin-induced resistant strain expressed the resistance forming a D zone near clindamycin. The presence of the *mecA* gene in CA-MRSA does not fulfill the identification criteria in itself for the expression of the inducible clindamycin resistance (Patel et al., 2006).

Boyle-Vavra et al. (2005) conducted a study with patients who had skin and soft tissue infections and another with colonized individuals with CA-MRSA, in order to test the resistance to various antibiotics and isolate those carrying the *mecA* gene. The results showed that 94% of the strains recovered from these infections and 85.3% of the strains that colonized healthy individuals showed resistance to three or more non-beta-lactam antibiotics. The *SCCmec* IV was present in 34% of the samples from individuals who had at least one risk factor for acquisition of MRSA and 14.7% of the isolates showed a different SCC*mec* called SCCmec VT (Boyle-Vavra et al., 2005).

6. Detection of phenotypic resistance to oxacillin

There are several tests that detect phenotypic resistance to oxacillin, such as the E-test with oxacillin agar screening test, or Kirb-Bauer disk diffusion test, cefoxitin disk diffusion, determining the minimum inhibitory concentration (MIC) (Felten et al., 2002), latex agglutination test to detect PBP2a (Bressler et al., 2005; Martins et al. 2010).

CHROMagar is used for the cultivation of *S. aureus* resulting in pink-colored colonies. Carricajo et al. (2001) tested the sensitivity and specificity of this medium compared with conventional (Columbia agar with 5% horse blood and chocolate agar). The CHROMagar allowed 22 strains of *S. aureus* grown from polymicrobial samples unlike conventional methods. Despite the high cost, this method had a sensitivity of 98% and specificity of 100% (Carricajo et al., 2001).

The latex agglutination test detects the PBP2a protein in the cell wall of staphylococci. To assess the effectiveness of this test, Bressler et al. (2005) compared it with PCR for *mecA* and determined the MIC of the MicroScan PC20 samples tested. The latex agglutination test had a 99% agreement with MicroScan; three strains that were false positive in the *mecA* agglutination had two strains that were resistant, and one presented sensitivity. The latter had a different aminoacid in PBP2a, the M483I that conferred susceptibile to oxacillin. This amino acid can increase the affinity for this antibiotic or eliminate the transpeptidase activity of PBP2a (Bressler et al., 2005).

The disk diffusion test in mannitol salt agar also showed favorable results in the detection of oxacillin resistance and a method almost as effective as the method of disk diffusion in Mueller-Hinton agar (Kampf et al., 1998).

The presence of heteroresistant strains can complicate the detection of the resistance by these methods due to the false-negative results. The disk diffusion test with cefoxitin is widely used due to the induction of *mecA* gene expression with the production of PBP2a, which promotes antibiotics in strains apparently sensitive to oxacillin (Feltenet al., 2002). Factors such as lower incubation temperature (30 to 35 ° C), osmolarity of the medium (2-4% NaCl), extended incubation period and inoculum density favor the detection of heteroresistant strains (Camarena & Sanchez, 2009).

The use of cefoxitin disk diffusion to detect strains carrying the *mecA* gene is widely applied, but there are laboratories that use only the broth dilution test to determine the MIC of a sample. One study showed correlation of the MIC of cefoxitin in the presence of the *mecA* gene for both *Staphylococcus aureus* and coagulase-negative *Staphylococcus* testing three brands of Mueller-Hinton broth. After testing, the strains were sent to the CDC for molecular detection of the *mecA* gene by PCR. For *mecA* negative *S. aureus* strains the MIC of cefoxitin was <4ug/ml and for *mecA* positive the MIC was $\geq$6 or 8 µg/ml when read in 18 hours of incubation, the result was highly sensitive and specific (99.7 and 100%). However, for coagulase-negative levels of cefoxitin were sensitive (at 24 hours, 94 to 99% for *S. epidermidis* and 91 to 100% non *S. epidermidis*), but not specific (24 hours, 85 to 91 % for *S. epidermidis* and 54 to 69% non *S. epidermidis*) to detect the presence of *mecA* (Swenson et al., 2009).

Screening with oxacillin agar supplemented with 4% NaCl proposed by CLSI, as well as the oxacillin agar dilution and broth microdilution with 2% NaCl is used with results close to 100% sensitivity for the detection of the *mecA* gene. However, when it comes to very diverse strains, detection of oxacillin resistance and the *mecA* gene are compromised, especially in disk diffusion testing, decreasing its specificity (classifying *mecA* negative strains as resistant) and agar screening, where low sensitivity values are obtained when more heterogenenous strains were tested (Swenson, 2002).

Experiments aimed at improving identification and detection MRSA strains, particularly heterogeneous strains, which are more difficult to detect by conventional methods. The sensitivity of disk diffusion testing using 1g oxacillin disk increased from 83.5% at 35 ° C to 91.7% when incubated at 30° C. Similarly, the sensitivity and specificity of the cefoxitin disk diffusion of 30 µg were 100% at a temperature of 30°C. Tests with cefoxitin are effective, because this antibiotic is able to detect strains inducing heterogeneous subpopulations expressing the *mec*A gene better than oxacillin. The sensitivity of the test screening at 6 µl oxacillin on Mueller-Hinton agar supplemented with 4% NaCl was 91.7% and specificity of 100% in 24 hours of incubation at 35°C. The latex agglutination test for detection of PBP2a can reach a sensitivity of 100%, being able to identify strains with low levels of PBP2a (Cauwelier et al. 2004).

Pereira et al. (2009) analyzed the sensitivity of the method of disk diffusion with oxacillin and cefoxitin disks, incubated for 24 h at 35°C in 100 samples of *S. aureus* isolated from pediatric and neonatal ICUs. They reported oxacillin disk sensitivity of 94.4% and specificity of 98%, while the cefoxitin disk presented 98% sensitivity and 100% specificity. The same authors also tested the screening method on Mueller Hinton agar with 6µg/ml of oxacillin and 4% NaCl and found a sensitivity of 98% and specificity of 100%.

Martins et al. (2010) compared the screening methods of disk diffusion and E-test for detection of oxacillin resistance. They found that approximately 45% of samples were positive for the *mecA* gene, and the disk diffusion method with oxacillin disk showed a sensitivity of 86.9% and specificity 91.1%, respectively. The screening method showed the same sensitivity and specificity of 91.3%, while the E-test showed the same specificity of other methods and a sensitivity of 97.8% (Martin et al., 2010).

The results found in several studies to determine the accuracy of these methods show that the results can vary depending on a number of factors especially the origin of the samples and the criteria used for its execution.

7. Characterization of strains of CA-MRSA

New typing multiplex PCR protocols have been proposed, which are fast, practical and economical for the differentiation of clones of CA-MRSA. Some techniques are able to differentiate the clone of the USA 300 from the USA 400, and detects the presence of the gene determining resistance to oxacillin the *mecA* gene target of the 16S rRNA that distinguish *Staphylococcus* spp. from other bacteria, the specific *nuc* gene of *S. aureus*, the PVL genes and other specific genes (Zhang et al., 2008). The multiplex PCR also allows the detection of genes encoding toxins and chromosomal cassettes responsible for antimicrobial resistance in a rapid and reliable manner compared to other methods (Oliveira & Lencastre, 2002).

The technique of Multilocus Sequence Typing (MLST) is widely used for typing of microorganisms and is based on amplification and sequencing of genes encoding proteins essential defining each strain based on the sequences of fragments of the seven loci of essential genes. As there are many allelic combinations for each of these genes, there are no identical profiles, and those that have, are considered members of a clone. This technique can be used to study evolutionary and population biology of bacteria (Enright et al., 2000).

Strains isolated in the United States were classified as pulsed-field types (PFT's) USA300, USA400, USA500, USA600, USA700, USA100 and USA800, USA900, USA1000, and USA1100 (Han et al., 2007). It is estimated that most CA-MRSA present the genetic profile of USA300, USA400, USA1000, and USA1100, which the predominant profile is USA300. Strains USA100, USA200 and USA500 are frequently associated with nosocomial infections, and mostly have chromosomal cassette multidrug resistance in type II (Klevens et al., 2007).

For MRSA typing techniques based on PCR, PFGE, ribotyping and plasmid typing, are widely used with successful results. The considerable genetic similarity between these microorganisms requires the use of more than one method for identifying more accurately (Oliveira et al., 2001).

spa typing involves sequencing the polymorphic region X of the gene of protein A (spa) that contains a variable number of repeated regions of 24 bp flanked by conserved regions as well. In addition to this grouping, based on the sequence of a locus, it is practical, inexpensive, fast, and has a lower probability of errors compared to PFGE and MLST techniques, and can be used in local and global epidemiological studies due to micro-and macro-variations that occur simultaneously in region X. The following types of protein A were characterized in CA-MRSA: t008, t019, t021, t044, T131, t216 (Hallin et al., 2007).

8. The role of the Panton-Valentine Leukocidin (PVL)

One of the most important common virulence mechanisms in CA-MRSA is PVL (Panton-Valentine Leukocidin) production. Strains that harbor the *SCCmec* element may simultaneously carry the *lukS* and *lukF* genes wich encode for PVL (Boyle-Vavra & Daum, 2007). Deep infections of skin and soft tissues such as skin boils and abscesses, and necrotizing pneumonia are attributed to the presence of PVL toxin in strains of *S. aureus* (Lina et al., 1999, Melles et al., 2006). The presence in the lungs causes hemorrhage, extensive necrosis of alveolar septa, destruction of the epithelium covering the bronchi and bronchioles (Zhang et al., 2005), and histological sections show necrotic lesions in the mucosa of the trachea (Lina et al., 1999). Due to these facts, studies have proposed that the propensity of CA-MRSA infections cause severe skin and soft tissue lesions, and possibly necrotizing pneumonia, is due to the presence of the gene encoding the production of PVL (Saïd-Salim et al. 2005).

PVL was first described as a "substance leukocidin" by Van deVelde in 1894 but was first associated with skin and soft tissue infections by Panton and Valentine in 1932. The acquisition of genes encoding PVL is made by transduction of a specific type of bacteriophage, phiSLT, which causes cytolysis in carrier gene cells and transport this gene to another cell. From its transcription two exoproteins , the Luks-PV and LukF-PV are produced, acting through the synergistic action of both subunits (Melles et al., 2006, Saïd-Salim et al., 2005). When secreted, LukS-PV initiates a connection to the membrane of the polymorphonuclear leukocyte (PMN) and is dimerized with LukF-PV, alternating one and another until the complete formation of a heptamer. Calcium channels are formed by inducing the production of interleukins and inflammatory mediators. Because of this evidence, probably the PVL is not directly associated with tissue necrosis, but related to lysosomal granules released by cytotoxic lysis of PMN, the release of granulocyte reactive oxygen or even the inflammatory cascade (Boyle-Vavra & Daum, 2007).

The main target of PVL is human and rabbit neutrophils, having little or no effect on non-human primates and mice (Löffler et al., 2010). The reason for differences in sensitivities to PVL is not yet fully known but may be related to receptor/signal transducers that are species-specific (Löffler et al., 2010). Its action is directly related to the concentration: at high concentrations, it causes cell lysis; at low concentrations, it mediates caspase dependent apoptosis by forming pores in the membrane of mitochondria (Boyle-Vavra & Daum, 2007; Lo & Wang 2011). Sub-lytic concentrations induce apoptosis of human neutrophils within 6 hours, and at high concentrations leads to cell death in only 1 hour (Lo & Wang, 2011).

9. Other virulence factors of MRSA

The pathogenicity of *S. aureus* depends on several determinants, among them, the production of toxins and extracellular membrane components (Jarraud et al., 2002; Gandhinagar & Silva, 2004). The molecular basis of pathogenicity of *S. aureus* depends on the expression of broad classes of accessory genes producing components of the cell wall and extracellular proteins. The expression of these virulence factors is regulated by genes in the operon *agr* (accessory gene regulator), which regulates the expression of genes for toxins and adhesins (Purcell & Fergie, 2005). Enzymes such as coagulase and catalase are responsible for its evasion of the immune system (Gandhinagar & Silva, 2004).

The toxins are related to staphylococcal toxic shock syndrome (TSS), staphylococcal scarlet fever (both due to the toxin of toxic shock syndrome 1 [TSST-1] and staphylococcal enterotoxins), scalded skin syndrome (SSS due to exfoliatins) and food poisoning (SE's, staphylococcal enterotoxins) (Santos et al., 2007; Jarraud et al., 2002; Johnson et al., 1991). Genetic sequencing of a strain called MW2, CA-MRSA, revealed the presence of genes responsible for specific virulence factors such as the PVL toxin, staphylococcal enterotoxin H (*seh*) and staphylococcal enterotoxin C (*sec*) (Saïd-Salim et al., 2005).

Toxic shock syndrome was related primarily to the use of a particular brand of tampons in 1980. The TSS can occur in patients of any age, with the main presenting symptoms being fever, rash, and toxicity, which often progresses to hypotension with a prior history of watery diarrhea, sore throat, nausea, vomiting and myalgia. A number of other symptoms involving dehydration and its effects are often related to the syndrome. Blood cultures may be negative for the pathogen. The strain that carries TSST-1 reacts with phage group I and is likely to produce toxins, including other enterotoxins, and exoproteins. It may also exhibit resistance to heavy metals, and proteolytic characteristics are not often haemolytic and usually tend to be pigmented. It is interesting that strains produce TSST-1 positive alpha-hemolysin in low quantities even if they have the gene, suggesting that certain genetic events leading to repression of some genes (e.g., hemolysin) at the same time the expression of other genes (i.e. TSST -1) is increased (Todd, 1988).

Scalded skin syndrome (SSS), better known as Ritter's disease was first described by German physician Baron Gotfried Ritter von Rittershain who observed the widespread phenomenon in 297 children calling it neonatal exfoliative dermatitis. This disease usually appears in children with clinical features ranging from localized to disseminated bullous impetigo, known for easily rupturing on the skin surface, releasing a fluid with features ranging from thin to thick, being opaque purulent yellowish, whitish or opaque. In neonates lesions are mainly located in the perineum, or both in the periumbilical region, and in older children the lesions are located near the umbilicus. This is the mildest form of the disease, in which the skin around the preserved area remains without systemic signs and symptoms. The generalized form of the disease is mainly spread across the surface of the skin and mucous membranes are usually spared. In infants, onset of symptoms begins between 3 to 16 days. Patients with systemic SSS present fever, malaise, lethargy, irritability, loss of appetite, followed by the appearance of erythematous papules that usually start in the head and neck and spread to the rest of the body in a few days (Ladhani et al., 1999).

Another mechanism of virulence that has often been identified in samples of CA-MRSA is phenol-soluble Moduline . PSM was first detected in cultures of *S. epidermidis*. Antimicrobial activity against Group A *Streptococcus* (Cogen et al., 2010) and activities that stimulate the immune system of NFkB nuclear factor kB in THP-1 cells and cytokines in THP-1 monocytes and its role in the infection still need to be clarified (Mehlin et al., 1999). In PVL-positive CA-MRSA samples, the PSM effect is to intensify the effects of the toxin in the presence of both units (LukS-and LukF-PV) (Hongo et al., 2009).

The detection of PSM in CA-MRSA strains was higher than in HA-MRSA strains showing that *S. aureus* PSM activate human neutrophils triggering an inflammatory response and thereby contributes to staphylococcal virulence. CA-MRSA PSM has an important role in leukocyte cytolysis by CA-MRSA primarily participating in evasion of the host defense system (Wang et al., 2007).

PVL, alpha-toxin and protein A, represent the virulence factors involved in pneumonia caused by *S. aureus.* Alpha-toxins and PVL form pores in the polymorphonuclear cells and thus causes an exaggerated response by the release of cytokines and reactive oxygen specimens and contributing to damage in lung tissue (Hayashida et al., 2009).

Studies in the United States report that the USA400 strain responsible for lethal pneumonia in three children, had cytotoxins, such as virulence factors alpha and gamma, PVL, phenol-soluble Moduline (PSMs), staphylococcal enterotoxin (SE) B or C. The profile of toxigenic strains of USA300 is similar, except for staphylococcal-like enterotoxin (SE-l) Q present in these strains. CA-MRSA USA 100 and 200 clones have emerged with alpha +/- and gamma-toxin +/-, PVL +/- PSM+ and TSST-1+ profiles. Probably the production of several cytotoxins combined with superantigen action culminates in a devastating disease (Schlievert, 2009).

Beta hemolysin was also related to lung injury as demonstrated by Hayashida et al. (2009). In this study, the hemolysin was attributed to the ability to increase the influx of neutrophils in the lung and alveolar spaces, causing leakage of serum proteins into the lung parenchyma and exudation of protein rich fluid into the air. The neutrophil migration is indirectly modulated by beta-hemolysin through the stimulation of other host factors. Thus, the virulence of hemolysin increases the regulation of various pro-inflammatory cytokines and generates an exaggerated response in the host (Hayashida et al., 2009)

10. Current antimicrobial drug choice

Given the great potential of CA-MRSA infections to develop into serious and/or systemic infections, there is an interest in reintroducing drugs such as trimethoprim/ sulfamethoxazole, tetracycline and clindamycin for treatment of CA-MRSA. In severe cases where there is need for hospitalization and intravenous therapy, antibiotics such as vancomycin, linezolid and daptomycin are reliable options (LaPlante et al., 2008).

The combination of trimethoprim/sulfamethoxazole (cotrimoxazole) has been considered a good therapeutic option for the treatment of patients affected by CA-MRSA. *In vitro* tests show that it has excellent bactericidal activity, but its activity can be reduced in the presence of rifampicin. Several antimicrobial combinations were tested, such as linezolid and cotrimoxazole, rifampicin,. Cotrimoxazole, minocycline, linezolid, clindamycin or moxifloxacin, cotrimoxazole alone proved to be more effective in *in vitro* tests (Kaka et al., 2006).

However, in another study with patients affected by CA-MRSA treated with trimethoprim/sulfamethoxazole, clindamycin and cephalexin resulted in a treatment failure rate of 26%, 25% and 33%, respectively. In addition, patients who received the drainage of abscesses in addition to antibiotic therapy had lower rates of treatment failure (25%) than patients who received only incision and drainage (60%) (Frei et al., 2010).

One of the main strains in the community, the USA300 had plasmid-mediated resistance to tetracycline, clindamycin, and mupirocin (Han et al., 2007). In addition, there is the possibility of clindamycin inducible resistant strains resulting in treatment failure. In places where there is high frequency of isolation of strains with this characteristic, it is necessary to choose alternative treatments. It is estimated that this phenomenon occurs in approximately 13% of CA-MRSA strains (LaPlante et al., 2007) and from 36% to 56% of HA-MRSA (Siberry et al., 2003). The treatment of clindamycin-sensitive strains was assessed showing that the best options were daptomycin, clindamycin, doxycycline, vancomycin, linezolid and trimethoprim/sulfamethoxazole, respectively, with the latter three being equally effective. Treatment with daptomycin was better than vancomycin and linezolid, the latter two having equal effect, but all three overcame the effects of clindamycin since these strains can show induced resistance and the treatment with clindamycin also induces the emergence of constitutive resistance (LaPlante et al., 2008).

Choosing the best option for treating infections caused by CA-MRSA has risks and benefits of each antimicrobial agent that must be considered before prescribing. The ideal antimicrobial agent would be one of low toxicity to the individual, the rapid bactericidal activity, excellent tissue penetration, consistent pharmacokinetics and pharmacodynamics that would allow a predetermined dose, low potential for development of resistance during therapy and a proven clinical efficacy and microbiological (Nguyen & Graber, 2010). Finding a single antimicrobial agent with these characteristics may be complex, whereas a combination of agents can be a successful alternative.

It is not enough to choose antimicrobials with these characteristics; it is also essential to observe antimicrobial participation in the various mechanisms of virulence of the microorganism. In several reports of infections caused by CA-MRSA, PVL appears simultaneously as a virulence factor. The use of antimicrobials may act in the synthesis of Leukocidin improving the patient's condition in cases of pneumonia caused by CA-MRSA PVL positive strains treated with linezolid and clindamycin which suggests that this is a good choice, acting on the protein production mechanism, these antibiotics prevent PVL production compared with vancomycin and nafcillin (Stevens et al., 2007).

11. Vancomycin resistance

Another concern is the emergence of resistance to the antibiotic of choice for treating MRSA, vancomycin. Few drugs are available to control MRSA, and vancomycin is one of them. Reports of resistance and low sensitivity to this antibiotic are present in nosocomial environments worldwide (Martins & Cunha et al., 2007).

The first case of reduced susceptibility to vancomycin was reported by Hiramatsu (1997) in a pediatric patient with positive culture for MRSA who was treated with glycopeptide. Phenotypic analysis showed that the MIC for this strain was 8 μg/mL in the microdilution test, and molecular analysis did not detect the presence of *vanA* or *vanB* genes. Strain Mu50, recovered from this patient, represents the first strain of *S. aureus* to demonstrate this level of resistance to vancomycin (Hiramatsu, 1997).

The first report of vancomycin resistance in the U.S. was described by Sievert et al. (2002). The patient was treated with several courses of antibiotics including vancomycin and subsequently developed MRSA bacteremia due to a hemodialysis catheter. He received vancomycin, rifampin and required removal of this catheter. The cultures of the catheter revealed the presence of *S. aureus* resistant to oxacillin and vancomycin. After one week, VRSA and vancomycin-resistant Enterococcus (VRE) were isolated. Cultures did not recovered VRSA from the patient being treated with trimethoprim/sulfamethoxazole, successfully. Molecular analysis revealed the presence of the *vanA* gene from enterococci, which explains the resistance to glycopeptides, and *mecA* (Sievert et al., 2002).

Cases of *S. aureus* with intermediate resistance to vancomycin (VISA) in addition to presenting heteroresistance are increasingly common in health centers where MRSA infections are treated with vancomycin (Trakulsomboon et al., 2001; Van Duijkeren et al., 2005; Kim et al., 2000).

Kim et al. (2000) observed that the vancomycin-resistant strains showed changes in the cell wall due to selective pressure caused by prolonged use of vancomycin in the treatment of infections caused by MRSA. On the other hand, *in vitro* gene transfer of *vanA* resistance was observed from vancomycin-resistant *Enterococcus* strains to *S. aureus* (Sievert et al., 2002).

The detection of resistance is a matter of controversy. Some authors Defend the idea that the disk diffusion method may not be effective in detecting resistance to glycopeptides, particularly vancomycin (Kim et al., 2000; Walsh et al., 2001).

In San Francisco, USA, a patient with subsequent complications was initially diagnosed with MRSA susceptible to trimethoprim-sulfamethoxazole. A more accurate survey was conducted showing that the strain belonged to the PFGE USA 300-0114 of community origin and had intermediate resistance to vancomycin. This strain is closely related to infections of skin and soft tissues as well as lung disease. Surveillance in the United States in San Francisco shows an explosive increase of infections by USA300 CA-MRSA, can also replace other strains (Graber et al., 2007).

12. Resistance in *Staphylococcus* spp.

Coagulase-negative staphylococci (CoNS) are part of the microbiota of the skin, most often presenting a benign relationship with the host. However, they are the major opportunistic pathogens of immunocompromised patients in hospitals (Bisno & Stevens, 1996; Cunha et al., 2004). Important infectious processes related to CoNS have been reported in recent decades. They are commonly isolated from blood cultures of patients undergoing invasive procedures such as prostheses, catheters, organ transplants, as well as from premature infants (Cunha et al., 2004).

The main species of CoNS that are involved in infections in humans are *S. epidermidis* (may cause bacteremia, osteomyelitis, peritonitis, surgical site infections, infections due to the installation of catheters and prostheses, endophthalmitis, etc.), *S. haemolyticus* (urinary tract infection, peritonitis, injuries, etc.) and *S. saprophyticus* (urinary tract infection and septicemia) (Cunha et al., 2004). Specifically regarded to the occurrence of bacteremia in hospitals, the species *S. epidermidis* was found to be the etiologic agent in 80% of cases (Gongora-Rubio et al., 1997).

Resistance to methicillin in species of CoNS (MRSCoN) colonizing healthy individuals can overcome MRSA in the same population as demonstrated by a Japanese study (Hisato et al., 2005). Analysis of 818 children revealed that 35 (4.3%) carried MRSA, while 231 (28.2%) MRSCoN. The fact that MRSCoN strains are prevalent in the community suggests that they are important reservoirs of SCC*mec* that can be carried to strains of *S. aureus* (Hisato et al., 2005).

Strains of vancomycin-resistant CoNS are common in hospitals due to this antibiotics' selective pressure in this environment, but few studies have been published on this community. A surveillance study assessed the cultures of saliva collected from employees of a private school and 37 hospital staff. The identification of specimens recovered from samples revealed that 98.5% were carriers of *Staphylococcus spp.* and 76.5% were carriers of more than one *Staphylococcus* spp. species. Four strains were resistant to vancomycin according to phenotypic tests isolated from two school officials and two hospital employees, and two identified as *S. capitis* and the other two as *S. haemolyticus* and *S. epidermidis.* All samples carried the *mecA* gene of resistance to oxacillin and were negative for the genes *vanA*, *vanB* and *vanC*. The samples relating to employees of the hospital were also resistant to other classes of antimicrobials (Palazzo et al., 2005).

MRSCoN may be involved in severe infections and present different resistances, as well as virulence factors able to offer health risks of individuals with impaired immune systems or in development as in the case of neonates. Despite its great importance in critically ill patients, its presence in healthy individuals deserves special attention mainly because they are both sources of genes for virulence and resistance.

13. Future prospects

The emergence of *S. aureus* resistant to methicillin in the community as the main agent of serious infections of skin and soft tissue is disturbing since oxacillin would be the drug of choice to treat infections caused by strains resistant to other antibiotics. Several techniques can be used to detect resistance to oxacillin, but PCR is the safest and most effective. In addition to PCR, other techniques allow genetic characterization of CA-MRSA detailing an arsenal of toxins and differentiation of clones involved in outbreaks. These techniques help epidemiologist determine correct measures in controlling the spread of this pathogen.

Studies in Epidemiology associated with molecular studies represent good tools for understand the distribution and inform treatment success. The detection of antimicrobial resistance in strains from patients living in the community reveals that the alternatives available to the medical community for successful treatment are decreasing gradually, thus, presenting an opportunity to research new drugs, and antimicrobial agents considered older and well established such as trimethoprim/sulfamethoxazole, which is re-emerging as an option for treating infections caused by CA-MRSA.

The presence of CA-MRSA strains involved in nosocomial infection implies the need for greater control of its spread among hospitalized patients, since the reports of strains of community origin suggest they are also more virulent compared to strains of nosocomial origin, and may lead to serious complications of rapid evolution. Treatment strategies that may delay or prevent the expression of these factors will need to be established, as well as administering the correct treatment quickly and effectively.

14. Conclusion

The presence of resistant strains in the community, especially *S. aureus*, poses a risk to public health since the treatment may fail, delaying the elimination of pathogens involved in these infections. This delay can result in serious complications leading to early death of the patient. New treatment alternatives and the rediscovery of antimicrobials that are no longer being used provide to the medical community a new opportunity for successful treatment.

In addition to antimicrobial resistance, community strains have become more virulent, which provides another challenge to the attending physician to choose the best treatment strategy possible. Attention should also be directed to CoNS strains resistant to methicillin, which can serve as reservoirs of resistance genes *S. aureus* that are more virulent. The detections of virulence factors and antimicrobial additional resistance can be truly challenging and lead to treatment failure if it is not detected quickly. Fortunately there are new approaches that are becoming affordable to microbiology laboratories that can detect as far as the patient is attended. But to reach the 100% of the treatment success it will need more than top notch technologies.

15. References

Alvarez, C.A.; Barrientes, O.J.; Leal, A.L.; Contreras, G.A.; Barrero, L.; Rincón, S.; Diaz, L.; Vanegas, N. & Arias, C.A. (2006). Community associated Methicillin-Resistant *Staphylococcus aureus*, Colombia. *Emerging Infectious Diseases*, Vol. 12, No. 12, pp. 2000-2001, ISSN 1080-6059.

Baba, T.; Takeuchi, F.; Kuroda, M.; Yuzawa, H.; Aoki, K.; Oguchi, A.; Nagai, Y.; Iwama, N.; Asano, K.; Naimi, T.; Kuroda, H.; Cui, L.; Yamamoto, K. & Hiramatsu, K. (2002). Genome and virulence determinants of high virulence community-acquired MRSA. *Lancet*, Vol. 359, No. 9320, (May 2002), pp. 1819-1827, ISSN 1474-547X.

Bisno, A.L. & Stevens, D.L. (1996). Streptococcal Infections of Skin and Soft Tissues. *England Journal of Medicine*, Vol. 334, No. 334, pp. 240-245, ISSN 1533-4406.

Bisognano, C.; Vaudaux, P.E.; Lew, D.P.; NG, E.Y.W. & Hooper D.C. (1997). Increased Expression of Fibronectin-Binding Proteins by Fluoroquinolone-Resistant *Staphylococcus aureus* Exposed to Subinhibitory Levels of Ciprofloxacin. *Antimicrobial Agents and Chemotherapy*, Vol. 41, No. 5, pp. 906–913, ISSN 1098-6596.

Boyle-Vavra, S.; Ereshefsky, B.; Wang, C.C. & Daum, R.S. (2005). Successful Multiresistant Community-Associated Methicillin-Resistant *Staphylococcus aureus* Lineage from Taipei, Taiwan, That Carries Either the Novel Staphylococcal Chromosome Cassette *mec* (*SCCmec*) Type VT or SCC*mec* Type IV. *Journal of Clinical Microbiology*, Vol. 43, No. 12, pp. 4719–4730, ISSN 1098-660X.

Boyle-Vavra, S. & Daum, R.S. (2007). Community-acquired methicillin-resistant *Staphylococcus aureus*: the role of Panton–Valentine leukocidin. *Laboratory Investigation*, Vol. 87, No. 1, pp. 3–9, ISSN 0023-6837.

Chambers, H.F. (1997). Methicillin Resistance in Staphylococci: Molecular and Biochemical Basis and Clinical Implications. *Clinical Microbiology Reviews*, Vol. 10, No. 4, pp. 781–791, ISSN 1098-6618.

Coates, T.; Bax, R. & Coates, A. (2009). Nasal decolonization of Staphylococcus aureus with mupirocin: strengths, weaknesses and future prospects. *Journal Antimicrobial and Chemotherapy*, Vol. 64, No. 1, pp. 9–15, ISSN 1460-2091.

Cogen, A.L.; Yamasaki, K.; Muto, J.; Sanchez, K.M.; Crotty, A.L.; Muto, J.; Tanios, J.; Lai, Y.; Kim, J.E.; Nizet, V. & Gallo R.L. (2010) *Staphylococcus epidermidis* Antimicrobial d-Toxin (Phenol-Soluble Modulin-c) Cooperates with Host Antimicrobial Peptides to Kill Group A *Streptococcus*. *PLoS ONE*, Vol. 5, No. 1, pp. e8557, ISSN 1932-6203.

Cunha, M.L.R.S.; Sinzato, Y.K. & Silveira, L.V.A. (2004). Comparison of Methods for the Identification of Coagulase negative Staphylococci. *Memórias do Instituto Oswaldo Cruz*, Vol. 99, No. 8, pp. 855-860, ISSN 1678-8060.

Cunha, M.L.R.S.; Peresi, E.; Calsolari, R.A.O & Araújo Jr, J.P. (2006). Detection of Enterotoxins genes in coagulase-negative Staphylococci isolated from foods. *Brazilian Journal of Microbiology*, Vol. 37, pp. 64-69, ISSN 1517-8382.

David, M.Z.; Crawford, S.E.; Boyle-Vavra, S.; Hostetler, M.A.; Kim, D.C. & Daum, R.S. (2006). Contrasting Pediatric and Adult Methicillin-resistant *Staphylococcus aureus* Isolates. *Emerging Infectious Diseases*, Vol. 12, No. 4, pp. 631-637, ISSN 1080-6059.

d'Azevedo, P.A.; Inoue, F.M.; Andrade, S.S.; Tranchesi, R. & Pignatari, A.C.C. (2009). Pneumonia necrotizante por *Staphylococcus aureus* resistente à meticilina. *Sociedade Brasileira de Medicina Tropical*, Vol. 42, No. 4, pp. 461-462, ISSN 0037-8682.

Dall'Antonia, M.; Coen, P.G.; Wilks, M.; Whiley, A. & Millar, M. (2005). Competition between methicillin-sensitive and -resistant *Staphylococcus aureus* in the anterior nares. *Journal of Hospital Infections*, Vol. 61, No. 1, pp. 62–67, ISSN 0195-6701.

Enright, M.C.; Day, N.P.J.; Davies, C.E.; Peacock, S.J. & Spratt, B.G. (2000). Multilocus Sequence Typing for Characterization of Methicillin-Resistant and Methicillin-Susceptible Clones of *Staphylococcus aureus*. *Journal of Clinical Microbiology*, Vol. 38, No. 3, pp. 1008–1015, ISSN 1098-660X.

Ellis M, Hospenthal D, Dooley D, Gray P, Murray C. (2004). Natural history of community acquired methicillin-resistant Staphylococcus aureus colonization and infection in soldiers. *Clin Infect Dis*. Vol. 39, No. 7, pp. 971–9, ISSN 1537-6591.

Euzéby, JP. List of Prokaryotic names with Standing in Nomenclature - Genus *Staphylococcus* [Internet]. [place unknown: publisher unknown]; [up dated 2010 june 4; cited 2011 august 31]. Available from: http://www.bacterio.cict.fr/s/staphylococcus.html

Fortes, C.Q.; Espanha, C.A.; Bustorff, F.P.; Zappa, B.C.; Ferreira, A.L.; Moreira, R.B.; Pereira, N.G.; Fowler V.G. Jr. & Deshmukh, H. (2008). First Reported Case of Infective Endocarditis Caused by Community-Acquired Methicillin-Resistant *Staphylococcus aureus* Not Associated With Healthcare Contact in Brazil. *Brazilian Journal of Infectious Diseases*, Vol. 12, No. 6, pp. 541-543, ISSN 1517-8382.

Frei, C.R.; Miller, M.L.; Lewis II, J.S.; Lawson, K.A.; Hunter, J.M.; Oramasionwu, C.U. & Talbert, R.L. (2010). Trimethoprim-Sulfamethoxazole or Clindamycin for Community-Associated MRSA (CA-MRSA) Skin Infections. *Journal of the American Board of Family Medicine*, Vol. 23, No. 6, pp. 714-719, ISSN 1558-7118.

Gelatti, L.C.; Sukiennik, T.; Becker, A.P.; Inoue, F.M.; Carmo, M.S.; Castrucci, F.M.S.; Pignatari, A.C.C.; Ribeiro, L.C.; Bonamigo, R.R.; Azevedo, P.A. (2009). Sepse por *Staphylococus aureus* resistente à meticilina adquirida na comunidade no sul do Brasil. *Sociedade Brasileira de Medicina Tropical*, Vol. 42, No. 4, pp. 458-460, ISSN 0037-8682.

Góngora-Rubio, F.; Pignatari, A.C.C.; Costa, L.M.D.; Bortolloto, V.I.; Machado, A.M. & De Góngora, D.V.N. (1997). Significância clínica, epidemiologia e microbiologia das bacteremias por estafilococos coagulase-negativos em Hospital de Ensino. *Revista da Associação Médica Brasileira*, Vol. 43, No. 1, pp. 9-14, ISSN 1806-9282.

Graber, C.J.; Wong, M.K.; Carleton, H.A.; Perdreau-Remington, F.; Haller, B.L. & Chambers, H.F. (2007). Intermediate Vancomycin Susceptibility in a Community-associated MRSA Clone. *Emerging Infectious Diseases*, Vol. 13, No. 3, pp. 491-493, ISSN 1080-6059.

Han, L.L.; Mcdougal, L.K.; Gorwitz, R.J.; Mayer, K.H.; Patel, J.B.; Sennott, J.M. & Fontana, J.L. (2007). High Frequencies of Clindamycin and Tetracycline Resistance in Methicillin-Resistant *Staphylococcus aureus* Pulsed-Field Type USA300 Isolates Collected at a Boston Ambulatory Health Center. *Journal of Clinical Microbiology*, Vol. 45, No. 4, pp. 1350–1352, ISSN 1098-660X.

Hanssen, A.M.; Kjeldsen, G. & Sollid, J.U.E. (2004). Local Variants of Staphylococcal Cassette Chromosome mec in Sporadic Methicillin-Resistant *Staphylococcus aureus* and Methicillin-Resistant Coagulase-Negative Staphylococci: Evidence of Horizontal

Gene Transfer? *Journal of Antimicrobial Chemotherapy*, Vol. 48, No. 1, pp. 285-296, ISSN 1460-2091.

Hanssen, A.M. & Sollid, J.U.E. (2007). Multiple Staphylococcal Cassette Chromosomes and Allelic Variants of Cassette Chromosome Recombinases in *Staphylococcus aureus* and Coagulase-Negative Staphylococci from Norway. *Journal of Antimicrobial Chemotherapy*, Vol. 51, No. 5, pp. 1671-1677, ISSN 1460-2091.

Hallin, M.; Deplano, A.; Denis, O.; De Mendonça, R.; De Ryck, R. & Struelens, M.J. (2007). Validation of Pulsed-Field Gel Electrophoresis and spa Typing for Long-Term, Nationwide Epidemiological Surveillance Studies of *Staphylococcus aureus* Infections. *Journal of Clinical Microbiology*, Vol. 45, No. 1, pp. 127-133, ISSN 1098-660X.

Hayashida, A.; Bartlett, A.H.; Foster, T.J. & Park, P.W. *Staphylococcus aureus* Beta-Toxin Induces Lung Injury through Syndecan-1. *The American Journal of Pathology*, Vol. 174, No. 2, (January 2009), pp. 509-518, ISSN 0002-9440.

Hiramatsu, K. (1997). Reduced Susceptibility of *Staphylococcus aureus* to Vancomycin Japan, 1996. *Morbidity and Mortality Weekly Report*, Vol. 46, No. 27, pp. 624-626, ISSN 1545-8601.

Hisata, K.; Kuwahara-Arai, K.; Yamanoto, M.; Ito, T.; Nakatomi, Y.; Cui, L.; Baba, T.; Terasawa, M.; Sotozono, C.; Kinoshita, S.; Yamashiro, Y. & Hiramatsu, K. (2005). Dissemination of Methicillin-Resistant Staphylococci among Healthy Japanese Children. *Journal of Clinical Microbiology*, Vol. 43, No.7, pp. 3364-3372, ISSN 1098-660X.

Hongo, I.; Baba, T.; Oishi, K.; Morimoto, Y.; Ito, T. & Hiramatsu, K. (2009). Phenol-Soluble Modulin a3 Enhances the Human Neutrophil Lysis Mediated by Panton-Valentine Leukocidin. *The Journal of Infectious Diseases*, Vol. 200, pp. 715-23, ISSN 1537-6613.

Huijsdens, X.W.; Van Santen-Verheuvel, M.G.; Spalburg, E.; Heck M.; Pluister, G.N.; Eijkelkamp, B.A.; Neeling, A.J. & Wannet, W.J.B. (2006). Multiple Cases of Familial Transmission of Community-Acquired Methicillin-Resistant *Staphylococcus aureus*. *Journal of Clinical Microbiology*, Vol. 44, No. 8, pp. 2994-2996, ISSN 1098-660X.

Ito, T.; Katayama, Y.; Asada, K.; Mori, N.; Tsutsumimoto, K.; Tiensasitorn, C. & Hiramatsu K. (2001). Structural Comparison of Three Types of Staphylococcal Cassette Chromosome *mec* Integrated in the Chromosome in Methicillin-Resistant *Staphylococcus aureus*. *Journal of Antimicrobial Chemotherapy*, Vol. 45, No. 5, pp. 1323-1336, ISSN 1460-2091.

Ito, T.; Katayama, Y. & Hiramatsu, K. (1999). Cloning and Nucleotide Sequence Determination of the Entire *mec* DNA of Pre-Methicillin-Resistant *Staphylococcus aureus* N315. *Journal of Antimicrobial Chemotherapy*, Vol. 43, No. 6, pp. 1449-1458, ISSN 1460-2091.

Ito, T.; Ma, X.X.; Takeuchi, F.; Okuma, K.; Yuzawa, H. & Hiramatsu, K. (2004). Novel Type V Staphylococcal Cassette Chromosome *mec* Driven by a Novel Cassette Chromosome Recombinase, *ccrC*. *Journal of Antimicrobial Chemotherapy*, Vol. 48, No. 7, pp. 2637-2651, ISSN 1460-2091.

IWG-SCCmec. International Working Group on the Staphylococcal Cassette Chromosome elements. [home page on the Internet]. [place unknown: publisher unknown]; [updated unknown; cited 2011 june 07]. Available from: http://www.sccmec.org/Pages/SCC_TypesEN.html

Jarraud, S.; Mougel, C.; Thioulouse, J.; Lina, G.; Meugnier, H.; Forey, F.; Nesme, X.; Etienne J. & Vandenesch, F. (2002). Relationships between *Staphylococcus aureus* Genetic Background, Virulence Factors, agr Groups (Alleles), and Human Disease. *Infection and Immunity*, Vol. 70, No. 2, pp. 631–641, ISSN 1098-5522.

Johnson, W.M.; Tylerm S.D.; Ewan, E.P.; Ashton, F.E.; Pollard, D.R. & Rozee, K.R. (1991). Detection of genes for enterotoxins, exfoliative toxins, and toxic shock syndrome toxin 1 in *Staphylococcus aureus* by the polymerase chain reaction. *Journal of Clinical Microbiology*, Vol. 29, No. 3, pp. 426-430, ISSN 1098-660X.

Kaka, A.S.; Rueda, A.M.; Shelburne III, S.A.; Hulten, K.; Hamill, R.J. & Musher, D.M. (2006). Bactericidal activity of orally available agents against methicillin-resistant *Staphylococcus aureus*. *Journal of Antimicrobial Chemotherapy*, Vol. 58, pp. 680–683. ISSN 1460-2091

Kallen, A.J.; Brunkard, J.; Moore, Z.; Budge, P.; Arnold, K.E.; Fosheim, G.; Finelli, L.; Beekmann, S.E.; Polgreen, P.M.; Gorwitz, R. & Hageman J. (2008). *Staphylococcus aureus* community-acquired pneumonia during the 2006 to 2007 influenza season. *Annals of Emergency Medicine*, Vol. 53, No. 3, pp. 358-365, ISSN 0196-0644.

Katayama, Y.; Ito, T. & Hiramatsu, K. (2001). Genetic organization of the chromosome region surrounding *mecA* in clinical staphylococcal strains: role of *IS431*-mediated *mecI* deletion in expression of resistance in *mecA*-carrying, lowlevel methicillin-resistant *Staphylococcus haemolyticus*. *Antimicrobial Agents and Chemotherapy*, Vol. 45, No. 7, pp. 1955–1963, ISSN 1098-6596.

Klevens, R.M.; Morrison, M.A.; Nadle, J.; Petit, S.; Gershman, K.; Ray, S.; Harrison, L.H.; Lynfield, R.; Dumyati, G.; Townes, J.M.; Craig, A.S.; Zell, E.R.; Fosheim, G.E.; McDougal, L.K.; Carey, R.B. & Fridkin, S.K. (2007). Invasive Methicillin-Resistant *Staphylococcus aureus* Infections in the United States. *JAMA*, Vol. 298, No. 15, pp. 1763-1771, ISSN 1538-3598.

Kim, M.N.; Pai, C.H.; Woo, J.H.; Ryu, J.S. & Hiramatsu, K. (2000). Vancomycin-Intermediate *Staphylococcus aureus* in Korea. *Journal of Clinical Microbiology*, Vol. 38, No. 10, pp. 3879–3881, ISSN 1098-660X.

Keuhnert, M.J.; Druszon-Moran, D.; Hill, H.; McQuillan, G.; McAllister, S.K.; Fosheim, G.; McDougal, L.K.; Chaitram, J.; Jensen, B.; Fridkin, S.K.; Killgore G.; Tenover, F.C. (2006). Prevalence of *Staphylococcus aureus* nasal colonization in the United States, 2001–2002. *Journal of Infectious Diseases*. Vol. 193, No. 2, pp 172–179, ISSN 1537-6613.

Ladhani, S.; Joannou, C.L.; Lochrie, D.P.; Evans, R.W. & Poston, S.M. (1999). Clinical, Microbial, and Biochemical Aspects of the Exfoliative Toxins Causing Staphylococcal Scalded-Skin Syndrome. *Clinical Microbiology Reviews*, Vol. 12, No. 2, pp. 224–242, ISSN 1098-6618.

LaPlante, K.L.; Leonard, S.N.; Andes, D.R.; Craig, W.A. & Rybak, M.J. (2008). Activities of Clindamycin, Daptomycin, Doxycycline, Linezolid, Trimethoprim-Sulfamethoxazole, and Vancomycin against Community-Associated Methicillin-Resistant *Staphylococcus aureus* with Inducible Clindamycin Resistance in Murine Thigh Infection and In Vitro Pharmacodynamic Models. *Antimicrobial Agents and Chemotherapy*, Vol. 52, No. 6, pp. 2156–2162, ISSN 1098-6596.

LaPlante, K.L.; Rybakn M. J.; Amjad, M. & Kaatz, G.W. (2007). Antimicrobial susceptibility and staphylococcal chromosomal cassette mec type in community- and hospital-associated methicillin-resistant *Staphylococcus aureus*. *Pharmacotherapy*, Vol. 27, No. 1, pp. 3–10, ISSN 1060-0280.

Layer, F.; Ghebremedhin, B.; Moder, K.A.; König, W. & König, B. (2006). Comparative Study Using Various Methods for Identification of *Staphylococcus* Species in Clinical Specimens. *Journal of Clinical Microbiology*, Vol. 44, No. 8, pp. 2824–2830, ISSN 1098-660X.

Lear, A.; McCord, G.; Peiffer, J.; Watkins, R.R.; Parikh, A. & Warrington, S. (2011). Incidence of *Staphylococcus aureus* Nasal Colonization and Soft Tissue Infection Among High School Football Players. *Journal of the American Board of Family Medicine*, Vol. 24, No. 4, pp. 429-435, ISSN 1558-7118.

Lina, G.; Piémont, Y.; Godail-Gamot, F.; Bes, M.; Peter, M.O.; Gauduchon, V.; Vandenesch, F. & Etienne, J. (1999). Involvement of Panton-Valentine Leukocidin–Producing *Staphylococcus aureus* in Primary Skin Infections and Pneumonia. *Clinical Infectious Diseases*, Vol. 29, pp. 1128–1132, ISSN 1537-6591.

Lo, W.T. & Wang, C.C. (2011). Panton-Valentine Leukocidin in the Pathogenesis of Community-associated Methicillin-resistant *Staphylococcus aureus* Infection. *Pediatrics and Neonatology*, Vol. 52, No. 2, pp. 59-65, ISSN 1875-9572.

Löffler, B.; Hussain, M.; Grundmeier, M.; Brück, M.; Holzinger, D.; Varga, G.; Roth, J.; Kahl, B.C.; Proctor, R.A. & Peters, G. (2010). *Staphylococcus aureus* Panton-Valentine Leukocidin Is a Very Potent Cytotoxic Factor for Human Neutrophils. *PLoS Pathogens*, Vol. 6, No. 1, pp. e1000715, ISSN 1553-7366.

Martins, A. & Cunha, M.L.R.S. (2007). Methicilin Resistance in *Staphylococcus aureus* and Coagulase-Negative Staphylococci: Epidemiological and Molecular Aspects. *Microbiology and Immunology*, Vol. 51, pp. 787-795, ISSN 1348-0421.

Martins, A.; Pereira, VC & Cunha, M.L.R.S. (2010). Oxacillin Resistance of *Staphylococcus aureus* Isolated from the University Hospital of Botucatu Medical School in Brazil. *Chemotherapy* Vol. 56, pp. 112-119 , ISSN 0009-3157 ISSN 1348-0421.

Mayhall, C.G. 2002. Control of Vancomycin-Resistant Enterococci: It Is Important, It Is Possible, and It Is Cost-Effective. *Infection Control and Hospital Epidemiology*, Vol. 3, No. 8, (August), pp. 420-423, ISSN 0899-823X.

Mehlin, C.; Headley, C.M. & Klebanoff, S.J. (1991). An Inflammatory Polypeptide Complex from *Staphylococcus epidermidis*: Isolation and Characterization. *Journal of Experimental Medicine*, Vol. 189, No. 6, pp. 907–917, ISSN 0022-1007.

Melles, D.C.; Van Leeuwen, W.B.; Boelens, H.A.M.; Peeters, J.K.; Verbrugh, H.A. & Van Belkum, A. (2006). Panton-Valentine Leukocidin Genes in *Staphylococcus aureus*. *Emerging Infectious Diseases*, Vol. 12, No. 7, pp. 1174-1175, ISSN 1080-6059.

Nouwen, J.L.; Ott, A.; Kluytmans-Vandenbergh, M.F.; Boelens, H.A.M.; Hofman, A.; van Belkum, A. & Verbrugh H.A. (2004). Predicting the *Staphylococcus aureus* nasal carrier state: derivation and validation of a "culture rule". *Clinical Infectious Diseases*, Vol. 39, pp. 806–11, ISSN 1537-6591.

Nguyen, H.M. & Graber, C.J. (2010). Limitations of antibiotic options for invasive infections caused by methicillin-resistant *Staphylococcus aureus*: is combination therapy the answer? *Journal of Antimicrobial Chemotherapy*, Vol. 65, pp. 24–36, ISSN 1460-2091.

Okuma, K.; Iwakawa, K.; Turnidge, J.D.; Grubb, W.B.; Bell, J.M.; O'brien, F.G.; Coombs, G.W.; Pearman, J.W.; Tenover, F.C.; Kapi, M.; Tiensasitorn, C.; Ito, T. & Hiramatsu, K. (2002). Dissemination of New Methicillin-Resistant *Staphylococcus aureus* clones in the community. *Journal of Clinical Microbiology*, Vol. 40, No. 11, pp. 4289–4294, ISSN 1098-660X.

Oliveira, G.A.; Faria, J.B.; Levy, C.E. & Mamizuka, E.M. (2001). Characterization of the Brazilian endemic clone of methicillin-resistant *Staphylococcus aureus* (MRSA) from hospitals throughout Brazil. *Braz J Infect Dis*, Vol. 5, No. 4, pp. 163-170, ISSN 1413-8670.

Oliveira, D.C. & de Lencastre, H. (2002). Multiplex PCR Strategy for Rapid Identification of Structural Types and Variants of the *mec* Element in Methicillin-Resistant *Staphylococcus aureus*. *Journal of Antimicrobial Chemotherapy*, Vol. 46, pp. 2155–2161, ISSN 1460-2091.

Palazzo, I.C.V.; Araujo, M.L.C. & Darini, A.L.C. (2005). First Report of Vancomycin-Resistant Staphylococci Isolated from Healthy Carriers in Brazil. *Journal of Clinical Microbiology*, Vol. 43, No. 1, pp. 179–185, ISSN 1098-660X.

Patel, M.; Waites, K.B.; Moser, S.A.; Cloud, G.A. & Hoesley, C.J. (2006). Prevalence of Inducible Clindamycin Resistance among Community and Hospital-Associated *Staphylococcus aureus* Isolates. *Journal of Clinical Microbiology*, Vol. 44, No. 7, pp. 2481–2484, ISSN 1098-660X.

Pereira, V.C.; Martins, A.; Rugolo, L.M.S.S. & Cunha, M.L.R.S. (2009). Detection of Oxacillin Resistance in *Staphylococcus aureus* Isolated from the Neonatal and Pediatric Units of a Brazilian Teaching Hospital. *Clinical Medicine Insights: Pediatrics*, Vol. 3, pp. 23–31, ISSN: 1179-5565.

Purcell, K. & Fergie, J. (2005). Epidemic of Community-Acquired Methicillin-Resistant *Staphylococcus aureus* Infections. *Archives of Pediatrics and Adolescent Medicine*, Vol. 159, pp. 980-985, ISSN 1538-3628.

Razera, F.; De Stefani, S.; Bonamigo, R.R.; Olm, G.S.; Dias, C.A.G. & Narvaez, G.A. (2009). CA-MRSA em furunculose: relato de caso do sul do Brasil. *Anais Brasileiros de Dermatologia*, Vol. 84, pp. 515-518, ISSN 0365-0596.

Reddy, P.; Qi, C.; Zembower, T.; Noskin, G.A. & Bolon, M. (2007). Postpartum Mastitis and Community-acquired Methicillin-resistant *Staphylococcus aureus*. *Emerging Infectious Diseases*, Vol. 13, No. 2, pp. 298-301, ISSN 1080-6059.

Reinert, C.; McCulloch, J.A.; Watanabe, S.; Ito, T.; Hiramatsu, K. & Mamizuka, E.M. (2008). Type IV *SCCmec* Found in Decade Old Brazilian MRSA Isolates. *Brazilian Journal of Infectious Diseases*, Vol. 12, No. 3, pp. 213-216, ISSN 1413-8670.

Ribeiro, A.; Dias, C.; Silva-Carvalho, M.C.; Berquó, L.; Ferreira, F.A.; Santos, R.N.S.; Ferreira-Carvalho, B.T. & Figueiredo, A.M. (2005). First Report of Infection with Community-Acquired Methicillin-Resistant *Staphylococcus aureus* in South America. *Journal of Clinical Microbiology*, Vol. 43, No. 4, pp. 1985–1988, ISSN 1098-660X.

Ricardo, S.B. (2004). Emergência de *S. aureus* Meticilina-Resistente (MRSA) na Comunidade. *Prática Hospitalar*, Vol. 4, No. 34, pp. 131-134, ISSN 1679-5512.

Rouzic, N.; Janvier, F.; Libert, N.; Javouhey, E.; Lina, G.; Nizou, J.Y.; Pasquier, P.; Stamm, D.; Brinquin, L.; Pelletier, C.; Vandenesch, F.; Floret, D.; Etienne, J.; Gillet, Y. (2010). Prompt and Successful Toxin-Targeting Treatment of Three Patients with Necrotizing Pneumonia Due to *Staphylococcus aureus* Strains Carrying the Panton-Valentine Leukocidin Genes. *Journal of Clinical Microbiology*, Vol. 48, No. 5, pp. 1952–1955, ISSN 1098-660X.

Rutland, B.E.; Weese, J.S.; Bolin, C.; Au, J. & Malani, A.N. (2009). Human-to-Dog Transmission of Methicillin-Resistant *Staphylococcus aureus*. *Emerging Infectious Diseases*, Vol. 15, No. 8, pp. 1328-1330, ISSN 1080-6059.

Saïd-Salim, B.; Mathema, B.; Braughton, K.; Davis, S.; Sinsimer, D.; Eisner, W.; Likhoshvay, Y.; DeLeo, F.R. & Kreiswirth, B.N. (2005). Differential Distribution and Expression of Panton-Valentine Leukocidin among Community-Acquired Methicillin-Resistant *Staphylococcus aureus* Strains. *Journal of Clinical Microbiology*, Vol. 43, No. 7, pp. 3373–3379, ISSN 1098-660X.

Salgado, C.D.; Farr, B.M. & Calfee, D.P. (2003). Community-Acquired Methicillin-Resistant *Staphylococcus aureus*: A Meta-Analysis of Prevalence and Risk Factors. *Clinical Infectious Diseases*, Vol. 36, pp. 131–139, ISSN 1537-6591 .

Santos, A.L.; Santos, D.O.; Freitas, C.C.; Ferreira, B.L.A.; Afonso, I.F.; Rodrigues, C.R. & Castro, H.C. (2007). *Staphylococcus aureus*: visitando uma cepa de importância hospitalar. *Jornal Brasileiro de Patologia e Medicina Laboratorial*, Vol. 43, No. 6, pp. 413-423, ISSN 1676-2444.

Sievert, D.M.; Boulton, M.L.; Stoltman, G.; Johnson, D.; Stobierski, M.G.; Downes, F.P.; Somsel, P.A.; Rudrik, J.T.; Brown, W.; Hafeez, W.; Lundstrom, T.; Flanagan, E.; Johnson, R.; Mitchell, J. & Chang, S. (2002). *Staphylococcus aureus* Resistant to Vancomycin — United States, 2002. *Morbity and Mortality Weekly Reports*, Vol. 51, No. 26, pp. 565-567, ISSN 1545-8601.

Schlievert, P.M. (2009). Cytolysins, Superantigens, and Penumonia due to Community-Associated Methicillin-Resistant *Staphylococcus aureus*. *Journal of Infectious Diseases*, Vol. 200, No. 5, pp. 676–678, ISSN 1537-6613.

Silva, W.P. & Gandra, E.A. (2004). Estafilococos coagulase positiva: patógeno de importância alimentar. *Higiene Alimentar*, Vol. 18, pp. 32-40, ISSN 0101-9171.

Siberry, G. K.; Tekle T.; Carroll K. & Dick J. (2003). Failure of clindamycin treatment of methicillin-resistant *Staphylococcus aureus* expressing inducible clindamycin resistance in vitro. *Clinical Infectious Diseases*, Vol. 37, pp. 1257–1260, ISSN 1537-6591.

Stemper, M.E.; Brady, J.M.; Qutaishat, S.S.; Borlaug, G.; Reed, J.; Reed, K.D. & Shukla, S.K. (2006). Shift in *Staphylococcus aureus* Clone Linked to an Infected Tattoo. *Emerging Infectious Diseases*, Vol. 12, No. 9, pp. 1444-1446, ISSN 1080-6059.

Stevens, D.L.; Ma, Y.; Salmi, D.B.; McIndoo, E.; Wallace, R.J. & Bryant, A.E. (2007). Impact of antibiotics on expression of virulence-associated exotoxin genes in methicillin-sensitive and methicillin-resistant *Staphylococcus aureus*. *Journal of Infectious Diseases*, Vol. 195, No. 2, pp. 202-211, ISSN 1537-6613.

Trakulsomboon, S.; Danchaivijitr, S.; Rongrungruang, Y.; Dhiraputra, C.; Susaemgrat, W.; Ito, T. & Hiramatsu, K. (2001). First Report of Methicillin-Resistant *Staphylococcus aureus* with Reduced Susceptibility to Vancomycin in Thailand. *Journal of Clinical Microbiology*, Vol. 39, No. 2, pp. 591–595, ISSN 1098-660X.

Tood, J.K. (1988). Toxic Shock Syndrome. *Clinical Microbiology Reviews*, Vol. 1, No. 4, pp. 432-446, ISSN 1098-6618.

Turabelidze, G.; Lin, M.; Wolkoff, B.; Dodson, D.; Gladbach, S. & Zhu, B.P. (2006). Personal Hygiene and Methicillin-resistant *Staphylococcus aureus* Infection. *Emerging Infectious Diseases*, Vol. 12, No. 3, pp. 422-427, ISSN 1080-6059.

Van Bambeke, F.; Laethem, Y.V.; Courvalin, P. & Tulkens, P.M. (2004) Glycopeptide antibiotics: from conventional molecules to new derivatives. *Drugs,* Vol. 64, No. 9, pp. 913-936, ISSN 1179-1950.

Van Belkum, A.; Verkaik, N.J.; Vogel, C.P.; Boelens, H.A.; Verveer, J.; Nouwen, J.L.; Verbrugh, H.A. & Wertheim, H.F.L. (2009). Reclassification of *Staphylococcus aureus* Nasal Carriage Types. *Journal of Infectious Diseases,* Vol. 199, pp. 1820 - 1826, ISSN 1537-6613.

Van Duijkeren, E.; Wolfhagen, M.J.H.M.; Heck, M.E.O.C. & Wannet, W.J.B. (2005). Transmission of a Panton-Valentine Leucocidin-Positive, Methicillin-Resistant *Staphylococcus aureus* Strain between Humans and a Dog. *Journal of Clinical Microbiology,* Vol. 43, No. 12, pp. 6209-6211, ISSN 1098-660X.

Walsh, T.R.; Howe, R.A.; Wootton, M.; Bennett, P.M. & MacGowan, A.P. (2001). Detection of glycopeptide resistence in *Staphylococcus aureus. Journal Antimicrobial and Chemotherapy,* Vol. 47, pp. 357-358, ISSN 1460-2091.

Wang, R.; Braughton, K.R.; Kretschmer, D.; Bach, T.H.L.; Queck, S.Y.; Li, M.; Kennedy, A.D.; Dorward, D.W.; Klebanoff, S.J.; Peschel, A.; DeLeo, F.R. & Otto, M. (2007). Identification of novel cytolytic peptides as key virulence determinants for community-associated MRSA. *Nature Medicine,* Vol. 13, No. 12, pp. 1510-1514, ISSN 1546-170X.

Wertheim, H.F.L.; Walsh, E.; Choudhurry, R.; Melles, D.C.; Boelens, H.A.M.; Miajlovic, H.; Verbrugh, H.A.; Foster, T. & van Belkum, A. (2008). Key Role for Clumping Factor B in *Staphylococcus aureus* Nasal Colonization of Humans. *PLoS Medicine,* Vol. 5, No. 1, (January), pp. e17, ISSN 1549-1676.

Wey, S.B.; Cardo, D.M.; Halker, E.; Carratu, F.P. & Saes, A.C. (1990). Distribution and analysis of 8,268 nosocomial infections at the Hospital São Paulo: 1985 to 1989. *Revista do Hospital São Paulo Escola Paulista de Medicina,* Vol. 1, pp. 169-174, ISSN 1806-9460.

Zhang, K.; McClure, J.A.; Elsayed, S.; Louie, T. & Conly, J.M. (2005). Novel Multiplex PCR Assay for Characterization and Concomitant Subtyping of Staphylococcal Cassette Chromosome *mec* Types I to V in Methicillin-Resistant *Staphylococcus aureus. Journal of Clinical Microbiology,* Vol. 43, No. 10, pp. 5026-5033, ISSN 1098-660X.

Zhang, K.; McClure, J.A.; Elsayed, S.; Louie, T. & Conly, J.M. (2008). Novel Multiplex PCR Assay for Simultaneous Identification of Community-Associated Methicillin-Resistant *Staphylococcus aureus* Strains USA300 and USA400 and Detection of *mecA* and Panton-Valentine Leukocidin Genes, with Discrimination of *Staphylococcus aureus* from Coagulase-Negative Staphylococci. *Journal of Clinical Microbiology,* Vol. 46, No. 3, pp. 1118-1122, ISSN 1098-660X.

Zhang, K.; McClure, J.A.; Elsayed, S.; Conly, J.M. (2009). Novel Staphylococcal Cassette Chromosome *mec* Type, Tentatively Designated Type VIII, Harboring Class A *mec* and Type 4 *ccr* Gene Complexes in a Canadian Epidemic Strain of Methicillin-Resistant *Staphylococcus aureus. Journal Antimicrobial and Chemotherapy,* Vol. 53, pp. 531-540, ISSN 1460-2091.

6

Epidemiological Aspects of Oxacillin-Resistant *Staphylococcus* spp.: The Use of Molecular Tools with Emphasis on MLST

André Martins and Maria de Lourdes Ribeiro de Souza da Cunha
UNESP- Univ. Estadual Paulista, Biosciences Institute, Botucatu, SP Brazil

1. Introduction

Studying infections caused by the *Staphylococcus* spp. genus is highly important for human health given that such organisms are causal agents of superficial infections, such as abscesses and impetigo, as well as of systemic infections, namely bacteremia and osteomyelitis. This genus is divided into two large groups. The first group is characterized by the production of enzyme coagulase, and its main representative is *S. aureus*, which is frequently associated with a large variety of infections. The second group, known as coagulase-negative staphylococci (CoNS), is usually associated with immunocompromised patients or those who use catheters. (Kloos & Bannerman, 1995). The main CoNS species associated with infection in humans are *S. epidermidis, S. haemolyticus, S. saprophyticus, S. cohnii, S. xylosus, S. capitis, S. warneri, S. hominis, S. simulans, S. saccharolyticus, S. auricularis, S. caprae, S. lugdunensis* and *S. schleiferi* (Kloos & Bannerman, 1995).

Several studies have reported increased prevalence of CoNS infection in hospitals, which is usually associated with resistance to the antibiotic of choice for treatment. Hence, this is a serious clinical and epidemiological problem (Jain et. al., 2008).

The use of methicillin and other semi-synthetic penicillins, such as oxacillin and penicillinase-resistant methicillin, which began in 1959, represented a significant phase in anti-staphylococcal therapy. The first report on methicillin resistance was in 1961, a short time after its use was implemented (Hiramatsu et al, 2001). In Brazil, it is estimated that the frequency of oxacillin resistance is high among *S. aureus* samples, particularly in large and in university hospitals. Gales (2009) described an oxacillin resistance rate of 31% in a multi-center study involving four Brazilian hospitals. As regards CoNS, 78.7% of the samples were resistant. At the Botucatu School of Medicine University Hospital - SP, approximately 45% of the *S. aureus* samples from hemocultures were positive for the *mecA* gene (Martins et al., 2010). In a study conducted at the neonatal intensive care unit of the same hospital, a total of 18% of MRSA samples was found (Pereira et al., 2009). According to a study by Sader et al. (2004) in Latin America and Brazil, respectively, 80.4% and 84.6% of the CoNS samples from hemocultures were oxacillin resistant.

Oxacillin resistance in CoNS samples varies significantly among the different species in the genus, a fact that reinforces the importance of their correct identification (Secchi et al., 2008).

Although *S. epidermidis* is the most frequently found species (Vuong & Otto, 2002), others are also associated with human infection, such as *S. haemolyticus*, which can be multi-resistant and present intermediate resistance to vancomycin (Secchi et al., 2008). The main resistance mechanism is the presence of the *mecA* gene, inserted in the chromosomal cassette, known as staphylococcal chromosomal cassette mec (SCC*mec*). The detection of this gene and the typing of the chromosomal cassette by means of various molecular methods are important tools for the diagnosis and epidemiology of oxacillin-resistant *Staphylococcus* spp.

There are eleven SCC*mec* types, with subtypes, which are characterized by molecular tools, such as Multilocus Sequence Typing (MLST), pulsed-field gel electrophoresis (PFGE), *spa* typing and Multiplex PCR for SCC*mec* detection. They are useful in the characterization and detection of alterations in molecular structure. By using these methods, it was possible to identify pandemic clones as well as to characterize strains causing outbreaks in hospitals. Among these methods, the MLST is noteworthy due to its high reproducibility and capacity of detecting pandemic clones. Given the fact that vancomycin is a therapeutic option for oxacillin-resistant samples, with the emergence of vancomycin-resistant *Staphylococcus* spp., the characterization of circulating strains and clones is highly important. This chapter aimed at addressing aspects related to the molecular epidemiology in *Staphylococcus* spp. since these microorganisms have been increasingly frequent as agents of nosocomial and community infection.

2. Epidemiological aspects

Oxacillin resistance in CoNS is a problem in hospitals around the world, and there are reports of oxacillin-resistant samples in all continents (Witte, 1999). The use of methicillin, a semi-synthetic penicillin, commenced in 1959, and only two years after its first use, the first report of a methicillin-resistant *Staphylococcus* spp. sample was published (Hiramatsu et al., 2001).

Oxacillin resistance rates vary among various studies, but they are usually high, above 50%. Chaudhury & Kumar (2007) reported that, in a study conducted in a tertiary Indian hospital, 64.6% of the CoNS samples were oxacillin resistant. The most prevalent species was *S. haemolyticus*, isolated from urine samples. Another study also performed in India, described resistance levels of approximately 63% (Jain et al., 2008).

In the European continent, several reports described high oxacillin resistance levels in hospital wards. In a study analyzing samples collected from various hospitals in Eastern Europe in 2005, Sader et al. (2007) reported oxacillin resistance levels in CoNS which varied from 54.8% in Sweden to 83.3% in Greece. A study conducted at a university hospital in Turkey found 54.4% of resistant samples from a total of 158 isolated samples (Ercis et al., 2008). The rates found by a multi-center study conducted in the USA in 2007 and 2008 were of 74% of CoNS oxacillin-resistant samples (Sader & Jones, 2009).

Nevertheless, in the last few years, resistance levels have stabilized. In Spain, a multi-center study on 146 hospitals detected oxacillin resistance in 61.3% of the samples in 2002 and 66.7% in 2006 (Cuevas et al., 2008). In Brazil, recent studies showed resistance rates of 69% (Caierão et al., 2004), 78.4% (Perez & d'Azevedo 2007) and even 88.1% (Antunes et al., 2007). In the case of non-*epidermidis* CNS, Secchi et al. (2008) reported 71% of resistant samples.

Based on the described reports, it is clear that oxacillin resistance is prevalent in hospital in all continents, a fact that reinforces the importance of good antibiotic therapy practices and of infection control measures in hospitals.

3. Oxacillin resistance

Oxacillin resistance is associated with the drug's reduced capacity to adhere to the penicillin-binding protein (PBP), thus also losing its capacity to lyse the bacterial cell. There are three mechanisms of resistance to semi-synthetic penicillinases, a group of drugs in which oxacillin is included. The first is related to the hyperproduction of β-lactamases, enzymes that cleave the drug's β-lactam ring, thus inactivating it (McDougal & Thornsberry, 1986). The second mechanism, known as MOD-SA, occurs when normal PBPs have reduced affinity with oxacillin (Tomasz et al., 1989). The third and most important mechanism is the presence of the *mecA* gene. This gene codifies a changed PBP, known as PBP 2a, thus preventing its binding to oxacillin (Zhang et al., 2009).

Although resistance mediated by the *mecA* gene is present in all cells of the population with intrinsic resistance, it can only be expressed by a small percentage of such cells, thus leading to the so-called heterogeneous resistance. Resistance expression in lineages with intrinsic resistance has been categorized into four phenotypic classes; classes 1 to 4, in which class 1 is the most heterogeneous and class 4 is the homogeneous one (Tomacz et al., 1991). The majority of cells (99.9 or 99.99%) in the culture of lineages with class-1 heterogeneous resistance show minimum inhibitory concentration (MIC) of 1.5 to 3 μg/ml, but such culture also contains a small number of bacteria (10^{-7} to 10^{-8}) that could form colonies even in the presence of 25 μg/ml or more of oxacillin. In class-2 lineage cultures, the majority of cells (≥ 99.9%) show MIC of 6 to 12 μg/ml, and in these cultures, the frequency of highly resistant cells (capable of growing in the presence of 25 μg/ml) is higher (10^{-5}) than in class-1 lineages (Tomacz et al. , 1991). Class-3 lineage cultures consist of bacteria (99 to 99,9%) that show high levels of oxacillin resistance (MIC = 50 to 200 μg/ml), but they usually have a subpopulation (10^{-3}) of highly resistant cells that are capable of forming colonies even in the presence of 300 to 400 μg de oxacillin/ml. Class-4 cultures comprise cells with homogeneous resistance, with all cells showing high resistance levels and MIC of 400 to 1,000 μg/ml (Tomacz et al., 1991).

The phenotypic expression codified by the *mecA* gene is affected by various factors, including pH, temperature and osmolarity (Swenson, 2002). When proper conditions are used for laboratory MRSA detection, including Mueller-Hinton agar supplementation with NaCl and adequate temperature and time, as recommended by CLSI (Clinical and Laboratory Standards Institute), detection is achieved without much difficulty. However, for more heterogeneous lineages, detection can be more difficult, even with reference methods (Swenson, 2002).

Adequate detection of oxacillin resistance mediated by the *mecA* gene is important for clinical laboratories. Although the recommended methods detect most of the oxacillin-resistant lineages, there are two situations that require additional phases to confirm sensitivity or resistance. The first is the occurrence of extremely heterogeneous lineages that are found to be sensitive by reference methods. The second is the occurrence of borderline resistance (MIC close to the sensitivity breakpoint), which must be differentiated from resistance mediated by the *mecA* gene as long as the clinical significance of the resistance determined by the *mecA* gene is greater.

The *mecA* gene is inserted in a transposable genetic element known as Staphylococcal Chromosomal Cassette *mec* (*SCCmec*). This element varies in its constitution and is divided into eleven types. The typing of *SCCmec* types is useful as an epidemiological tool (Mombach Pinheiro Machado et al., 2007) given that the different types are more prevalent in hospital and community environments. The SCC*mec* types (IWG-SCC, 2009) differ from one another in relation to the number of genes that they carry in their gene architecture (Hiramatsu et al., 2001). Some of these types are carriers of resistance genes that are determinant for multiple antibacterial drugs. In addition to beta-lactam antibiotics, macrolides, lincosamides, streptogramins, aminoglycosides and tetracycline are noteworthy. Hence, when a bacterial cell acquires such SCC*mec*, it at once acquires a multiple-resistance phenotype (Ito et al., 2003).

The SCC*mec* types have been defined by the combination of two parts: the *ccr* complex and the *mec* complex, with three phylogenetically distinct *ccr* genes classified as: *ccrA, ccrB* and *ccrC*. Additionally, there are five classes of *mec* gene complexes (classes *A, B, C1, C2* and class *D*) (Ito et al., 2004; IWG-SCC, 2009). The different SCC*mec* types are classified as: type-I SCC*mec* (class *B* and *ccrA1B1 mec* gene complex), type-II SCC*mec* (class *A* and *ccrA2B2 mec* gene complex), type-III SCC*mec* (class *A* and *ccrA3B3 mec* gene complex), type-IV SCC*mec* (class *B* and *ccrA2B2 mec* gene complex), type-V SCC*mec* (class *C2* and *ccrC mec* gene complex), type-VI SCC*mec* (class *B* and *ccrA4B4 mec* gene complex), type-VII SCC*mec* (class *C1* and *ccrC mec* gene complex) and type-VIII SCC*mec* (class *A* and *ccrA4B4 mec* gene complex). The remaining region of SCC*mec* is called the J region (Joining region), which constitutes non-essential components of the cassette that can carry additional antimicrobial resistance determinants (Hanssen & Sollid, 2006; IWG-SCC, 2009). Recently, types IX (class C2, ccr1 *mec* gene complex), X (class C1, ccr7 *mec* gene complex) and XI (class E, ccr8 *mec* gene complex) have been described (IWG-SCC, 2011) (Table 1).

SCC*mec* type	*mec* gene complex	*ccr* gene complex
I	B	1 (A1B1)
II	A	2 (A2B2)
III	A	3 (A3B3)
IV	B	2 (A2B2)
V	C2	5 (C1)
VI	B	4 (A4B4)
VII	C1	5 (C1)
VIII	A	4 (A4B4)
IX	C2	1 (A1B1)
X	C1	7 (A1B6)
XI	E	8 (A1B3)

Source: http://www.sccmec.org/Pages/SCC_TypesEN.html. Accessed on 06/20/2011

Table 1. SCC*mec* types identified in *S.aureus*

The first three types were detailed by Ito et al. in 2001, and the same author also reported and described type V in 2004. Ma et al. (2002) described type IV, which is mainly found in community samples. Types I, II and III are mainly responsible for nosocomial infections, and they are significantly larger than the last types IV and V. Type-I cassette was described with a size of 34.364 bp, and it is the largest of the three. This cassette does not feature any inserted transposons or plasmids that provide resistance to other drugs besides methicillin or to heavy metals. It has a sub-type known as IA, which differs from type I for having an integrated plasmid, pUB110 (Shore et al., 2005).

The second cassette, referred to as II, has 53.017 bp, and in addition to the *mecA* and *mecRI* genes, which cause methicillin resistance, it contains transposon Tn 554. The latter is responsible for the resistance of this sample type to erythromycin and streptomycin. This cassette has a sub-type that is referred to as IIA, with a size of 40 Kb, thus being a little smaller than type II (Shore et al., 2005).

Type-III cassette, the largest of the five types, has a size of 66.896 bp and contains genes *mecA, mecRI*, transposons Tn 554 and ψTn 554 and plasmid pt 181. Transposon ψTn 554 induces cadmium resistance, and plasmid pt 181 is responsible for tetracycline and mercury resistance. In addition to the information described above, the authors also mentioned differences between the *ccr* gene types, by describing, in type-III *SCCmec,* a gene that is not present in the other types and is referred to as *ψccr*. They also suggested that some of the resistance characteristics in type III can be used as selective markers. This cassette type presents two sub-types: IIIA, which does not have plasmid pt 181 and flanks with element IS 431, and IIIB, where there are no copies of plasmids pt 181 or tn 554 (Shore et al., 2005).

Type-IV SCC*mec* is mainly responsible for community infections. It is a small element that does not carry other resistance genes, except for *mecA*. It is also divided into multiple sub-types, which suggests that type-IV SCC*mec* is highly transmittable (Ito et al., 2004). The four sub-types of type-IV, -IVA, -IVB, -IVC and -IVD cassettes differ for presenting different sequences on the left extremity of the *ccr* complex, which is known as L – C Region (Shore et al., 2005).

Type-V SCC*mec* was identified by Ito et al. (2004) in an Australian isolate. It has the size of 27.624 bp, and it is a little larger than SCC*mec* IV although smaller than the other existing types. Similarly to type IV, it has only genes that codify methicillin resistance; however, differently from the other elements in this family, type V has a new *ccr* gene type that is characterized as type c and is individually found, contrarily to other elements, which have a pair of such genes. Another new element found only in type V is a restriction and modification system codified by genes V22 and V23. Recent studies associate the presence of this *mec* cassette type with community infections (O'Brien et al., 2005; Ho et al., 2007).

Oliveira et al. (2006) characterized type-VI SCC*mec*, which is found in samples belonging to the pediatric clone of MRSA (Methicillin Resistant *S.aureus*) samples and previously typed as SCC*mec* IV. The authors described differences in the *ccrAB* complex, identified as type 4, and the presence of the type-B *mec* complex, which does not have the *mecl* gene.

Type-VII SCC*mec* was identified by Higuchi et al. (2008) through a detailed analysis of community *S.aureus* samples isolated in Taiwan. It has a size of 41.347 bp, and its *mec* complex is homologous to that found in type V, but presents substitutions, insertions and rearrangements that differentiate it. The main characteristics of this cassette type are the presence of the *ccrC* complex, of transposon ΨIS431 and of a unique sequence on the right side of the cassette which is referred to as *orf*35.

Recently, Zhang et al. (2009) have described a new SCC*mec* type which has been denominated as SCC*mec* VIII and was found in an MRSA sample from a hospital. This new cassette has a size of 32.168 base pairs, and genes *mecA mecR1 mecI* of the *mec* complex and *ccrA4 ccrB4* of the *ccr* complex are present in addition to transposon Tn554, which is also present in type II.

4. Molecular epidemiology

In addition to the characterization of SCC*mec* types as an epidemiological tool, other methods are available for molecular epidemiology studies, such as Pulsed Field Gel Electrophoresis (PFGE), Multilocus Sequence Typing (MLST) and *spa* typing, which allow for the identification of circulating bacterial clones in hospitals and in the community.

PFGE is a method that uses restriction enzymes to cleave the extracted DNA, and in the case of the *Staphylococcus* genus, the enzyme used is *Sma*I. The fragments are separated in agarose gel. The direction of the electrical field is periodically changed, forming a 120° angle. This allows for fragments of up to 12mb to be separated, contrarily to conventional electrophoresis, which is not capable of separating fragments that are larger than 50kb (Herschleb et al., 2007). This method is generally used in local studies, such as in hospital outbreaks, which allows for identifying the circulating type.

The sequencing of constitutive bacterial genes can also be used as an important epidemiological tool. The method known as *spa* typing investigates polymorphisms on a single locus. It can discriminate between PFGE and MLST and is also applied in local studies and for detecting pandemic clones (Malachowa et al., 2005).

Another methodology that uses the sequencing and analysis of genetic polymorphisms is MLST. It analyzes the sequence of seven constitutive genes (*gmk, pta, dfp, gtr, mutS, pyrR,* and *xpt*) and compares them with the sequences of each allele in the locus, which are previously numbered. The combination of the alleles identified in each gene determines the profile of the sample. (Aanensen & Spratt, 2005). It is the most adequate methodology for detecting pandemic clones given that the investigated genes are constitutive, with low mutation rates when compared to the analysis of the whole chromosome, in the case of PFGE (Miragaia et al., 2007).

5. Pandemic clones of MRSA samples

Currently, *Staphylococcus spp.* samples have been typed in numerous epidemiological studies by means of the methods described above. By using these tools, 05 large pandemic clones have been described. These are the Brazilian clone, characterized by *SCCmec* IIIA, MLST 2-3-1-4-4-3 (ST 239); the Iberian clone with type-IA *SCCmec,* and MLST 3-3-1-1/12-4-4-16 (ST 247); the clone known as New York / Japan, with type-III SCC*mec,* pattern MLST 1-4-1-4-12-1-10 (ST 05); the Hungarian clone, with SCC*mec III,* MLST 2-3-1-1-4-4-3 (ST 239); the pediatric clone, with type-IV SCC*mec,* MLST 1-4-1-4-12-1-10 (ST 05) and the last large clone known as EMRSA-16, *SCCmec* II MLST 15-12-16-02-16-02-25-17-24-24-24 (ST 36) (Oliveira et al., 2002; Melter et al., 2003; Velásquez-Meza et al. 2004; Aires de Souza & De Lencastre, 2004, Aires Ribeiro et al., 2005).

In our scenario, the predominant MRSA samples belong to the Brazilian clone (Oliveira et al., 2001). The first report on the emergence of this clone dates to 1992-93 in various hospitals in Brazil. The samples were characterized as belonging to the same clone by methods such as PFGE and by showing patterns of transposon *Tn554* and the polymorphism of the *mecA* gene (Teixeira et al., 1995). In other countries, the Brazilian clone is also disseminated, as is the case of the Czech Republic, where the isolation of this clone represented 80% of the MRSA samples found in 1996-1997 (Melter et al., 2003). The Brazilian clone was also described in India, in two hospitals in the region of Bengalore, conjointly with the Hungarian clone (*SCCmec III*) (Arakere et al., 2005)

Other clones are distributed in several parts of the world. The Iberian clone was firstly described in samples from hospitals in Barcelona and Madrid, Spain, and in Lisbon, Portugal. These samples were typed by the PFGE method and probe hybridization, producing a pattern that characterized them as belonging to the same clone. This clone is also described in other countries, such as the Czech Republic (Melter et al., 2003). The clone known as New York - Japan, firstly isolated in the USA in 1994-98 and in Japan in 1997-98 (Oliveira et al., 2002), was also predominant in Mexico during a study on 98 MRSA samples, thus replacing the local clone, known as Mexican (PFGE M, type-IV SCC*mec*), in nosocomial infections (Velasquez-Meza et al., 2004).

The Hungarian clone, firstly identified in Hungary in 1993-94, was characterized by the same methods used for the clones described above in studies on MRSA samples from hospitals in 06 provinces in that country (De Lencastre, 1997). The pediatric clone was isolated in large numbers in 1996-98 in Colombia, and it is also found in Argentina and Poland in 1994-98 and 1990-98 (Oliveira et al., 2002).

The last of the large pandemic clones, referred to as EMRSA-16, is prevalent in hospitals in the United Kingdom, Mexico and Greece, in addition to being responsible for an outbreak in Sweden from 1997 to 2000 (Aires de Souza & De Lencastre, 2004).

6. Epidemiology and MLST

The MLST method was developed by Maiden et al. (1998) by the sequencing and analysis of the loci of eleven constitutive genes of *Neisseria meningitidis*, and it is presently applied in molecular epidemiology studies on various pathogens, among which are *S. aureus* and *S. epidermidis*.

This methodology has been used in numerous studies on molecular epidemiology with good results due its good reproducibility, thus allowing for the detection of pandemic clones from circulating *S. aureus* and *S. epidermidis* samples.

Geng et al. (2010) reported the presence of clone ST59-MRSA-IV in China in community samples isolated from 47 children with impetigo and abscesses. In Malaysia, a study on 36 samples isolated from a hospital in Klang Valley for a five-month period reported a rate of 83.3% of samples belonging to clone ST 239 *SCCmec* III (Neela et al., 2010).

MLST has been used for studies in which circulating clones are identified in replacement of another already established clone. Sola et al. (2006) reported the emergence of a new clone identified as ST5 in hospitals in Cordoba, Argentina, in replacement of the Brazilian clone (ST239), which circulates in that region. In that study, 103 MRSA samples isolated from April to June 2001 and 31 MSSA samples isolated from 1999 to 2002 were used.

Previous studies have used MLST for comparison between samples and the prevalence between different pandemic clones. Campanille et al. (2009) analyzed 301 MRSA samples isolated from 19 Italian hospitals from 1990 to 2001. An increase of clone ST228, known as Italian clone, was observed from 2000 to 2007, conjointly with the decrease of clone ST247 (Iberian clone) when compared to the 1990-1999 period.

Clone ST228 is also associated with patients with cystic fibrosis. A study conducted on 93 MRSA samples isolated from patients with that disease at a treatment center in Madrid, Spain, identified 15 different PFGE patterns. A sample of each of these patterns was typed by MLST, with clone ST228 showing higher prevalence, with eight pulsetypes, followed by ST5, with two pulsetypes, and ST247, ST72 and ST255 with one pulsetype each (Molina et al., 2008).

In addition to epidemiological studies in hospitals and the detection of these pandemic clones from MRSA samples, the MLST method has been used to detect the transmission of oxacillin-resistant samples from animal reservoirs to humans, including its detection in hospitals. Some studied have detected the presence of MRSA clones in swines, thus emphasizing the importance of such animals as reservoirs. Smith et al. (2009) reported the presence of ST398 samples in swines and farmers in the mid-western region of the United States, which suggests transmission between animals and their breeders. In Germany, 1,600 swabs from swines from 40 farms were analyzed in a study where samples typed as ST398 were also identified (Köck et al., 2009).

MLST is usually used for detecting pandemic clones with good results. But this method can also be utilized for characterizing samples involved in hospital outbreaks.

Peacock et al. (2002) compared the MLST and PFGE methods in a study conducted on 104 *S. aureus* samples isolated from nasal swabs from patients under renal therapy. The isolated samples were typed by the MLST and PFGE methods with a similar discriminatory power between the two techniques for identification of circulating samples in hospitals.

Vindel et al. (2009) analyzed 463 *S.aureus* samples isolated from 145 Spanish hospitals in 2006. In addition to MLST, several methodologies such as PFGE, spa typing, *SCCmec* characterization and *agr* typing were used. MLST showed good correlation with the methodologies used for detecting circulating samples, with applicability in localized nosocomial studies.

The combination of the two molecular epidemiology techniques can increase discriminatory power for analysis of different clones. Cookson et al. (2007) reported that the combination of the MLST and *SCCmec* methods are more appropriate for multi-center studies. The authors analyzed MRSA samples from various European countries by means of PFGE, MLST, *SCCmec* analysis and *spa* typing.

7. Vancomycin-resistant *S. aureus* (VRSA)

Detection of oxacillin resistant staphylococci is important to guide therapies and also to avoid use of vancomycin, which is an antimicrobial agent with therapeutic complications, and can lead to selection of resistant strains. Acquired microbial resistance to vancomycin is a growing problem, in particular, within healthcare facilities such as hospitals. The widespread use of vancomycin makes resistance to the drug a significant worry, especially for individual patients if resistant infections are not quickly identified and the patient continues the ineffective treatment. Vancomycin-resistant Enterococcus (VRE) emerged in 1987 and the transfer potential of such resistance to other bacteria, vancomycin resistance surveillance has been an object of great scientific interest worldwide. Vancomycin resistance emerged in more common pathogenic organisms during the 1990s and 2000s, including vancomycin-intermediate *Staphylococcus aureus* (VISA) and vancomycin-resistant *Staphylococcus aureus* (VRSA).

In 1996, the first clinical *S. aureus* isolate with reduced vancomycin sensitivity, with MIC value in the intermediate range (MIC = 8 μg/ml) and referred to as VISA was reported in Japan (Hiramatsu et al. 1997). Additionally, in June 2002 [44], eight patients with infections caused by *S. aureus* with reduced vancomycin sensitivity were confirmed in the United States. One month later, the Centers for Disease Control and Prevention (CDC) published the first reported on vancomycin-resistant *S. aureus* (VRSA, with MIC = or ≥ 32 μg/ml) in a patient in Michigan, United States. The sample isolated from the patient contained the *vanA* gene as well as the *mecA* gene for oxacillin resistance. The presence of the *vanA* gene in this VRSA suggests that resistance may have been acquired through the passage of genetic material from vancomycin-resistant enterococci to *S. aureus.* In October of the same year [44], the second clinical isolate of VRSA was reported in a patient in Pennsylvania. The VRSA isolate also contained the *vanA* and the *mecA* genes. The presence of the *vanA* gene suggests that the resistance determinant was acquired from vancomycin-resistant *Enterococcus* isolated from the same patient. April 2004, the third VRSA isolated from a patient in New York was reported. The isolate also contained the oxacillin- and vancomycin-resistance *mecA* and *vanA* genes, respectively. According to CDC, the three VRSA isolated did not seem to be epidemiologically related (CDC 2002; CDC 2004). The CDC (2010) has recently confirmed the 11th case of vancomycin resistant *Staphylococcus aureus* (VRSA) infection since 2002 in the United States (Table 2). This serves as a reminder about the

Case	State	Year	Age	Source
1	Michigan	2002	40	Plantar ulcers & Catheter tip
2	Pennsylvania	2002	70	Plantar ulcer
3	New York	2004	63	Urine from a nephrostomy tube
4	Michigan	2005	78	Toe wound
5	Michigan	2005	58	Surgical site wound after panniculectomy
6	Michigan	2005	48	Plantar ulcer
7	Michigan	2006	43	Triceps wound
8	Michigan	2007	48	Toe wound
9	Michigan	2007	54	Surgical site wound after foot amputation
10	Michigan	2009	53	Plantar foot wound
11	Delaware	2010	64	Wound drainage

Source: CDC (2010)

Table 2. Vancomycin resistant *Staphylococcus aureus* (VRSA) infection in the United States

important role of clinical laboratories in the diagnosis of VRSA cases to ensure prompt recognition, isolation, and management by infection control personnel. Appropriate antimicrobial prescribing by healthcare providers, adherence to recommended infection control guidelines, and, ultimately, the control of both MRSA and VRE are necessary to prevent further emergence of VRSA strains.

8. Conclusions and perspectives

Given the high rates of oxacillin resistance reported in various countries and the emergence of vancomycin-resistant MRSA samples, further detailed studies on the characteristics of circulating strains in hospitals and the characterization of clones prevailing in larger regions are necessary since the different MRSA clones vary in virulence and antimicrobial resistance. The molecular epidemiology methods are useful tools in these types of study, and the MLST technique is especially useful due to its versatility, easy performance and high reproducibility, with applications in localized studies, such as in the characterization of outbreaks and in the detection of circulating clones in large regions.

9. Acknowledgements

The support by FAPESP is gratefully acknowledged.

10. References

Aanensen, D.M.; Spratt, B.G. (2005) The multilocus sequence typing network: mlst.net. *Nucleic Acids Research*. Vol.33, pp. 728-33. ISSN 1362-4962

Aires de Sousa, M.; De Lencastre, H. (2004) Bridges from hospitals to the laboratory: genetic portraits of methicillin-resistant *Staphylococcus aureus* clones. *FEMS Immunology and Medical Microbiology*, Vol 40, pp. 101-111. ISSN: 0928-8244

Arakere, G.; Nadig, S.; Swedberg, G.; Macaden, R.; Amarnath, S.K.; Raghunath, D. (2005) Genotyping of methicillin-resistant *Staphylococcus aureus* strains from two hospitals in Bangalore, South India. *Journal of Clinical Microbiology*. Vol. 43, pp.3198-3202. ISSN 1098-660X

Antunes, A.L.S.; Secchi, C.; Reiter, K.C.; Perez, L.R.R.; Freitas, A.L.P.; d'Azevedo, P.A. (2007) Evaluation of oxacillin and cefoxitin disks for detection of resistance in coagulase negative staphylococci. *Memórias do Intituto Oswaldo Cruz*. Vol 102, pp. 719-23 ISSN 0074-0276

Caierão, J.; Musskopf, M., Superti, S., Roesch, E., Dias, C.G., d'Azevedo, P.A. (2004) Evaluation of phenotypic methods for methicillin resistance characterization in coagulase-negative staphylococci (CNS). *Journal of Medical Microbiology*. Vol. 53, pp.1195-1199, ISSN 0022-2615

Campanile, F.; Bongiorno, D.; Borbone, S.; Stefani, S. (2009) Hospital-associated methicillin-resistant *Staphylococcus aureus* (HA-MRSA) in Italy. *Annals of Clinical Microbiology and Antimicrobials*. Vol. 24, pp. 8-22. ISSN 1476-0711

CDC. Centers for Disease Control and Prevention. (2002) *Staphylococcus aureus* resistant to vancomycin-United States. *Morbity and Mortality Weekly Reports*.Vol. 51, pp. 565-567. ISSN 0892-3787

CDC. Centers for Disease Control and Prevention. (2004) Brief Report: Vancomycin-Resistant *Staphylococcus aureus*- New York. *Morbity and Mortality Weekly Reports.* Vol. 53, pp. 322-323. ISSN 0892-3787

CDC. Centers for Disease Control and Prevention. CDC Reminds Clinical Laboratories and Healthcare Infection Preventionists of their Role in the Search and Containment of Vancomycin-Resistant *Staphylococcus aureus* (VRSA), May 2010. Available at: http://www.cdc.gov/HAI/settings/lab/vrsa_lab_search_containment.html. Accessed June 18, 2011.

Chaudhury, A.; Kumar, A.G. (2007) In vitro activity of antimicrobial agents against oxacillin resistant staphylococci with special reference to *Staphylococcus haemolyticus. Indian Journal of Medical Microbiology*.Vol.25, No.1, pp.50-52. ISSN 0255-0857

Cuevas, O.; Cercenado, E.; Goyanes, M.J.; Vindel, A.; Trincado, P.; Boquete, T.; Marín, M.; Bouza, E. (2008) *Staphylococcus spp.* in Spain: present situation and evolution of antimicrobial resistance (1986-2006). *Enfermidades Infecciosas y Microbiología Clínica.* Vol.26, pp.269-77. ISSN 1578-1852

Cookson, B.D.; Robinson, D.A.; Monk, A.B.; Murchan, S.; Deplano, A.; de Ryck, R.; Struelens, M.J.; Scheel, C.; Fussing, V.; Salmenlinna, S.; Vuopio-Varkila, J.; Cuny, C.; Witte, W.; Tassios, P.T.; Legakis, N.J.; van Leeuwen, W.; van Belkum, A.; Vindel, A.; Garaizar, J.; Haeggman, S.; Olsson-Liljequist, B.; Ransjo, U.; Muller-Premru, M.; Hryniewicz, W.; Rossney, A.; O'Connell, B.; Short, B.D.; Thomas, J.; O'Hanlon, S.; Enright, M.C. (2007) Evaluation of molecular typing methods in characterizing a European collection of epidemic methicillin-resistant *Staphylococcus aureus* strains: the HARMONY collection. *Journal of Clinical Microbiology.* Vol. 45, pp.1830-1837. ISSN 1098-660X

De Lencastre, H.; Severina, E.P.; Milch, H.; Thege, M.K.; Tomasz, A. (1997) Wide geographic distribution of a unique methicillin-resistant *Staphylococcus aureus* clone in Hungarian hospitals. *Clinical Microbiology and Infection.* Vol. 3, pp. 289-296. ISSN:1198-743X

Ercis, S.; Sancak, B.; Hasçelik, G. (2008) A comparison of PCR detection of mecA with oxacillin disk susceptibility testing in different media and sceptor automated system for both *Staphylococcus aureus* and coagulase-negative staphylococci isolates. *Indian Journal of Medical Microbiology.* Vol. 26, pp. 21-4. ISSN 0255-0857

Gales, A.C.; Sader, H.S.; Ribeiro, J.; Zoccoli, C.; Barth, A.; Pignatari, A.C. (2009) Antimicrobial susceptibility of gram-positive bacteria isolated in Brazilian hospitals participating in the SENTRY Program (2005-2008). *Brazilian Journal Infectious Diseases*. 2009; 13: 90-8. ISSN 1413-8670

Geng, W.; Yang, Y.; Wang, C.; Deng, L.; Zheng, Y.; Shen, X. (2010) Skin and soft tissue infections caused by community-associated methicillin-resistant *Staphylococcus aureus* among children in China. *Acta Paediatrica*. Vol. 99, pp. 575-580. ISSN 1651-2227

Herschleb, J.; Ananiev, G.; Schwartz, D.C. (2007) Pulsed-field gel electrophoresis. *Nature Protocols*. Vol. 2, pp.677-84. ISSN: 1754-2189

Higuchi, W.; Takano, T.; Teng, L.J.; Yamamoto, T. (2008) Structure and specific detection of staphylococcal cassette chromosome *mec* type VII. *Biochemical and Biophysical Research Communications*. Vol. 377, pp.752-756. ISSN: 0006-291X

Hiramatsu, K.; Hanaki, H.; Ino, T.; Yabuta, K.; Oguri, T.; Tenover, F.C. (1997) Methicillin-resistant *Staphylococcus aureus* clinical strain with reduced vancomycin susceptibility. *Journal of Antimicrobial Chemotherapy*. Vol. 40, pp.135-136. ISSN 1460-2091

Hiramatsu, K.; Chui, L.; Kuroda, M.; Ito, T. (2001) The emergence and evolution of methicilin resistant *Staphylococcus aureus*. *Trends Microbiology* Vol. 9, pp. 486-93. ISSN: 0966-842X

Ho, P.L.; Wang, T.K.; Ching, P.; Mak, G.C.; Lai, E.; Yam, W.C.; Seto, W.H. (2007) Epidemiology and genetic diversity of methicillin-resistant *Staphylococcus aureus* strains in residential care homes for elderly persons in Hong Kong. *Infection Control and Hospital Epidemiology*. Vol. 28, pp. 671-678. ISSN:0899-823X

International Working Group on the Classification of Staphylococcal Cassette Chromosome Elements (IWG-SCC). Classification of Staphylococcal Cassette Chromosome *mec* (SCC*mec*): Guidelines for Reporting Novel SCC*mec* Elements. *Antimicrobial Agents Chemotherapy*. Vol. 53, pp. 4961–4967. ISSN 0066-4804

International Working Group on the Staphylococcal Cassette Chromosome elements (IWG-SCC). [Accessed on June 20, 2011]. SCC*mec* up to date. Available at: http://www.sccmec.org/Pages/SCC_TypesEN.html

Ito, T.; Okuma, K.; Ma, X.X.; Yuzawa, H.; Hiramatsu, K. (2003) Insights on antibiotic resistance of *Staphylococcus aureus* from its whole genome: genomic island SCC. *Drug Resistance Update*, Vol. 6, pp. 41-52. ISSN 1368-7646

Ito, T.; Ma, X.X.; Takeuchi, F.; Okuma, K.; Yuzawa, H.; Hiramatsu, K. (2004) Novel type V staphylococcal cassette chromosome *mec* driven by a novel cassette chromosome recombinase, *ccrC*. *Antimicrobial Agents and Chemotherapy*. Vol. 48, pp. 2637-2651. ISSN 0066-4804

Jain, A.; Agarwal, A.; Verma, R.K. (2008) Cefoxitin disc diffusion test for detection of meticillin-resistant staphylococci. *Journal of Medical Microbiology*. Vol. 57, p. 957-961. ISSN 0022-2615

Kloos, W.E.; Bannerman, T.L. (1995). *Staphylococcus* and *Micrococcus*, In: *Manual of Clinical Microbiology*, Murray, P.R., Baron, E.J., Pfaller, M.A., Tenover, F.C., Yolken, R.H., (Ed.), 282-298, ASM press, ISBN 13: 978-1555811266, Washington DC.

Köck, R.; Harlizius, J.; Bressan, N.; Laerberg, R.; Wieler, L.H.; Witte, W.; Deurenberg, R.H.; Voss, A.; Becker, K.; Friedrich, A.W. (2009) Prevalence and molecular characteristics of methicillin-resistant *Staphylococcus aureus* (MRSA) among pigs on German farms and import of livestock-related MRSA into hospitals. *European*

Journal of Clinical Microbiology & Infectious Diseases. Vol. 28, pp. 1375-1382. ISSN 0934-9723

Ma, X.X.; Ito, T.; Tiensasitorn, C.; Jamklang, M.; Chongtrakool, P.; Boyle-Vavra, S.; Daum, R.S.; Hiramatsu, K. (2002) Novel type of staphylococcal cassette chromosome *mec* identified in community-acquired methicillin-resistant *Staphylococcus aureus* strains. *Antimicrobial Agents and Chemotherapy*. Vol. 46, pp. 1147-52. ISSN 0066-4804

Maiden, M.C.; Bygraves, J.A.; Feil, E.; Morelli, G.; Russell, J.E.; Urwin, R.; Zhang, Q.; Zhou, J.; Zurth, K.; Caugant, D.A.; Feavers, I.M.; Achtman, M.; Spratt, B.G. (1998) Multilocus sequence typing: a portable approach to the identification of clones within populations of pathogenic microorganisms. *Proceedings of the National Academy of Sciences, USA*. Vol. 95, pp. 3140-3145. ISSN: 0027-8424.

Malachowa, N.; Sabat, A.; Gniadkowski, M.; Krzyszton-Russjan, J.; Empel, J.; Miedzobrodzki, J.; Kosowska-Shick, K.; Appelbaum, P.C.; Hryniewicz, W. (2005) Comparison of multiple-locus variable-number tandem-repeat analysis with pulsed-field gel electrophoresis, *spa* typing, and multilocus sequence typing for clonal characterization of *Staphylococcus aureus* isolates. *Journal of Clinical Microbiology*. Vol. 43, pp. 3095-100. ISSN 1098-660X.

Martins, A.; Pereira, V.C.; Cunha, M.L.R.S. (2010) Oxacillin resistance of *Staphylococcus aureus* isolated from the university hospital of Botucatu Medical School in Brazil. *Chemotherapy*. Vol. 56, pp. 112-9. ISSN 0009-3157.

McDougal, L.K.; Thornsberry, C. (1986) The role of beta-lactamase in staphylococcal resistance to penicillinase-resistant penicillins and cephalosporins. *Journal of Clinical Microbiology*. Vol. 23, pp. 832-839. ISSN 1098-660X.

Melter, O.; Aires De Sousa, M.; Urbaskova, P.; Jakubu, V.; Zemlickova, H.; De Lencastre, H. (2003) Update on the major clonal types of methicillin-resistant *Staphylococcus aureus* in the Czech Republic. *Journal of Clinical Microbiology*. Vol. 41, pp.4998-4905. ISSN 1098-660X.

Miragaia, M.; Thomas, J.C.; Couto, I.; Enright, M.C.; de Lencastre, H. (2007) Inferring a population structure for *Staphylococcus epidermidis* from multilocus sequence typing data. *The Journal of Bacteriology*. Vol. 189, pp. :2540-2552. ISSN 1098-5530

Molina, A.; Del Campo, R.; Máiz, L.; Morosini, M.I.; Lamas, A.; Baquero, F.; Cantón, R. (2008) High prevalence in cystic fibrosis patients of multiresistant hospital-acquired methicillin-resistant *Staphylococcus aureus* ST228-SCCmecI capable of biofilm formation. *Journal of Antimicrobial Chemotherapy*. Vol 62, pp. 961-967. ISSN 1460-2091

Mombach Pinheiro Machado A.B.; Reiter, K.C.; Paiva, R.M.; Barth, A.L. (2007) Distribution of staphylococcal cassette chromosome mec (SCC*mec*) types I, II, III and IV in coagulase-negative staphylococci from patients attending a tertiary hospital in southern Brazil. *Journal of Medical Microbiology*. Vol. 56, pp.1328-1333. ISSN 0022-2615

Neela, V.; Ghasemzadeh Moghaddam, H.; van Belkum, A.; Horst-Kreft, D.; Mariana, N.S.; Ghaznavi Rad, E. (2010) First report on methicillin-resistant *Staphylococcus aureus* of Spa type T037, Sequence type 239, SCC*mec* type III/IIIA in Malaysia. *European Journal of Clinical Microbiology & Infectious Diseases*. Vol. 29, pp. 115–117. ISSN 0934-9723

O'Brien, F.G.; Zaini, Z.; Coombs, G.W.; Pearson, J.C.; Christiansen, K.; Grubb, W.B.; Macrolide, lincosamide and streptogramin B resistance in a dominant clone of Australian community methicillin-resistant *Staphylococcus aureus*. *Journal of Antimicrobial Chemotherapy*, Vol. 56; pp. 985-986. ISSN 1460-2091.

Oliveira, G.A.; Faria, J.B.; Levy, C.E.; Mamizuka, E.M. (2001) Characterization of the Brazilian endemic clone of methicillin-resistant *Staphylococcus aureus* (MRSA) from hospitals throughout Brazil. *Brazilian Journal of Infectious Diseases*.Vol. 5, pp. 163-170. ISSN 1413-8670

Oliveira, D.C.; Tomasz, A.; De Lencastre, H. (2002) Secretes of sucess of a human pathogen: molecular evolution of pandemic clones of methicilin-resistant *Staphylococcus aureus*. *The Lancet Infectious Disease*. Vol. 2, pp. 180-189. ISSN 1473-3099

Oliveira, D.C.; Milheiriço, C.; de Lencastre, H. (2006) Redefining a structural variant of staphylococcal cassette chromosome *mec, SCCmec* type VI. *Antimicrobial Agents and Chemotherapy*. Vol. 50, pp. 3457-3459. ISSN 0066-4804

Peacock, S.J., de Silva, G.D.; Justice, A.; Cowland, A.; Moore, C.E.; Winearls, C.G.; Day, N.P. (2002) Comparison of multilocus sequence typing and pulsed-field gel electrophoresis as tools for typing *Staphylococcus aureus* isolates in a microepidemiological setting. *Journal of Clinical Microbiology*. Vol. 40, pp. 3764-70. ISSN 1098-660X

Pereira, V.C.; Martins, A.; Rugolo, L.M.S.S.; Cunha, M.L.R.S. (2009)Detection of Oxacillin Resistance in *Staphylococcus aureus* Isolated from the Neonatal and Pediatric Units of a Brazilian Teaching Hospital. *Clinical Medicine: Pediatrics*. Vol. 3, pp. 23–31. ISSN: 1179-5565

Perez, L.R.R.; d'Azevedo, P.A. (2008) Evaluation of the Accuracy of Various Phenotypic Tests to Detect Oxacillin Resistance in Coagulase-Negative Staphylococci. *Brazilian Journal Infectious Diseases*. Vol. 12, pp.210-212. ISSN 1413-8670

Sader, H.S.; Jones, R.N.; Gales, A.C.; Silva, J.B.; Pignatari, A.C. (2004) SENTRY antimicrobial surveillance program report: Latin American and Brazilian results for 1997 through 2001. *Brazilian Journal of Infectious Diseases*. Vol. 8, pp.25-79. ISSN 1413-8670

Sader, H.S.; Watters, A.A.; Fritsche, T.R.; Jones, R.N. (2007) Daptomycin antimicrobial activity tested against methicillin-resistant staphylococci and vancomycin-resistant enterococci isolated in European medical centers (2005). *BMC Infectious Disease*. Vol. 18, pp.7-29. ISSN 1471-2334

Sader, H.S.; Jones, R.N. (2009) Antimicrobial susceptibility of Gram-positive bacteria isolated from US medical centers: results of the Daptomycin Surveillance Program (2007-2008). *Diagnostic Microbiology and Infectious Disease*. 2009, Vol. 65, pp.158-162. ISSN: 07328893.

Secchi, C.; Antunes, A.L.; Perez, L.R.; Cantarelli, V.V.; d'Azevedo, P.A. (2008) Identification and detection of methicillin resistance in non-epidermidis coagulase-negative staphylococci. *Brazilian Journal of Infectious Diseases*. Vol. 12, pp. 316-320. ISSN 1413-8670

Shore, A.; Rossney, A.S.; Keane, C.T.; Enright, M.C.; Coleman, D.C. (2005) Seven novel variants of the staphylococcal chromosomal cassette mec in methicillin-resistant *Staphylococcus aureus* isolates from Ireland. *Antimicrobial Agents and Chemotherapy* 2005; Vol. 49, pp. 2070-2083. ISSN 0066-4804

Smith, T.C.; Male, M.J.; Harper, A.L.; Kroeger, J.S.; Tinkler, G.P.; Moritz, E.D.; Capuano, A.W.; Herwaldt, L.A; Diekema, D.J. (2009) Methicillin-resistant *Staphylococcus aureus* (MRSA) strain ST398 is present in midwestern U.S. swine and swine workers. *PLoS One*. Vol. 4, pp. e4258. ISSN 1932-6203Sola, C.; Cortes, P.; Saka, H.A.; Vindel, A.; Bocco, J.L. (2006) Evolution and molecular characterization of methicillin-resistant *Staphylococcus aureus* epidemic and sporadic clones in Cordoba, Argentina. *Journal of Clinical Microbiology*. Vol. 44, pp.192-200. ISSN 1098-660X

Swenson, J.M. (2002) New tests for the detection of oxacillin-resistant *Staphylococcus aureus*. *Clinical Microbiology Newsletter*, Vol. 24, pp. 159-163. ISSN: 0196-4399

Teixeira, L.A.; Resende, C.A.; Ormonde, L.R.; Rosenbaum, R.; Figueiredo, A.M.; De Lencastre, H.; Tomasz, A. (1995) Geographic spread of epidemic multiresistant *Staphylococcus aureus* clone in Brazil. *Jounal of Clinical Microbiology*. Vol. 33, pp. 2400-2404. ISSN 1098-660X

Tomasz, A.; Drugeon, H.B., de Lencastre, H.M.; Jabes, D.; McDougall, L.; Bille, J. (1989) New mechanism for methicillin resistance in *Staphylococcus aureus*: clinical isolates that lack the PBP 2a gene and contain normal penicillin-binding proteins with modified penicillin-binding capacity. *Antimicrobial Agents and Chemotherapy*. Vol. 33, pp. 1869-1874. ISSN 0066-4804

Tomasz, A.; Nachman, S.; Leaf, H. (1991) Stable classes of phenotypic expression in methicillin-resistant clinical isolates of staphylococci. *Antimicrobial Agents and Chemotherapy*. Vol. 35, pp. 124-129. ISSN 0066-4804.

Velazquez-Meza, M.E.; Aires De Sousa, M.; Echaniz-Aviles, G.; Solorzano-Santos, F.; Miranda-Novales, G.; Silva-Sanchez, J.; De Lencastre, H. (2004) Surveillance of methicillin-resistant *Staphylococcus aureus* in a pediatric hospital in Mexico City during a 7-year period (1997 to 2003): clonal evolution and impact of infection control. *Journal of Clinical Microbiology*, Vol. 42, pp. 3877-80. ISSN 1098-660X

Vindel, A.; Cuevas, O.; Cercenado, E.; Marcos, C.; Bautista, V.; Castellares, C.; Trincado, P.; Boquete, T.; Pérez-Vázquez. M.; Marín, M.; Bouza, E. (2009) Methicillin-resistant *Staphylococcus aureus* in Spain: molecular epidemiology and utility of different typing methods. *Journal of Clinical Microbiology*. Vol. 47, pp. 1620-1627. ISSN 1098-660X

Vuong, C.; Otto, M. (1999) *Staphylococcus epidermidis* infections. *Microbes and Infection*. Vol. 4, pp. 481-489. ISSN:1286-4579

Witte, W. (1999) Antibiotic resistance in gram-positive bacteria: epidemiological aspects. *Journal of Antimicrobial Chemotherapy*. Suppl A:1-9. ISSN 1460-2091

Zhang, K.; McClure, J.A.; Elsayed, S.; Conly, J.M. (2009) Novel staphylococcal cassette chromosome *mec* type, tentatively designated type VIII, harboring class A *mec* and type 4 *ccr* gene complexes in a Canadian epidemic strain of methicillin-resistant *Staphylococcus aureus*. *Antimicrobial Agents and Chemotherapy*. Vol. 53, pp. 531-540. ISSN 0066-4804

Section 3

Neuro-Psychiatric Epidemiology

7

The Epidemiology of Child Psychopathology: Basic Principles and Research Data

Kuschel Annett
Humboldt Universität zu Berlin
Germany

1. Introduction

Epidemiological information is needed for developing public policies to improve children's mental health. In particular, epidemiological research could provide answers to questions such as 1) How many children in the community have mental health problems; 2) What is the distribution of mental health problems across age, sex, levels of socio-economic status, and neighbourhood disadvantage; 3) What is the information about mental health problems from different informants (parents, teachers, and the child); and 4) What is the developmental course of mental health problems in childhood (Costello & Angold, 2006)? Answers to such questions may assist policy-makers and clinicians in designing strategies for improving mental health in children.

After briefly explaining epidemiological concepts and strategies, a selective review of epidemiological research relevant to child mental health policies is given. The purpose of the second part of this chapter is to report on results of two studies. The studies were performed in order to assess the prevalence of emotional and behavioural problems from different informants, to investigate factors which may be associated with prevalence, and to determine the prevalence and incidence rates of ADHD and ODD from preschool to primary school. Of additional concern was the developmental course of externalizing behaviour problems. Finally, the implication of the epidemiological outcomes for future research and mental health services are discussed.

2. Aims of epidemiological research

The epidemiology of childhood psychopathology includes the following aims (Costello & Angold, 1995):

- to identify the onset, frequency and distribution of mental disorders and the occurrence of psychological symptoms in different population groups and regions,
- the risk-increasing factors that determine the onset and course of disorder, to determine in different population groups,
- to determine the risk mitigation factors that protect individuals at increased risk of interference from mental disorders,
- to examine the mechanisms of disturbance in individuals with increased risk for mental disorders,

- to determine the need for psychosocial support facilities and possible costs that burdens the healthcare system due to mental disorders and their consequences.

Epidemiology does not refer to a single scientific discipline or the use of one specific methodology. Instead, epidemiology derives and integrates concepts and methods from other areas such as biology, statistics, and sociology. In epidemiology, the combination of measurement principles and statistics is used for the development and testing of diagnostic assessment procedures. When applied to psychological concepts, the combination of measurement and statistics is called psychometrics. In epidemiology of child psychopathology, psychometric principles play an important role. A number of specialized areas that are derived from classical epidemiology are relevant to child psychopathology, including clinical epidemiology, genetic epidemiology, and pharmaco-epidemiology. Clinical epidemiological studies concern the development and application of diagnostic and screening tests, the prognosis of disorders, the effects of treatment and clinical decision-making.

3. Epidemiological concepts and strategies

Epidemiology is concerned with the study of the distribution and determinants of disease frequency in human populations. The quantification of the occurrence of psychopathology in populations, can be regarded the central task of epidemiology. Well-known measures of frequency are *prevalence* (see 4.1) or *incidence*. Incidence quantifies the number of new cases with a disorder that develop in a population during a specified period of time. *Cumulative incidence* is the proportion of individuals who become disordered during a specified period of time (Verhulst, 1995). The distribution of disorders, involves comparisons between different populations or subpopulations. The examination of factors that are associated with variations in the distribution of psychopathology is essential for testing etiological hypotheses. Measures of association and risk are quantifications of the influence of certain factors on the occurrence of disorder. In follow-up studies measures of risk for developing a disorder using categorical data are *relative risk*, and *attributable risk*. In case-control studies the measure often used is the *odds ratio* which reflects the likelihood for developing a disorder in the group with a possible aetiological factor versus the group without this factor (Verhulst, 1995). For a more detailed discussion, see Verhulst and Koot (1992).

Epidemiological studies can be divided into prospective and retrospective studies, depending respectively on whether the measurement of exposure to a risk factor was done before or after the disorder occurred. A study, in which the presence or absence of a disorder and the presence or absence of associated factors are assessed at the same time, is called a cross-sectional study. If the aim of the cross-sectional study is limited to the determination of the prevalence, the study is called prevalence study.

4. Prevalence studies

4.1 Basics

Prevalence can be defined as the proportion of a population that has mental health problems at a specific point in time; it is often defined as *point prevalence*. Prevalence is calculated by dividing the number of cases by the total population. It is also possible to quantify the number of cases known to have the disorder at any time during a specified period. This so-called *period prevalence* (e.g. 6-month prevalence or lifetime prevalence) is frequently used in prevalence studies of child psychiatric conditions. There are two types of studies determining the prevalence of child psychopathology: (1) those that produce prevalence rates of psychiatric diagnoses, usually based on DSM (Diagnostic and Statistical Manual of Mental Disorders) criteria, and (2) those that generate scores on psychiatric symptom rating scales.

Many studies that determined prevalence rates of DSM diagnoses in general population samples of children have been conducted. Costello, Egger and Angold (2005), Roberts, Attkisson and Rosenblatt (1998), Verhulst (1995), and Waddell et al. (2002) provided reviews. Despite huge research efforts and many children involved, comparisons between these studies are seriously hampered by large differences in design and methodology including differences in sample size, age of children, assessment and sampling procedures, and case definition. Even for studies conducted in countries comparable in language, culture, and availability of services, differences in prevalence rates were extremely large and ranged from 10% to 20% (Waddell et al., 2002). It is more likely that these differences reflect variations in methodology than differences in true prevalence. Methodological variations and the lack of standardization among studies seriously limit the value of prevalence figures of categorical diagnoses.

The second approach, the use of rating scales for assessing parent- or self-reported emotional and behavioural problems of children in representative general population samples, is less vulnerable to methodological differences. This approach produces problem scores on continuous scales and does not generate prevalence rates for categorical diagnoses. Often, statistical criteria are used for distinguishing between cases and non-cases. Although dividing lines for caseness may be rather arbitrary, there are epidemiological methods for selecting effective cut-off points. However, prevalence figures will vary with the statistical criterion and cannot be used as absolute population prevalence measures without relating them to similar measures for other populations or subpopulations (Verhulst, 1995). In two recent multicultural prevalence studies, parents' reports and youths' self-reports of problems for children using the Child Behavior Checklist (CBCL) in 31 cultures, and the Youth Self-Report (YSR) in 24 cultures, were compared (Rescorla et al., 2007a; b). It was found that, when the same standardized assessment procedures are used for assessing children from different cultures, cultural differences per se do not lead to big differences in reported problems. Instead, individual differences within each cultural group are bigger than differences between the average scores obtained in different cultures. Assessment procedures with good cross-cultural track records and appropriate translations that capture individual differences in reliable and valid ways are apt to reflect the mental health needs of children that are robust across cultures (Achenbach & Rescorla, 2007).

4.2 Methodological Issues

A number of methodological issues of child psychiatric prevalence studies will be considered for better understanding the results of these studies. Issues that pertain to general epidemiological methodology, such as sampling and data analysis, will not be discussed here. The focus will be on issues that are specific to child psychopathology, such as assessment, diagnostic principles, and morbidity criteria.

Assessment: All assessment procedures are subject to error due to variations in the phenomena being assessed and in the procedures themselves. To reduce variations in the data obtained and to improve precision is the use of standardized assessment procedures. Epidemiological researchers in child psychiatry were among the first to use standardized assessment procedures (Rutter et al., 1970). Rating scales were developed because they could easily be applied in a cost effective way in large-scale epidemiological studies, and standardized psychiatric interviews were developed for more in-depth assessments of the prevalence of psychiatric diagnoses. Conversely, epidemiological data are indispensable for obtaining norms and for testing the validity of these instruments (Shaffer et al., 1999). Epidemiological comparisons of normal and disordered children are needed to determine how childhood disorders are actually distributed and for identifying optimal cut-offs for distinguishing between children who will most likely benefit from particular interventions versus those who will not (Fombonne, 2002; Verhulst, 1995).

There are two main approaches, the *empirical* and the *a priori* approach, to determine the level of psychopathology in individuals. The empirical approach employs multivariate statistical techniques, such as factor analysis and principal components analysis that are used to identify sets of problems that tend to occur together. These co-occurring items constitute empirical syndromes. This approach starts with empirical data derived from informants who describe the behaviour of children, without any assumptions about whether these syndromes reflect predetermined diagnostic categories. The empirical-quantitative approach forms the basis of the empirical syndromes of rating scales such as the Child Behavior Checklist (CBCL; Achenbach, 2009) or the Conners' Rating Scales (Conners, 1997). Prevalence studies using the empirical approach generate quantitative scores reflecting the level of problems of a child. Imposing cut points to the quantitative scores can make categorical distinctions between disordered and normal individuals. The second approach refers to the diagnostic categories employed by of one of the two international nosological systems, the fourth edition of the American Psychiatric Association's *Diagnostic and Statistical Manual of Mental Disorders (DSM-IV)* or the World Health Organization's *International Classification of Diseases (ICD)*. This approach starts with assumptions about which disorders exist and about which symptoms define them. Some prevalence studies generating DSM diagnoses for general population samples as discussed above used combinations of both approaches with rating scales for screening the total sample and psychiatric interviews used for assessing a selected subsample of children scoring in the problem range of the rating scales.

Multiple informants: To obtain a comprehensive picture of a child's functioning, information from different informants is needed. Many prevalence studies used information from usually parents, teachers, and the child. The reason for this is because agreement among informants is far from perfect, and because no one informant can substitute for all others. Different informants having different relations to the child and seeing the child under different conditions, often vary in their response to the child's behaviour. In a first meta-analytic study, Achenbach et al. (1987) computed the average correlation between different informants' ratings of problem behaviours in a large number of published samples. The mean correlation between pairs of adult informants who played different roles with respect to the children was 0.28 (e.g., parents versus teachers). The mean correlation between self-reports and reports by parents, teachers, and mental health workers was even lower (0.22). In contrast, the mean correlation between pairs of similar informants (e.g., father and mother; teacher and teacher aide) was 0.60. These findings were confirmed by more recent studies (Duhig et al. 2000; Grietens et al. 2004). There are several possible explanations for cross-informant discrepancies in parent and teacher reports of child behaviour problems, including issues related to informant bias, the demands of the context in which the child's behaviour is being assessed and poor measurement reliability (De Los Reyes & Kazdin, 2005). For reasons of comparability, it is recommended that prevalence studies report prevalence rates based on specific informants separately, and that procedures for combining information from different informants will be well documented in ways that can be easily replicated.

Disagreement among informants can be valuable (Jensen et al., 1999). As example, Ferdinand et al. (2003) studied problem behaviour in adolescents from the Dutch general population, aged 15 to 18 years, across a 4-year period. Initially, parent information was obtained with the CBCL and self-reports with the Youth Self-Report. Signs of poor outcome, including police contacts and drug use, were assessed four years later. Discrepancies between information from parents and adolescents added significantly to the prediction of poor outcome based on information from each informant separately. For instance, scores on the Delinquent Behavior syndrome based on parent information or on adolescents´ self-reports separately did not predict future police contacts. However, if parents reported scores in the deviant range on the Delinquent Behavior scale, while adolescents reported scores in the normal range on this scale, adolescents were at increased risk for later police or judicial contacts (Verhulst & Koot, 1995).

Morbidity criteria: Most problem behaviours in children can best be regarded as quantitative variations rather than present/absent categories. This approach allows for inter-individual differences that are normal. Abnormality can be regarded as the quantitative extreme of the normal distribution. This quantitative approach makes it possible to assess the degree to which an individual child's problems deviate from those that are typical of the individual's age and sex. In order to make such comparisons, we need data on large, representative samples of boys and girls of different ages from the general population. Despite the fact that many psychopathological phenomena in children can best be regarded as quantitative variations, for identifying individuals in the general population with mental health problems, we need to dichotomise quantitative information into categories that are defined by cut points for distinguishing between cases and non-cases. There is as yet little basis for perfect categorical distinctions between psychopathology and normality. For most problem rating scales this is done by comparing the distribution of scores for non-cases with the distribution of scores for cases. In the absence of an ultimate criterion for caseness, the most frequently used morbidity criterion is whether a child has been referred for specialist mental health services. However, caution is needed because this approach is fallible; some children who are not referred may have significant problems, while not all children who are referred really need professional help.

DSM diagnostic criteria can also be used for deciding who is disordered and who is not. These criteria are the result of negotiations among expert panels and often lack firm empirical evidence. Prevalence studies that use DSM diagnostic criteria to define caseness run into the problem that DSM criteria are overinclusive, often resulting in extremely high prevalence rates. As example, Bird et al. (1988) found that 49.5% of children in Puerto Rico met criteria for DSM-III disorders. As a result studies using DSM criteria often combine

DSM diagnostic criteria with impairment measure, for example the Children's Global Assessment Scale (CGAS; Shaffer et al., 1999). The newest versions of some psychiatric interviews such as the Diagnostic Interview Schedule for Children (DISC; Shaffer et al., 2000) and the Child and Adolescent Psychiatric Assessment (CAPA; Angold & Costello, 2000) have included impairment criteria. Because many children who meet criteria for DSM disorders are not greatly impaired in their everyday functioning, the addition of impairment measures results in a decrease of prevalence rates. In a Dutch prevalence study, for example, the prevalence of 21.8 % of children who met criteria for any DSM-III-R disorder based on parent interview information dropped to 5.9 % when combined with a CGAS score indicating definite impairment (Verhulst et al., 1997). Conversely there are also many children who can be regarded functionally impaired but do not meet criteria for DSM diagnoses. Some 50% of children attending clinics in the Great Smoky Mountains Study do not reach DSM or ICD criteria for a diagnosis and yet half of these are significantly impaired in their social functioning (Angold et al., 1999).

4.3 Factors associated with prevalence

Of many factors that have been tested for association with prevalence in general population studies, findings for gender, age, SES, and degree of urbanization will be discussed here, because those are factors with findings that have been replicated across studies (Achenbach & Rescorla, 2007).

Gender: Gender differences in prevalence are very robust across cultures, informants and across types of studies, in particular those that used rating scales and those that used DSM diagnostic criteria. Girls score higher than boys on internalizing psychopathology such as anxiety, depression and somatic complaints, and boys score higher than girls on externalizing behaviours such as attention and hyperactivity problems and aggressive and delinquent behaviours. These gender differences are found for both parent- and self-reported problems. Despite the range in cultural, economic, political and genetic differences, there is consistency in population-based findings that boys have more externalizing and girls have more internalizing problems.

Age of children and adolescents: From a developmental perspective, the effects of age on levels of psychopathology in individuals can best be studied through longitudinal studies. For public policy purposes, cross-sectional data on prevalence with age can be important for service planning. Age interacts with gender as a factor associated with prevalence. Boys show more problems than girls when they are younger, whereas girls show more problems than boys in adolescence (Achenbach & Rescorla, 2007). In a multicultural study of self-reported problems across 7 countries, both internalizing and externalizing behaviours increased with ages 11 to 18 years. In another multicultural study of parent-reported problems of children aged 6 through 11 years across 12 countries, and aged 6 through 17 years in 9 countries, externalizing problems decreased and internalizing problems increased with age (Achenbach & Rescorla, 2007). Although parents and adolescents agreed in reporting increases with age of internalizing problems, they disagreed about externalizing problems. Apparently parents are increasingly unaware of their child's externalizing behaviours with increasing age. This is probably caused by a developmental shift in type of externalizing problems, with overt physically aggressive and oppositional behaviours decreasing with age and status violations such as truancy, running away from home, and substance abuse increasing with age (Bongers et al., 2003).

Socio-economic status: Previous studies have shown that rates of psychopathology are higher among individuals with lower socioeconomic status (SES) than those with higher SES (e.g. Schonberg & Shaw 2007). Published findings regarding associations between parents' marital status, immigration, and child behaviour problems are rare, and fewer studies still have reported on these associations in early childhood (Javo et al., 2004). Achenbach and Rescorla (2007) summarize studies from 15 cultures that tested associations between scores on empirically based scales and measures of socio-economic status (SES) in large population samples. Measures of SES varied across studies, but most used the occupation and/or education of the child's parents and grouped participants into low-, medium-, and high-SES groups. A few studies also used measures of family income. Although the studies varied in statistical details, they were consistent in reporting higher problem scores for children from lower-SES than from higher SES (Verhulst, 1995; Waddell, 2002). Although this finding was consistent across studies, the effects were rather small. There are a number of reasons that may be responsible for the finding that children from lower SES are somewhat disadvantaged.

Degree of urbanization: Most studies investigating differences in prevalence rates between urban and rural populations did not find significant differences (Waddell et al., 2002). Achenbach and Rescorla (2007) conducted a detailed comparison of varying degrees of urbanization while controlling for sex, age, referral status, SES, region and ethnicity in a US national sample. Children from the most urban areas showed a slight tendency to obtain higher parent reported problem scores than children from the most rural areas. However, unexpectedly, the greatest contrast in problem scores was found between children in the intermediate categories versus those in the most rural areas, with highest scores for children in the intermediate categories.

5. Behavioural and emotional problems of kindergarten children

5.1 Background

Behavioural and emotional disturbance are very common among children and adolescents. Approximately 20 % of children in Western, industrialized countries experience the signs and symptoms that constitute internalizing (e.g. anxiety/depression, withdrawal) or externalizing (e.g. oppositional defiance, aggression) DSM-IV disorders (Tolan & Dodge, 2005). Recently, epidemiological research has begun to focus on children younger than six and to consider the clinical significance of behavioural and emotional problems of this period of the life span (Angold & Egger, 2007). A review on the epidemiology of emotional and behavioural disorders in preschool children estimated the overall prevalence of 'problematic' behaviour as lying at somewhere between 7 % and 25 % (Egger & Angold, 2006). Empirical findings illustrate a first peak in multi modal distribution of mental health service utilization in childhood in 6-9-year-old children (e.g. Campbell, 2006). This raises the question of whether child psychiatric disturbance pre-exists school attendance, but remains undetected.

In a study in the US, Wadsworth and Achenbach (2005) reported differential incidence by SES for elevated scores on internalizing and externalizing disorders. It is not yet clear whether these findings can be generalized outside of the US, and to preschool age and other informants. From a multicultural perspective, Achenbach and Rescorla (2007) specified in their comprehensive review the need for comparable data on preschool-aged instruments. The aims of the study were 1) to assess the prevalence of emotional and behavioural problems from different informants in children aged 3-6 years old, and 2) to investigate factors which may be associated with prevalence such as demographic and socio-economic factors.

5.2 Methods

5.2.1 Participants

The study population comprised 474 families and their children attending preschools in the city of Braunschweig (Germany), a moderately sized city with 250,000 inhabitants. Families were recruited for universal and selective prevention efficacy studies of child behaviour problems. Study details for recruitment were described by Hahlweg et al. (2010) and Heinrichs (2006). Data reported here were collected at the first (pre) assessment point. The age of the parents ranged between 23 and 47 years (mothers: M = 34.5, SD = 5.3; fathers: M = 36.4, SD = 6.1). The families had between one and four children (M = 2.0, SD = 0.9). The average age of the target children was 4.5 years (SD = 1.0), and 53% (n = 253) were boys. Seventy-eight percent (n = 219) of the couples were married, and 27 % (n = 127) were single parents. 200 fathers (91 % participation rate) completed the questionnaire assessment at pre-test. Forty-two percent of mothers (51 % of fathers) had a higher-track school school leaving qualification (= 13 years of schooling), and 37 % (22 %) had completed medium-track school (= 10 years of schooling). The net family income was equivalent to the German average; 35 % of the families were receiving social security benefits, and 7 % of mothers (5 % of fathers) were immigrants.

5.2.2 Measures

To assess psychopathology in children the German translation of the ASEBA Preschool Forms & Profiles (Achenbach & Rescorla, 2000) was used. The CBCL/1½-5 and the C-TRF are similarly constructed to cover an empirical range of behavioural, emotional and social function problems. Both forms comprise 99 items, and the respondent is requested to rate each item, based on the preceding two months, as 0 for *not true,* 1 for *somewhat or sometimes true* or 2 for *very true or often true*. The CBCL/1½-5 was completed by the mothers and fathers, whereas the kindergarten teachers completed the C-TRF.

The CBCL/1½-5 consists of three problem scales (Internalizing, Externalizing, and Total Problems) and seven syndrome subscales (Emotionally Reactive, Anxious/Depressed, Somatic Complaints, Withdrawn, Sleep Problems, Attention Problems, and Aggressive Behavior). The C-TRF consists also of three problem scales (Internalizing, Externalizing, and Total Problems) and six syndrome subscales (Emotionally Reactive, Anxious/Depressed, Somatic Complaints, Withdrawn, Attention Problems, and Aggressive Behavior). Studies on the German versions of the ASEBA Preschool Forms have supported the psychometric properties, showing good reliability and validity in both clinical and non-clinical populations (e.g. Plück et al., under review). Since there are no German norms available for the ASEBA Preschool Forms & Profiles, we used the norms provided by Achenbach and Rescorla (2000).

5.2.3 Statistical analysis

Prevalence rates of problem scales and syndrome subscales were calculated for mothers, fathers and caregivers based on the norms provided by Achenbach and Rescorla (2000). Prevalence rates were calculated as a proportion of children with *subclinical* behaviour

(T = 60 - 63 for problem scales, T = 65 - 69 for syndrome subscales) and *clinically relevant* behaviour (T ≥ 64 for problem scales, T ≥ 70 for syndrome subscales). Associations between problem scale prevalence and demographic and socio-economic factors (e.g. child´s age and gender, single parenthood, parents' education, family income, migration status) were carried out with Chi square statistics, and the significance level was set at $p < .01$. To determine whether children who had deviant problem scores (T ≥ 60) were at higher risk of having a demographic (economic) factor, odds ratios (OR) and 95 % confidence intervals were calculated.

5.3 Results

Table 1 reports the prevalence rates of problem scales and syndrome subscales for different informants. In this sample, the prevalence rate of *Internalizing* problems varied from 7.3 % (fathers) to 12.0 % (mothers) in the borderline range. Across informants, about 12 - 13% of the children met the criterion of the clinical range. For internalizing syndrome scales, 5 - 6 % prevalence rates were obtained for predominantly clinically relevant somatic complaints, anxious depressive behaviour, and withdrawn behaviour. Prevalence rates of *Externalizing* problems ranged from 4.9 % (fathers) to 9.7 % (caregivers) in the borderline range. Across informants, 6 - 9% of the children met the criterion of the clinical range. For externalizing syndrome scales, marginally higher rates of aggressive behaviour (4 - 5% clinically relevant) than attention problems were found. In summary, the results indicate higher prevalence rates on internalizing than externalizing problem behaviour across informants. For *Total Problems,* rates varied from 6.9 % (mothers) to 10.8 % (caregivers) in the borderline range. For the clinical range, 5.8 % (fathers) to 11.0 % (caregivers) of the children met the criterion. Overall, total problems were more frequently indicated by caregivers compared to parents.

Scales	Borderline Range			Clinical Range		
	Mother	Father	Caregiver	Mother	Father	Caregiver
Internalizing	*12.0*	*7.3*	*8.8*	*12.4*	*11.6*	*12.8*
Emotionally Reactive	8.4	9.2	6.8	4.1	2.4	2.9
Anxious/Depressed	5.6	6.4	5.3	3.0	0.6	6.4
Somatic Complaints	10.1	7.3	4.0	4.3	3.1	6.4
Withdrawn	3.9	3.1	5.3	5.6	5.2	2.2
Sleep Problems	2.4	0.6	only parents	3.9	2.4	only parents
Externalizing	*8.6*	*4.9*	*9.7*	*7.3*	*5.5*	*8.6*
Attention Problems	3.9	2.4	4.2	3.0	2.1	3.1
Aggressive Behavior	4.5	4.3	5.5	2.8	1.2	2.6
Total Problems	*6.9*	*7.0*	*10.8*	*10.3*	*5.8*	*11.0*

Table 1. Prevalence rates in percentage for syndrome scales and *broad-band scales,* and different informants.

For all informants, there were no significant associations between children's age and gender in terms of prevalence of problem and syndrome subscales. Odds ratios ranged between 0.99 and 1.28 and were not significant. Chi-square analysis showed that *Internalizing* problems reported by mothers were overrepresented among mothers with lower education (< 9 years) compared to those with higher education levels (35.1% vs. 26.4 and 16.9%; $\chi^2(2) = 12.31$, $p < .01$). Fathers reported significantly more *Total Problems* with lower maternal education compared to higher maternal education (28.3% vs. 6.5 %; χ^2 (2) = 15.82, $p < .001$). Rates of total problem behaviour were also significantly more common with lower education of fathers (< 9 years) in comparison to fathers with a higher education level (24.7% vs. 8.6 %; χ^2 (2) = 12.72, $p < .01$). Caregivers reported no significant associations between parents' education and child behaviour problems.

The prevalence of *Internalizing* problems reported by both parents was higher in low-income families (mothers: 35.5 %, fathers: 32.7 %) than in the group with an income of over 3,000 € per month (10.8 % and 9.2 %; χ^2 (2) = 20.71, $p < .001$; χ^2 (2) = 12.14, $p < .01$). The prevalence of *Total Problems* reported by mothers is comparable in this context: Children from low-income households (24.3 %) were overrepresented compared to children from higher-income families (3.2 %; χ^2 (2) = 18.67, $p < .001$). In contrast to these findings, caregivers reported more *Externalizing* problems for children from lower-income families. The results narrowly failed to reach statistical significance.

The immigrant children's adjustment reported by informants was as follows: Non-German children (rated by their mothers) had higher prevalence rates on internalizing problems than those reported for native-German preschool children (48.5 % vs. 20.3 %; χ^2 (2) = 24.23, $p < .001$). The odds ratio was 3.0 (95 %-CI 1.82-4.96). There were no significant associations between immigrant status, problem behaviour and other informants. There were also no significant discrepancies between parental marital status and prevalence rates of problem scales. The odds ratio for *Internalizing* problems in single-parent families versus dual-parent households was 1.96 (95 %-CI 1.07-2.68). The odds ratio for scoring $T \geq 60$ on *Total Problems* was 1.80 (95 %-CI 1.08-3.00) for children with single parent versus dual-parent families.

5.4 Discussion

This study was designed to determine the prevalence rates of behavioural and emotional problems for different informants among 3-6-year-old preschool children and to evaluate demographic factors which may be associated with prevalence.

In conclusion, 5 - 6 % predominantly clinically relevant internalizing problems were found. From the total of 447 children, 12 – 13 % met the criterion of the clinical range of internalizing mental health problems. Thus, an important finding across informants was higher prevalence for internalizing than externalizing problems in preschool children. Other studies in this age group have found higher rates of externalizing as opposed to internalizing problems (Bongers et al., 2003; Campbell, 2006). Therefore, this result was unexpected and might be important in understanding mental health in the preschool years. Such discrepancies may result from different assessment measures, procedures, and normative data. The use of the CBCL ASEBA preschool forms (Achenbach & Rescorla, 2000) is a particular strength of the study, as the CBCL is a well-established measure of mental health morbidity. While this advantage is important, the study was limited by the lack of representativeness. So far, no comparable studies using ASEBA preschool instruments have been published. When interpreting the results, it should be taken into account that the child mental health status was assessed by a symptom checklist questionnaire. Given a large number of subjects and multiple informants, the questionnaire approach is economical and offers useful information, but lacks the specificity and additional depth that structured psychiatric interviews might provide.

When compared with other studies of older children, many similarities are seen concerning the associations between prevalence and demographic factors. In the current study, parental education, income, and immigrant status were also significantly associated with mental health problems of preschool children. In contrast to earlier studies, we observed effects specific to internalizing problem behaviour. In this context, it is essential to underline the fundamental longitudinal results of Wadsworth and Achenbach (2005), who found more interactions of SES over time, indicating increasing socioeconomic differences for child behaviour problems. The results for odds ratios are consistent with those reported by Harland et al. (2002) for a larger range of children's age.

The results of the present study revealed that the psychopathology of preschool children was already as high as has been found in studies of school children and adolescents. An increased utilization of child mental health services by older children, who already show disturbance in preschool years, has important implications for early preschool recognition of child mental health problems and indicates the need for the prevention and development of a differentiated delivery of child mental health services for preschool children. Clinicians working in primary care, day care, or school systems need to be attentive to opportunities for early detection and intervention regarding preschoolers' emotional and behavioural problems, particularly since efficacious prevention and treatment exists for the psychopathology of young children (e.g. Weisz et al., 2005).

6. Continuity and change of externalizing behaviour

6.1 Background

Within the last century, considerable changes in the health and illness patterns of young children have been observed. One characteristic of this phenomenon, which is referred as the "new morbidity', is the growing importance of mental health concerns (Palfrey et al., 2005). Externalizing problem behaviours are the most common and persistent forms of childhood maladjustment (Campbell, 2006). Kraemer et al. (2000) reported that, at the same time, externalizing behaviours change so much in expression and frequency over the course of development that studies at any single point in development will provide only limited information or misrepresent the phenomenon. Therefore, there is a growing agreement that externalizing behaviour must be studied from a developmental perspective (Costello & Angold, 2006). The present article aims to describe the development of externalizing behaviours from preschool age to primary school.

Previous studies have investigated the development of externalizing behaviour in the general population (e.g. Bongers et al., 2004; Hofstra et al., 2000; Loeber et al., 2000). However, these studies used two different diagnostic approaches to describe externalizing problem behaviour. The *empirical approach* utilized multivariate statistical techniques to identify sets of problems that tend to occur together. This approach starts with empirical data derived from different informants who describe the behaviour of children and forms the basis of the empirical syndromes of rating scales such as the Child Behavior Checklist (CBCL; Achenbach, 2009) or the Conners' Rating Scales (Conners, 1997). The *diagnostic approach* is to take the diagnostic categories of one of the international nosological systems, the fourth edition of the American Psychiatric Association's Diagnostic and Statistical Manual of Mental Disorders (DSM-IV) or the World Health Organization's International Classification of Diseases (ICD). Instead of disregarding one approach for the other,

Verhulst and Koot (1995) hold the view that both approaches are needed, and that combining both by adding information from one approach that is not captured by the other may increase our knowledge of children's psychopathology (Ferdinand et al., 2004).

A classification scheme of externalizing behaviours developed by Frick and colleagues (1993) distinguishes four types of externalizing behaviour problems based on a meta-analysis of 60 studies involving more than 28,000 youth. The four behavioural clusters that emerged may be ordered along two independent dimensions (overt vs. covert; destructive vs. non-destructive) and were labelled opposition, aggression, property violations, and status violations. These behaviour clusters were also confirmed in independent studies of adolescents. Most mental health practitioners and researchers distinguish between two types of childhood conduct problems based on the age at which children show first symptoms and the persistence of the symptoms across development (Moffitt, 2003). The differentiation between childhood-onset and adolescent-onset conduct problems is based on results from the Dunedin Multidisciplinary Health and Development Study, a 30-year longitudinal study of 1,000 New Zealand youths (Moffitt et al., 2001). Moffitt et al. (2001) identified two developmental pathways for childhood conduct problems: the life-course persistent path and the adolescence-limited path. Children with life-course persistent conduct problems first show symptoms in preschool or early primary school. Partly consistent with this theory, four developmental trajectories were identified for boys' externalizing problems from ages 2 to 8 and 6 to 15 years in two samples (Nagin & Tremblay, 1999): a *persistent problem* trajectory, a *high-level desister* trajectory, a *moderate-level desister* trajectory, and a *persistent low* trajectory. In addition, Campbell et al. (2006) identified for physical aggression from 24 months to age 9 the following trajectories: very-low, low-stable, moderate-decreasing, moderate-stable, and high stable aggression. Schaeffer et al. (2003) identified four somewhat different pathways of antisocial behaviour from first to seventh grade within an epidemiological sample of boys: *chronic high, moderate* (and stable), and *increasing aggression* trajectories as well as a *nonaggressive* trajectory. Early, persistent externalizing problems (e.g. aggression), however, predicts a range of negative outcomes including poor emotion regulation and impulsive behaviour, school failure and dropout, peer problems, and adolescent delinquency (Patterson et al., 1989; Tremblay, 2000).

Studies, in which researchers employed the empirical approach, have shown that between ages 2 and 9 children generally decline on externalizing behaviour measures (NICHD Early Child Care Research Network ECCRN; Shaw et al., 2003). Bongers et al. (2003) also found a decline in mother-reported externalizing behaviour problems for both boys and girls between ages 4 and 18 in a representative sample of over 2,000 Dutch children. The aims of the study were 1) to assess the prevalence and incidence of externalizing behavioural problems in children from kindergarten to primary school, and 2) to investigate the developmental course of externalizing behaviours.

6.2 Methods

6.2.1 Sample and design

In the present study, families with children aged 3 to 6 years were recruited in preschools in the city of Braunschweig (Germany), a moderately sized city with 250,000 inhabitants. Families were recruited for a universal prevention efficacy study of child behaviour problems. Study details for recruitment were described by Hahlweg et al. (2010). We first contacted all potentially eligible preschools (*N* = 33). Project staff members were present at preschool teacher meetings and explained the project. Twenty-three preschools (70 %) expressed interest in participating in the project. Seventeen of these preschools were then randomly selected to participate in the project, and then preschools were randomly assigned to either the intervention or control condition.

The study population comprised 136 control preschool children. The baseline demographic characteristics of the 136 children and their families were follows: The age of the mothers ranged between 23 and 57 years (*M* = 35.0, *SD* = 5.4). The families had between one and five children (*M* = 2.0, *SD* = 0.9). The average age of the target children was 4.1 years (*SD* = 1.1), and 51% (*n* = 69) were girls. 33 % (*n* = 46) of the children lived with single parents. Fifty-three percent of mothers had a higher-track school qualification (= 13 years of schooling), and 32 % had completed a medium-track school (= 10 years of schooling). The net family income was equivalent to the German average; 33 % of the families were receiving social security benefits, and 8 % of mothers were immigrants.

The developmental course of child behaviour problems was established with self-report measures from mothers at pre, 1, 2, 3 and 4 years after the first assessment (follow-up 1 - 4). Across the four years after pre-test, 2 - 4 % of the families dropped out of the study, leaving 122 families (retention rate 90 %). The sample size at the 4-year follow-up assessment (primary school) consisted of 62 boys (50.8 %) and 60 girls. The mean age of the children was 8;8 years (*SD* = 1;1; range 6;3 – 10;8 years).

6.2.2 Measures

At pre-assessment, families provided information regarding their age, nationality, relationship to the child, education level, employment, receipt of social welfare assistance, and household income. They also provided data on the age and gender of the child of interest and any siblings.

Child mental health was measured during the preschool years by the German version of the Child Behavior Checklist (CBCL/1½-5; Achenbach & Rescorla, 2000; see 5.2.2). A recent study tested the generalizability of the seven-syndrome model in 23 societies (Ivanova et al., 2010). Findings from this study indicate that researchers (clinicians) can use the syndromes to assess preschool psychopathology. For the 2-year follow-up and after, the Child Behavior Checklist 4-18 (Arbeitsgruppe Deutsche Child Behavior Cheklist, 1998) was used. The scores from the parent-report were classified according to the manual into age- and sex-dependent categories which are based on the percentiles of the normative study.

The German ADHD Rating scale (FBB-HKS) is part of the comprehensive Diagnostic System for Mental Disorders in Childhood and Adolescence (DISYPS-KJ; Döpfner & Lehmkuhl, 1998) and can be rated by parents and teachers. This ADHD rating scale includes 20 items addressing symptom criteria of both ICD-10 and DSM-IV as well as additional criteria assessing symptom onset, symptom duration, pervasiveness and functional impairment. Internal consistencies were satisfactory to very good in the different representative samples (Döpfner et al., 2008). The DSM-IV recognizes three subtypes of the disorder - the predominantly inattentive type, the predominantly hyperactive-impulsive type and the combined type. Children were diagnosed with any ADHD if parents reported that six or more symptoms had persisted for at least 6 months.

The German Conduct Disorder Rating scale (FBB-SSV) is also part of the comprehensive Diagnostic System for Mental Disorders in Childhood and Adolescence (DISYPS-KJ). The rating scale includes 23 items using the symptom criteria of both the ICD-10 and DSM-IV, as well as additional criteria (e.g. symptom onset). Studies have supported the instrument's psychometric properties, showing good reliability and validity in both clinical and non-clinical populations (Döpfner et al., 2008). Children were diagnosed with oppositional defiant disorder (ODD) if parents reported that four or more symptoms had persisted for at least 6 months. All questionnaire assessments were conducted at five assessment points: pre-test, and 1, 2, 3 and 4 years after the first assessment (follow-up 1- 4).

6.2.3 Statistical analysis

Prevalence rates of the Externalizing problem scale during the preschool years were calculated for mothers based on the norms provided by Achenbach and Rescorla (2000). Prevalence rates were calculated as a proportion of children with *subclinical* behaviour (T = 60 - 63) and *clinically relevant* behaviour (T ≥ 64). From the 2-year follow-up, the CBCL 4-18 with representative German norms was used. Percentages of ADHD and ODD mental health problems were calculated for all assessment points. Incidence rates are based on cumulative incidence for time periods as follows: pre-FU1, pre-FU2, pre-FU3, and pre-FU4.

6.3 Results

Figure 1 reports the prevalence rates of the CBCL-Externalizing problem scale and DSM-IV ADHD- and DSM-IV ODD-disorders for each assessment point. In this sample, the prevalence rate of *Externalizing* problems in the borderline and clinical range varied from 7.5 % (FU1) to 30.8 % (FU2). In primary school, about 22 % of the children were identified as having clinically significant externalizing behaviour problems. There was an increase over time in prevalence of 11 %. Significantly more children had externalizing problems during the primary school years than in the preschool years: 11.3 % vs. 30.8 % (FU2; χ^2 (1) = 12.3, $p < .001$), 22.0 % (FU3; χ^2 (1) = 16.3, $p < .001$, and 22.9 % (FU4; χ^2 (1) = 10.4, $p < .001$). For *ADHD disorders*, prevalence rates between 6 % and 10 % were obtained. Chi-square analysis showed that the gain of prevalence in attention deficit-/hyperactivity disorder over time failed to reach statistical significance. Prevalence rates of *ODD disorder* ranged from 7.4 % (FU3) to 10.5 % (FU1). There were no significant increases in prevalence rates.

The incidence rates for the CBCL-Externalizing problems and DSM-IV ADHD- and DSM-IV ODD-disorders are shown in Figure 2. This represents the *cumulative incidence* for the time periods from first assessment (pre) to each follow-up (FU1-FU4). Incidence for externalizing problems ranged from 4.5 % to 22.5 %. The highest incidence was present in the period two years after the pre-assessment. Infants had an incidence of 15-16 %. Lower rates in the DSM-IV-ODD were found, ranging from 3.5 % to 6.1%. Incidence for oppositional defiant disorder decreased from kindergarten to primary school. These findings are comparable to the incidence of DSM-IV-ADHD. The lowest incidence was 2.3 % (pre-FU2), the highest incidence was 4.8 % (pre-FU4). In summary, the results indicate higher incidence rates on externalizing behaviour problems established by the empirical approach than externalizing behaviour problems based on diagnostic categories of DSM-IV.

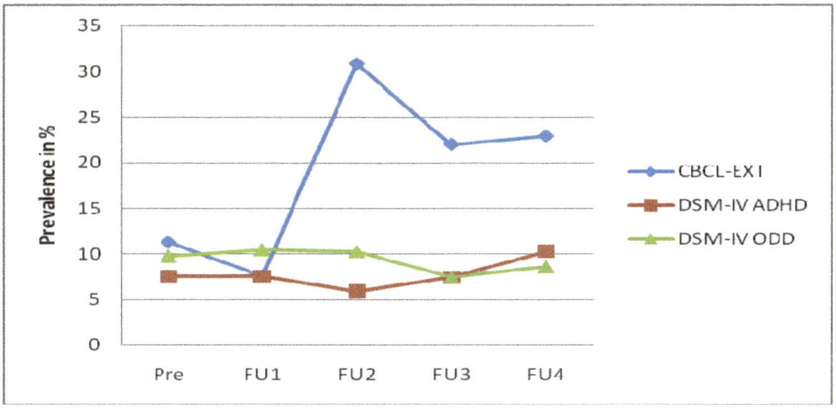

Fig. 1. Prevalence rates of externalizing problems and DSM-IV-disorders

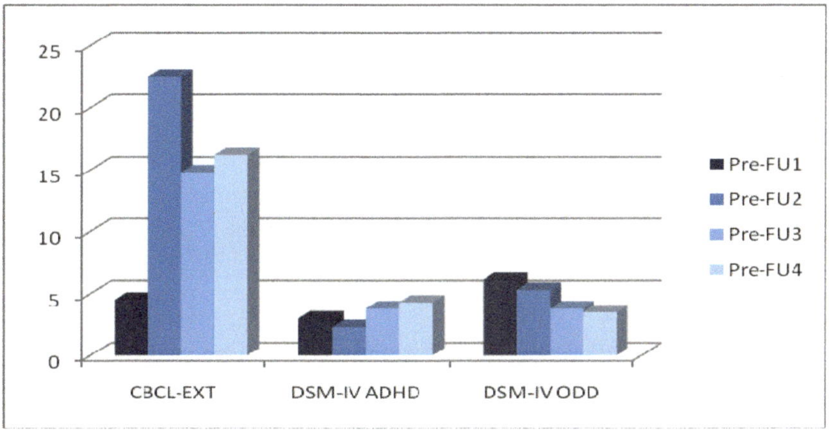

Fig. 2. *Incidence rates of externalizing problems and DSM-IV-disorders*

The developmental course of externalizing behaviour problems is presented in Table 2. Table 2 includes the developmental patterns of CBCL-Externalizing problems, DSM-IV ADHD- and DSM-IV ODD-disorders. Overall, we found three different patterns: the first group is *stable normal* - for each of the five assessments no borderline and clinical scores on the Child Behavior Checklist or no diagnoses of ADHD or no diagnoses of ODD were obtained. The second group of children is *temporary clinical* - for at least one assessment borderline and clinical scores on the Child Behavior Checklist or a diagnosis of ADHD or a diagnosis of ODD was seen. The third group (*stable clinical*) showed relevant externalizing symptoms on the Child Behavior Checklist or ADHD-diagnoses or ODD-diagnoses for at least four of five assessments.

On the CBCL Externalizing scale 61.0 % of the sample was stable normal; from preschool to primary school, mother's report resulted in T-scores < 60. In addition, 31.6 % of the children had deviant CBCL scores for at least one assessment point. The stable clinical-pattern (remaining deviant at least four times) occurred in 7.4 % of the sample. In comparison with rates of ADHD- and ODD-disorders in childhood, the percentage of children in the group "temporary clinical" was relatively high. Regarding the ADHD-disorders and as shown in Figure 3, 83.8 % of our sample was stable normal and showed no clinical relevant ADHD-symptoms over the course. Overall, 12 % of children met at least at one assessment time the criteria for a disorder of ADHD. For 3.7 % of the sample the *stable clinical* pattern was observed. These children met on at least four occasions the criteria for a DSM-IV ADHD disorder. We found similar results in terms of oppositional deviant disorder: Stable normal behaviour was seen in 80.1 % of the sample. The percentage of the *stable clinical* pattern (3.7 %) corresponds with that for the rate of attention deficit-/hyperactivity. Only in relation to the temporary clinical course was a slightly higher rate (16.2 % to 12.5 %) observed.

Developmental pattern	CBCL-EXT	DSM-IV ADHD	DSM-IV ODD
Stable normal	61.0	83.8	80.1
Temporary clinical	31.6	12.5	16.2
Stable clinical	7.4	3.7	3.7

Table 2. Developmental course of externalizing problem (CBCL EXT) behaviour and DSM-IV-disorders. Data in percent.

In summary, the results showed that about 80 % to 84 % of the preschool children were stable normal with regard to the development of ADHD- and ODD-disorders. However, when only CBCL externalizing scores were taken into consideration the rate decreased from 80 % to 60 %. In about one third of the sample temporary clinical CBCL Externalizing scores were observed. In contrast to results for the diagnostic categories of DSM-IV these rates are two-fold higher. Regarding the stable clinical pattern from preschool to primary school, 4 % of the children fulfilled the criteria for an ADHD- or an ODD-DSM-IV disorder.

6.4 Discussion

In summary, with regard to the empirical approach a considerable variation and a significant increase in the prevalence of externalizing problems were found. The results for preschool aged children correspond with other German findings reported by Beyer and Furniss (2007). Within the BELLA study, a representative national sample of children and adolescents was surveyed (Ravens-Sieberer et al., 2008). Parent's report on externalizing problems in children aged 7-10 indicated a slightly lower prevalence than in the current sample. In a multicultural study on the CBCL, Externalizing scores generally decreased with age (Achenbach & Rescorla, 2007). A review by Rescorla et al. (2007a) included data from 31 societies. Therefore, our findings were unexpected and might be important in understanding mental health in the preschool and primary school years. Discrepancies were attributed to different assessment instruments, sample procedures, use of cut-off points, and normative data. In this study, prevalence rates of 7 - 10% for the diagnoses of ADHD according to DSM-IV symptom criteria were found. When compared with a representative German sample (Döpfner, Breuer, et al., 2008), similarities are seen concerning the prevalence in the age group 7 -10 years. Our prevalence rates are also in line with results found in other countries and cultures and with other assessment instruments. In their international review, Polanczyk et al. (2007) found an overall rate of 5.3 % and a rate of 4.6 %

for Europe in general. The findings of this study support the assumption that studies without a definition of impairment had significantly higher prevalence rates than those with a definition of impairment. Besides, the diagnostic approach on oppositional defiant disorder in the preschool and primary school years has yielded prevalence rates ranging from 7.4 to 10.5 %. These results are consistent with the lifetime prevalence of ODD reported by Nock et al. (2007), who found a rate of 10.2 %. Prevalence estimates in previous studies have yielded a wide range from 2 - 15% (e.g. Loeber, Burke et al., 2000). Our prevalence is concordant with those of another European study on preschool children. Furthermore, although considerable research exists on ADHD and conduct disorder, information regarding ODD is limited.

So far, no comparable studies reporting incidence rates on externalizing behaviour have been published. In the absence of sufficient comparison studies it is not yet clear whether the findings reported here can be generalized. Further research is urgently called for to answer this important question. Therefore, incidence rates and the developmental course of externalizing problem behaviour are considered together.

On the CBCL about 7 % of preschool and primary school children showed a stable pattern of relevant externalizing problem behaviour. A recent study by van Lier et al. (2007) assessed the trajectories of parent-rated symptoms of conduct problems from age 4 to 18 years old also in a general population sample. In this broader age group slightly lower rates (4 - 5 %) of a high trajectory of ODD- and ADHD-symptoms were found. A thorough statistical analysis of trajectories through growth mixture modelling on a large sample size of Dutch children yielded these results. The discrepancies in findings from those in the present study were attributable to different age groups, data collection and recruitment procedures, and CBCL-versions. The results on the stable normal pattern are in line with data from the literature (Bongers et al., 2003; Keiley et al., 2000).

The study had several strengths. First, it is one of the rare studies with preschool children conducted in a universal setting with a 4-year follow-up over that time span. Second, the time intervals between the assessments were shorter compared with other longitudinal studies examining the same topic. Third, we used two different diagnostic approaches to describe externalizing problems: one of the best-studied instruments for the evaluation of children´s psychopathology (Achenbach, 2009) and DSM-IV ADHD- and ODD-diagnostic criteria. In this context, the study met for the most part the methodological criteria previously suggested by Robins and Rutter (1990), since it investigated behavioural problems in a sample of the population assessed longitudinally through standardized procedures. The present study is not without limitations. A main limitation is the generalizability of findings. Our sample is relatively advantaged with only 1/3 of all potentially eligible families participating. This finding corresponds to the fact that the rates of families and children recruited for family-focused preventions are typically very low (e.g. Spoth & Redmond, 2000). When interpreting the results, it should be taken into account that the child mental health status was assessed by symptom checklist questionnaires and disorder rating scales. The use of maternal self-report on child behaviour ratings may have been affected by the mother's experience of stress, depressive symptomatology, or marital problems. Given a large number of subjects, the questionnaire approach is economical and offers useful information, but lacks the specificity and additional depth that structured psychiatric interviews might provide.

Furthermore, a teacher perspective could add valuable information about problem behaviour at school, which might possibly result in reports of more externalizing problems. Due to principles of data collection, frequent change of teachers, and the transition from kindergarten to primary school it was only possible to obtain the parental report. For international comparison of the results, the age at school entry in Germany, generally at the age of 6 years, needs to be taken into account.

To sum up, the study contributes to a more complete understanding of externalizing behaviour problems and their continuity from kindergarten to primary school. The results point to the need for early child psychiatric research on child mental health beginning in infancy and the preschool years. The development of problem behaviour in specific clinical or risk groups may differ from the pattern found in the present data. An increased utilization of child mental health services by older children, who already show disturbances in the preschool years, has important implications for early preschool recognition of child mental health problems and indicates the need for the prevention and development of a differentiated delivery of child mental health services. Clinicians working in primary care, day care, or school systems need to be attentive to opportunities for early detection and intervention regarding preschoolers' externalizing behavioural problems, particularly since efficacious prevention and treatment exists for the psychopathology of young children (e.g. Weisz et al., 2005).

7. Conclusion

Since the first child psychiatric epidemiological studies in the 1950´s and 1960´s, epidemiological research has provided a wealth of empirical findings that may aid develop strategies for improving the mental health outcomes of children. Descriptive epidemiological data on prevalence rates, historical trends, and outcomes of mental health problems can help planning mental health services for children and provide evidence for setting priorities when resources are limited. Etiologic epidemiological research forms the basis for prevention interventions by unravelling the causative mechanisms in the development of psychopathology. Clinical epidemiological strategies are important for more evidence-based approaches to diagnostic assessment and intervention strategies, and outcome research may help improving the quality of mental health services. Finally, more efforts should be put into improving partnerships between epidemiological researchers and prevention specialists and between epidemiological researchers and policy-makers for improving strategies for preventing and treating mental health problems in children.

8. Acknowledgment

The research was supported by the Deutsche Forschungsgemeinschaft (DFG; German Research Foundation, HA 1400/14-1-4) and the Jacobs Foundation, Zürich (Switzerland). I am very grateful to the families for participating in the studies and to Mrs Joswig-Gröttrup and Mrs Hamilton Kohn, Jugendamt der Stadt Braunschweig, Department of Preschools, as well as to all preschool teachers for their very good cooperation. My warmest thanks also to Dr. Kurt Hahlweg, PhD Frank C. Verhulst and Dr. Nina Heinrichs for their comments on earlier versions of this manuscript.

9. References

Achenbach, T. M. (2009). *ASEBA: Development, findings, theory, and applications*. University of Vermont Research Center for Children, Youth and Families, ISBN 978-1932975130, Burlington, VT

Achenbach, T. M., McConaughy, S. H. & Howell, C. T. (1987). Child/adolescent behavioral and emotional problems: implications of cross-informant correlations for situational specificity. *Psychological Bulletin*, Vol.101, 213–232, ISSN 0033-2909

Achenbach, T. M. & Rescorla, L. A. (2000). *Manual for the ASEBA preschool forms and profiles*. University of Vermont, ISBN 978-0938565680, Burlington

Achenbach, T. M., & Rescorla, L. A. (2007). *Multicultural understanding of child and adolescent psychopathology: Implications for mental health assessment*. Guilford Press, ISBN 978-1593853488, New York, NY

Angold, A. & Costello, E. J. (2000). The Child and Adolescent Psychiatric Assessment (CAPA). *Journal of the American Academy of Child and Adolescent Psychiatry, 39*, 39-48, ISSN 0890-8567

Angold, A., Costello, E. J., Farmer, E. M., Burns, B. J. & Erkanli, A. (1999). Impaired but undiagnosed. *Journal of the American Academy of Child and Adolescent Psychiatry*, Vol.38, 129-137, ISSN 0890-8567

Angold, A., & Egger, H. L. (2007). Preschool psychopathology: Lessons for the lifespan. *Journal of Child Psychology & Psychiatry*, Vol. 48, 961–966, ISSN 0021-9630

Arbeitsgruppe Deutsche Child Behavior Checklist (1998). *Elternfragebogen über das Verhalten von Kindern und Jugendlichen, deutsche Bearbeitung der Child Behavior Checklist (CBCL/4-18)*. Köln: Arbeitsgruppe Kinder-, Jugend- und Familiendiagnostik (KJFD).

Beyer, T., & Furniss, T. (2007). Child psychiatric symptoms in primary school. *Social Psychiatry and Psychiatric Epidemiology*, Vol.42, No.9, 753-758, ISSN 0933-7954

Bird, H. R., Canino, G., Rubio-Stipec, M., Gould, M. S., Ribera, J., Sesman, M., Woodbury, M., Huertas-Goldman, S., Pagan, A., Sanchez-Lacay, A. & Moscoso, M. (1988). Estimates of the prevalence of childhood maladjusment in a community survey in Puerto Rico: The use of combined measures. *Archives of General Psychiatry*, Vol.45, 1120-1126, ISSN 0003-990X

Bongers, I., Koot, H. M., van der Ende, J., & Verhulst, F. C. (2003). The normative development of child and adolescent problem behavior. *Journal of Abnormal Psychology*, Vol.112, 179–192, ISSN 0021-843X

Bongers, I. L., Koot, H. M., van der Ende, J., & Verhulst, F. C. (2004). Developmental trajectories of externalizing behaviors in childhood and adolescence. *Child Development*, Vol.75, 1523-1537, ISSN 0009-3920

Campbell, S. B. (2006). *Behavior problems in preschool children: Clinical and developmental issues* (2. ed.). Guilford Press, ISBN 978-1593853778, New York, NY

Campbell, S. B., Spieker, S., Burchinal, M., & Poe, M. D. (2006). Trajectories of aggression from toddlerhood to age 9 predict academic and social functioning through age 12. *Journal of Child Psychology and Psychiatry*, Vol.47, No.8, 791–800, ISSN 0021-9630

Conners, C. K. (1997). *Conners' Rating Scales-Revised*. Multi-Health Systems, ISBN 978-0158046396, North Tonawanda, NY

Costello, E. J., & Angold, A. (2006). Developmental epidemiology. In D. Cicchetti & D. J. Cohen (Eds.), *Developmental Psychopathology: Theory and method* (2nd ed., pp. 41-65). John Wiley & Sons, ISBN 978-0471237365, New Jersey

Costello, E. J., Egger, H., & Angold, A. (2005). 10-Year Research Update Review: The Epidemiology of Child and Adolescent Psychiatric Disorders: I. Methods and Public Health Burden. *Journal of the American Academy of Child & Adolescent Psychiatry*, Vol.44, No.10, 972–986, ISSN 0890-8567

De Los Reyes, A. & Kazdin, A. E. (2005). Informant discrepancies in the assessment of childhood psychopathology: a critical review, theoretical framework, and recommendations for further study. *Psychological Bulletin*, Vol. 131, 483–509, ISSN 0033-2909

Duhig, A. M., Renk, K., Epstein, M. K. & Phares, V. (2000). Interparental agreement on Internalizing, Externalizing, and Total problems: A meta-analysis. *Clinical Psychology: Science and Practice*, Vol.7, 435–453, ISSN 0969-5893

Döpfner, M., & Lehmkuhl, G. (1998). *DISYPS-KJ. Diagnostik-System für psychische Störungen im Kindes- und Jugendalter nach ICD-10 und DSM-IV* [DISYPS-KJ. Diagnostic system for psychiatric disorders in children and adolescents in ICD-10 and DSM IV]. Huber, ISBN 978-3456830063, Bern

Döpfner, M., Breuer, D., Wille, N., Erhart, M., & Ravens-Sieberer, U. (2008). How often do children meet ICD-10/DSM-IV criteria of attention deficit-/hyperactivity disorder and hyperkinetic disorder? Parent-based prevalence rates in a national sample - results of the BELLA study. *European Child & Adolescent Psychiatry*, Vol.17, No.0, 59-70, ISSN 1018-8827

Döpfner, M., Görtz-Dorten, A., & Lehmkuhl, G. (2008). Diagnostik-System für Psychische Störungen im Kindes- und Jugendalter nach ICD-10 und DSM-IV, DISYPS-II. [DISYPS-II. Diagnostic system for psychiatric disorders in children and adolescents in ICD-10 and DSM IV 2nd Edition]. Huber, ISBN 978-1111155401, Bern

Egger, H. L. & Angold, A. (2006). Common emotional and behavioral disorders in preschool children: Presentation, nosology, and epidemiology. *Journal of Child Psychiatry and Psychology*, Vol.47, 313–337, ISSN 0021-9630

Ferdinand, R. F., Visser, J. H., Hoogerheide, K. N., van Der Ende, J., Kasius, M. C., Koot, H. M. & Verhulst, F. C. (2004). Improving estimation of the prognosis of childhood psychopathology: Combination of DSM-III-R/DISC diagnoses and CBCL scores. *Journal of Child Psychology and Psychiatry*, Vol.45, No.3, 599-608, ISSN 0021-9630

Fombonne, E. (2002). Case identification in an epidemiological context. In M. Rutter & E. Taylor (eds.), *Child and Adolescent Psychiatry* (pp 52-69), Blackwell, ISBN 978-0865428805, Oxford, England

Frick, P. J., Lahey, B. B., Loeber, R., Tannenbaum, L., van Horn, Y., Christ, M. A. G. et al. (1993). Oppositional defiant disorder and conduct disorder: A meta-analytic review of factor analyses and cross-validation in a clinic sample. *Clinical Psychology Review*, Vol.13, No.4, 319-340, ISSN 0272-7358

Grietens, H., Onghena, P., Prinzie, P., Gadeyne, E., van Assche, V., Ghesquiere, P. & Hellinckx, W. (2004). Comparison of mothers', fathers', and teachers' reports on problem behavior in 5- to 6-year-old children. *Journal of Psychopathology and Behavioral Assessment*, Vol.*26*, 137–146, ISSN 0882-2689

Hahlweg, K., Heinrichs, N., Kuschel, A., Bertram, H. & Naumann, S. (2010) Long-term outcome of a randomized controlled universal prevention trial through a Positive Parenting Program: Is it worth the effort? *Child and Adolescent Psychiatry and Mental Health*, Vol.4, No.14, ISSN 1753-2000

Harland, P., Reijneveld, S. S., Brugman, E., Verloove-Vanhorick, S. P. & Verhulst, F. C. (2002) Family factors and life events as risk factors for behavioural and emotional problems in children. *European Child & Adolescent Psychiatry*, Vol.11, 176–184, ISSN 1018-8827

Heinrichs, N. (2006) The effects of two different incentives on recruitment rates of families into a prevention program. *Journal of Primary Prevention*, Vol.27, 345-365, ISSN 0278-095X

Ivanova, M. Y., Achenbach, T. M., Rescorla, L. A., Harder, V. S., Ang, R. P., Bilenberg, N. et al. (2010). Preschool psychopathology reported by parents in 23 societies: Testing the seven-syndrome model of the Child Behavior Checklist for ages 1.5-5. *Journal of the American Academy of Child & Adolescent Psychiatry*,Vol.49, No.12, 1215-1224, ISSN 0890-8567

Javo, C., Ronning, J. A., Heyerdahl, S. & Rudmin, F. W. (2004).Parenting correlates of child behavior problems in a multiethnic community sample of preschool children in northern Norway. *European Child & Adolescent Psychiatry*, Vol.13, 8–18, ISSN 1018-8827

Jensen, P. S., Rubio-Stipec, M., Canino, G., Bird, H., Dulcan, M., Schwab-Stone, M. E. & Lahey, B. (1999). Parent and child contributions to diagnosis of mental disorder: Are both informants necessary? *Journal of the American Academy of Child and Adolescent Psychiatry*, Vol.3, 1569-1579. ISSN 0890-8567

Keiley, M. K., Bates, J. E., Dodge, K. A., & Pettit, G. S. (2000). A cross-domain growth analysis: Externalizing and internalizing behaviors during 8 years of childhood. *Journal of Abnormal Child Psychology*, Vol.28, 161-179, ISSN 0091-0627

Kraemer, H. C., Yesavage, J. A., Taylor, J. L., & Kupfer, D. (2000). How can we learn about developmental processes from cross-sectional studies, or can we? *American Journal of Psychiatry*, Vol.157, 163-171, ISSN 0002-953X

Loeber, R., Burke, J. D., Lahey, B. B., Winters, A. & Zera, M. (2000). Oppositional defiant and conduct disorder: A review of the past 10 years. Part I. *Journal of the American Academy of Child & Adolescent Psychiatry*, Vol.39, 1468-1484, ISSN 0890-8567

Moffitt, T. E. (2003). Life course persistent and adolescence-limited antisocial behavior: A 10-year research review and research agenda. In B. B. Lahey, T. E. Moffitt & A. Caspi

(Eds.), *Causes of conduct disorder and juvenile delinquency* (pp. 49-75). Guilford Press, ISBN 978-1572308817, New York

Moffitt, T. E., Caspi, A., Rutter, M., & Silva, P. A. (2001). *Sex differences in antisocial behavior: Conduct disorder, delinquency, and violence in the Dunedin Longitudinal Study*. Cambridge University Press, ISBN 0521010667, Cambridge, UK

Nagin, D. S. & Tremblay, R. E. (1999). Trajectories of boys' physical aggression, opposition, and hyperactivity on the path to physically violent and nonviolent juvenile delinquency. *Child Development*, Vol.70, 1181–1196, ISSN 0009-3920

Nock, M. K., Kazdin, A. E., Hiripi, E. & Kessler, R. C. (2007). Lifetime prevalence, correlates, and persistence of oppositional defiant disorder: Results from the National Comorbidity Survey Replication. *Journal of Child Psychology and Psychiatry*, Vol.48, No.7, 703-713, ISSN 1469-7610

Palfrey J. S., Tonniges, T. F., Green, M., & Richmond, J. (2005). Introduction: addressing the millennial morbidity-the context of community. *Pediatrics*, Vol.115, 1121-1123, ISSN 0031-4005

Patterson, G. R., DeBaryshe, B. D., & Ramsey, E. (1989). A developmental perspective on antisocial behavior. *American Psychologist*, Vol. 44, 329–335, ISSN 0003-066X

Plück, J., Döpfner, M., Kuschel, A., Heinrichs, N., Denner, C. & Schmeck, K. (under review). *Zur Reliabilität und faktoriellen Validität der Fragebögen für Eltern und ErzieherInnen von Klein- und Vorschulkindern (CBCL/1½ - 5; C-TRF1½ - 5).*

Polanczyk, G., de Lima, M. S., Horta, B. L., Biederman, J., & Rohde, L. A. (2007). The worldwide prevalence of ADHD: A systematic review and metaregression analysis. *American Journal of Psychiatry*, Vol.164, 942–948, ISSN 0002-953X

Ravens-Sieberer, U., Wille, N., Erhart, M., Bettge, S., Wittchen, H.-U., Rothenberger, A. et al. (2008). Prevalence of mental health problems among children and adolescents in Germany: results of the BELLA study within the National Health Interview and Examination Survey. *European Child & Adolescent Psychiatry*, Vol.17, Suppl. 1, 22-33, ISSN 1018-8827

Rescorla, L., Achenbach, T., Ivanova, M. Y., Dumenci, L., Almqvist, F., Bilenberg, N., et al. (2007a). Behavioral and emotional problems reported by parents of children ages 6 to 16 in 31 societies. *Journal of Emotional and Behavioral Disorders*, Vol.15, No.3, 130–142, ISSN 1063-4266

Rescorla, L., Achenbach, T. M., Ivanova, M. Y., Dumenci, L., Almqvist, F., Bilenberg, N., et al. (2007b). Epidemiological comparisons of problems and positive qualities reported by adolescents in 24 countries. *Journal of Consulting and Clinical Psychology*, Vol.75, No.2, 351–358, ISSN 0022-006X

Roberts, E. E., Attkisson, C. C. & Rosenblatt, A. (1998). Prevalence of psychopathology among children and adolescents. *American Journal of Psychiatry, 155*, 715-725. ISSN 0002-953X

Robins, L. N., & Rutter, M. (1990). *Straight and devious pathways from childhood to adulthood.* The Free Press, ISBN 978-0521427395, New York

Rutter, M., Tizard, J. & Whitmore, K. (1970). *Education, health and behaviour.* Longman, ISBN 9780582320987, London

Schaeffer, C. M., Petras, H., Ialongo, N., Poduska, J., & Kellam, S. (2003). Modeling growth in boys' aggressive behavior across elementary school: Links to later criminal involvement, conduct disorder, and antisocial personality disorder. *Developmental Psychology*, Vol.39, 1020–1035, ISSN 0012-1649

Schonberg, M. A. & Shaw, D. S. (2007). Do the predictors of child conduct problems vary by high- and low-levels of socioeconomic and neighborhood risk? *Clinical Child and Family Psychology Review*, Vol.10, 101–136, ISSN 1096-4037

Shaffer, D., Fisher, P., Lucas, C. P., Dulcan, M. K., & Schwab-Stone, M. E. (2000). NIMH Diagnostic Interview Schedule for Children Version IV (NIMH DISC-IV): description, differences from previous versions, and reliability of some common diagnoses. *Journal of the American Academy of Child and Adolescent Psychiatry, 39*, 28-38, ISSN 0890-8567

Shaffer, D., Lucas, C. P. & Richters, J. E. (1999). *Diagnostic Assessment in Child and Adolescent Psychopathology*. Guilford Press, ISBN 978-1572305021, New York

Shaw, D. S., Gilliom, M., Ingoldsby, E. M., & Nagin, D. S. (2003). Trajectories leading to school-age conduct problems. *Developmental Psychology*, Vol.39, 189–200, ISSN 0012-1649

Spoth, R. & Redmond, C. (2000). Research on family engagement in preventive interventions: Toward improved use of scientific findings in primary prevention practice. *Journal of Primary Prevention*, Vol.21, 267-284, ISSN 0278-095X

Tolan, P. H. & Dodge, K. A. (2005). Children´s mental health as a primary care and concern. *American Psychologist*, Vol.60, 601–614, ISSN 0003-066X

van Lier, P. A. C., van Der Ende, J., Koot, H. M. & Verhulst, F. C. (2007). Which better predicts conduct problems? The relationship of trajectories of conduct problems with ODD and ADHD symptoms from childhood into adolescence. *Journal of Child Psychology and Psychiatry*, Vol.48, No.6, 601-608, ISSN 0021-9630

Verhulst, F. C. (1995). The epidemiology of child and adolescent psychopathology: Strengths and limitations. In F. C. Verhulst & H. M. Koot (Eds.), *The epidemiology of child and adolescent psychopathology* (pp. 1–21). Oxford University Press, ISBN 978-0192623409, Oxford

Verhulst, F. C. & Koot, H. M. (1992). *Child Psychiatric Epidemiology: Concepts, Methods and Findings*. Sage, ISBN 978-0803939974, Newbury Park

Verhulst, F. C. & Koot, H. M. (1995). *The epidemiology of child and adolescent psychopathology*. Oxford University Press, ISBN 978-0192623409, Oxford

Verhulst, F.C., van der Ende, J., Ferdinand, R. F. & Kasius, M. C. (1997). The prevalence of DSM-III-R diagnoses in a national sample of Dutch adolescents. *Archives of General Psychiatry*, Vol.54, 329-336, ISSN 0003-990X

Waddell, C., Offord, D. R., Shepherd, C. A., Hua, J. M. & McEwan, K. (2002). Child psychiatric epidemiology and canadian public policy-making: The state of the science and the art of the possible. *Canadian Journal of Psychiatry*, Vol.47, 825-832, ISSN 0703-7437

Wadsworth, M. E. & Achenbach, T. M. (2005). Explaining the link between low socioeconomic status and psychopathology: Testing two mechanisms of the social causation hypothesis. *Journal of Consulting and Clinical Psychology*, Vol.73, 1146–1153, ISSN 0022-006X

Weisz, J. R., Sandler, I. N., Durlak, J. A. & Anton, B. S. (2005). Promoting and protecting youth mental health through evidence-based prevention and treatment. *American Psychologist*, Vol.60, 628-648, ISSN 0003-066X

8

Impact of Epidemiology on Molecular Genetics of Schizophrenia

Nagafumi Doi[1], Yoko Hoshi[2], Masanari Itokawa[2], Takeo Yoshikawa[3] and Tomoe Ichikawa[2]
[1]*Ibaraki Prefectural Medical Center of Psychiatry*
[2]*Tokyo Metropolitan Institute of Medical Science*
[3]*RIKEN Brain Science Institute*
Japan

'To grasp the full meaning of the *obvious* is a better basis for the understanding than the confused knowledge of the *obscure*.'
(Engels)

1. Introduction

Schizophrenia is a common deleterious psychosis that begins typically in late adolescence or early adulthood (Gottesman, 1991; Jablensky, 1995). Although it has a strong genetic component in its etiology, no susceptibility genes conferring a large proportion of heritability have been identified (Allen et al., 2008; Need et al, 2009). Results of association studies including genome-wide scans have been inconsistent, and schizophrenia-associated genes including copy number variations differ across populations or even across individuals of a same ethnicity (Allen et al., 2008; Xu et al., 2008; Need et al, 2009). Thus, situation of molecular genetics of schizophrenia has become rather perplexing just contrary to our expectation.

In this chapter, we describe the consistent major epidemiological findings of schizophrenia, and show how these evident macroscopic aspects shed light to the confused microscopic aspects of schizophrenia genetics today, proposing a new hypothesis for this puzzling disorder.

2. Devil's triangle of human genetics – Epidemiological facts of schizophrenia

We describe here three epidemiological facts of schizophrenia - high prevalence, high heritability and low reproductive fitness. These properties form a Devil's triangle; any combination of the two tends to exclude the third, and in this triangle most diseases vanish except for schizophrenia, suggesting that schizophrenia has a unique etiological basis among the many human diseases.

2.1 Schizophrenia as a common disease

Substantial evidence of epidemiology shows that schizophrenia crosses all cultures and tribes in different continents at a relatively high prevalence (approximately 0.7%; 95%

Confidence Interval 0.3% - 2.7%) (Saha et al., 2005); the prevalence of schizophrenia, at the macro-level, varies within narrow limits (Jablensky, 1995), and appears to be stable across generations in several countries (Harrison et al., 1991; Osby et al., 2001). This epidemiological fact suggests that schizophrenia has an ancient origin.

2.2 Schizophrenia as a heritable disease

It has long been known that schizophrenia runs in families (McGue & Gottesman, 1991). Adoption studies demonstrate an increased risk of schizophrenia in biological relatives of adoptees with schizophrenia, suggesting that genetic components play an important role in the etiology of schizophrenia (Kendler & Dichl, 1993). Now it has been established by twin studies that heritability of schizophrenia is ~0.85 (Cannon et al., 1998; Cardno et al., 1999).

Although the mode of transmission of schizophrenia is still unknown, several reports suggest a higher maternal transmission of schizophrenia (Shimizu et al., 1987; Goldstein et al., 1990; Valero et al., 1998; Li et al., 2007).

2.3 Schizophrenia as a low fitness disease

It has been well documented that the fertility of patients with schizophrenia, particularly of males, is remarkably reduced compared to healthy individuals (Böök, 1953; Larson & Nyman, 1973; Ødegård, 1980; Nanko & Moridaira, 1993; Fãnanás & Bertranpetit, 1995; Nimgaonkar, 1998; McGrath et al., 1999; Haukka et al., 2003; Svensson et al., 2007). The latest meta-analysis (Bundy et al., 2011) shows that fertility ratio (patients/controls) is ~0.39 and that the reduction of fertility is more pronounced in males (male/female ratio is ~0.54).

Because schizophrenia is an early onset disease (late adolescence ~ early adulthood), psychotic symptoms of the disease such as autistic way of life and abnormal behaviors may make mating unsuccessful. This tendency may be more pronounced in males because the age at onset is significantly lower in males than in females (Jablensky, 1995; Kulkarni & Fink, 2000). Thus, unsuccessful mating, coupled with an increased mortality (McGrath et al., 2008), may remarkably reduce the fertility of patients with schizophrenia.

2.4 Schizophrenia and the Devil's triangle of human genetics

The three epidemiological characteristics of schizophrenia - high prevalence, high heritability and low fitness - form a Devil's triangle; any combination of the two tends to exclude the third, and in this triangle most diseases vanish except for schizophrenia (**Fig. 1**). Diseases with high prevalence and high heritability such as type 2 diabetes and adult cancers are late-onset diseases and exhibit almost normal reproductive fitness. Diseases with high heritability and low reproductive fitness such as most harmful Mendelian diseases in childhood are rare. Diseases with low reproductive fitness and high prevalence such as poor nutrition, severe injuries and infections in childhood or early adulthood are mainly due to the environmental factors.

This may lead us to strongly suspect that schizophrenia has a unique etiological basis among the many human diseases.

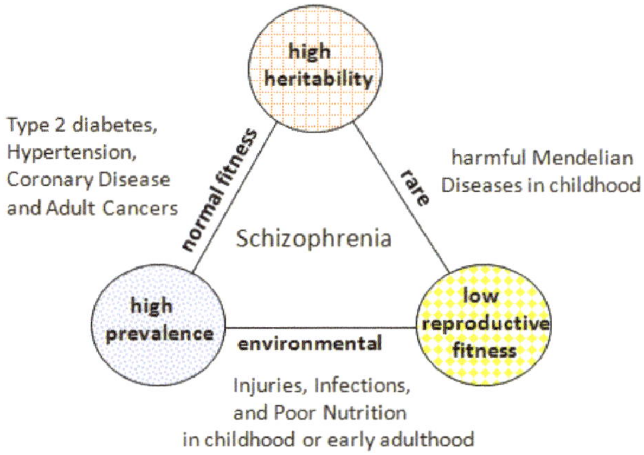

Fig. 1. Devil's triangle of human genetics (Doi et al., 2009)

3. Persistence problem and mutation-selection balance in schizophrenia

The three epidemiological characteristics of schizophrenia mentioned above give a paradox. How has a highly heritable disease associated with a remarkable biological disadvantage never been extinct in the long human history? And how can it persist at a relatively high prevalence? This 'persistence problem of schizophrenia' (or 'schizophrenia paradox') has puzzled scientists for long years (Huxley et al., 1964; Crow, 1995; Brüne, 2004; Keller & Miller, 2006).

In this section, we discuss that the only plausible mechanism for the persistence is mutation-selection balance with or without heterozygote advantage. Based on the consistent epidemiological findings on the fertility of patients with schizophrenia and their family members, we show that heterozygote advantage works in the mitochondrial genome model but not in the nuclear genome model.

3.1 Mutation-selection balance is the only plausible mechanism for the persistence

From an evolutionary viewpoint, four explanations are possible for the persistence: (i) ancestral neutrality, (ii) negative frequency-dependent selection, (iii) heterozygote advantage (balancing selection or pleiotropy), and (iv) mutation-selection balance.

'Ancestral neutrality' assumes that reproductive fitness of affected individuals and/or their relatives was higher in ancient environments and that selection coefficients of pathogenic alleles were close to zero. Because the effective population size in ancient times might be much smaller than now, pathogenic but neutral or almost neutral alleles could be fixed by genetic drift. While this hypothesis explains that schizophrenia has not been extinct in the long human history, ancestral neutrality itself provides no explanation for the apparently stable prevalence of the disease across generations today; although 'ancestral neutrality' might be plausible, it needs another mechanism to account for the persistence in modern environments, where the effective population size has been expanded and the influence of negative selection pressure may be much stronger than ever before.

'Negative frequency-dependent selection' explains the persistence only when the fitness of the affected individuals increases as the prevalence in the general population decreases, which seems not to be the case with schizophrenia.

Thus, the remaining possibility for persistence mechanism is mutation-selection balance with or without heterozygote advantage.

3.2 Heterozygote advantage works in the mitochondrial genome model but not in the nuclear genome model for schizophrenia

'Heterozygote advantage' assumes that the susceptibility alleles increase the fitness of the unaffected gene carriers, thereby sustaining the gene frequencies. This line of explanations may include: (i) physiological advantage (resistance to shock, infections, and poor nutrition etc.), (ii) a higher sexual activity and/or attractiveness, and (iii) creative intelligence or a higher trait creativity including 'everyday creativity'.

This hypothesis needs two lines of confirmation: (a) that unaffected gene carriers have such advantages, and (b) that such advantages really contribute to sufficiently increase their reproductive fitness.

It seems to gain the confirmation (a). For example, Erlenmeyer-Kimling (1968) reported an increased survival rate of *female* children of parents with schizophrenia, proposing a possible physiological advantage associated with schizophrenia. Kinney et al. (2001), in a well-designed and methodologically sophisticated study, showed that an advantage of everyday creativity was linked to a subtle clinical picture (schizotypal signs) in a non-psychotic sample of schizophrenia offspring.

However, it lacks the confirmation (b) in the nuclear genome model. This hypothesis, although theoretically plausible and fascinating, has not been supported by most epidemiological studies, which show a decreased reproductive fitness of unaffected siblings of patients with schizophrenia. Although recent large-sampled epidemiological studies (Bassett et al., 1996; McGrath et al., 1999; Haukka et al., 2003; Svensson et al., 2007) have consistently shown that the reproductive fitness of unaffected *female* siblings of patients with schizophrenia is slightly but significantly increased (1.02-1.08), it is not large enough to compensate for the gene loss due to the decreased reproductive fitness of patients (0.2-0.3 in males and 0.4-0.5 in females) and their unaffected male siblings (0.9-1.0) in the nuclear genome model. On the other hand, the latest meta-analysis (Bundy et al., 2011) shows no significant difference between the fertility of parents of patients with schizophrenia and healthy controls, although there is a trend towards parents having more offspring. Therefore, heterozygote advantage seems not to work in the nuclear genome model.

On the other hand, it works in the mitochondrial genome model because mitochondrial DNA (mtDNA) is transmitted to the next generation only through females. Indeed, we can see that this slightly elevated reproductive fitness of the unaffected female siblings, coupled with the less pronounced decreased reproductive fitness of female patients, is sufficient to compensate for the gene loss; when we calculate $-\Delta$, the cross-generational reduction of the frequency of females with a putative pathogenic mtDNA in the general population, using the data in the largest-sampled cohort study to date (Haukka et al., 2003), we have $-\Delta < 5.06 \times 10^{-3}$ (**Note**). This figure implies that the gene loss can be balanced by *de novo* mutation in the mtDNA which occurs at a rate of $8.8\times10^{-4}\sim1.3\times10^{-2}$ per locus per generation (4.3×10^{-3} on average) (Sigurđardóttir et al., 2000).

4. Persistence criterion for nuclear susceptibility genes for schizophrenia

As is shown in the previous section, putative pathogenic genes, if located in the mtDNA, are sustained by mutation-selection balance with heterozygote advantage. On the other hand, if located in the ncDNA, they should be sustained by mutation-selection balance without heterozygote advantage. In this section, we introduce our previous work (Doi et al., 2009), in which we carefully re-examined the necessary conditions for putative nuclear susceptibility genes for schizophrenia and deduced a criterion (persistence criterion, or 'P-criterion') that every nuclear susceptibility gene should fulfill for persistence of the disease, and present its applications to association studies for schizophrenia.

4.1 Three basic assumptions

At first we describe our three basic assumptions.

4.1.1 An ideal human population

We assume here a random-mating human population with a sufficiently large effective population size at equilibrium, where negative selection pressures on the susceptibility alleles for schizophrenia are predominant and the effect of genetic drift is negligibly small. The prevalence p of schizophrenia in this ideal human population is assumed to be stable across generations by mutation-selection balance. Therefore, the gene frequency in the general population (m_G) is given in terms of the gene frequencies in the affected population (m_A) and in the unaffected population (m_U):

$$m_G = pm_A + (1-p)m_U \text{ , or } m_A - m_G = (1-p)d \text{ . } d \equiv m_A - m_U \text{)} \quad (1)$$

4.1.2 Mutation-selection balance in each risk locus

We assume here that the total of the population frequencies of the pathogenic alleles at *each risk locus* is preserved by mutation-selection balance. Therefore, $-\Delta m_G$,the cross-generational reduction of the frequency of a pathogenic allele should not be more than the rate of mutations that produce pathogenic variants at the locus. On the other hand, since mutations at the locus include mutations of two directions that produce pathogenic or non-pathogenic variants, the mutation rate at the locus (μ) should be greater than the rate of mutations that produce pathogenic variants at the locus.

Thus we have:

$$\mu > -\Delta m_G . \quad (2)$$

4.1.3 Multifactorial threshold model

We assume the multifactorial threshold model, in which quantitative traits such as liability to the disease are determined by multiple genetic and non-genetic factors including a stochastic and/or an epigenetic effect. Under this assumption, the relative fitness as a quantitative trait in the affected population is determined by multiple factors and approximately follows a gamma distribution with a mean $(1-s)$. (s is the selection coefficient of schizophrenia; the mean relative fitness in the normal population is 1.)

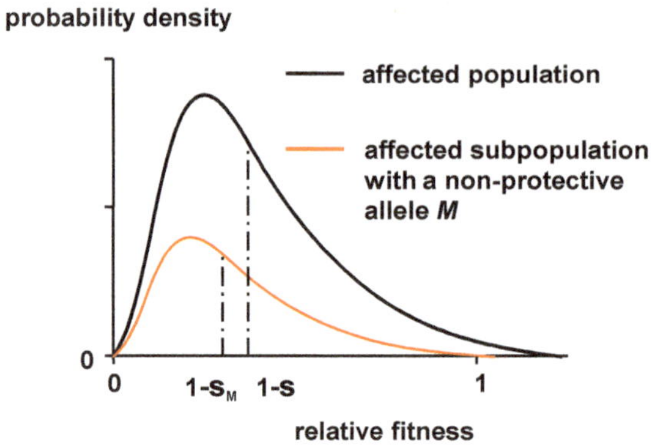

Fig. 2. Distribution curve of the reproductive fitness in the affected population

Distribution curve of the reproductive fitness in the affected subpopulation with a schizophrenia-associated allele M never shifts to the right unless M has a strong protective effect (i.e. an effect of elevating carrier's reproductive fitness by reducing severity of and liability to the disease). Therefore, we can assume that s_M, the selection coefficient in the affected subpopulation with a schizophrenia-associated allele M, is not smaller than s ($s \le s_M < 1$) for a susceptibility allele (**Fig. 2**). The inequality $s > s_M$ implies that M is a resistance gene that reduces severity and risk of the disease.

No special assumptions else are required on the allelic structure in each locus, penetrance of each susceptibility gene, and possible interactions among the loci.

4.2 Deduction of the P-criterion

Now we proceed to deduce the P-criterion. From the assumptions, m'_G, the population frequency of the schizophrenia-associated allele M in the next generation, is given by:

$$m'_G = \frac{p \cdot m_A \cdot (1-s_A) + (1-p) \cdot m_U \cdot 1}{p \cdot (1-s_M) + (1-p) \cdot 1} = \frac{m_G - s_M p m_A}{1 - s_M p}.$$

Therefore the reduction of the population frequency of the schizophrenia-associated allele M per generation is:

$$-\Delta m_G = m_G - m'_G = \frac{s_M p (m_A - m_G)}{1 - s_M p} = p(1-p)d \cdot \frac{s_M}{1 - s_M p}. \quad (3)$$

From (2) and (3) we have:

$$\mu > p(1-p)d \cdot \frac{s_M}{1-s_M p} \quad (4)$$

Since $\frac{s_M}{1-s_M p}$ is monotonically increasing for s_M ($0 < s_M < 1$) and $s \le s_M < 1$ holds for the susceptibility allele M, we have:

$$\mu > p(1-p)d \cdot \frac{s}{1-sp}, \text{ or } \frac{(1-sp)\mu}{(1-p)sp} > d. \quad (5)$$

On the other hand, the principle of association studies demands: $0 < d$.

Thus we have the criterion for a susceptibility gene:

$$0 < d < \nu, \text{ where } \nu \text{ is defined as } \nu \equiv \frac{(1-sp)\mu}{(1-p)sp}. \quad (6)$$

From the observation (5), we can see that $d \ge \nu$ implies $s > s_M$ for any schizophrenia-associated variant M which is sustained by mutation-selection balance.

4.3 Parameter estimate for schizophrenia

Mutation rates on autosomes and the X chromosome almost always fall within the range between 10^{-6} and 10^{-4} per locus per generation (usually < 10^{-5}; one generation = 20 years) (Nachman & Crowell, 2000) and can be approximated by a linear function of the parental age at least under 30 years for maternal age and under 40 years for paternal age (Risch et al., 1987). Large-sampled cohort studies in Israel, Sweden and Denmark show that the mean age of parents in the general population is ~ 28 years for mothers and ~31 years for fathers; the mean age of both parents is < 29.6 years (Malaspina et al., 2001; El-Saadi et al., 2004). Therefore we assume here:

$$10^{-6} < \mu < \frac{29.6}{20} \times 10^{-4} = 1.48 \times 10^{-4}.$$

According to the epidemiological data by Haukka et al. (2003), the estimated values for p and s are $p = 1.29 \times 10^{-2}$ and $s = 6.54 \times 10^{-1}$. Therefore, we have $\nu = 1.76 \times 10^{-3}$ for the average mutation rate (1.48×10^{-5}), $\nu = 1.76 \times 10^{-2}$ for the highest mutation rate (1.48×10^{-4}), and $\nu = 1.76 \times 10^{-4}$ for a relatively low mutation rate (1.48×10^{-6}).

4.4 Implications for association studies of schizophrenia

We present here some applications of the P-criterion to association studies of schizophrenia. The results suggest that common disease/common variant hypothesis is unlikely to fit schizophrenia and that an enormous sample size is required to detect a nuclear susceptibility gene for schizophrenia.

4.4.1 Calculation of an upper bound of the effect size of a putative susceptibility gene of a given frequency

Using the P-criterion, we can calculate an upper bound of the effect size of a putative susceptibility gene of a given frequency.

Effects size of a susceptibility gene M is expressed by odds ratio defined as

$$OR = \frac{m_A(1-m_U)}{(1-m_A)m_U},$$

which is monotonically increasing for m_A and monotonically decreasing for m_U. Since the criterion demands $m_U < m_A < m_U + \nu$, we have

$$\frac{m_U(1-m_U)}{(1-m_U)m_U} < OR < \frac{(m_U+\nu)(1-m_U)}{(1-m_U-\nu)m_U}, \text{ or } 1 < OR < 1 + \frac{\nu}{m_U(1-\nu-m_U)} \quad (7)$$

for $0 < m_U < 1-\nu$.

And since the criterion demands $m_A - \nu < m_U$, we have

$$1 < OR < \frac{m_A(1-m_A+\nu)}{(1-m_A)(m_A-\nu)} = 1 + \frac{\nu}{(1-m_A)(m_A-\nu)} \quad (8)$$

for $1-\nu \le m_U < 1$.

Thus, we have an upper bound of the effect size for a given frequency.

From the above we can easily see that the common disease/ common variant hypothesis, which proposes that common alleles at a handful of loci interact to cause a common disease, is unlikely to fit schizophrenia. No common alleles with population frequency between 0.05 and 0.95 can have large effects for schizophrenia: the odds ratio of every common risk allele is less than 1.04 for the average mutation rate, less than 1.58 for the highest mutation rate, and less than 1.004 for a relatively low mutation rate (**Table 1**).

4.4.2 Calculation of range of the frequency of a putative susceptibility gene of a given effect size

By solving the inequality (7) or (8), we can estimate the range of gene frequency for a given effect size. Thus, we can see that susceptibility genes of the average mutation rate and a moderate effect that meet the criterion are limited to 'very rare variants' or 'very common variants'. For example, suppose $\mu = 1.48 \times 10^{-5}$ and *OR*=5.0, then we have: $\nu = 1.76 \times 10^{-2}$ and

$$4 < \frac{\nu}{m_U(1-\nu-m_U)}.$$

Solving this inequality, we get either $0 < m_U < 0.00044$ (that is, $0 < m_A < m_U + 0.00176 < 0.0022$) or $m_U > 0.9977$.

m_U	$\mu = 1.48 \times 10^{-6}$	$\mu = 1.48 \times 10^{-5}$	$\mu = 1.48 \times 10^{-4}$
0.01	< 1.02	< 1.18	< 2.81
0.02	< 1.009	< 1.09	< 1.92
0.05	< 1.004	< 1.04	< 1.38
0.1	< 1.002	< 1.02	< 1.20
0.3	< 1.0009	< 1.009	< 1.09
0.5	< 1.0008	< 1.008	< 1.08
0.7	< 1.0009	< 1.009	< 1.09
0.9	< 1.002	< 1.02	< 1.24
0.95	< 1.004	< 1.04	< 1.58
0.98	< 1.009	< 1.10	< 8.49

Table 1. Upper bounds of odds ratio for given allele frequencies in the unaffected population

4.4.3 Calculation of the required sample size and the power of an association study

Using the P-criterion we can calculate a lower bound of sample size required in an association study of a given power as well as an upper bound of the power of an association study of a given sample size.

Concerning the required sample size $2N$ (N case-control pairs) and the power $1-\beta$ of an association study, we have the well-established formulae (Ohashi & Tokunaga, 2002):

$$N \cong \frac{1}{2}\left(\frac{z^*_\alpha \sqrt{2x(1-x)} + z_\beta \gamma}{d}\right)^2,$$

and

$$1-\beta \cong \Phi\left(\frac{\sqrt{2N}d - z^*_\alpha \sqrt{2x(1-x)}}{\gamma}\right).$$

Here, Φ, z^*_α, and z_β denote the cumulative distribution function of the standard normal curve, the two sided a point (a: a significant level) and the upper β point of the standard normal curve, and x (population frequency of the allele) and γ^2 are defined as follows.

$$x \equiv \frac{1}{2}(m_A + m_U) \qquad \gamma^2 \equiv m_A(1-m_A) + m_U(1-m_U) = 2x(1-x) - \frac{1}{2}d^2$$

For the average mutation rate $\mu = 1.48 \times 10^{-5}$, we have $\nu = 1.76 \times 10^{-3}$. Suppose $0.0005 < x < 0.9995$, then we have $2x(1-x) > 0.9995 \times 10^{-3}$. From the P-criterion, we have:

$$\frac{1}{2}d^2 < \frac{1}{2}\nu^2 < 1.6 \times 10^{-6} < 2x(1-x) \times 0.002.$$

Therefore, we have the following approximation with an error smaller than 0.2 %:

$$\gamma^2 = 2x(1-x) - \frac{1}{2}d^2 \cong 2x(1-x) \text{, or } \gamma \cong \sqrt{2x(1-x)} .$$

Thus, we have:

$$N \cong \frac{1}{2}\left(\frac{z^*_\alpha \sqrt{2x(1-x)} + z_\beta \gamma}{d}\right)^2 \cong \left(\frac{z^*_\alpha + z_\beta}{d}\right)^2 x(1-x) > \left(\frac{z^*_\alpha + z_\beta}{\nu}\right)^2 x(1-x)$$

$$1-\beta \cong \Phi\left(\frac{\sqrt{2N}d - z^*_\alpha \sqrt{2x(1-x)}}{\gamma}\right) \cong \Phi\left(\sqrt{\frac{N}{x(1-x)}}d - z^*_\alpha\right) < \Phi\left(\sqrt{\frac{N}{x(1-x)}}\nu - z^*_\alpha\right).$$

Let us calculate the required sample size in a genome-wide association study ($\alpha = 2.5 \times 10^{-7}$, $1-\beta = 0.95$). Since we have $z^*_{0.00000025} + z_{0.05} = 6.79$,

$$N > \left(\frac{z^*_\alpha + z_\beta}{\nu}\right)^2 x(1-x) = \left(\frac{6.79}{1.76 \times 10^{-3}}\right)^2 x(1-x) = 3.72 \times 10^6$$

for $x = 0.5$. Therefore, more than 3.7 million case-control pairs are required in a genome-wide association study with a power 0.95 to detect a susceptibility variant of the average mutation rate and a population frequency between 0.0005 and 0.9995.

Similarly we can see that more than 37,000 case-control pairs are required in a genome-wide association study with a power 0.95 to detect a susceptibility variant of the highest mutation rate ($\mu = 1.48 \times 10^{-4}$) and a population frequency between 0.005 and 0.995.

Finally, let us consider the case with a relatively low mutation rate $\mu = 1.48 \times 10^{-6}$, which corresponds to $\nu = 1.76 \times 10^{-4}$. In this case, more than 370 million case-control pairs are required in a genome-wide association study with a power 0.95 to detect a susceptibility variant of a population frequency between 0.000005 and 0.999995. Therefore it would take more than several hundred years to gather the required number of samples even if all of the affected individuals in the world were to be recruited to the study.

5. Mitochondrial DNA (mtDNA) hypothesis of schizophrenia

In this final section, we discuss on the nature of those schizophrenia-associated genes that do not meet the P-criterion, suggesting that these genes should be resistance genes that reduce the morbid risk and severity of the disease. We show that the results of association studies to date is compatible with the mitochondrial genome model but not with the nuclear genome model and propose a new hypothesis which assumes that the risk loci are in the mtDNA. We present eight major predictions of this hypothesis, and discuss that these predictions seem to accord with the other epidemiological findings and the results of the genetic and the pathophysiological studies to date.

5.1 Nature of schizophrenia-associated genes that do not meet the P-criterion

Now, let us consider the nature of those schizophrenia-associated genes that do not meet the persistence criterion. The inequality $d \geq \nu$ implies $s_M < s$, where s_M and s denote the selection coefficient in the affected subpopulation with an allele M and in the affected population respectively. Therefore, such genes, if sustained by mutation-selection balance, cannot be susceptibility genes but resistance genes that reduce severity and risk of the disease (see 4.2). If they were not resistance genes, their frequencies in the affected population must have been reduced to the same level in the unaffected population.

5.2 The results of association studies to date accord with the mitochondrial genome model but not with the nuclear genome model

Since a resistance gene in the nuclear genome model cannot be associated with the disease unless it is linked with a susceptibility gene, resistance genes in the nuclear model should be located in the vicinity of susceptibility genes, which disagrees with the results of association studies to date.

For example, on the chromosome 1, all of the schizophrenia-associated genes that could meet the criterion (*RGS4, PLXNA2, DISC1*) are located on 1q, while four resistance genes (*MHTFR, GRIK3, PDE4B, GSTM1*) are on 1p (**Table 2**). Fifteen resistance genes are located on 2q, 5q, 7q, 10q, 11p, 12p, 12q, 13p, 13q, 16p, 17p, and 19q, where no schizophrenia-associated variants that could meet the criterion are located (data: not shown). Therefore, the results of association studies to date argue against the nuclear genome model.

A possible interpretation which accords with the nuclear genome model might be that many nuclear susceptibility genes of less than the highest mutation rates have not been detected by association studies to date due to lack of power. In this case, however, an enormous sample size (more than 3.7~370 million case-control pairs) would be required to identify them as was mentioned above. In other words, such an enormous sample size is required to prove the nuclear genome model.

On the other hand, every resistance gene on *any* chromosome can be associated with schizophrenia in the mitochondrial genome model; since mtDNA is transmitted only via females and there is no link between the nuclear genome and the mitochondrial genome, every nuclear genome which interacts with a pathogenic mitochondrial genome to alter severity and risk of the disease is subject to natural selections in the predisposed maternal lineage that succeeds to a same pathogenic mitochondrial genome. Therefore, every resistance gene for schizophrenia in the mitochondrial genome model is to be subject to a positive selection in the predisposed maternal lineage, thereby associating with schizophrenia.

Thus, the mitochondrial genome model is compatible with the results of the association studies to date.

It should be noted that in the mitochondrial genome model every facilitating gene (a gene that increases the severity and morbid risk in the predisposed population) on any chromosome may diminish in the predisposed matrilineal pedigrees by negative selection, thereby negatively associating with the disease.

Schizophrenia-associated variants listed in the top 45 in the SZGene Database (the version of 10th December, 2010) were selected. Based on the genotype distributions in meta-analyses, allele frequencies and the case-control differences were calculated. 4 variants at the 3 loci (*RGS4, PLXNA2, DISC1*) could meet the criterion under the assumption that the mutation rates at those loci are near the upper limit in the autosomes. All of them are located on 1q, while 4 resistance genes (*MHTFR, GRIK3, PDE4B, GSTM1*) are on 1p. * schizophrenia-associated alleles; variants that could meet the criterion are shown in bold characters

Genes and SNPs	Location	Allele (minor/major)	m_A	m_U	*OR*	*d*
MHTFR	1p36.22					
rs1801133		T*/C	0.3532	0.3211	1.15	0.032
GRIK3	1p34.3					
rs6691840		G*/T	0.2600	0.2226	1.25	0.037
PDE4B	1p31.3					
rs910694		C/T*	0.5780	0.5477	1.30	0.030
GSTM1	1p13.3					
GSTM1*0		ins-allele/del-allele*	0.7546	0.7140	1.35	0.041
RGS4	**1q23.3**					
rs2661319		A/**G***	0.4920	0.4744	**1.08**	**0.0176**
IL10	1q32.1					
rs1800896		G*/A	0.3056	0.2657	1.42	0.040
PLXNA2	**1q32.2**	A/G				
rs841865		A/G*	0.8434	0.8001	1.32	0.043
rs1327175		G/**C***	0.92840	0.91243	1.32	**0.016**
DISC1	**1q42.3**					
rs3737597		**A***/G	0.03069	0.01735	1.80	**0.013**
rs999710		**A***/G	0.3989	0.3819	1.07	**0.0170**

Table 2. Schizophrenia-associated genes on the chromosome 1 that could meet the criterion

5.3 The mtDNA hypothesis for schizophrenia and its predictions

Thus we propose here a new hypothesis which insists that the risk loci for schizophrenia are in the mtDNA.

Mitochondria are involved in a variety of major cellular events such as oxidative phosphorylation, free radical production and Ca^{2+} buffering, and play an active role in apoptosis. They possess two classes of antioxidant defense system (non-enzymatic and enzymatic), and structurally and functionally intact mitochondria serve as a *net sink* rather than a *net source* of reactive oxygen species (ROS) (Andreyev et al., 2005). ROS-defenses are severely undermined in structurally compromised mitochondria (Andreyev et al., 2005). Thus, mitochondrial dysfunction, presumably through imbalance of ROS production and removal (Andreyev et al., 2005), raises ROS emission (Esposito et al., 1999; Senoo-Matsuda et al., 2001) and causes intracellular oxidative stress.

Because abnormal mtDNA may cause mitochondrial dysfunction, the hypothesis predicts: (1) enhanced oxidative stress and disturbed energy metabolism in predisposed individuals, which may cause various pathogenic alterations such as genomic instability, aberrations in neurodevelopment, and the brain dysfunction. Furthermore, because mtDNA can be transmitted only through females and there is no link between the nuclear genome and the mitochondrial genome, the mtDNA hypothesis predicts: (2) a higher maternal transmission of schizophrenia, and (3) positive associations between resistance genes and schizophrenia as well as negative associations between facilitating genes and schizophrenia (see 5.2). These predictions seem to be consistent with other major epidemiological findings and the results of the genetic and the pathophysiological studies to date.

5.3.1 Mitochondrial dysfunction and enhanced oxidative stress in affected individuals

The hypothesis predicts that patients with schizophrenia show mitochondrial dysfunction and enhanced oxidative stress.

Indeed, in the past decade, mitochondrial dysfunction and oxidative stress in schizophrenia has been suggested by several independent lines of evidence (for review, see Marchbanks et al., 1995; Ben-Shaffer, 2002; Wood et al., 2009); those include mitochondrial hypoplasia, disturbed oxidative phosphorylation, and altered mitochondrial-related gene expression in several cell lines.

The pioneering works in this field may be noteworthy (Utena & Niwa, 1992). As early as 1950, Hayashi, in a longitudinal study on glucose metabolites in blood sampled from the superior bulb of the internal jugular vein of schizophrenics, observed a decreased carbonic dioxide production in the brain and a higher level of lactate and glutathione, the brain's dominant free radical scavenger, in patients in an acute exacerbation of the illness. Utena and Ezoe (1951) reported a decreased glucose consumption *in vitro* in cortical brain tissues sampled from patients with schizophrenia who underwent prefrontal leukotomy. Takahashi (1953) confirmed this finding and emphasized the necessity of further investigations on oxidative phosphorylation in the brain tissue of schizophrenics. In line with those findings was the report by Stabenau et al. (1969), who observed, in a biochemical study of discordant monozygotic twin pairs, that lactate production and the lactate-pyruvate ratio were higher in the affected twins than the unaffected cotwins. More recently, Prabakaran et al. (2004), in a large-scale functional genomics study, suggested a state of intermittent or chronic hypoxic stress and mitochondrial dysfunction in the brain of patients with schizophrenia.

5.3.2 The mode of transmission

The hypothesis predicts a higher maternal transmission of schizophrenia. Although there has been no convincing evidence for maternal transmission of schizophrenia, several reports suggest a higher maternal transmission of schizophrenia (Shimizu et al., 1987; Goldstein et al., 1990; Valero et al., 1998; Li et al., 2007).

Some researchers have proposed the hypothesis that schizophrenia is associated with *de novo* mutations arising in paternal germ cells (Malaspina et al., 2001; Zammit et al., 2003; Byrne et al., 2003; El-Saadi et al., 2004; Sipos et al., 2004). It is based on the observation ('paternal age effect') that the risk of schizophrenia in the offspring seems to increase as the paternal age advances from 20 years to over 50 years.

However, the difference in the mean ages of fathers between affected and unaffected individuals are not very large (< 1.7 years) (Malaspina et al., 2001; El-Saadi et al., 2004). Furthermore, the risk of schizophrenia was also increased in the offspring of younger men

(< 21 years) (Malaspina et al., 2001; El-Saadi et al., 2004; Sipos et al., 2004) as well as in the offspring of younger women (< 20 years) (El-Saadi et al., 2004). Therefore, major roles of paternally derived mutations in schizophrenia seem to remain unsubstantiated.

Indeed, no available data can exclude the possibility that the 'paternal age effect' has a 'maternal origin'; while women in many countries today may be usually supposed to bear children after the age of 20 years and not to marry much older men or too young men unless the men have special socio-economic benefits, a certain proportion of predisposed women might behave differently.

It should be noted that in the famous twin study by Gottesman and Bertelsen (1989) which included almost equal number of male and female monozygotic twins, most schizophrenic twins whose offspring are affected are females (12 out of 14), implying that the transmission was mainly via females ($p = {}_{14}C_{12} \times 0.5^{14} + {}_{14}C_{13} \times 0.5^{14} + {}_{14}C_{14} \times 0.5^{14} < 0.007$). While this gender effect might be due to non-genetic factors such as stronger psychological interactions between mother and child, we must also consider the possibility that it is due to the closer genetic relationship between mother and child, i.e. the mtDNA.

5.3.3 Sex difference and a protective effect of estrogen in schizophrenia

The hypothesis predicts that endogenous antioxidants exhibit a protective effect against schizophrenia, and may give a plausible explanation for sex difference of the disease.

A consistent and specific finding for schizophrenia is that the age at onset is significantly lower in males than in females (Jablensky, 1995; Kulkarni & Fink, 2000); schizophrenia starts earlier on average in males and reaches its peak between 15 and 25 years of age, whereas in females it occurs almost between 20 and 30 years of age and shows a less steep curve after that age. It also appears that women are vulnerable to relapses or first episode of schizophrenia in the perimenoposal period (the second peak of onset for females) (Kulkarni & Fink, 2000), when estrogen production diminishes. A close association between premenstrual or menstruation phase and exacerbation of the illness in females has been well documented (Kulkarni & Fink, 2000). In addition, less negative symptoms, less brain morphological changes, and better response to neuroleptic medication are relatively consistent finding in female patients with schizophrenia (Jablensky, 1995; Goldstein & Lewine, 2000).

These observations lead to the concept that estrogen protects predisposed females (Kulkarni & Fink, 2000), which seems to accord with the hypothesis; estrogen has been shown to have antioxidant activity due to its intrinsic antioxidant structure that lies in the phenolic moiety of the steroidal compound (Behl, 2002), to increase antioxidant enzyme activities (Strehlow et al., 2003; Pajović et al., 2003), and to have neuroprotective effect against oxidative stress (Behl, 2002; Brann et al., 2007). Furthermore, mitochondrion has estrogen binding sites (Monje & Boland, 2001; Chen et al., 2004) and estrogen increases mitochondrial efficiency and reduces intracellular oxidative stress (Stirone et al, 2005).

5.3.4 Low comorbidity between schizophrenia and rheumatoid arthritis

The hypothesis predicts that diseases predisposed by facilitating genes, if present, would be negatively associated with schizophrenia. Rheumatoid arthritis could be one of such candidates.

A role of oxidative stress in the pathogenesis of rheumatoid arthritis has been suggested by several lines of evidence (for review, see Hitchon et al, 2004). In addition, it has been shown that chronic oxidative stress in the synovial T lymphocytes is not secondary to exposure to environmental free radicals but originates from intracellularly produced reactive oxygen species (Remans et al, 2005). Therefore, a presumptive susceptibility gene for rheumatoid arthritis, which may cause intracellular oxidative stress in several cell lines, could be a facilitating gene for schizophrenia in this model and is likely to be subject to a negative selection in the predisposed matrilineal pedigrees.

Indeed, robust evidence shows a negative association between schizophrenia and rheumatoid arthritis while the exact mechanism is still unknown (Vinogradov et al., 1991; Jablensky, 1995; Rubinstein, 1997; Oken 1999). According to the nuclear genome model, several hypotheses have been proposed such that pathogenic genes for schizophrenia may be protective genes for rheumatoid arthritis and vice versa.

Thus the mitochondrial genome model may offer a new explanation for the low comorbidity between schizophrenia and rheumatoid arthritis and the additional prediction: most of patients with both of the diseases would be females because the survival rate of males in early life stage must be remarkably reduced due to lack of the antioxidant defense by estrogen, and show more negative symptoms, poorer response to neuroleptic medication, and/or more morphological changes in the brain.

5.3.5 Prenatal risk factors for schizophrenia

The hypothesis predicts that early-life exposure to environments which induce strong oxidative stress can increase the risk of later development of schizophrenia in the predisposed population.

Indeed, prenatal environmental factors such as severe nutritional deficiency (Susser, et al., 1996), exposure to increased homocysteine (Brown et al., 2007) or lead (Opler & Susser, 2005), and infection of influenza virus (Limosin et al., 2003; Brown et al., 2004; Opler & Susser, 2005) and Toxoplasma gondii (Brown et al., 2005) have been suggested to increase the risk for schizophrenia. More recently, it has been suggested that central nervous system infections of cytomegalovirus or mumps virus in childhood may also increase the risk for schizophrenia (Dalman et al., 2008). All of these factors have been shown to affect mitochondria, inducing strong intracellular oxidative stress and/or apoptosis (Akaike et al., 1990; Edlund et al., 1994; Speir et al., 1998; He et al., 2003; Berger et al., 2004; Zaki et al., 2005; Gupta et al., 2004; Kruman et al., 2006; Wang et al., 2006; Poncet et al., 2006; Chang et al., 2007; Nishikawa et al., 2007).

5.3.6 Increased obstetric complications in the birth of patients with schizophrenia

It has been suggested that mitochondrial dysfunction may be involved in the etiology of preeclampsia (Shanklin et al., 1990; Barton et al., 1991; Furui et al., 1994). In addition, a high incidence of preeclampsia, eclampsia, and stillborn infants has been observed in a family with a known mitochondrial disorder (Torbergsen et al. 1989). Folgero et al. (1996) demonstrated two separate mtDNA point mutations in two families having a high incidence of preeclampsia and eclampsia.

Therefore, the hypothesis predicts that the risk of preeclampsia, eclampsia, or stillbirth may be increased in the birth of patients with schizophrenia as well as in the pregnancies of women with schizophrenia. Indeed, an excess of stillbirths and neonatal deaths among women with schizophrenia has been reported by several investigators (Sobel, 1961; Rieder et al., 1975; Modrzewska, 1980; Webb et al., 2005).

Furthermore, there has been a body of evidence for an increased risk of obstetric complications in the birth of patients with schizophrenia (Dalman et al., 1999; Cannon et al., 2002). A meta-analysis of population-based data (Cannon et al., 2002) found significant estimates for three main categories of obstetric complications: (1) complications of pregnancies, (2) abnormal fetal growth and development, and (3) complications in delivery. Among all, preeclampsia was the strongest individual risk factor detected in the largest single population-based cohort study to date (Dalman et al., 1999).

Although obstetrical events in schizophrenia are often considered as having a direct causative effect, none of the available data can refute the hypothesis that they are merely markers of some other causal process (Rapoport et al., 2005), such as mitochondrial dysfunction which is implicated in this hypothesis.

5.3.7 An apparent signature of positive selection in schizophrenia-associated genes

Since the positive selection of the schizophrenia-associated alleles mentioned above occurs only in the predisposed matrilineal pedigrees, a ubiquitous subpopulation in humans, frequencies of those alleles may not be so high in the general population as if the selection had occurred *recently* in the general population.

Thus, the hypothesis predicts that every schizophrenia-associated nuclear gene shows an apparent signature as if it had been subject to a positive selection in the recent evolutionary history of humans. Recent two reports (Lo et al, 2007; Crespi et al., 2007) seem to be in line with this prediction.

On the other hand, the nuclear genome model predicts that every schizophrenia-associated nuclear gene shows an apparent signature of negative selection due to the strong negative selection pressure.

5.3.8 Genomic instability

It is generally thought that a major cause of DNA damage that leads to mutations is reactive oxygen species, which are generated as a normal part of oxygen metabolism but are also produced by ionising radiation, metabolism of exogenous compounds (Hussain et al., 2003; Finkel, 2003). It has been shown that endogenous mitochondrial oxidative stress can induce many types of DNA damage including double strand breaks, end-to-end fusions, base and sugar modifications, DNA-protein cross-links, and gross chromosomal rearrangements (Ragu et al., 2007; Samper et al., 2003).

Therefore, the hypothesis predicts that the enhanced oxidative stress may cause genomic instability during meiosis and/or early phase of ontogeny, producing increased rates of random point mutations and/or structural variants of the nuclear genome in the predisposed population. In addition, genomic instability may be more pronounced in males due to lack of antioxidant protection by estrogen.

There have been numerous reports of associations between schizophrenia and chromosomal abnormalities including fragile sites, reciprocal translocations, inversions, insertions, deletions, disomy and trisomy in many autosomes, and sex chromosome aneuploidies (Macintyre et al, 2003). However, with an exception of 22q11 deletion, none of these have been consistently replicated, and with another exception of (1,11) (q42;q14.3) balanced translocation, none provides convincing evidence for the location of a 'susceptibility' gene (Kirov et al., 2005).

A popular explanation in the nuclear genome model may be that most of these structural variants are coincidental findings of no clinical significance. Alternatively, those alterations may indicate genomic instability in schizophrenia. An increased risk of schizophrenia in individuals with 22q11 deletion (Pulver et al., 1994; Murphy et al., 1999) might be due to haplodeficiency of presumptive resistance genes of gain-of-function type and/or presumptive facilitating genes of loss-of-function type aggregated on 22q11.

More recently, it has been reported that rare structural variants such as microdeletions or microduplications of sizes ranging from 100kb to 15MB throughout the genome are more frequent among individuals with schizophrenia than unaffected individuals (Walsh et al., 2008). While many of those structural variants duplicate or delete genes in neurodevelopmental pathways, one third of those do not disrupt genes, leaving their role in causation of the disease unwarranted. Another recent report (Xu et al., 2008) has shown that *de novo* copy number mutations are increased in sporadic schizophrenia. However, the cytobands of those copy number mutations are diverse among the affected individuals and their roles in the pathogenesis still remain unclear. Therefore, no available data can refute the possibility that those structural variants and copy number mutations are not the causes of schizophrenia but the results of the genomic instability in schizophrenia predicted by our hypothesis.

Indeed, direct measure of the de novo mutation rates shows an increased mutation rate in schizophrenia (Awadalla et al., 2010), and genomic and epigenomic instability has been suggested in schizophrenia (Smith et al., 2010). Furthermore, it has been shown that blood cells from patients with schizophrenia present a higher rate of folate-sensitive fragile sites, and that male patients exhibit twice as many fragile sites as females while there are no age effects (Demirhan et al., 2006). This sex difference may indicate that increased fragile sites expression (genomic instability) is the results of enhanced oxidative stress in patients with schizophrenia.

6. Conclusion

Genetic research of schizophrenia based on the nuclear genome model has been one of the most active areas in psychiatry for the past two decades. Although this effort is ongoing, results of association studies have been inconsistent and the situation of molecular genetics of schizophrenia today has become much confused just contrary to our expectation. The consistent major epidemiological findings of schizophrenia, coupled with the results of association studies to date, argue against the nuclear genome model for schizophrenia.

Rather, they seem to argue in favor of the mitochondrial genome model, suggesting a necessity of paradigm shift from the nuclear genome model to the mitochondrial genome model in genetic research of schizophrenia in the coming years.

Note: Cross-generational reduction of females with pathogenic genes in the mitochondrial genome model

At first we define several notations. N_1: the number of normal females in the first generation; N_2: number of female offspring of normal females; S_1: the number of unaffected female siblings of patients in the first generation; S_2: the number of female offspring of unaffected female siblings of patients; P_1: the number of female patients; P_2: the number of female offspring of female patients; r ($0 < r < 1$): the proportion of gene carriers in normal females in the first generation. Then the number of female gene carriers in the first generation is ($rN_1 + S_1 + P_1$) and the frequency of female gene carriers in the first generation is given by:

$$f_1 = \frac{rN_1 + S_1 + P_1}{N_1 + S_1 + P_1} = r + \frac{S_1 + P_1}{N_1 + S_1 + P_1} \cdot (1 - r) .$$

And the frequency of female gene carriers in the second generation is given by:

$$f_2 = \frac{rN_2 + S_2 + P_2}{N_2 + S_2 + P_2} = r + \frac{S_2 + P_2}{N_2 + S_2 + P_2} \cdot (1 - r) .$$

Thus we have (**Table 3**):

$$-\Delta = f_1 - f_2 = \left(\frac{S_1 + P_1}{N_1 + S_1 + P_1} - \frac{S_2 + P_2}{N_2 + S_2 + P_2} \right) \times (1 - r) < 5.06 \times 10^{-3} .$$

	N	S	P	Total	$(S+P)/\text{Total}$
# of females	410,093	11,873	4,784	426,750	0.03903
# of female children	366,460	10,969	1,917	379,346	0.03397
$-\Delta$					$0.00506 \times (1 - r) < 5.06 \times 10^{-3}$

Table 3. Epidemiological data by Haukka et al. (2003)

In this largest-sampled cohort study to date, Haukka et al. comprised all births in Finland during 1950-1959 (N=870,093) and followed up through the National Hospital Discharge Register for Hospitalizations between 1969 and 1992. N: normal females; S: unaffected female siblings of patients; P: female patients with schizophrenia

7. References

Akaike, T., Ando, M., Oda, T., Doi, T., Ijiri, S., Araki, S. & Maeda, H. (1990). Dependence on O_2^- generation by xanthine oxidase of pathogenesis of influenza infection in mice. *J Clin Invest*, Vol. 85, (Mar 1990), pp. 739-745, ISSN 0021-9738

Allen, N.C., Bagades, S., McQueen, M.B., Ioannidis, J.P.A., Kavvoura, F.K., Khoury, M.J., Tanzi, R.E. & Bertram, L. (2008). Systematic Meta-Analyses and Field Synopsis of Genetic Association Studies in Schizophrenia: The SZGene Database. *Nat Genet*, Vol. 40, No. 7, (July 2008), pp. 827-834, ISSN 1061-4036 http://www.schizophreniaforum.org/res/szgene/default.asp

Andreyev, A.Y., Kushnareva, Y.E. & Starkov, A.A. (2005). Mitochondrial metabolism of reactive oxygen species. *Biocemistry (Moscow)*, Vol. 70, No. 2, (Feb 2005), pp. 200-214, ISSN 0006-2979

Awadalla, P., Gauthier, .J, Myers, R.A., Casals, F., Hamdan, F.F., Griffing, A.R., Côté, M., Henrion, E., Spiegelman, D., Tarabeux, J., Piton, A., Yang, Y., Boyko, A., Bustamante, C., Xiong, L., Rapoport, J.L., Addington, A.M., DeLisi, J.L.E., Krebs, M-O., Joober, R., Millet, B., Fombonne, É., Mottron, L., Zilversmit, M., Keebler, J., Daoud, H., Marineau, C., Roy-Gagnon, M-H., Dubé, M-P., Eyre-Walker, A., Drapeau, P., Stone, E.A., Lafrenière, R.G., Rouleau, G.A. (2010). Direct measure of the de novo mutation rate in autism and schizophrenia cohorts. *Am J Hum Genet* Vol. 87, No. 3, (Sep 2010), pp.316–324, ISSN 0002-9297

Barton, J.R., Hiett, A.K., O'Connor, W.M., Nissen, S.E. & Greene, J.W. (1991). Endomyocardial ultrastructural findings in preeclampsia. *Am J Obstet Gynecol*, Vol. 165, No. 2, (Aug 1991), pp. 389-391, ISSN 0002-9378

Bassett, A.S., Bury, A., Hodgkinson, K.A. & Honer, W.G. (1996). Reproductive fitness in familial schizophrenia. *Schizophr Res*, Vol. 21, No. 3, (Sep 1996), pp. 151-160, ISSN 0920-9964

Behl, C. (2002). Oestrogen as a neuroprotective hormones. *Nat Rev Neurosci*, Vol. 3, No. 6 , (Jun 2002),pp. 433-442, ISSN 1471-003X

Ben-Shachar, D. (2002). Mitochondrial dysfunction in schizophrenia: a possible linkage to dopamine. *J Neurochemistry*, Vol. 83, No. 6, (Dec 2002), pp. 1241-1251, ISSN 1471-4159

Berger, M.M., Jia, X.Y., Legay, V., Aymard, M., Tilles, J.G. & Lina, B. (2004). Nutrition- and virus-induced stress repress the expression of manganese superoxide dismutase *in vitro*. *Exp Biol Med*, Vol. 229, No. 8, (Sep 2004), pp. 843-849, ISSN 1535-3702

Böök, J.A. (1953). A genetic and neuropsychiatric investigation of a North-Swedish population. *Acta Genet et Stat Med*, Vo. 4, No. 1, (Jan 1953), pp. 1-100, ISSN 0576-7440

Brann, D.W., Dhandapani, K., Wakade, C., Mahesh, V.B. & Khan, M. (2007). Neurotrophic and neuroprotective actions of estrogen: basic mechanism and clinical implications. *Steroids*, Vol. 72, No. 5, (May 2007), pp. 381-405, ISSN 0039-128X

Brown, A.S., Begg, M.D., Gravenstein, S., Schaefer, C.A., Wyatt, R.J., Bresnahan, M., Babulas, V.P. & Susser, E.S. (2004). Serologic evidence of prenatal influenza in the etiology of schizophrenia. *Arch Gen Psychiatry*, Vol. 61, No. 8, (Aug 2002), pp. 774-780, ISSN 0003-990X

Brown, A.S., Shaefer, C.A., Quesenberry, Jr. C.P., Liu, L., Babulas, V.P. & Susser, E. (2005). Maternal exposure to toxoplasmosis and risk of schizophrenia in adult offspring. *Am J Psychiatry*, Vol. 162, No. 4, (Apr 2005), pp. 767-773, ISSN 0002-953X

Brown, A.S., Bottiglieri, T., Shaefer, C.A. , Quesenberry, Jr. C.P., Liu, L. Bresnahan, M. & Susser, E.S. (2007). Elevated prenatal homocysteine levels as a risk factor for schizophrenia. *Arch Gen Psychiatry*, Vol. 64, No. 1, (Jan 2007), pp. 31-39, ISSN 0003-990X

Brüne, M. (2004). Schizophrenia - an evolutionary enigma? *Neurosci Biobehav Rev*, Vol. 28, No. 1, (Mar 2004), pp. 41-53, ISSN 0149-7634

Bundy, H., Stahl, D. & McCabe, J.H. (2011). A systemic review and meta-analysis of the fertility of patients with schizophrenia and their unaffected relatives. *Acta Psychiatr Scand*, Vol. 123, No. 2, (Feb 2011), pp. 98-106, ISSN 1600-0447

Byrne, M., Agerbo, E., Ewald, H., Eaton, W.W. & Mortensen, P.B. (2003). Parental age risk of schizophrenia. A case-control study. *Arch Gen Psychiatry*, Vol. 60, No. 7, (Jul 2003), pp. 673-678, ISSN 0003-990X

Cannon, T.D., Kaprio, J., Lönnqvist, .J, Huttunen, M. & Koskenvuo, M. (1998). The genetic epidemiology of schizophrenia in a Finnish twin cohort. A population-based modeling study. *Arch Gen Psychiatry*, Vol. 55, No. 1, (Jan 1998), pp. 67-74, ISSN 0003-990X

Cannon, M., Jones, P.B. & Murray, R.M. (2002).Obstetric complications and schizophrenia: historical and meta-analytic review. *Am J Psychiatry*, Vol. 159, No. 7, (July 2002), pp. 1080-1092, ISSN 0002-953X

Cardno, A.G., Marshall, E.J., Coid, B., Macdonald, A.M., Ribchester, T.R., Davies, N.J., Venturi, P., Jones, L.A., Lewis, S.W., Sham, P.C., Gottesman, I.I., Farmer, A.E., McGuffin, P., Reveley, A.M. & Murray, R.M. (1999). Heritability estimates for psychotic disorders. Maudsley twin psychosis series. *Arch Gen Psychiatry*, Vol. 56, No.2 , (Feb 1999), pp. 162-168, ISSN 0003-990X

Chang, C.M., Yu, C.C., Lu, H.T., Chou, Y.F. & Huang, R.F. (2007). Folate deprivation promotes mitochondrial oxidative decay : DNA large deletions, cytochrome c oxidase dysfunction, membrane depolarisation and superoxide overproduction in rat liver. *Br J Nutr*, Vol. 97, No. 5, (May 2007), pp. 855-863, ISSN 0007-1145

Chen, J.Q., Delannoy, M., Cooke, C. & Yager, J.D. (2004). Mitochondrial localization of ERalpha and ERbeta in human MCF7 cells. *Am J Physiol Endocrinol Metab*, Vol. 286, No. 6, (Jun 2004), E1011-E1022, ISSN 0193-1849

Crepsi, B., Summers, K., Dorus, S. (2007). Adaptive evolution of genes underlying schizophrenia. *Proc R Soc B* 2007, Vol. 274, No. 1627, (Nov 2007), pp. 2801-2810, ISSN 1471-2954

Crow, T.J. (1995). A Darwinian approach to the origin of psychosis. *Brit J Psychiatry*, Vol. 167, No. 1, (July 1995), pp. 12-25, ISSN 0007-1250

Dalman, C., Allebeck, P., Gunnell, D., Harrison, G., Kristensson, K., Lewis, G., Lofving, S., Rasmussen, F., Wicks, S. & Karlsson, H. (2008). Infections in the CNS during childhood and the risk of subsequent psychotic illness: a cohort study of more than one million Swedish subjects. *Am J Psychiatry*, Vol. 165, No. 1, (Jan 2008), pp. 59-65, ISSN 0002-953X

Dalman, C., Allebeck, P., Cullberg, J., Grunewald, C. & Köster, M. (1999). Obstetric complications and the risk of schizophrenia. A longitudinal study of a national birth cohort. *Arch Gen Psychiatry*, Vo. 56, No. 3, (Mar 1999), pp. 234-240, ISSN 0003-990X

Demirhan, O., Tastemir, D. & Sertdemir, Y. (2006). Chromosomal fragile sites in schizophrenic patients. *Genetika*, Vol. 42, No. 7, (July 2006), pp. 985-92, ISSN 0016-6758

Doi, N., Hoshi, Y., Itokawa, M., Usui, C., Yoshikawa, T., & Tachikawa, H. (2009). Persistence criteria for susceptibility genes for schizophrenia - a discussion from an evolutionary view point. *PLoS One*, Vol. 4, No.11, (Nov 2009), e7799, ISSN 1932-6203

Edlund, C., Holmberg, K., Dallnen, G., Norrby, E. & Kristensson, K. (1994). Ubiquinone-10 protects neurons from virus-induced degenerations. *J Neurochem*, Vol. 63, No. 2, (Aug 1994), pp. 634-639, ISSN 1471-4159

El-Saadi, O., Pedersen, C.B., McNeil, T.F., Saha, S., Welham, J., O'Callaghan, E., Cantor-Graae, E., Chant, D., Mortensen, P.B. & McGrath, J. (2004). Paternal and maternal age as risk factors for psychosis: findings from Denmark, Sweden and Australia. *Schizophr Res*, Vol. 67, No. 2-3, (April 2004), pp. 227-236, ISSN 0920-9964

Erlenmeyer-Kimling, L. (1968). Mortality rates in the offspring of schizophrenic parents and a physiological advantage hypothesis. *Nature*, Vol. 5169, 220, (Nov 1968), pp. 798-800, ISSN 0028-0836

Esposito, L.A., Melov, S., Panov, A., Cottrell, B.A. & Wallace, D.C. (1999). Mitochondrial disease in mouse results in increased oxidative stress. *Proc Natl Acad Sci USA*, Vol. 96, No. 9, (Apr 1999), pp. 4820-4825, ISSN 0027-8424

Fãnanás, L. & Bertranpetit, J. (1995). Reproductive rates in families of schizophrenic patients in a case-control study. *Acta Psychiatr Scand*, Vol. 91, No. 3, (Mar 1995), pp. 202-204, ISSN 1600-0447

Finkel, T. (2003). Oxidant signals and oxidant stress. *Curr Opin Cell Biol*, Vol. 15, No.2 , (Apr 2003), pp. 247-254, ISSN 0955-0674

Folgero, T., Storbakk, N., Torbergsen, T. & Oian, P. (1996). Mutations in mitochondrial transfer ribonucleic acid genes in preeclampsia. *Am J Obstet Gynecol*, Vol. 174, No. 5, (May 1996), pp. 1626-1630, ISSN 0002-9378

Furui, T., Kurauchi, O., Tanaka, M., Mizutani, .S, Ozawa, T. & Tomoda, Y. (1994). Decrease in cytochrome c oxidase and cytochrome oxidase subunit I messenger RNA levels in preeclamptic pregnancies. *Obstet Gynecol*, Vol. 84, No. 2, (Aug 1994), 283-288, ISSN 0029-7844

Goldstein, J.M., Faraone, S.V. & Chen, W.J., Tolomiczencko, G.S. & Tsuang, M.T. (1990). Sex differences in the familial transmission of schizophrenia. *Br J Psychiatry*, Vol. 156, No. 6, (Jun 1990), pp. 819-826, ISSN 0007-1250

Goldstein, J.M. & Lewine, R.R.J. (2000). Overview of sex differences in schizophrenia: where have we been and where do we go from? In: *Women and schizophrenia*, Castle, D.L., McGrath, J. & Kulkarni, J. eds., pp. 111-143, Cambridge University Press, ISBN 978-0521786171, Cambridge

Gottesman, I.I. & Bertelsen, A. (1989). Confirming unexpressed genotypes for schizophrenia. Risks in the offspring of Fischer's Danish identical and fraternal discordant twins. *Arch Gen Psychiatry*, Vol. 46, No. 10, (Oct 1989), pp. 867-872, ISSN 0003-990X

Gottesman, I.I. (1991). *Schizophrenia Genesis; The Origin of Madness.* Freeman & Company, ISBN 978-0716721475, New York, NY

Gupta, P., Narang, M., Banerjee, B.D. & Basu, S. (2004). Oxidative stress in term small for gestational age neonates born to undernourished mothers: a case controlled study. *BMC Pediatrics*, Vol. 4, No. 4, (July 2004), pp. 14-20, ISSN 1471-2431

Harrison, G., Cooper, J.E. & Gancarczyk, R. (1991). Changes in the administrative incidence of schizophrenia. *Br J Psychiatry*, Vol. 159, No. 6, (Dec 1991), pp. 811-816, ISSN 0007-1250

Haukka, J., Suvisaari, J., & Lonnqvist, J. (2003). Fertility of patients with schizophrenia, their siblings, and the general population: a cohort study from 1950 to 1959 in Finland. *Am J Psychiatry*, Vol. 160, No. 3, (Mar 2003), pp. 460-463, ISSN 0002-953X

Hayashi, M. (1950). A study of schizophrenia. (in Japanese) *Psychiatr Neurol Japonica*, Vol. 51, No. 3, (Mar 1950), pp.193-245, ISSN 0033-2658

He, L., Perkins, G.A., Poblenz, A.T., Harris, J.B., Hung, M., Ellisman, M.H. & Fox, D.A. (2003). Bcl-x_L overexpression blocks bax-mediated mitochoncrial contact site formation and apoptosis in rod photoreceptors of lead-exposed mice. *Proc Natl Acd Sci USA*, Vol. 100, No. 3, (Feb 2003), pp. 1022-1027, ISSN 0027-8424

Hitchon, C.A. & El-Gabalawy, H.S. (2004). Oxidation in rheumatoid arthritis. *Arthritis Res Ther*,Vol. 6, No. 6, (Oct 2004), pp. 265-278, ISSN 1473-6362

Hussain, S.P., Hofseth, L.J. & Harris, C.C. (2003). Radical causes of cancer. *Nat Rev Cancer*, Vol. 3, No. 4, (Apr 2003), pp. 276-285, ISSN 1474-175X

Huxley, J., Mayr, E., Osmond, H. & Hoffer, A. (1964). Schizophrenia as a genetic morphism. *Nature*, Vol. 204, No. 4955, (Oct 1964), pp. 220-221, ISSN 0028-0836

Jablensky, A.V. (1995). Schizophrenia: the Epidemiological Horizon. In: *Schizophrenia* Hirsch, S.R. & Weinberger, D.R., eds., pp. 206-252, Blackwell Science, ISBN 0-632-03276-6, London

Keller, M.C. & Miller, G. (2006). Resolving the paradox of common, harmful, heritable mental disorders: Which evolutionary genetic models work best? *Behav Brain Sci*, Vol. 29, No. 4, (Aug 2006), pp. 385-404, ISSN 0140-525X

Kendler, K.S. & Dichl, S.R. (1993). The genetics of schizophrenia: a current, genetic-epidemiologic perspective. *Schizophr Bulletin*, Vol. 19, No. 2, (Apr 1993), pp. 261-285 ISSN 0586-7614

Kinney, D.K., Richards, R., Lowing, P.A., LeBranc, D., Morris, E., Zimbalist, M.E., & Harlan, P. (2001). Creativity in offspring of schizophrenic and control parents: an adoption study. *Creativity Research Journal*, Vol. 13, No. 1, (Jan 2001), pp.17-25, ISSN 1532-6934

Kirov, G., O'Donovan, M.C., Owen, M.J. (2005). Finding schizophrenia genes. *J Clin Invest*, Vol. 115, No. 6, (Jun 2005), pp. 1440-1448, ISSN 0021-9738

Kruman, I.I., Culmsee, C., Chan, S.L., Kruman, Y., Guo, Z., Penix, L. & Mattson, M.P. (2006). Homocysteine elicits a DNA damage response in neurons that promotes apoptosis and hypersensitivity to excitotoxicity. *J Neurosci*, Vol. 20, No. 18, (Sep 2006), pp. 6920-6026, ISSN 1529-2401

Kulkarni, J. & Fink, G. (2000). Hormones and psychosis. In: *Women and schizophrenia*, Castle, D.L., McGrath, J. & Kulkarni, J. eds., pp. 51-66, Cambridge University Press, ISBN 978-0521786171, Cambridge

Larson, C.A. & Nyman, G.E. (1973). Differential fertility in schizophrenia. *Acta Psychiatr Scand*, Vol. 49, No. 3, (Jun 1973), pp. 272-280, ISSN 1600-0447

Limosin, F., Rouillon, F., Payan, C., Cohen, J-M. & Strub, N. (2003). Prenatal exposure to influenza as a risk factor for adult schizophrenia. *Acta Psychiatr Scand*, Vol. 107, No. 5, (May 2003), pp. 331-335, ISSN 1600-0447

Li, X., Sundquist, J. & Sundquist, K. (2007). Age-specific familial risks of psychotic disorders and schizophrenia: a nation-wide epidemiological study from Sweden. *Schizophr Res*, Vol. 97, No. 1-3, (Dec 2007), pp. 43-50, ISSN 0920-9964

Lo, W.S., Xu, Z., Yu, Z., Pun, F.W., Ng, S.K., Chen, J., Tong, K.L., Zhao, C., Xu, X., Tsang, S.Y., Harano, M., Stöber, G., Nimgaonkar, V.L., & Xue, H. (2007). Positive selection within the schizophrenia-associated $GABA_A$ receptor β_2 gene. *PLoS One*, Vol. 2, No. 5, (May 2007), e462, ISSN 1932-6203

Macintyre, D.J., Blackwood, D.H.R., Porteous, D.J., Pickard, B.S. & Muir, W.J. (2003). Chromosomal abnormalities and mental illness. *Mol Psychiatry*, Vol. 8, No. 3, (Mar 2003), pp. 275-287, ISSN 1359-4184

Malaspina, D., Harlap, S., Fennig, S., Heiman, D., Nahon, D., Feldman, D. & Susser, E.S. (2001). Advancing paternal age and the risk of schizophrenia. *Arch Gen Psychiatry*, Vol. 58, No. 4, (Apr 2001), pp. 361-367, ISSN 0003-990X

Marchbanks, R.M., Mulcrone, J. & Whatley, S.A. (1995) Aspects of oxidative metabolism in schizophrenia. *Brit J Psychiatry*, (1995), Vol. 167, No. 3, (Sep 1995), pp.293-298, ISSN 0007-1250

McGrath, J.J., Hearle, J., Jenner, L., Plant, K., Drummond, A. & Barkla, J.M. (1999). The fertility and fecundity of patients with psychoses. *Acta Psychiatr Scand*, Vol. 99, No. 6, (Jun 1999), pp. 441-446, ISSN 1600-0447

McGrath, J., Saha, S., Chant, D. & Welham, J. (2008). Schizophrenia: A concise overview of incidence, prevalence, and mortality. *Epidemiologic Reviews*, Vol. 30, No. 1, (Nov 2008), pp. 67-76, ISSN 0193-936X

McGue, M. & Gottesman, I.I. (1991). The genetic epidemiology of schizophrenia and the design of linkage studies. *Eur Arch Psychiatry Clin Neurosci*, Vol. 240, No. 3, (Feb 1991), pp. 174-181, ISSN 0940-1334

Modrzewska, K. (1980). The offspring of schizophrenic parents in a North Swedish isolate. *Clin Genet*, Vol. 17, No. 3. (Mar 1980), pp. 191-201, ISSN 1399-0004

Monje, P. & Boland, R. (2001). Subcellular distribution of native estrogen receptor alpha and beta isoforms in rabbit uterus and ovary. *J Cell Biochem*, Vol. 82, No. 3, (Sep 2001), pp. 467-479, ISSN 1097-4644

Murphy, K.C., Jones, L.A. & Owen, M.J. (1999). High rates of schizophrenia in adults with velo-cardio-facial syndrome. *Arch Gen Psychiatry*, Vol. 56, No. 10, (Oct 1999), pp. 940-945, ISSN 0003-990X

Nachman, M.W. & Crowell, S.L. (2000). Estimate of the mutation rate per nucleotide in humans. *Genetics*, Vol. 156, No. 3, (Sept 2000), pp. 297-304, , ISSN 0016-6731

Nanko, S. & Moridaira, J. (1993). Reproductive rates in schizophrenic outpatients. *Acta Psychiatr Scand*, Vol. 87, No. 6, (Jun 1993), pp. 400-404, ISSN 1600-0447

Need, A.C., Ge, D., Weale, M.E., Maia, J., Feng, S., Heinzen, E.L., Shianna, K.V., Yoon, W., Kasperaviciūte, D., Gennarelli, M., Strittmatter, W.J., Bonvicini, C., Rossi, G., Jayathilake, K., Cola, P.A., McEvoy, J.P., Keefe, R.S., Fisher, E.M., St Jean, P.L., Giegling, .I, Hartmann, A.M., Möller, H.J., Ruppert, A., Fraser, G., Crombie, C., Middleton, L.T., St Clair, D., Roses, A.D., Muglia, P., Francks, C., Rujescu, D., Meltzer, H.Y. & Goldstein, D.B. (2009). A Genome-Wide Investigation of SNPs and CNVs in Schizophrenia. *PLoS Genet* Vol. 5, No. 2, (Feb 2009), e1000373, ISSN 1553-7404

Nimgaonkar, V.L. (1998). Reduced fertility in schizophrenia: here to stay? *Acta Psychiatr Scand*, Vol. 98, No. 5, (Nov 1998), pp. 348-353, ISSN 1600-0447

Nishikawa, Y., Kawase, O., Vielemeyer, O., Suzuki, H., Joiner, K.A., Xuan, X. & Nagasawa, H. (2007). Toxoplasma gondii infection induces apoptosis in noninfected macrophages: role of nitric oxide and other soluble factors. *Parasite Immunol*, Vol. 29, No. 7, (July 2007), pp.375-385, ISSN 0141-9838

Ohashi, J & Tokunaga, K. (2002). The expected power of genome-wide linkage disequilibrium testing using single nucleotide polymorphism markers for detecting a low-frequency disease variant. *Ann Hum Genet*, Vol. 66, No. 4, (July 2002), pp. 297-306, ISSN 0003-4800

Ødegård, Ø. (1980). Fertility of psychiatric first admissions in Norway, 1936-1975. *Acta Psychiatr Scand*, Vol. 62, No. 3, (Sep 1980), pp. 212-220, ISSN 1600-0447

Oken, R.J. & Schulzer, M. (1999). At issue: schizophrenia and rheumatoid arthritis: the negative association revised. *Schizophr Bull*, Vol. 25, No.4 , (Oct 1999), pp. 625-638, ISSN 0586-7614

Opler, M.G.A. & Susser, E.S. (2005). Fetal environment and schizophrenia. *Environment Health Perspectives*, Vol. 113, No. 9, (Sep 2005), pp. 1239-1242, ISSN 0091-6765

Osby, U., Hammer, N., Brandt, L., Wicks, S., Thinsz, Z., Ekbom A, Sparén P. (2001). Time trends in first admissions for schizophrenia and paranoid psychosis in Stockholm County, Sweden. *Schizophr Res*, Vol. 47, No. 2-3, (Mar 2001), pp. 247-254, ISSN 0920-9964

Pajović, S.B., Saičić, Z.S., Spasić, M.B. & Petrović, V.M. (2003).The effect of ovarian hormones on antioxidant enzyme activities in the brain of male rats. *Physiol Res*, Vol. 52, No. 2, (Mar2003), pp. 189-194, ISSN 0826-8404

Poncet, D., Pauleau, A.L., Szabadkai, G., Vozza, A., Scholz, S.R., Le Bras, M., Brière, J.J., Jalil, A., Le Moigne, R., Brenner, C., Hahn, G., Wittig, I., Schägger, H., Lemaire, C., Bianchi, K., Souquère, S., Pierron, G., Rustin, P,. Goldmacher, V.S., Rizzuto, R., Palmieri, F. & Kroemer G. (2006). Cytopathic effects of cytomegalovirus-encoded apoptosis inhibitory protein vMIA. *J Cell Biol*, Vol. 174, No. 7, (Sep 2006), pp. 985-996, ISSN 0021-9525

Prabakaran, S., Swatton, J.E., Ryan, M.M., Huffaker, S.J., Huang, J.T-J., Griffin, J.L., Wayland, M., Freeman, T., Dudbridge, F., Lilley, K.S., Karp, N.A., Hester, S., Tkachev, D., Mimmack, L., Yolken, R.H., Webster, M.J., Torrey, E.F., & Bahn, S. (2004). Mitochondrial dysfunction in schizophrenia: evidence for compromised brain metabolism and oxidative stress. *Molecular Psychiatry*, Vol. 9, No. 7, (July 2004), pp. 684-697, ISSN 1359-4184

Pulver, A.E., Nestadt, G., Goldberg, R., Shprintzen, R.J., Lamacz, M., Wolyniec, P.S., Morrow, B., Karayiorgou, M., Antonarakis, S.E., Housman, D. et al. (1994). Psychotic illness in patients diagnosed with velo-cardio-facial syndrome and their relatives. *J Nerv Ment Dis*, Vol. 182, No. 8, (Aug 1994), pp. 476-478, ISSN 0022-3018

Ragu, S., Faye, G., Iraqui, I., Masurel-Heneman, A., Kolodner, R.D. & Huang, M-E. (2007). Oxygen metabolism and reactive oxygen species cause chromosomal rearrangements and cell death. *Proc Natl Acad Sci USA*, Vol. 104, No. 23, (Jun 2007), pp. 9747-9752, ISSN 0027-8424

Rapoport, J.L., Addington, A.M. & Fragnau, S. (2005). The neurodevelopmental model of schizophrenia: update 2005. *Mol Psychiatry*, Vol. 10, No. 5, (May 2005), pp. 434-449, ISSN 1359-4184

Remans, P.H., van Oosterhout, M., Smeets, T.J., Sanders, M., Frederiks, W.M., Reedquist, K.A., Tak, P.P., Breedveld, F.C. & van Laar, J.M. (2005). Intracellular free radical production in synovial T lymphocytes from patients with rheumatoid arthritis. *Arthritis & Rheumatism*, Vol. 52, No. 7, (July 2005), pp. 2003-2009, ISSN 0004-3591

Rieder, R.O., Rosenthal, D., Wender, P. & Blumenthal, H. (1975). The offspring of schizophrenics, I: fetal and neonatal deaths. *Arch Gen Psychiatry*, Vol. 32, No. 2, (Feb 1975), pp. 200-211, ISSN 0003-990X

Risch, N., Reich, E.W., Wishnick, M.M. & McCarthy, J.G. (1987). Spontaneous mutation and parental age in humans. *Am J Hum Genet*, Vol. 41, No. 2, (Aug 1987), pp.218-248, ISSN 0002-9297

Rubinstein, G. (1997). Schizophrenia, rheumatoid arthritis and natural resistance genes. *Schizophr Res*, Vol. 25, No. 3, (Jun 1997), pp. 177-181, ISSN 0920-9964

Samper, E., Nicholls, D.G. & Melov, S. (2003). Mitochondrial oxidative stress causes chromosomal instability of mouse embryonic fibroblasts. *Aging Cell*, Vol. 2, No. 5, (Oct 2003), pp. 277-285, ISSN 1474-9718

Senoo-Matsuda, N., Yasuda, K., Tsuda, M., Ohkubo, T., Yoshimura, S., Nakazawa, H., Hartman, P.S. & Ishii, N. (2001). A defect in the cytochrome b large subunit in complex II causes both superoxide anion overproduction and abnormal energy metabolism in *Caenorhabditis elegans*. *J Biol Chem*, Vol. 276, No. 45, (Nov 2001), pp. 41553-41558, ISSN 0021-9258

Shanklin, D.R., Sibai, B.M. (1990). Ultrastructural aspects of preeclampsia. II. Mitochondrial changes. *Am J Obstet Gynecol*, Vol. 163, No. 3, (Sep 1990), pp.943-953, ISSN 0002-9378

Shimizu, A., Kurachi, M., Yamaguchi, N., Torii, H. & Isaki K. (1987). Morbidity risk of schizophrenia to parents and siblings of schizophrenic patients. *Jpn J Psychiatry Neurol*, Vol. 41,No. 1, (Mar 1987), pp. 65-70, ISSN 0912-2036

Sigurđardóttir, S., Helgason, A., Gulcher, J.R., Stefansson, K. & Donnely, P. (2000). The mutation rate in the human mtDNA control region. *Am J Hum Genet*, Vol. 66, No. 5, (May2000), pp. 1599-1609, ISSN 0002-9297

Sipos, A., Rasmussen, F., Harrison, G., Tynelius, P., Lewis, G., Leon, D.A. & Gunnell, D. (2004). Paternal age and schizophrenia; a population based cohort study. *BMJ*, Nov 6; 329(7474):1070. Epub 2004 Oct 22, ISSN 1468-5833

Smith, C.L., Bolton, A. & Nguyen, G. (2010). Genomic and epigenomic instability, fragile sites, schizophrenia and autism. *Current Genomics*, Vol. 11, No. 6, (Sep 2010), pp. 447-469, ISSN 1389-2029

Sobel, D. E. (1961). Infant mortality and malformations in children of schizophrenic women. *Psychiatr Q*, Vol. 35, No. 1, (Mar 1961), pp. 60-65, ISSN 0033-2720

Speir, E., Yu, Z.X., Ferrans, V.J., Huang, E.S. & Epstein, S.E. (1998). Aspirin attenuates cytomegalovirus infectivity and gene expression mediated by cyclooxigenase-2 in coronary artery smooth muscle cells. *Circ Res*, Vol. 83, No. 2, (July 1998), pp. 210-216, ISSN 0009-7330

Stabeneau, J.R., Pullin, W., Moshe, R.L.R., Froman, C., Friedhoff, A.J., & Turner, W. (1969). Study of monozygotic twins discordant for schizophrenia. Some biologic variables. *Arch Gen Psychiatry*, Vol. 20, No. 2, (Feb 1969), pp. 145-158, ISSN 0003-990X

Stirone, C., Duckles, S.P., Krause, D.N. & Procaccio, V. (2005). Estrogen increases mitochondrial efficiency and reduces oxidative stress in cerebral blood vessels. *Mol Pharmacol*, Vol. 68, No. 4, (Oct 2005), pp.959-965, ISSN 0026-895X

Strehlow, K., Rotter, S., Wassmann, S., Adam, O., Grohé, C., Laufs, K., Böhm, M. & Nickenig, G. (2003). Modulation of antioxidant enzyme expression and function by estrogen. *Circ Res*, Vol. 93, No. 2, (July 2003), pp. 170-173, ISSN 0009-7330

Susser, E., Neugebauer, R., Hoek, H.W., Brown, A.S., Lin, S., Labovitz, D. & Gorman, J.M. (1996). Schizophrenia after prenatal famine. Further evidence. *Arch Gen Psychiatry*, Vol. 53, No. 1, (Jan 1996), pp. 25-31, ISSN 0003-990X

Svensson, A.C., Lichtenstein, P., Sandin, S. & Hultman, C.M. (2007). Fertility of first-degree relatives of patients with schizophrenia: A three generation perspective. *Schizophr Res*, Vol. 91, No. 1-3, (Mar 2007), pp. 238-245, ISSN 0920-9964

Takahashi, Y. (1953). An enzymological study on brain tissue of schizophrenic patients. Carbohydrate metabolism. *Folia Psychiatrica Neurologica Japonica*, Vol. 7, No. 3, (Dec 1953), pp. 214-269, ISSN 0015-5721

Torbergsen, T., Oian, P., Mathiesen, E. & Borud, O. (1989). Pre-eclampsia - A mitochondrial disease? *Acta Obstet Gynecol Scand*, Vol. 68, No. 2, (Feb 1989), pp. 145-148, ISSN 0001-6349

Utena, H. & Ezoe, T. (1951). Studies on the carbohydtrate metabolism in brain tissues of schizophrenic patients. II. Report. (in Japanese, with English abstract) *Psychiatr Neurol Japonica*, Vol. 52, No. 3, (Mar 1951), pp. 216-232, ISSN 0033-2658

Utena, H. & Niwa, S. (1992). The history of schizophrenia research in Japan. *Schizophr Bull*, Vol. 18, No. 1, (Jan 1992), pp. 67-73, ISSN 0586-7614

Valero, J., Martorell, L., Marine, J., Vilella, E., & Labad, A. (1998). Anticipation and imprinting in Spanish families with schizophrenia. *Acta Psychiatr Scand*, Vol. 97, No. 5, (May 1998), pp. 343-350, ISSN 1600-0447

Vinogradov, S., Gottesman, I.I., Moises, H.W. & Nicol, S. (1991). Negative associaton between schizophrenia and rheumatoid arthritis. *Schizophr Bull*, Vol. 17, No. 4, (Oct 1991), pp. 669-678, ISSN 0586-7614

Wang, J., Wu, J. & Zhang, Z. (2006). Oxidative stress in mouse brain exposed to lead. *Ann Occup Hyg*, Vol. 50, No. 4, (Jun 2006), pp. 405-409, ISSN 0003-4878

Walsh, T., McClellan, J.M., McCarthy, S.E., Addington, A.M., Pierce, S.B., Copper, G.M., Nord, A.S., Kusenda, M., Malhortra, D., Bhandari, A., Stray, S.M., Rippery, C.F., Roccanova, P., Makarov, V., Lakshmi, B., Finling, R.L., Sikich, L., Stromerg, T., Merriman, B., Gogtay, N., Butler, P., Eckstrand, K., Noory, L., Gochman, P., Long, R., Chen, Z., Davis, S., Baker, C., Eichler, E.E., Meltzer, P.S., Nelson, S.F., Singleton, A.B., Lee, M.K., Rapoport, J.L., King, M.C., Sebat, J. (2008). Rare structural variants disrupt multiple genes in neurodevelopmental pathways in schizophrenia. *Science*, Vol. 320, No.5875 , (Apr 2008), pp. 539-43, ISSN 0036-8075

Webb, R., Abel, K., Pickles, A. & Appleby, L. (2005). Mortality in offspring of parents with psychotic disorders: a critical review and meta-analysis. *Am J Psychiatry*, Vol. 162, No.6, (Jun 2005), pp. 1045-56, ISSN 002-953X

Wood, S.J., Yücel, M., Pantelis, C., & Berk, M. (2009). Neurobiology of schizophrenia spectrum disorders: the role of oxidative stress. Ann Acad Med Singapore, Vol. 38, No. 5, (May 2009), pp. 396-401, ISSN 1145745

Xu, B., Roos, J.L., Levy, S., van Rensburg, E.J., Gogos, J.A. & Karayiorgou, M. (2008). Strong association of de novo copy number mutations with sporadic schizophrenia. *Nat Genet*, Vol. 40, No. 7, (July 2008),pp. 880-885, ISSN 1546-1718

Zaki, M.H., Akutu, T., & Akaike, T. (2005). Nitric oxide-induced nitrative stress involved in microbial pathogenesis. J Pharmacol Sci, Vol. 98, No. 2, (Jun 2005), pp. 117-129, ISSN 1347-8613

Zammit, S., Allebeck, P., Dalman, C., Lundberg, I., Hemmingson, T., Owen, M.J, & Lewis, G. (2003). Paternal age and risk for schizophrenia. *Brit J Psychiatry*, Vol. 183, No. 5, (Nov 2003), pp. 405-408, ISSN 0007-1250

9

Epidemiology of Tics

Blair Ortiz, William Cornejo and Lucía Blazicevich
Universidad de Antioquia, Child Neurology Group,
Child and Adolescent Diseases Research Group PEDIACIENCIAS
Colombia

1. Introduction

Tics are the most frequent movement disorders during childhood; their highest prevalence occurs at scholar and adolescence-ages. Most tics are transient but some of them become chronic having educational, familial and social negative implications.

Moreover, some tics are related to disorders with significant impact, like attention-deficit hyperactivity disorder (ADHD), obsessive-compulsive (OCD) and affective disorders. Epidemiological studies are the initial approach to diagnose them and properly begin treatment.

In this chapter, we explained the clinical bases of tics, review the more representative epidemiological studies that assess the prevalence of tics and make a critical standpoint of these studies about epidemiology applicable to clinical practice.

2. Content

2.1 Definition of tics and their practical ways to characterize them since clinical view

As we described elsewhere, tics are defined as "sudden, rapid, recurrent, nonrhythmic, stereotyped motor movements or vocalizations"and have clinical concerns[1].Tics are likely to differ in terms of the body location, number, frequency, complexity, intensity or forcefulness, noticeable and resulting social consequences[2]. Intervals between tics can range from seconds, hours or even days. The forcefulness with which a tic is performed can range from slight and barely noticeable to intense and obvious. Over time, the frequency and intensity of tics may wax and wane and maybe influenced by a variety of internal and external stimuli including private events, contextual variables and social reinforcement contingencies[3].

Tics can also vary considerably in their complexity. Tics that involve the contraction of a single muscle group are typically referred as simple tics and those that involve the contraction of multiple muscle groups are typically considered complex. Simple tics are typically of very short duration (*i.e.* 1 second) and include such behaviors as eye blinking; jerking of the face, head, torso, or limbs; coughing; sniffing; throat clearing and making singles syllable sounds. Complex tics are often sustained for longer durations or occur in paroxysms and can include virtually any orchestrated pattern of behavior otherwise meeting the definition of a tic. Common examples include picking, tapping, gesturing, mimicking the gestures of others (echopraxia), repeating one's own speech (palilalia), mimicking the speech of others (echolalia) and the production of inappropriate words or sentences.

Tics comprise a group of movement disorders. Thus, transient tics, the most common form of the disorder, consists of single or multiple motor and/or vocal tics that occur for at last four weeks but no longer than 12 months. GTS has onset before 18 years of age, characterized by motor and vocal tics over more than a year, there is never a tic-free period of more than 3 consecutive months, not produced by Huntington disease neither viral encephalitis and produces a negative personal impact. The disorder is called chronic motor tics if the criteria of GTS are present but vocal tics are absent. By contrast, if there are vocal tics but no motor tics the disorder is called chronic vocal tics[4].

2.1.1 Differential diagnosis

Simple motor tics may need to be differentiated from myoclonic jerks, which are not typically repetitive in the same body part like tics. Tics are commonly associated with premonitory sensations and suppressibility. Complex motor tics need to be distinguished from stereotypies that are longer lasting, more stereotyped movements (*eg*, body rocking, head nodding, and hand/wrist flapping) or sounds (eg, moaning, yelling) that occur over and over again in a more continuous, less paroxysmal fashion. Stereotypies are typically seen in patients with autism, mental retardation, Down syndrome, Rett syndrome, psychosis, or congenital blindness and deafness.

Some tics are slow or twisting in character resembling dystonia and are termed "dystonic tics". Contrary to dystonic tics, dystonia *per se* tends to beslower and leads to more sustained disturbances in posture of a limb, the neck, or trunk. Compulsions frequently occur in association with tics, can sometimes be difficult to distinguish from complex motor tics but typically differ by being done in response to an obsession, being performed to avoid future problems or being done according to ritualistic rules[5] [6] With very high comorbidity rates of both ADHD and OCD, GTS may represent a multifaceted developmental neuropsychiatric brain disorder[7].

2.1.2 Secondary tic disorders

A secondary cause for tics should be considered if it is accompanied by other movement disorders or neurologic abnormalities. Tics often indicate the presence of a global brain developmental disorder in conditions like mental retardation, autism and pervasive developmental disorder. Similarly, a variety of genetic and neurodegenerative conditions can cause tics, including Wilson disease, neuroacanthocytosis[8] [9], neurodegeneration with brain iron accumulation[10] [11]and Huntington disease[12].Other potential causes of tics include lesions involving frontal-subcortical circuits like trauma[13], carbon monoxide poisoning[14], hypoxic-ischemic encephalopathy and stroke[15]; central nervous system (CNS) infections (neuroborreliosis[16], viral encephalitis[17]) and central nervous system immune disorders (like antiphospholipid antibody syndrome[18], Sydenham'schorea[19]). Tics can be a manifestation of neuroleptic drug-related tardive dyskinesia[20] or withdrawal emergent syndrome[21]. Induction or exacerbation of tics has been reported with antiepileptic drugs[22] [23], cocaine[24], caffeine[25]and stimulants[26].

3. Biological frame to understand the base of tics and related comorbidities

3.1 Mechanism and pathways of tics and comorbidities

Figure 1 is a practical schema explaining the mechanism and pathways of tics and related disorders based in experimental models resulting of neuroanatomy and neurobiology grounds.

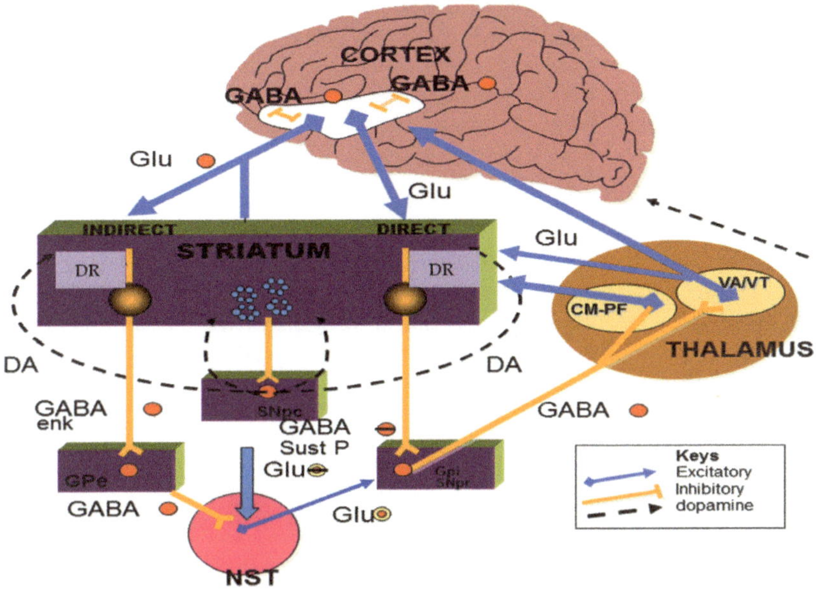

Fig. 1. Cerebral cortex giving glutamatergic excitatory projections to striatum. Abbreviations: Glu: glutamate, DR: dopamine receptors, DA: dopamine, GABA: gamma aminobutiric acid, enk: encephaline K, SNpc: substantia nigra pars compacta, SNpr: substantia nigra pars reticulata, Sust P: susbstantia P, GPe: external globus pallidus, GPi: internal globus pallidus, NST: nucleus subthalamic, VA: ventral anterior, VT: ventral nuclei, CM-PF: centromedian -parafascicular nuclear complex.

The cerebral cortex provides excitatory glutamatergic projections to striatum. The striatum has a topographic distribution as follows: somatosensorial dorsolateral, intermediate / associative and a centromedial / limbic.

Five parallel circuits connecting the cortex to the striatum[27 28]:

1. Motor circuit: gives origin to motor tics and arises in the supplementary motor area.
2. Oculomotor circuits: is the potential source for ocular tics and connects the frontal eye field with the caudate nucleus.
3. Dorsolateral prefrontal circuit: related to difficulties in executive functions, motor planning, cognition and attention. It is connected to Brodmann areas 9 and 10 and caudate head.
4. Lateral orbitofrontal circuit: It is associated with OCD, irritability and mania. It originates from the inferolateral prefrontal cortex and projects to ventromedial caudate.

5. Anterior cingulate circuit: is part of limbic system and is associated to silence, apathy and tics. This circuit is originated in anterior cingulate gyrus and connects with ventral striatum, which is formed by olfactory tubercle, nucleus accumbens, caudate and putamen. Moreover, the striatum receives additional inputs of hippocampus, amygdala and entorhinal cortex.

Although the hypothesis of neural circuit was developed for tics and movement disorders, it is possible that this fundamental principle works for limbic and cognitive aspects. Gangliobasal outputs to frontal lobe via thalamus provide an anatomical substrate for the production of simple and complex tics and compulsions. Thus, abnormal activation of the motor cortex via thalamocortical circuit can cause motor and vocal tics. Abnormal activation of the supplementary area and gyrus cinguli can cause complex tics. Abnormal activation of orbitofrontal cortex can cause compulsions.

3.1.1 Stratium

Striatum has three anatomical divisions: caudate, putamen and ventral striatum or limbic[29]. It has bony neurons with the inhibitory neurotransmitter GABA and another subgroup which uses substance P and dynorphin. Striatum projects to globus pallidus and substantia nigra pars reticulata[30]. By the way, neurons with encephalin projects to external globus pallidus and subthalamic nucleus.

Boneless interneurons are divided into five subgroups: cholinergic and GABAergic neurons expressing parvualbumin; those expressing somatostatin; neuropeptide Y; nicotinamide adenine dinucleotide phosphatase and nitric oxide[31].

3.1.2 Striatotalamhic and thalamocortical tracts

There are two different striatal pathways: one is direct and projects to the internal pallidus globus and substantia nigra pars reticulata; and the indirect going to the external globus pallidus. Both are inhibitory and mediated by GABA and neuroactive peptide. Integration of pathways inhibitory direct and indirect excitatory takes place at the internal globus pallidus and substantia nigra pars reticulata. Internal globus pallidus projects to thalamus through inhibitors GABA fibers.

The effects of facilitation played by the direct route or suppression maintained by the indirect on the outputs of the thalamus to the cortex influences movement and cognitive processing. Deinhibition of thalamic neurons results in hyperexcitability of the projections from the thalamus to the motor cortex leading to tics.

4. Initial treatment considerations

The critical first step in making treatment decisions in patients with tics or GTS is select the most appropriate target symptoms, the ones causing the most problemsin a patient's daily functioning. In one patient it maybe the tics themselves, in another it may be comorbid ADHD or OCD and in another it may be a combination of targets. Because psychosocial stresses can worsen symptoms, it is important to probe for these and consider interventions such as individual or family counseling. For patients with mild symptoms, educational and psychological interventions may be sufficient to bringing down symptoms to a tolerable level. Clinicians should remember that tics characteristically wax and wane in severity, so sometimes just waiting for some period of time can result in a lessening of tics and avoid medication use or increases.

Tics that interfere with school or other daily activities or are disabling because of social embarrassment, physical discomfort or self-injury must be treated. Tic-suppressing medications should be dosage titrated to identify the lowest one that will produce resolution of disability.

4.1 Tic-suppressing drugs

Usual medication treatment for tics centers in alpha agonists and antipsychotics. However, other types of drugs may be of benefit for patients having an inadequate response or problems with tolerability. Clonazepam has had reported modest tic-suppressing effects in published case series[32].This drug may be particularly useful in patients with an associated anxiety disorder. The dopamine-depleting drug tetrabenazine has possible efficacy. The drug is marketed with restriction in some countries. In an open-label study the drug showed sustained moderate to marked reduction in tics over an average of 2 years' follow-up[33]. However, only 22% of subjects were free of side effects. The most common side effects are sedation, depression, insomnia, and parkinsonism. Children may tolerate higher doses of tetrabenazine than adults[34]. Tetrabenazine does not cause tardive phenomena but dopamine-depleting agents can cause neuroleptic malignant syndrome even after years of use[35].

Local injections of botulinum toxin can be considered when one or a few dystonic tics are present in patient's repertoire, such as holding of a sustained neck posture or sustained eye closure[36], cervical tics associated with myelopathy[37] and laryngeal injections for severe vocal tics, including copralalia[38].

4.2 Deep brain stimulation surgery

Deep brain stimulation surgery (DBS) is an approach used to treat other movement disorders including tremor and may be effective for selected patients with severe, disabling and medication-refractory tics. Have been open-label reports of tic reduction following transcranial magnetic stimulation (TMS) of the supplementary motor area[39 40]. To date, most reported cases involve bilateral targeting of the centro-median parafascicular and ventralis oralis complex or central nuclei of the thalamus[41], the globus pallidus internus[42] and nucleus accumbens/anterior limb of the internal capsule[43].

Although sustained benefit has been reported to at least 17 months and most patients continue to require some medication for tics[44], more careful investigation of their efficacy, safety, and tolerability of DBS for the treatment of tics is needed.

4.3 Treatment of tics associated with streptococcal infection

The "Pediatric autoimmune neuropsychiatric disorders associated with streptococcal infection (PANDAS)" hypothesis suggested that chronic, recurrent tics and OCD can arise as an autoimmune sequel of infection with group A beta-hemolytic streptococcus[45]. Actually, there is insufficient evidence to conclude that streptococcal infection has a true etiological role in causing tics. Children with documented streptococcal infections be treated with an appropriate course of antibiotics, but that treatment with chronic antibiotics or immune-modifying therapies like plasma exchange or intravenous immuneglobulin are not justified based on existing evidence.

4.4 Treatment of secondary tic disorders

Tic disorders secondary to CNS lesions or infection may improve with antipsychotic drug therapy. Tics are not commonly a disabling feature of neurodegenerative diseases such as Huntington's disease and antipsychotics have the potential to worsen overall motor function. In tardive phenomena patients including tics, discontinuation of the offending agent is suggested as first-line treatment and improvement can be attained with use of clonazepam, clozapine, an alpha-2-agonist[46] or reintroduction of an antipsychotic[47].

4.5 Behavioral treatment

Behavioral therapies have not been particularly beneficial for patients with disabling tics. Behavioral approaches have included operant conditioning models, rewarding tic suppression and discouraging disruptive tics and massed practice, repeated, voluntarily performance of a tic until fatigue occurs. Habit reversal therapy (HRT) can be considered if a single tic or small subset of tics is unduly disruptive or causing self-injury or pain. HRT trains patients to recognize their tics and to perform a volitional movement different from the tic each time a problem tic occurs. Open-label assessments have identified sustained benefit from HRT for up to 10months[48]. However, current trials will include raters blinded to treatment assignment lacking in previous trials.

In the school setting, approaches often include preferential classroom seating, extra time for tests, an opportunity to take tests in a separate quiet room and assistance with organizing schoolwork. An alpha-2-agonist, such as guanfacine, is a good first choice medication for patients experiencing problematic tics and ADHD because this type of drug can improve both conditions.

4.6 Treatment of ADHD

For patients with tics and ADHD without response to behavioral therapies, options of treatment including the use of the norepinephrine reuptake inhibitor atomoxetine. This drug has documented efficacy for ADHD and has been associated with either no change or a slight reduction in tics[49]. Stimulants remain the most potent and most predictably effective medications for treating ADHD in children with tics and they are well tolerated by the majority of patients. It does seem that upon initiation of therapy stimulants can worsen tics in some patients but this effect is temporary and tic severity usually returns to baseline or even declines from baseline within a few weeks[50]. The efficacy and good tolerability of the stimulant methylphenidate in children with tics and ADHD has been well documented in placebo-controlled trials[51]. Methylphenidate may be less likely to exacerbate tics than some other stimulant preparations, such as mixed amphetamine salts and dextroamphetamine[52]. Newer extended release preparations of methylphenidate tend to provide good coverage of ADHD during the school day and have been very well tolerated by patients with tics. Supplemental use of short-acting methylphenidate formulations can be useful, particularly for college students who have unpredictable study hours.

4.7 Treatment of OCD

Associated OCD can be more disabling than the tics themselves and may create a state of tension and anxiety that heightens tic severity. Cognitive behavioral therapy performed by a well-trained and experienced therapist can be a very effective non-pharmacological treatment for OCD. Selective serotonin reuptake inhibitors (SSRIs) are considered the first-line medications for OCD. Combination with an atypical antipsychotic may be helpful for cases resistant to an SSRI alone. DBS involving the internal capsule/nucleus accumbens is under investigation as a therapy more severe and medication-refractory cases of OCD.

The Tourette Syndrome Association (TSA) is an informative reference guide to patients, parents, and teachers, because it clearly outlines many home and school psychoeducational modifications and interventions that may be effective for children with ADHD and tics. There are local support groups in many cities that can provide information, guidance, and support.

The optimum management of patients with tics involves a comprehensive approach that focuses not only on the tics themselves, but also on neuropsychiatric comorbidities (particularly ADHD and OCD) and existing psychosocial stressors. For young patients, major goals of treatment include helping the child to develop self-confidence, personal resilience, and positive psychosocial skills. A critical goal is to reduce obstacles to successful learning and socialization. The ultimate management usually requires a spectrum of interventions that may include education, cognitive-behavioral therapies, counseling, and medications. DBS might prove to be a useful therapy for patients with severe, disabling tics, or OCD.

4.8 Educating the patient, family and school

Education of parents, teachers and peers is a critical initial intervention. Patients and their parents should be informed that it is appropriate explain to others that they have tics, that they cannot control certain movements or sounds, provide patients and parents with current information about the causes of tics such as genetic factors, brain neurochemical imbalances, emphasize that they are not signs of psychological or emotional illness, a common misperception, explain how tics change in type over time and that they naturally fluctuate in severity.

A majority of GTS patients experience improvement of tics in late adolescence or early adulthood. So the prognosis of TS could be quite good.

Education is often needed for school personnel because there are many misperceptions of tics as being voluntary, attention-seeking or purposely disruptive behaviors. It is recommended that special accommodations be considered in the school setting, like excusing the child, at his or her request, to the nurse's office to release tics or providing additional time in a separate room when taking school tests. Such provisions should be mandated in the countries under laws protecting individuals with disabilities.

5. Studies about tics

As expected in behavior-analytic research, direct observation has been the preferred method for quantifying tic severity. However, researchers in psychiatry, neurology, and even the broader field of behavior therapy have preferred indirect measures, such as clinical impression, self-report inventories and clinician-rated scales. The most commonly cited reasons for not using direct observation include concerns about generalization of observations made in clinic or research settings to other relevant settings, such as home or school[53] and disagreement about the best methods for collecting and scoring direct observation data[54]. Although the empirical basis for these concerns is not firmly established, acquisition of data supporting the use of direct observation methods may encourage those outside behavior analysis to use direct observation as a primary assessment method rather than relying on potentially biased verbal self-reports.

Studies in tics may be divided into three groups: 1) Studies made in clinical grounds, 2) Large-scale screenings and 3) Studies involving selectively school population.

Studies of in-hospital population comprise patients with most severe symptoms, in different age groups and different methods of final diagnosis confirmation are used. Procedures used in large-scale screening studies make possible the elimination of potential selection bias. Large populations are studied using transparent and repetitive confirmation of diagnoses. Their validity is additionally checked in parallel validity studies. The highest prevalence of tics is obtained in studies involving schoolchildren. Data are gathered from multiple sources: from parents, teachers, and children, as well as videos, from classroom observation and diagnoses made by experienced clinicians. Epidemiological surveys of school-age children have shown tic rates ranging from 4% to 50%[55]. This instability in reported rates is perplexing and is probably more artifact than truth. For example, prevalence of tics increases if transient tics are taken into account[56], if studies were made just in public awards and when children attending special education schools were studied[57]. Inversely, prevalence of tics lowers after direct observation extends for a wide time[58].

5.1 Indirect observations

Majority of the studies regarding prevalence of tics based in indirect measures employs questionnaires for parents, teacher and patient; instruments self-administered for detect and draw characteristics of tics, as follows in Table 1.

Tics are abnormal movements with the following characteristics:
They are sudden, brief, and rapid
They are repetitive
They can be controlled voluntarily during short periods of time
They can change and affect other body parts periodically
They improve and worsen from time to time
The most common tics are eye blinking, elevating the eyebrows, twitching the nose and the mouth and shoulder shrugging, shaking the head, twitching the neck, touching objects, other people, or body parts (hair, nose, etc.), kicking the legs, throat clearing, sniffing, barking, and verbalizations.
According to these characteristics:
Do you believe that your son/daughter has had tics? (yes or no)
Do you believe that your son/daughter (or pupil) has tics? (yes or no)

Table 1. General structure used in questionnaires for tics detection.

The indirect measures of tic severity could seem inadequate and, as such, research that has relied exclusively on instruments designed for collection of indirect measures should be interpreted with caution.

5.2 Direct observation

One of the hallmarks of behavior analysis is the use of direct observation to quantify behavior. This preference is based on the premise that direct observation is more objective than indirect methods such as self-report or clinician ratings of tic severity. Several studies, published in behavior-analytic outlets, demonstrate the value of using direct observation to quantify changes in tic frequency when evaluating behavioral treatments for tics[59]. Still, many researchers outside behavior analysis have largely preferred indirect measures over direct observation[60]. Among the foremost concerns raised by these researchers is that observations conducted within a clinical or research context may not generalize to other settings such as school or home. Generalization between settings is an important issue in both research and clinical practice. Indeed, it is not uncommon for parents to report that a child's tics are more or less severe while at the clinic compared to when the child is at home[61] Such reactivity to setting has been attributed to several factors including natural fluctuation, reinforcement contingencies, children's ability to volitionally suppress or temporarily withhold tics, reactivity to observation and internal states such as anxiety[62].

Regardless of the reason for contextual variation in tics, such fluctuations have important implications for the measurement of tics. If the scientific and clinical community is to have confidence in the results of behavior-analytic work utilizing direct observation methodology, observations conducted within a research setting must be generalizable to other settings. Clinic- and homebased observations are highly related, suggesting that, in general, clinic observations correspond well with home observations[63]. However, examination of individual data shows that generalization should not necessarily be assumed; many children exhibited differential tic frequencies across the two settings, suggesting that, whenever possible, observations should be conducted in multiple settings. Lack of consensus regarding the most reliable, valid and feasible methods for collecting and coding direct observation data has also been cited as a reason for the preference of indirect measures over direct observation[64]. Practitioners and researchers in disciplines outside behavior analysis may be more likely to use direct observation methods if the effort associated with their use can be reduced, without any sacrifice of their validity and capacity to generate representative samples of target behaviors.

Direct observation to longer samples and event-frequency coding to a less arduous time-sampling method (*i.e.* partial-interval coding) have been used to evaluate outcomes in tic research[65], although partial-interval coding is more user-friendly because it does not require the observer to record each occurrence of the tic; thus, it might be preferred over the event frequency method. However, partial-interval coding cannot be recommended as an alternative if it does not yield a reliable measure of the behavior. Because simulation studies have suggested that partial-interval coding may underestimate the frequency of high-rate short duration responses, especially if they occur in rapid succession or as bouts, as is the case with many tics[66].

5.3 Yale global tic severity scale

Yale global tic severity scale (YGTSS) is a clinician-completed rating scale used to rate tic severity along several dimensions based on parent and child reports and clinician observations during the interview[64]. Each dimension is represented by a subscale designed to quantify the number, frequency, duration, intensity and complexity of both motor and vocal tics. Each subscale includes several descriptions to help the clinician make his or her ratings. Guided by these descriptions, each subscale is issued a rating between 0 and 5, with higher scores indicating greater severity. Examples of descriptions included on the number subscale are single tic, multiple discrete tics and multiple discrete tics plus several orchestrated paroxysms of multiple simultaneous or sequential tics where it is difficult to distinguish discrete tics. Examples of items on the frequency subscale are "rarely—specific tic behaviors have been present during the previous week; these behaviors occur infrequently, often not on a daily basis; if bouts of tics occur, they are brief and uncommon and "always—specific tic behaviors are present virtually all the time". Examples of items on the intensity subscale include "minimal intensity—tics not visible or audible (based solely on patient's private experience) or tics are less forceful than comparable voluntary actions and are typically not noticed because of their intensity" and "severe intensity— tics are extremely forceful and exaggerated in expression; these tics call attention to the individual and may result in risk of physical injury because of their forceful expression". Examples on the complexity subscale include "borderline—some tics are not clearly 'simple in character" and "severe—some tics involve lengthy bouts of orchestrated behavior or speech that would be impossible to camouflage or successfully rationalize as normal because of their duration or extremely unusual, inappropriate, bizarre or obscene character". Examples of interference items include "minimal—when tics are present, they do not interrupt the flow of behavior of speech" and "severe—when tics are present, they frequently disrupt intended action or communication". Finally, examples of items on the impairment subscale include "minimal—tics associated with subtle difficulties in self-esteem, family life, social acceptance or school or job functioning" and "severe—tics associated with extreme difficulties in self-esteem, family life, social acceptance or school or job functioning". The five subscales are rated separately for motor and vocal tics. The motor subscales are then summed to produce an overall motor tic severity rating and the vocal tic subscales are summed to provide an overall vocal tic severity rating; each ranges from 0 to 25. The motor and vocal tic severity ratings are then summed to produce an overall tic severity score that ranges from 0 to 50. Studies have shown the YGTSS total tic score to have acceptable internal consistency, good inter-rater reliability and acceptable convergent and divergent validity in samples of adults and children.

5.4 Gross-site procedural training

Prior to the beginning of the study, a face-to-face meeting between personnel for tic assessment must held to review the standardized observation protocol and to conduct training on YGTSS administration and scoring. Sample tapes of children with tics may be used to conduct cross site YGTSS training and direct observation coding. Tapes included an interview and YGTSS administration conducted by the primary investigators with a child and his or her parents, along with a while direct observation segment of the child (at least 10 minutes). YGTSS training has to continue until the clinicians obtained agreement of at least 90% on the training. Disagreements during training have to be resolved by discussion between the primary investigators and coders and recoding of videotapes until agreement criterion is reached.

5.5 Not clinical studies of tics

A key factor in understanding these divergent results of epidemiological studies concerns the sample size, randomization, stratification, steps in epidemiological assessment and clinical aspects to warrant quality of databases[67]. Most relevant studies about prevalence are showed in Table 2, including their methodological aspect.

Author	Year	Population	Methodology	Prevalence	Strenghts	Limitations
Kurlan R, Como PG, Miller B, Palumbo D, Deeley C, Andresen EM, et al5.	2002	Community-based study of school children 12.5 to 15.7 years old.	1596 children assessed using interviews to determine the prevalence of tics and psychopathological disorders.	21.2% had tics.	Community sample should minimize problems with ascertainment bias, controlled study.	Data obtained from the Child Behavior Checklist (CBCL) can be influenced by which parent or teacher completed the scale, tic severity and psychotropic medication, factors that were not included in analyses.
Khalifa N, Knorring ALV[68].	2003	4479 Swedish school children aged 7 to 15 years	Total population and their parents were asked to fill in a questionnaire covering both motor and vocal tics. A three- stage procedure was used: screening, interview and clinical investigation. SGT were diagnosed according to DSM-IV criteria.	6.63% were found to have tics, 4.24% were male and 2.43% female. Further, 4.8% of the children had transient tics. All together, 6.6% of 7 to 15 year old children currently had or had experienced some kind of tic disorder during the last year.	Investigators used the DSM-IV instead DSM-III-R criteria. The first one requires that the tics cause a marked disturbance or significant functional impairment. Inclusion criteria were that tics had occurred sometime during the last 12 months. Same physician performed both the telephone interview and the clinical assessment.	As a result of a decision from the ethics committee, investigators were not allowed to ask the teachers about their pupils´ tics in the main study and some cases may have been missed. Some parents were no Swedish and the screening questionnaire could be not easy to complete in its language. However, in these cases a professional translator helped the parents. If the child refused further participation, the telephone

						interview was expanded to make a correct diagnosis. Thus it is plausible that misdiagnoses were minimized. The study has not focused on the severity of the disorders, functional impairment as well as comorbid disorders, school problems and learning disabilities.
Lanzi G, Zambrino CA, Termine C, Palestra M, Ferrari O, Orcesi S, et al[69].	2004	The study population comprised 2347 primary school children from the city of Pavia, Northern Italy, 5-12 years from 15 primary schools.	Using trained school teachers as the source of cases, all children with motor or vocal tics occurring intermittently and unpredictably out of a background of normal motor activity were accepted. The type, frequency, and circumstances of tic disorders were noted. School performance was correlated to the presence of tics. Diagnostic criteria for a tic disorder were those of the Tourette Syndrome Classification Study Group.	A total of 68 children (56 boys, 12 girls) aged 6–11 years were identified with tic disorders. The period prevalence was 2.9% (95% CI 2.3 to 3.7). The prevalence was 4.4% in boys and 1.1% in girls, with no detectable trends at age 6–11. Situation related tics were noted in 37 cases. A significant correlation was found between the presence of tic disorders and impaired school performance.	The purposes of the study, the definition and characteristics of the tic disorders were illustrated by authors to all the school teachers, with the support of videotaped interviews. Investigators used stringent and different diagnostic criteria; data sources and movement disorders were excluded. Different sources have been used to identify subjects with tic disorders, including direct observations at school, parents´ interview/questionnaire, teachers´ interview/quiestionnaire and clinical examination. A pilot study was conducted on 232 children from one school, evenly distributed across school years (two classes for each school year). This sample served to test the validity and reliability of the school teachers as a source for the ascertainment of patients with tics. In each class, one investigator with experience in the field of movement disorders	Case ascertainment was no attempt to verify the teachers´ observations through direct examination of all the affected children.

					spent four morning hours observing the students and noted any symptoms resembling tics.	
Linazasoro G, Blercom NV, Ortiz C[58].	2006	867 Children of two schools, 4 to 16 years.	The study was conducted in three successive steps: information to parents and teacher by way of speeches and projection of videotapes; anonymous fulfilling of specified questionnaire by teachers and parents and identification of children as possible tic disorder according to questionnaire; and confirmation of presence of tics by 20 minutes direct observation of children at school.	57 cases were identified after direct observation in the classroom, thereby prevalence was 6.5%. The vast majority of tics were mild in severity and duration. Most of identified cases were quite mild, not leading to major functional disability.	High participation rate and collaboration offered by parents and teachers data highly reliable. Investigators chose one private and one public school to exclude possible selection bias related to the socioeconomic status. Blind observation phase of the study.	Investigators decided not to interview directly parents and children, but some children could be identified during direct observation phase. Diagnosis of tics was not confirmed. Investigators emphasize the convenience of including a later step in the methodology to confirm the diagnosis. Length of direct observation in the classroom was 20 min, which could be quite limited. To observe children during their routine school activity requires a considerable degree of mental concentration.
Stefanoff P, Wolanczyk T, Gawrys A, Swirszcz K, Stefanoff E, Kaminska A, et al[70].	2008	12-15 year old Warsaw schoolchildren attending 24 randomly selected schools.	Children were screened by inquiring their parents and teachers. Children indicated as tic-positive by the screening procedure were investigated using semi-structured questionnaires and the Polish version of YGTSS scale. A validity study involved random selection and investigation of 130 non indicated subjects. Screening procedure had	Lifetime prevalence of 9.9% (95%CI 7.1-12.6%) and a point prevalence of 6.7% (4.3-9.1%). Lifetime prevalence of ICD-10 tic disorders was 2.6% (95% CI 1.2-4.1%) for transient tic disorder (TTD).	The schools were chosen randomly and should not differ systematically from other mainstream schools.	Reference group differed significantly from the total study population in terms of gender distribution. The number of subjects with tics found in this group could be even higher, leading to lower positive predictive value. Teachers interviewed in the study protocol knew their students for

		high sensitivity (92%) and low positive predictive value (18%). International Classification of Diseases-10 (ICD-10) criteria were used for tic disorders.		3-4 years and were coping with them on a daily basis as their formal tutors. A relatively high proportion of false negative subjects in the reference group is the result of poor knowledge of involuntary movements in the polish population and indicates a possible underestimation of prevalence estimates. classification of tic disorders based on the ICD-10 criteria could yield misdiagnosing of tic disorders. The ICD classification reflects the current concepts of tic disorders as a behavioral continuum, and two most severe syndromes—chronic tic disorders and GTS—differ only in terms of duration of tic symptoms. The use of ICD criteria should not constitute a problem in terms of comparability with previous epidemiological studies, especially that most of them that utilized DSM-III-R criteria, very similar toICD-10.

Schlander M, Schwarz O, Rothenberger A, Roessner V[71].	2009	2.2 million live records during 2003 covered by Statutory Health Insurace (SHI) in Norbaden, Germany, 0 to 50 years old.	12-months administrative prevalence rates as well as rates of co-occurrence of tics and ADHD based upon the number of diagnosed cases of tics disorders.	Prevalence of any tic disorder was 0,8%. Both tics and ADHD were diagnosed most often in the age group 7-12 years. Tic disorders were observed in 2,3% of patients with ADHD.	Prevalence rates within this large sample established the remitting course of tics. The study confirms the co-ocurrence of tics and ADHD in children and adolescents, presenting both perspectives: the rate of ADHD in patients with tics as well the rate of tics in patients with ADHD.	These outpatients have no detailed information about the exact diagnostic procedures. Short time of follow-up. Diagnoses in children made more often by a medical specialist and by a primary care physician in adults. The study is difficult to compare with previous reports, which is related to different study design. The absolute administrative prevalence rates should be interpreted cautiously. Some people could not be assisted to SHI.
Ortiz B, David M, Sánchez Y, Mira J, Sierra JM, Cornejo JW[72].	2011	346 students of public basic school.	Students were assessed by structured questionnaire, interview and 20 minutes of clinical examination. Comorbidity with ADHD was detected by DSM-IV criteria. Severity and interference produced by tics was determined by apply **YGTSS**.	Tics were present in 17.97% and GTS in 3.4% of scholars. According to time onset, 27.6% had transient tics and 72.4% had chronic tic disorder. 53.4% of patients with tics agree with DSM-IV ADHD criteria. Mean age to tics presentation was 9 years old. There was no difference in tics frequency between children studying in public and private schools.	First study in South America establishing prevalence of tics in children. Wide clinical sample that includes training to teachers and parents, structured questionnaire, clinical assessment and direct observation in the classroom by experts in tics detection. Percentage of children with GTS was higher than other studies probably because evaluators considered milder cases and depicting that the disorder was not as rare as previously was believed.	Authors detected that hyperactivity was confused with tics by parents and teachers on parents and teachers questionnaires

Table 2. Not clinical studies of tics.

5.6 Clinical studies of tics

Clinic-based studies are believed to underestimate the frequency of tics, as only a small fraction of children and adults with tics are brought to a health care provider for evaluation[73]. There is evidence of a reporting bias in community studies with 50% of the children with observed tics reported to have tics by their parents. Results of investigations also support the previously reported findings that tics wax and wane in severity and frequency over time, as individual shad fluctuating symptoms over the observation period[74]. Most relevant clinical studies about prevalence are showed in Table 3.

Authors	Year	Patients	Methodology	Results	Strenghts	Limitations
Chouinard S, Ford B[75].	2000	411 adults with tic disorders who presented between 1988 and 1998 to the movement disorders clinic at Columbia-Presbyterian Medical Center after the age of 21.	Patients' charts were retrospectively reviewed for demographic information, age of onset of tics, tic phenomenology, distribution, the presence of premonitory sensory symptoms and tic suppressibility, family history and associated psychiatric features. These patients' videotapes were reviewed for diagnostic confirmation and information was obtained about disability, course, and response to treatment in a structured follow up interview.	5.35% presented for the first time with tic disorders after the age of 21. 2.18% of patients had a history of previous childhood transient tic disorder, but in 3.16% of patients, the adult onset tic disorder was new. Among the new onset cases, 1.45% of patients developed tics in relation to an external trigger, secondary tic disorders. The remaining patients had idiopathic tic disorders. The categorical breakdown among 22 patients was: idiopathic new onset tics in seven (32%), new onset secondary tic disorder in six (27%) and recurrent childhood tic disorder in nine (41%).The appearance of the tic disorder, the course and prognosis, the family history of tic disorder and the prevalence of obsessive-compulsive disorder were found to be similar in adult patients with recurrent childhood tics and those with new onset adult tics. Adults with new	The study shows that adult onset tic disorders represent an underrecognised condition that is more common than generally appreciated or reported and clinical evidence suggesting that adult tic disorders are part of a range of illness that includes childhood onset tics and GTS. Authors propose a new classification of tic disorders in adult age category that is subdivided by disease course into tic disorders that persist from childhood, tic disorders that represent a recurrence of transient childhood tics and genuine new onset adult tic disorders.	The study cannot estimate the prevalence of adult onset tic disorders in general population. Establishing that an adult patient with apparent new onset tics did not have tics during childhood can rarely be done with certainty because some patients are unaware of their tics and reliable observers who knew the patient as a child may not be available. All patients were self referred for tics, a referral bias that usually selects for more severely affected people.

				onset tics were more likely to have a symptomatic or secondary tic disorder, likely caused by infection, trauma, cocaine use, and neuroleptic exposure.		
Eapen V, Lees A, Lakke JPWF, Trimble MR; Robertson MM[76].	2002	Study about report of eight adult patients with adult-onset motor tics and vocalizations.	All the cases were evaluated using the National Hospital Interview Schedule for the assessment of GTS and related behaviors; this is a standardized, semistructured instrument that includes systematic assessment of personal and family history of GTS, ADHD and OCB.	All patients there were a potential trigger event, such as drug exposure, viral or bacterial infection, physical trauma, cerebrovascular disease or psychiatric illness prior to the onset of tic symptoms. These may have acted as a trigger to unmask the symptoms in a constitutionally predisposed individual. 50% of cases, there was either a personal or family history of GTS-related behavior. The symptoms were severe in 75% and 50% suffered extreme occupational or social disadvantage as a direct result of tics.	The interview was conducted with the patient and a family member (usually a parent) who knows the patient well enough to give relevant details about childhood.	Further study of the phenomenology and natural history of these adult-onset cases is needed.
Prior AC, Tavares S, Figueiroa S, Temudo T[77].	2006	78 Children and teenagers with tics diagnosed based by DSM-IV criterions.	Retrospective analyses from clinical archives of child neurology outpatients of Hospital General de Santo Antonio, Spain.	84.6% were boys. Family history of tics, depression and OCD occurred in 30%. ADHD was the most frequent neuropsychologycal disorder (67.9%). In more than two thirds of the patients, tics were simple. Mean age for tics was 7 years old. 59.7% of tics were chronic and 45.7% of those were GTS.	Wide clinical sample.	Boys were derived to the clinic because symptoms of ADHD instead of tics. Descriptions were extracted of patients untreated. Sex selection bias may take place (male:female ratio was 5.5:1) because ADHD was more frequent in boys. Neurobehavioral and family aspects may be overestimated by the type retrospective of study.

Table 3. Clinical warding studies of tics.

5.7 Clinical characterization of tics

Author	Year	Population	Methodology	Motor (%)	Vocal (%)	SGT (%)
Khalifa N, Knorring ALV[78].	2003	4479 Swedish school children aged 7 to 15 years.	Total population and their parents were asked to fill in a questionnaire covering both motor and vocal tics. A three- stage procedure was used: screening, interview and clinical investigation. SGT were diagnosed according to DMS-IV criteria.	0,8	0,5	0,6
Himle, M. B., & Woods, D. W[63].	2006	43 children, ages 8 to 17 years	Patients recruited through print advertisement, physician referrals and Tic Disorder Clinics. The assessment consisted of a structured diagnostic interview, including intelligence quotient (IQ), videotape and patient, parent and clinics-reports. Monetary compensation was given to children.	15,4	10	95,3
Prior AC, Tavares S, Figueiroa S, Temudo T[77].	2006	78 Children and teenagers with tics diagnosed based by DSM-IV criterions.	Retrospective analyses from clinical archives of child neurology outpatients of Hospital General de Santo Antonio, Spain.	NA	NA	45,7
Stefanoff P, Wolanczyk T, Gawrys A, Swirszcz K, Stefanoff E, Kaminska A, et al[70].	2008	12-15 year old Warsaw schoolchildren attending 24 randomly selected schools.	Students were screened by inquiring their parents and teachers. Children indicated as tic-positive by the screening procedure were investigated using semi-structured questionnaires and the Polish version of YGTSS scale. A validity study involved random selection and investigation of 130 non indicated subjects. Screening procedure had high sensitivity (92%) and low positive predictive value (18%).	NA	NA	0,6
Ortiz B, David M, Sánchez Y, Mira J, Sierra JM, Cornejo JW[72].	2011	346 students of public elementary school.	Assessment by structured questionnaire, interview and 20 minutes of clinical examination.	63,8	12	19

Table 4. Clinical characteristics of tics.

6. Related problems in tic disorders along life

Oftenly, presence of tics are associated with messing conditions that impair the performance at work, familiar and social environments. Prevalence studies should consider these entities because detection is a first step to diagnose and treat them. We illustrate studies of tic disorders and related morbidities in Table 3.

6.1 Studies of comorbidity in tics

Author	Year	Methodology	Results	Strenghts	Limitations
Kurlan R, Como PG, Miller B, Palumbo D, Deeley C, Andresen EM, Eapen S, *et al*5.	2002	Community-based study of school children since 12,5 to 15,7 years old using interviews to determine the prevalence of tics and psychopathological disorders. A standard psychiatric interview and standardized rating scales were utilized to diagnose childhood behavioral disorders.	1596 children interviewed, 21.2% had tics, 38.4% with ADHD, 10.9% with OCD, 29.2% with social phobia, 9.4% with agoraphobia, 14.8% with separation anxiety, 21.2% with anxiety disorder, 1.2% with mania and 17.4% oppositional defiant disorder (ODD).	Community sample is intended to minimize problems with ascertainment bias, controlled study.	Data obtained from the CBCL can be influenced by which parent or teacher completed the scale, tic severity and psychotropic medication, factors that were not included in analyses.
Snider LA, Seligman LD, Ketchen BR, Levitt SJ, Bates LR, Garvey et al[79].	2002	553 children of kindergarten through sixth grade, observed monthly from November 1999 to June 2000 by 3 raters. Problem behaviors were rated as absent, subclinical or clinical in following categories: disruptive, hyperactive, impulsive, aggressive, anxious and distracted.	One quarter of all children exhibited problem behaviors. The monthly point prevalence was significantly higher during winter months compared with the spring months. Behavior comorbidity is associated with the more persistent tic symptoms versus all tic symptoms, as children with isolated tics lasting only 1 to 2 months did not have increased rates of problem behaviors, whereas those with a more persistent course did.	Children were followed by three independent raters and problem behaviors were classified by their impact.	Conclusions about seasonal prevalence are limited because the children were not observed from July through October. It's possible that clinic-based studies overestimate the frequency of comorbid behavior problems, in part because the behavior problems can be more troublesome than the tic symptoms and become the motivating factor for seeking treatment. It is also possible that clinic-based studies estimate accurately the prevalence of comorbid conditions and that the discrepancy came from the inappropriate generalization of clinic based data to community populations.
Prior AC, Tavares S, Figueiroa S, Temudo T[77].	2006	78 Children and teenagers with tics diagnosed based by DSM-IV criterions. Retrospective analyses from clinical archives of child neurology outpatients of Hospital General de Santo Antonio, Spain.	ADHD was present in 67.9%, learning difficulties in 59%, sleep disorders in 23.1%, developmental delay in 21.8%, unspecified mental retardation in 16.7%, ODD in 10.3%, obsessive compulsive symptoms (OCS) in 7.7%, epilepsy in 6.4%, autism in 3.8%, migraine/headache in 3.8% and depression in 2.6%	Wide clinical sample. DSM-IV criteria were used for tics, which allow comparison with other studies.	Data was extracted from clinic archives and patients were selected by an unknown and not-validated questionnaire.

Table 5. Related disorders in tics.

6.2 Adults with tics and comorbidities

Tics and vocalizations developing in later life in association with neuroacanthocytosis[80], Sydenham's chorea and L-dopa-treated postencephalitic parkinsonian syndrome[81]. There are a few reports of isolated and spontaneous adult-onset tics disorders.

Chouinard and colleagues reported on 7 cases of idiopathic tic disorder that presented after the patients were 21 years of age[75]. Adult-onset tic disorder in the absence of any other primary neurological disorder has onset of tic symptoms from 23 to 52 years[76].

Adult-onset cases need to be evaluated using a wide screening, like the National Hospital Interview Schedule for the assessment of GTS and related behavior[82]; this is a standardized, semistructured instrument that includes systematic assessment of personal and family history of GTS, ADHD, and obsessive compulsive behavior (OCB). The interview is conducted with the patient and a family member (usually a parent) who knows the patient well enough to give relevant details about childhood.

Several cases of secondary tourettism have been described in the literature. The causes have included postencephalic syndrome and carbon monoxide intoxication, and other causes have been degenerative or vascular[75]. Tourettism has also occurred secondary to trauma[83], infection[84], alcohol withdrawal[85], or intake of certain drugs such as stimulants, anticholinergics, or antipsychotics[86 87]. In almost all patients there was a potential trigger event, such as drug exposure, viral or bacterial infection, physical trauma, cerebrovascular disease, or psychiatric illness prior to the onset of tic symptomatology. These may have acted as a trigger to unmask the symptoms in a constitutionally predisposed individual. In this regard, it is interesting to note that in 50% of cases there is either a personal or family history of GTS-related behavior. However, it is also possible that these represented secondary tics. It is now recognized that GTS has a genetic cause, with some studies suggesting an autosomal dominant transmission and others a mixed model[88].

Goetz and coworkers in a study of 58 adult GTS patients diagnosed during childhood observed that childhood tic severity had no predictive value and that coprolalia did not increase the risk for severe tics in adult life[89]. Features predictive of mild tics in adulthood were mild tics during the patients' worst preadulthood function and mild tics during adolescence. The phenomenology of tics encountered in later life may also be somewhat different from those in early-onset GTS. For example, it has been reported reduced response to treatment (31%), a high degree of social morbidity (89%) and a low frequency of spontaneous complete remission in adult-onset cases. It seems that adult-onset tic disorder, whether idiopathic, secondary or a recurrence of childhood tics, may be different from younger-onset GTS.

A majority of patients exhibit OCB in childhood and have a positive family history of tics or OCB. It may also be noted that childhood rheumatic chorea may resolve only to return in late adult life[89]. Linazasoro and colleagues described a patient who had presented with only OCD since childhood but developed GTS symptoms at the age of 72 years and suggested that the expression of the gene may be different in the same patient during the course of his life[90].

7. Conclusions

Data from tics research prompt significant variations in prevalence. Future research should, at minimum, supplement indirect measures with direct methods. Nolan demonstrated that correspondence between direct observation scores and YGTSS ratings may be lower for low-frequency tics than for high-frequency tics[91].

Whether tic frequency is the most important dimension of tic severity (*e.g.* best predicts psychosocial functioning) is an empirical issue that warrants investigation. Studies should evaluate methods capable of quantifying multiple dimensions of tics including overt physical dimensions (*e.g.* frequency, intensity, complexity), social dimensions (*e.g.* social reinforcement and punishment contingencies, functional interference) and the concomitant private dimensions commonly reported to accompany tics (*e.g.* sensory events). The research will likely require novel direct observation techniques used in combination with other measurement methods (*e.g.* functional assessment, self-report, clinician ratings, social acceptability ratings, physiological measures, neuroimaging techniques, etc.) and research strategies (*e.g.* functional analysis, group research designs, inferential statistical analyses).

The use of not traditional measurement techniques to complement direct observation is likely to increase in popularity within the broader field of clinical behavior analysis. Clinical researchers are increasingly concerning themselves with the study of behavior that is complex, highly variable and not easily accessible by traditional direct-observation techniques (*e.g.* the private behaviors of individuals who suffer from anxiety and mood disorders). If behavior analysts are to continue to be at the forefront for understanding and treating clinical problems (including tic disorders), they must systematically determine which dimensions of specific target behaviors are socially relevant and must be diligent not to restrict themselves by investigating only those aspects that are easily quantifiable with traditional direct observation methods[92]. This will require researchers both to refine their current measurement techniques and to incorporate techniques that have not traditionally been employed in behavior-analytic research (*e.g.* clinician ratings, self-report, physiological and neuroimaging techniques, etc). This is not to suggest that clinical behavior analysts abandon direct observation in favor of other measurement techniques. On the contrary, it is a call to behavior analysts to develop, investigate and incorporate new direct and indirect measurement techniques that will enhance scientific investigation of the environment-behavior relations involved in clinical problems.

8. References

[1] Cornejo JW. (2008). Tics y síndrome de Gilles de la Tourette. In: *Manual de pediatría ambulatoria.* Marín A; Jaramillo JC; Gómez JF; Gómez LF. Pp. 151-153. Editorial Médica Panamericana. ISBN 978-958-4410-19-9. Bogotá.

[2] Leckman, J. F.; King, R. A. & Cohen, D. J. (1999). Tics and tic disorders. In: *Tourette's syndrome – Tics, obsessions, compulsions: Developmental psychopathology and clinical care,* J. F. Leckman & D. J. Cohen, pp. 23–42, Wiley, ISBN 0-471-16037-7, New York.

[3] Carr, J. E., Taylor, C. C., Wallander, J. J., & Reiss, M. L. (1996). A functional analytic approach to the diagnosis of transient tic disorder. *Journal of Behavior Therapy and Experimental Psychiatry*, 27, 291–297, ISSN 0005-7916.

[4] Cornejo W, Posada C, Uribe A. (2001). Caracterización clínica de pacientes con trastorno de Gilles de la Tourette. *Acta Neurológica Colombiana*; 17: 97-102, ISSN 0120-8748.

[5] Kurlan R, Como PG, Miller B, Palumbo D, Deeley C, Andresen EM, Eapen S, McDermott MP. (2002). "The behavioral spectrum of tic disorders: a community-based study." *Neurology*; 59(3):414-20, ISSN 0028-3878.

[6] Robertson MM. (2000). Tourette syndrome, associated conditions and the complexities of treatment. *Brain*;123(pt 3):425–462. ISSN 1460-2156.
[7] Palumbo D, Maughan A, Kurlan R. (1997). Hypothesis III. Tourette syndrome is only one of several causes of a developmental basal ganglia syndrome. *Arch Neurol*;54:475–483, ISSN 1538-3687.
[8] Ruiz-Sandoval JL, Garcia-Navarro V, Chiquete E, et al. (2007). Choreoacanthocytosis in a Mexican family. *Arch Neurol*;64: 1661–1664, ISSN 1538-3687.
[9] Hardie RJ, Pullon HW, Harding AE, et al. (1991). Neuroacanthocytosis. A clinical, haematological and pathological study of 19 cases. *Brain*;114 (pt 1A):13–49, ISSN 1460-2156.
[10] Scarano V, Pellecchia MT, Filla A, Barone P. (2002). Hallervorden-Spatz syndrome resembling a typical Tourette syndrome. *Mov Disord*;17:618–620, ISSN 0885-3185.
[11] Pellecchia MT, Valente EM, Cif L, et al. (2005). The diverse phenotype and genotype of pantothenate kinase-associated neurodegeneration. *Neurology*;64:1810–1812, ISSN 0028-3878.
[12] Angelini L, Sgro V, Erba A, Merello S, Lanzi G, Nardocci N. (1998). Tourettism as clinical presentation of Huntington's disease with onset in childhood. *Ital J Neurol Sci*;19:383–385, ISSN 0392-0461.
[13] Krauss JK, Jankovic J. (1997). Tics secondary to craniocerebral trauma. *Mov Disord*;12:776–82, ISSN 0885-3185.
[14] Pulst SM, Walshe TM, Romero JA. (1983). Carbon monoxide poisoning with features of Gilles de la Tourette's syndrome. *Arch Neurol*;40:443–444, ISSN 1538-3687.
[15] Kwak CH, Jankovic J. (2002). Tourettism and dystonia after subcortical stroke. *Mov Disord*;17:821–825, ISSN 0885-3185.
[16] Riedel M, Straube A, Schwarz MJ, Wilske B, Muller N. (1998). Lyme disease presenting as Tourette's syndrome. *Lancet*;351: 418–419, ISSN 0140-6736.
[17] Northam RS, Singer HS. (1991). Postencephalitic acquired Tourette-like syndrome in a child. *Neurology*;41:592–593, ISSN 0028-3878.
[18] Martino D, Chew NK, Mir P, Edwards MJ, Quinn NP, Bhatia KP. (2006). Atypical movement disorders in antiphospholipid syndrome. *Mov Disord*;21:944–949, ISSN 0885-3185.
[19] Moore DP. Neuropsychiatric aspects of Sydenham's chorea: a comprehensive review. (1996). *J Clin Psychiatry*;57:407–414, ISSN 1555-2101.
[20] Bharucha KJ, Sethi KD. (1995). Tardive tourettism after exposure to neuroleptic therapy. *Mov Disord*;10:791–793, ISSN 0885-3185.
[21] Polizos P, Engelhardt DM, Hoffman SP, Waizer J. (1973). Neurological consequences of psychotropic drug withdrawal in schizophrenic children. *J Autism Child Schizophr*;3:247–253, ISSN 0021-9185.
[22] Lombroso CT. (1999). Lamotrigine-induced tourettism. *Neurology*; 52:1191–1194, ISSN 028-3878.
[23] Neglia JP, Glaze DG, Zion TE. (1984). Tics and vocalizations in children treated with carbamazepine. *Pediatrics*;73:841–844, ISSN 1098-4275.
[24] Cardoso FE, Jankovic J. (1993). Cocaine-related movement disorders. *Mov Disord*;8:175–78, ISSN 0885-3185.
[25] Davis RE, Osorio I. (1998). Childhood caffeine tic syndrome. *Pediatrics*;101:E4, ISSN 1098-275.

[26] Lowe TL, Cohen DJ, Detlor J, Kremenitzer MW, Shaywitz BA. (1982). Stimulant medications precipitate Tourette's syndrome. *JAMA*;247:1729–1731, ISSN 1538-3598.

[27] Harris K, Singer HS. (2006). Tic disorders: neural circuits, Neurochemistry, and Neuroimmunology. *J Child Neurol*; 21 (8) :678-89, ISSN 1708-8828.

[28] Langen M, M JH Kas,. Staal WG, Engeland HV, Durston S. (2011). The neurobiology of repetitive behavior: Of mice. *Neuroscience and Biobehavioral Reviews*; 345-355, ISSN 0149-7634.

[29] Y. Kawaguchi. (2003). Local circuit neurons in the frontal Cortico-striatal system. In: *Excitatory-Inhibitory Balance: Synapses, Circuits, Systems,* Hensch T.K.; Fagiolini M, pp. 125-148, KluwerAcademic/Plenum Publishers, ISBN 0-306-47962-1, New York.

[30] Ouyer J.J., Park D.H., Joh T.H., Pickel V.M. (1984). Chemical and structural analysis of the relation between tyrosine hydroxyl cortical inputs and terminals in rat-containing neostriatum. *Brain Research;* 302 (2), pp. 267-275, ISSN 1872-6240.

[31] Kalanithi PS, Zheng W, Kataoka Y, DiFiglia M, Grantz H, Saper CB, Schwartz ML, Leckman JF, Vaccarino FM. (2005). Altered parvalbumin-positive neuron distribution in basal ganglia of individuals with Tourette syndrome. *Proc Natl Acad Sci U S A*; 13;102(37):13307-12, ISSN 1091-6490.

[32] Steingard RJ, Goldberg M, Lee D, DeMaso DR. (1994). Adjunctive clonazepam treatment of tic symptoms in children with comorbid tic disorders and ADHD. *J Am Acad Child Adolesc Psychiatry*;33:394–399, ISSN 0890-8657.

[33] Kenney C, Jankovic J. (2006). Tetrabenazine in the treatment of hyperkinetic movement disorders. *Expert Rev Neurother*;6:7–17, ISSN 1473-7175.

[34] Jain S, Greene PE, Frucht SJ. (2006). Tetrabenazine therapy of pediatric hyperkinetic movement disorders. *Mov Disord*;21: 1966–1972, ISSN 0885-3185.

[35] Petzinger GM, Bressman SB. (1997). A case of tetrabenazine-induced neuroleptic malignant syndrome after prolonged treatment. *Mov Disord*;12:246–248., ISSN 0885-3185.

[36] Jankovic J. (1994). Botulinum toxin in the treatment of dystonic tics. *Mov Disord*;9:347–349, ISSN 0885-3185.

[37] Salloway S, Stewart CF, Israeli L, et al. (1996). Botulinum toxin for refractory vocal tics. *Mov Disord*;11:746–748, ISSN 0885-3185.

[38] Trimble MR, Whurr R, Brookes G, Robertson MM. (1998). Vocal tics in Gilles de la Tourette syndrome treated with botulinum toxin injections. *Mov Disord*;13:617–619., ISSN 0885-3185.

[39] Mantovani A, Lisanby SH, Pieraccini F, Ulivelli M, Castrogiovanni P, Rossi S. (2006). Repetitive transcranial magnetic stimulation (rTMS) in the treatment of obsessive-compulsive disorder (OCD) and Tourette's syndrome (TS). *Int J Neuropsychopharmacol*;9:95–100, ISSN 1461-1457.

[40] Mantovani A, Leckman JF, Grantz H, King RA, Sporn AL, Lisanby SH. (2007). Repetitive transcranial magnetic stimulation of the supplementary motor area in the treatment of Tourette syndrome: report of two cases. *Clin Neurophysiol*;118:2314–2315, ISSN 1388-2457.

[41] Servello D, Porta M, Sassi M, Brambilla A, Robertson MM. (2008). Deep brain stimulation in 18 patients with severe Gilles de la Tourette syndrome refractory to treatment: the surgery and stimulation. *J Neurol Neurosurg Psychiatry*;79:136–142, ISSN 0022-3050.

[42] Dehning S, Mehrkens JH, Muller N, Botzel K. (2008). Therapy-refractory Tourette syndrome: beneficial outcome with globus pallidus internus deep brain stimulation. *Mov Disord*;23: 1300–1302, ISSN 0885-3185.

[43] Flaherty AW, Williams ZM, Amirnovin R, et al. (2005). Deep brain stimulation of the anterior internal capsule for the treatment of Tourette syndrome: technical case report. *Neurosurgery*; 57:E403; discussion E403, ISSN 0148-396X.

[44] Servello D, Porta M, Sassi M, Brambilla A, Robertson MM. (2008). Deep brain stimulation in 18 patients with severe Gilles de la Tourette syndrome refractory to treatment: the surgery and stimulation. *J Neurol Neurosurg Psychiatry*;79:136–142, ISSN 0022-3050.

[45] Swedo SE, Leonard HL, Garvey M, et al. (1998). Pediatric autoimmune neuropsychiatric disorders associated with streptococcal infections: clinical description of the first 50 cases. *Am J Psychiatry*;155:264–271, ISSN 0002-953X.

[46] Jaffe E, Tremeau F, Sharif Z, Reider R. (1995). Clozapine in tardive Tourette syndrome. *Biol Psychiatry*; 38:196–197, ISSN 0006-3223.

[47] Reid SD. (2004). Neuroleptic-induced tardive Tourette treated with clonazepam: a case report and literature review. *Clin Neuropharmacol*;27:101–104, ISSN 0362-5664.

[48] Wilhelm S, Deckersbach T, Coffey BJ, Bohne A, Peterson AL, Baer L. (2003). Habit reversal versus supportive psychotherapy for Tourette's disorder: a randomized controlled trial. *Am J Psychiatry*;160:1175–1177, ISSN 0002-953X.

[49] Allen AJ, Kurlan RM, Gilbert DL, et al. (2005). Atomoxetine treatment in children and adolescents with ADHD and comorbid tic disorders. *Neurology*;65:1941–1949, ISSN 0028-3878.

[50] Tourette's Syndrome Study Group. (2002). Treatment of ADHD in children with tics: a randomized controlled trial. *Neurology*; 58: 527–536, ISSN 0028-3878.

[51] Gadow KD, Sverd J, Nolan EE, Sprafkin J, Schneider J. (2007). Immediate- release methylphenidate for ADHD in children with comorbid chronic multiple tic disorder. *J Am Acad Child Adolesc Psychiatry*;46:840–848, ISSN 0890-8567.

[52] Castellanos FX, Giedd JN, Elia J, et al. (1997). Controlled stimulant treatment of ADHD and comorbid Tourette's syndrome: effects of stimulant and dose. *J Am Acad Child Adolesc Psychiatry*;36:589–596, ISSN 0890-8657.

[53] Goetz, C. G., Leurgans, S., & Chmura, T. A. (2001). Home alone: Methods to maximize tic expression for objective videotape assessments in Gilles de la Tourette syndrome. *Movement Disorders*, 16, 693–697, ISSN 0885-3185.

[54] Chappell, P. B., McSwiggan-Hardin, M. T., Scahill, L., Rubenstein, M., Walker, D. E., Cohen, D. J., et al. (1994). Videotape tic counts in the assessment of Tourette's syndrome: Stability, reliability, and validity. *Journal of the American Academy of Child and Adolescent Psychiatry*, 33, 386–393, ISSN 0890-8657.

[55] Nomoto F, Machiyama Y. (1990). An epidemiological study of tics. *Jpn J Psychiatry Neurol*;44:649–655, ISSN 0912-2036.

[56] Wang HS, Kuo MF. (2003). Tourette's syndrome in Taiwan: an epidemiological study of tic disorders in an elementary school at Taipei County. *Brain Dev*;25(Suppl. 1):S29 -S31, ISSN 0387-7604.

[57] Saccomani L, Fabiana V, Manuela B, Giambattista R. (2005). Tourette syndrome and chronic tics in a sample of children and adolescents. *Brain Dev*;27:349 -352, ISSN 0387-7604.

[58] Linazasoro G, Blercom NV, Ortiz C. (2006). Prevalence of tic disorder in two schools in the Basque Country: results and methodological caveats. *Movement disorders;* 21: 2106-2109, ISSN 0885-3185.

[59] Peterson, A. L., & Azrin, N. H. (1992). An evaluation of behavioral treatments for Tourette syndrome. *Behaviour Research and Therapy,* 30, 167–174, ISSN 0005-7967.

[60] Bruun, R. D., & Budman, C. L. (1996). Risperidone as a treatment for Tourette's syndrome. *Journal of Clinical Psychiatry,* 57, 29–31, ISSN 1555-2101.

[61] Comings, D. E. (1990). *Tourette syndrome and human behavior,* Hope Press, ISBN 1-878267-27-2, Durante, CA:.

[62] Himle, M. B., & Woods, D. W. (2005). An experimental evaluation of tic suppression and the tic rebound effect. *Behaviour Research and Therapy,* 43, 1443–1451, ISSN 0005-7967.

[63] Himle MB, Chang S, Woods DW, Pearlman A, Buzzella B, Bunaciu L, Piacentini JC. (2006). Establishing the feasibility of direct observation in the assessment of tics in children with chronic tic disorders. *Journal of applied behavior analysis,* 39, 429–440, ISSN 0021-8855.

[64] Leckman, J. F., Riddle, M. A., Hardin, M., Ort, S. I., Swartz, K. L., & Stevenson, J., et al. (1989). The Yale global tic severity scale: Initial testing of a clinicianrated scale of tic severity. *Journal of the American Academy of Child and Adolescent Psychiatry,* 28, 566–573, ISSN 0890-8657.

[65] Azrin, N. H., & Peterson, A. L. (1988). Behavior therapy for Tourette's syndrome and tic disorders, In: *Tourette syndrome and tic disorders: Clinical understanding and treatment,* D. J. Cohen, J. F. Leckman, & R. D. Bruun (Eds.), pp. 237–255, Wiley, ISBN 978-0471629245, New York.

[66] Harrop, A., & Daniels, M. (1986). Methods of time sampling: A reappraisal of momentary time sampling and partial interval recording. *Journal of Applied Behavior Analysis,* 19, 73–77, ISSN 0021-8855.

[67] Stefanoff P, Mazurek J. (2003). Epidemiological methods used in studies in the prevalence of Tourette syndrome. *Psychiatr Pol;*37: 97–107, ISSN 0033-2674.

[68] Khalifa N, Knorring ALV. (2003). Prevalence of tic disorders and Tourette syndrome in a Swedish school population. *Developmental medicine and child neurology;* 45 (5): 315-319, ISSN 0012-1622.

[69] Lanzi G, Zambrino CA, Termine C, Palestra M, Ferrari O, Orcesi S, et al. (2004). Prevalence of tic disorders among primary schools students in the city of pavia, Italy. *Arch Dis Child;* 89: 45-47, ISSN 1468-2044.

[70] Stefanoff P, Wolanczyk T, Gawrys A, Swirszcz K, Stefanoff E, Kaminska A, et al. (2008). Prevalence of tic disorders among schoolchildren in Warsaw, Poland. *Eur Child Adolesc psychiatry;* 17: 171-178, ISSN 1018-8827.

[71] Schlander M, Schwarz O, Rothenberger A, Roessner V. (2010). Tic disorders: administrative prevalence and co-occurrence with attention-definit/hyperactivity disorder in a German community sample. European Psychiatry. *Eur Psychiatry.* 26(6):370-4, ISSN 0924-9338.

[72] Ortiz B, David M, Sánchez Y, Mira J, Sierra JM, Cornejo W. (2011). Prevalencia de tics en población escolar de 6 a 12 años de edad en el municipio de itagüi - colombia en el año 2010. *In press.*

[73] Mason A, Banerjee S, Eapen V, Zeitlin H, Robertson MM. (1998). The prevalence of Tourette syndrome in a mainstream school population. *DevMed Child Neurol;*405:292–296, ISSN 0012-1622.

[74] Saunders-Pullman R, Braun I, Bressman S. (1999). Pediatric movement disorders. *Child Adolesc Psychiatry Clin North Am*;8:747–765, ISSN 1056-4993.

[75] Chouinard S, Ford B. (2000). Adult onset tic disorders. *J Neurol Neurosurg Psychiatry*; 68: 738-743, ISSN 0022-3050.

[76] Eapen V, Lees AJ, Lakke J.P.W.F., Trimble MR, Robertson MM. (2002). Adult-Onset Tic Disorders. *Movement Disorders* Vol. 17, No. 4, pp. 735–740, ISSN 0885-3185.

[77] Prior AC, Tavares S, Figueiroa S, Temudo T. (2007). Tics in children and adolescents: a retrospective analysis of 78 cases. *An Pediatr (Barc)*; 66(2):129-34, ISSN 1695-4033.

[78] Khalifa N, Knorring ALV. (2003). Prevalence of tic disorders and Tourette syndrome in a Swedish school population. *Developmental medicine and child neurology*; 45 (5): 315-319. ISSN 1469-8749.

[79] Snider LA, Seligman LD, Ketchen BR, Levitt SJ, Bates LR, Garvey et al. (2002). Tics and problem behaviors in schoolchildren: prevalence, characterization and associations. *Pediatrics*; 110: 331-336, ISSN 0031-4005

[80] Hardie RJ, Pullon HW, Harding AE, et al. (1990). Neuroacanthocytosis. *Brain*;114:13–49, ISSN 1460-2156.

[81] Sacks OW. (1982). Acquired Tourettism in adult life. In: *Advances in neurology: Gilles de la Tourette syndrome*, Friedhoff AJ, Chase TN, editors, Raven Press, ISBN 0091-3952, New York.

[82] Robertson MM, Eapen V. (1996). The National Hospital Interview Schedule for the assessment of Gilles de la Tourette syndrome and related behaviours. *Int J Methods Psychiat Res*;6:203–226, ISSN 1557-0657.

[83] Goetz CG, Pappert EJ. Trauma and movement disorders. *Neurol Clin* 1992;10:907–919, ISSN 0733-8619.

[84] Swedo SE, Leonard HL, Garvey M, Mittleman B, Allen AJ, Perlmutters, Longee L, Dow S, Zamkoff J, Dubbert BK. (1998). Pediatric autoimmune neuropsychiatric disorders associated with streptococcal infections: clinical description of the first 50 cases. *Am J Psychiatry*;155:264–271, ISSN 0002-953X.

[85] Cardoso F, Vargas AP. (1996). Persistent dyskinesia and obsessive compulsive behaviour following alcohol withdrawal. *Neurology*; 47:844, ISSN 0028-3878.

[86] Stahl SM. (1980). Tardive Tourette's syndrome in an autistic patient after long term neuroleptic administration. *Am J Psychiatry*;137: 1267–1269, ISSN 0002-953X.

[87] Fog R, Pakkenberg H, Regeur L, Pakkenberg B. (1982). "Tardive" Tourette syndrome in relation to long term neuroleptic treatment multiple tics. *Adv Neurol*;35:419–421, ISSN 0091-3952.

[88] Walkup JT, LaBuda MC, Singer HS, Brown J, Riddle MA, Hurko O. (1996). Family study of segregation analysis of Tourette syndrome. *Am J Hum Genet*;59:684–693, ISSN 0002-9297.

[89] Goetz CG, Tanner CM, Stebbins GT, Leipzig G, Carr WC. (1992). Adult tics in Gilles de la Tourette syndrome. *Neurology*;42:784–788, ISSN 0028-3878.

[90] Linazasoro G, Olsagasti B, Marti Masso JF. (1992). Atypical presentation of Gilles de la Tourette syndrome. *Br J Psychiatry*;160:426, ISSN 1472-1465.

[91] Nolan EE, Gadow KD, Sverd J. (1994). Observations and ratings of tics in school settings. *J Abnorm Child Psychol*;22(5):579-93, ISSN 1573-2835.

[92] Baer, D. M., Wolf, M. M., & Risley, T. R. (1987). Some still-current dimensions of applied behavior analysis. *Journal of Applied Behavior Analysis*, 20, 313–327, ISSN 0021-8855.

10

A Review of the Etiology Delirium

Nese Kocabasoglu[1], Gul Karacetin[2], Reha Bayar[1] and Turkay Demir[3]
[1]*Cerrahpasa Medical School, Department of Psychiatry*
[2]*Department of Child and Adolescent Psychiatry*
[3]*Cerrahpasa Medical School, Department of Child and Adolescent Psychiatry*
Turkey

1. Introduction

Delirium, also called as organic brain syndrome, acute brain syndrome, acute brain failure, acute confusional episode and reversible or masked dementia, as a concept, stretches back to the age of Hypocrates (Burns et al., 2004). Delirium is described as a condition characterized by a disturbance of consciousness with reduced ability to focus, sustain, or shift attention according to the Diagnostic and Statistical Classification of Mental Disorders, Fourth Edition, Text Revision (DSM-IV-TR) criteria (American Psychiatric Association, 2000). Also, delirium involves a change in cognition (such as memory deficit, disorientation, language disturbance) or the development of a perceptual disturbance that is not better accounted for by a preexisting, established, or evolving dementia (American Psychiatric Association, 2000). In addition to these, impairment in the brain's ability to integrate perceptions correctly, coupled with memory deficits and confusion may result in psychotic symptoms in delirium. Hallucinations (especially visual and tactile), delusions, paranoia, illusions, and bizarre behavior are the commonly encountered psychotic symptoms in delirium (Leigh, 2008).

Delirium is associated with longer hospital stay, poorer functional outcome, and cognitive decline in addition to an elevated morbidity and mortality. Despite these adverse outcomes, delirium recognition rates are low (12–43%) and its management remains inadequate in up to 80% of patients (Morrison et al., 2003). These findings suggest lack of preventive and screening activities, missed diagnoses, and inappropriate management of diagnosed delirium (Michaud et al., 2007).

2. Epidemiology

2.1 Prevalence

The prevalence of delirium varies with the population that is being studied (Fong et al., 2009). Delirium is a relatively common disorder, especially in older people with physical illness (Saxena & Lawley, 2009). Community rates of delirium are reported to vary from 0.4% to 2% (Saxena & Lawley, 2009, Fong et al., 2009). In general hospital setting prevalence of delirium has been reported to range from 11% to 33% on admission (Lindesay et al., 2002) and its incidence during hospital stay ranges between 3% and 56% (Inouye, 2006; Michaud L et al., 2007).

Delirium rates depend on the setting in which the patient belong; for example, delirium prevalence has been reported to be between 7-10% in emergency department, whereas it has been reported to be as high as 33% in the orthopedic surgery patients (Samuels & Neugroschl, 2005). Postoperative delirium is reported to be in 15% to 62% of elderly patients (Saxena & Lawley, 2009, Fong et al., 2009). Higher rates of delirium have been reported in elderly patients in intensive care units (ICU), which ranges from 70% to 87% (Saxena & Lawley, 2009, Fong et al., 2009).

Children are also are at risk of delirium. There is a paucity of data on the rates of delirium in children, but delirium was reported to be seen in 10 to 40 percent of preschool children during emergence from anesthesia. Children with severe burns and fever are at risk for delirium (Saxena & Lawley, 2009).

3. Etiology

Delirium is divided into subtypes according to the etiological factors. When there is evidence from the history, physical examination, or laboratory findings that the disturbance is caused by the direct physiological consequences of a general medical condition, it is called as *Delirium due to a general medical condition.* When the symptoms of delirium are due to substance intoxication, it is called as *Substance intoxication delirium.* When the delirium is due to substance withdrawal, it is called as *Substance withdrawal delirium.* When there is evidence from the history, physical examination, or laboratory findings that the delirium has more than one etiology, it is called as *Delirium due to multiple etiologies.* Delirium that is of unclear etiology is called as *Delirium not otherwise specified* (American Psychiatric Association, 2000).

Delirium usually has a multifactorial etiology. It has been reported that 90% of patients with delirium had three to four identifiable etiologic factors, 27% had two factors, and only 16% had one identifiable etiologic factor (Camus et al., 2000). The etiology of delirium is complex and multifactorial, with the interaction of precipitating factors (acute insults) on a vulnerable patient with predisposing conditions (Inouye, 1999).

3.1 Predisposing factors

The predisposing factors are those that place patients vulnerable to develop delirium. Older age, neurological disorders, male sex, sensory impairment, , depression, functional dependence, immobility, hip fracture, dehydration, alcoholism, severity of physical illness, stroke, metabolic abnormalities are among the predisposing factors that increase an individual's vulnerability to delirium (Inouye, 1999; Burns et al., 2004; Fong et al., 2009; Staus, 2011). The National Clinical Guideline Center (in the UK) has published a data synthesis on this topic commissioned by the National Institute for Health and Clinical Excellence (NICE). In this analysis, the risk factors for delirium were reported as age 65 years or older, cognitive impairment (past or present) and/or dementia, hip fracture on admission, severe illness (a clinical condition that is deteriorating or is at risk of deterioration) (National Clinical Guideline Center).

3.1.1 Age

One of the most important predisposing factors is age (Inouye, 1999). Both the geriatric and pediatric populations are at risk of developing delirium (Dulcan, 2010). The elderly are more vulnerable to delirium because of the age-related loss of cholinergic reserve that is necessary for memory, learning, attention, and wakefulness (Maclullich et al., 2008).

Among this age group, one of the most common risk factors for delirium is dementia, with two-thirds of elderly cases of delirium having comorbid dementia (Fong et al., 2009). Delirium and dementia are both associated with cholinergic deficiency (Hshieh et al., 2008) and decreased cerebral blood flow or metabolism (Fong et al., 2006, Yokota et al., 2003); these common properties might explain the relationship between these two conditions (Eikelenboom and Hoogendijk, 1999; Fong et al., 2009).

As mentioned above, the main mechanism that predisposes elderly to delirium is diminished cholinergic reserve; on the other extremes of age are children who are also prone to delirium because of the immature and evolving structural brain development (Williams, 2007). According to the study of Leentijens et al., 2008, etiological factors differed among pediatric, adult and geriatric populations; for children neurological, respiratory and circulatory disorders were among the most important causes of delirium (with ratios of 39%, %26, %17 in order), whereas for adults the most common factors were medication intoxication or withdrawal (24%), brain metastases/CNS neoplasms (24%) and metabolic and endocrine causes(20%), for elderly patients metabolic and endocrine causes (26%), systemic effects of a neoplasm (19%),medication intoxication or withdrawal (19%) were most important factors (Leentijens et al., 2008).

3.1.2 Neurological disorders

Dementia is a major predisposing factor for delirium, a meta-analysis suggesting a relative risk of 5.2 (Elie et al., 1998). Fick et al. reported that approximately 45% of patients with dementia develop delirium during hospitalization (2002). Elderly patients with dementia are at higher risk for developing delirium not only because they have the usual age-related decrease in acetylcholine described previously, but also have a focal loss of acetylcholine due to death of the cholinergic cells in the nucleus basalis of Meynert as a result of the disease process (Tune & Egeli, 1999).

In a study that included patients over the age of 65 years admitted to hospital with a fractured neck of femur, cognitive impairment which was measured by the Mini-Mental State Examination (MMSE), has been found to be the most significant predisposing factor for the development of delirium (Freter et al., 2005).

Other neurological causes are cerebrovascular diseases (thrombosis, embolism, arteritis, hemorrhage, hypertensive encephalopathy), degenerative disorders (multiple sclerosis), epilepsy, head trauma, space-occupying lesions (tumor, subdural hematoma, abscess, aneurysm) and encephalitis (Michaud et al., 2007; Fong et al., 2009).

3.1.3 Hip fracture

Hip fracture patients are at increased risk of delirium because of the trauma associated with the injury and the rapid progression to hospitalization and surgery, in addition to the pain and loss of function (Schor et al., 1992; Williams et al., 1985). Delirium has been reported to be seen in 20%-40% of patients with hip fracture at the time of hospital admission (Magaziner et al., 1989; Gustafson et al., 1991; Marcantonio et al., 2002).

The most common of delirium in hip fracture patients were reported as drugs that have central nervous system effects, infections, fluid-electrolyte disturbances, metabolic/ endocrine disturbances, intracranial processes, cardiopulmonary compromise and/or drug withdrawal and sensory/environmental causes (Brauer et al., 2000).

3.1.4 Severe, traumatic or systematic illnesses

Medical comorbidities such as burns (Palmu, 2011), cancer (Bond et al., 2011), cardiovascular disease (Branco et al., 2011), and alcoholism (Pompei et al., 1994) are among the predisposing factors for delirium. Sensory impairments like visual impairment and functional dependence also predispose individuals to delirium (Burns et al., 2004). In a study investigating a multifactorial model of delirium etiology, a predictive model was formed and 4 predisposing factors were identified for delirium: vision impairment, severe illness, cognitive impairment and BUN/creatinine ratio of ≥18 (Inouye, 1999).

Having a severe illness and staying in intensive care unit are also predisposing factors for delirium. Delirium has been reported in up to 80% of critically ill patients (Ouimet et al., 2007). Delirium is an independent predictor of adverse intensive care unit outcomes, including increased risk of death, longer hospital stay, and higher costs (Ely et al., 2004; Milbrandt et al., 2004; Thomason et al., 2005).

3.1.5 Male gender

Male gender was found to be a risk factor in some of the studies of delirium (Williams-Russo et al., 1992; Fisher & Flowerdew, 1995; Kolbeinsson & Jonsson, 1993; Schor et al., 1992; Edlund et al., 2001). In the meta-analysis of Elie et al., a statistically significant relative risk of 1.9 was found for the male gender (1998). In a study that investigated the differences between preoperative and postoperative delirium regarding predisposing, precipitating factors and outcome in older patients admitted to hospital with femoral neck fractures, it was found that the men with femoral neck fractures were in poorer health than the women, except that more female patients had hypertension and were treated with diuretics (Edlund et al., 2001). In the same study, male patients were reported to suffer more postoperative complications and have higher long-term mortality (Edlund et al., 2001). These factors might have contributed to the increased risk of delirium in men.

Another factor contributing to the increased risk of delirium in men might be reluctance of men to consult a doctor. Men with health problems were found to be more likely than women to have had no recent contact with a doctor regardless of income or ethnicity (Courtenay, 2000). This reluctance means that men often do not seek help until a disease has progressed (Banks, 2001).

3.1.6 Depression

Depression has been reported to be a predisposing factor for delirium in the elderly (Elie et al., 1998) and in non-cardiac surgical patients (Dasgupta and Dumbrell, 2006). The reduced functional connectivity in the human brain which is associated with depression (Anand et al., 2005) was hypothesized to be one of the mechanisms that predispose depressive patients to delirium (Sanders, 2011). On the other hand, the authors of the data synthesis commissioned by the National Institute for Health and Clinical Excellence (NICE) reported uncertainty for depression as a precipitating factor for delirium (National Clinical Guideline Center; Steiner, 2011).

3.2. Precipitating factors

Precipitating factors are the acute insults that trigger the mechanisms resulting in delirium (Fong et al., 2009; Inouye, 1999). Factors that have been reported to precipitate delirium are: anemia (Joosten et al., 2006), hypoxaemia (Kazmierski et al., 2010), Intensive Care Unit admission (Branco et al., 2011), electrolyte abnormalities (Korevaar et al., 2005), sleep deprivation (Weinhouse et al., 2009), pain, bladder catheter use, drugs and surgery (Burns et al., 2004). Biochemical abnormalities such as hyponatremia and hypokalemia and hyperuricemia and low body mass index and sensory impairment reflects the severity of the underlying precipitating cause of delirium (Elie et al., 1998; Mussi et al., 1999).

Inouye and Charpentier performed a study to establish a predictive model for development of delirium and identified 5 independent precipitating factors for delirium in the elderly: use of physical restraints, malnutrition, more than 3 medications added, use of bladder catheter and any iatrogenic event (Inouye & Charpentier, 1996). Among the predisposing factors, surgery and drugs will be discussed in this section.

3.2.1 Surgery

The incidence of post-operative delirium ranges from 5% to 15%(Deiner& Silverstein, 2009). Certain high-risk groups have increased rates of delirium. Delirium has been reported in 16.3% after cardiac surgery (Kazmierski et al., 2010). Rates as high as 30.2% after hip surgery (Lee et al., 2011) and 50% have been reported in elderly patients (Inouye et al., 1993; Dasgupta & Dumbrell, 2006). Factors that increase the risk of delirium in surgical patients include electrolyte disturbances, increased age, dementia, low cardiac output, perioperative hypotension, postoperative hypoxia, and use of anticholinergic drugs. (Michaud et al., 2007; Norkiene et al., 2007). Pandharipande et al. found that 70% of the combined surgical and trauma ICU patients had at least one episode of delirium (Pandharipande et al., 2007).

3.2.2 Drugs

Delirium is characterised by a global cerebral dysfunction resulting in a generalized reduction in cerebral oxidative metabolism and an imbalance of several neurotransmitters in the brain. Any drug that interferes with these neurotransmitter systems or with the supply or use of substrates for metabolism of the central nervous system can cause delirium (Gray et al., 1999; Moore & O'Keeffe, 1999; Nayeem & O'Keeffe, 2003). For a drug to be clearly implicated as an etiological factor in delirium, the administration of the drug should precede the onset of symptoms of delirium within a short time duration and withdrawal of the drug should result in a return to baseline cognitive functioning (Moore & O'Keeffe, 1999).

3.2.2.1 Anticholinergic drugs

The causal association of drugs to delirium is most clear for anticholinergic drugs with muscarine receptor affinity (White et al., 2007). Antihistaminics, antipsychotics, tricyclic antidepressants, digoxin, frusemide, isosorbide dinitrate, warfarin, dipyridamole, codeine, and captopril are among the mostly used durs that have primary or secondary anticholinergic effects contributing to risk of delirium (Burns, 2004,). Many commonly used drugs in the elderly, that are the principal treatments of clinical conditions, such as urinary incontinence and cardiovascular disease, have anticholinergic properties (Scheife & Takeda, 2005; Uusvaara et al., 2011). Older patients and those with mental illness are particularly vulnerable to the adverse neuropsychiatric effects of anticholinergics as they may already have cognitive impairment (Gerretsen & Pollock, 2011).

3.2.2.2 Opioids

Delirium has been reported to be associated with opioid use (Gray et al., 1999, Brouquet, 2010). The association of delirium with opioids is dose-related (Burkhart et al., 2010). Persistent delirium has been reported to be associated with use of opioids at doses greater than 54mg/day (Pisani et al., 2010). On the other hand, there are studies reporting no association between opioid use and delirium (Pandharipande et al., 2006; Pisani et al., 2007). In a systemic review which aimed to determine medications to avoid in people at risk of delirium, it was concluded that, although use of opioids should be prescribed with caution in people at risk of delirium, as untreated severe pain can itself trigger delirium, this caution should be tempered (Clegg & Young, 2011).

3.2.2.3 Antidepressants

All tricyclic antidepressants have an anticholinergic effect, with amitryptiline having the strongest and nortriptyline the weakest (White et al., 2007). Delirium has been reported to develope after abrupt discontinuation of fluoxetine (Blum et al., 2008) and with concominant use of fluoxetine and lamotrigine (Chistyakova & Amos, 2008). In addition, concomitant use of low-dose bupropion sustained release and fluoxetine has been reported to be associated with delirium (Chan et al., 2006).

3.2.2.4. Other drugs

Benzodiazepines (Sanders, 2011), antipsychotics with strong anticholinergic effects (e.g. clozapine) (Centorrino et al., 2003), antiparkinson medications (i.e. levodopa) (Delmas et al., 2008) are among the other drugs that were erorted to be associated with delirium. A systematic review of prospective studies that investigated the association between medications and risk of delirium reported that delirium risk appears to be increased with opioids, benzodiazepines, dihydropyridines and possibly antihistamine. The authors conluded that there appears to be no increased risk with neuroleptics or digoxin and there is uncertainty regarding H(2) antagonists, tricyclic antidepressants, antiparkinson medications, steroids, non-steroidal anti-inflammatory drugs and antimuscarinics (Clegg, A. & Young, 2011).

3.3. Pathophysiology

The pathophysiology of delirium is still poorly understood. The risk factors described above may act by similar mechanisms, leading to a common pathway that interferes with neurotransmitter function or with the supply or use of substrates to the brain (Maldonado, 2008). Imbalance in neurotransmitter systems is the leading hypothesized mechanism for delirium (Inouye, 2006). Other hypothesized mechanisms are neural injury, inflammation, and stress response (Hshieh et al., 2008).

3.3.1 Imbalance in neurotransmitter systems

3.3.1.1 Cholinergic deficiency

Cholinergic neurons play an important role in cognition and memory (Kopelman, 1986). Evidence from electroencephalographic and pharmacologic studies supports the role of cholinergic deficiency in genesis of delirium. Electroencephalographic studies have shown that delirium is associated with occipital slowing, peak power and alpha decrease, delta and theta power increase and slow wave ratio increase during active delirious states (Thomas et al., 2008). Cholinergic thalamo-cortical pathways responsible for attention, alertness and vigilance regulation modulate the basic EEG alpha rhythm (Nunez et al., 2001). Centrally acting anticholinergics result in a pattern very similar to the electroencephalographic findings in delirium (Renner et al., 2005; Sloan et al., 1992).

Pharmacologic studies have shown an association between delirium and administration of anticholinergic drugs and serum anticholinergic activity (Inouye, 2006). High serum anticholinergic activity is associated with severity of delirium (Mussi et al., 1999; Trzepacz, 1999). Also, the importance of cholinergic deficiency in pathophysiology of delirium is supported by studies showing that acetylcholine neurotransmission decreases with age, which is consistent with the finding that increasing age is a risk factor for delirium (Flacker & Lipsitz, 1999). Several mechanisms can result in cholinergic deficiency and predispose to delirium, including impairment in acetylcholine synthesis and cholinergic synaptic mechanisms, ischemia and global stressors and neurotransmitter imbalance (Hshieh et al., 2008).

3.3.1.2 Monoamine neurotransmitter system

Another neurotransmitter system supposed to have a role in pathogenesis of delirium is monoamine neurotransmitter system (Gaudreau & Gagnon, 2005). Dopamine, norepinephrine and serotonin have roles in arousal and sleep-wake cycle, they modulate physiological responses to stimuli (Robbins & Arnsten, 2009). This system, which is composed of three monoamine neurotransmitters, dopamine, norepinephrine and serotonin, has a balancing role for the cholinergic activity. The development of delirium involves interaction between these two neurotransmitter systems (Cole, 2004; Trzepacz & van der Mast, 2002). But instead of deficiency, dopamine excess has been reported to play a role in delirium (Moyer, 2011). It is suggested that dopamine increase during the stress of surgery can cause postoperative agitation and delusions in the patient. In laboratory studies, stress has been shown to elevate levels of mesocortical dopamine (Cassem et al., 2004). Haloperidol, a dopamine blocking agent has been used successfully to treat delirium for years (Moore & O'Keeffe, 1999).

Depending on the serotonin receptor bound, both serotonin excess and deficiency may be associated with cholinergic deficiency and predispose to delirium (Hshieh et al., 2008). Selective serotonin reuptake inhibitors like fluoxetine and buproprion have been reported to cause delirium (Chan et al., 2006). Delirium has been reported in a patient taking paroxetine preoperatively, the authors have contributed that postoperative delirium was indicating an adverse drug interaction involving, paroxetine (Stanford & Stanford, 1999).

3.3.2 Neural injury, inflammation, and stress response

Delirium has been hypothesized to result from increased release of proinflammatory cytokines in cases of trauma, infection or surgery (Eikelenboom et al., 2002; Rudolph et al.,

2008). Proinflammatory cytokines can affect the synthesis or release of acetylcholine, dopamine, noradrenaline and serotonin, and thereby increase the risk of delirium (Dunn, 2006). Also, these cytokines can stimulate responses from microglia, by this way cause inflammation in the brain (Dilger & Johnson, 2008). The effect of these proinflammatory cytokines do not appear to affect younger individuals with healthy brains, while the aging brain is more susceptible to the memory impairments produced by immune system activation (Staus, 2011).

4. Conclusion

Delirium is a common condition, especially in the elderly and in patients with severe illness. Delirium is associated with longer hospital stay, poorer functional outcome, and cognitive decline. Also, it is associated with elevated morbidity and mortality. Understanding etiology of delirium is important because treatment of delirium is identification and reversal of etiological factors. Etiological factors are of two types: predisposing and precipitating factors. The risk of delirium should be kept in mind when approaching to a patient with predisposing factors like increased age, cognitive impairment, hip fracture on admission and severe illness are among the most common ones. The presence of precipitating factors (the acute insults that trigger the mechanisms resulting in delirium) like anemia, hypoxaemia, electrolyte abnormalities, sleep deprivation, pain, bladder catheter use and drugs should be evaluated and be treated promptly if possible.

5. References

American Psychiatric Association., 2000. Diagnostic and Statistical Manual of Mental Disorders, Text Revision, 4th ed. American Psychiatric Press, Washington, DC.

Anand, A.; Li,Y.; Wang, Y.; Wu, J.; Gao, S.; Bukhari, L.; Mathews, V.P.; Kalnin, A. & Lowe, M.J. (2005). Activity and connectivity of brain mood regulating circuit in depression: a functional magnetic resonance study. *Biological Psychiatry,* Vol. 57, No. 10, (May 2005), pp. 1079-1088. ISSN 0006-3223.

Banks, I. (2001). No man's land: men, illness, and the NHS. *British Medical Journal,* Vol. 323, No. 7320, (November 2001), pp. 1058-1060. ISSN 0959-8138.

Blum, D.; Maldonado, J.; Meyer, E. & Lansberg, M. (2008). Delirium following abrupt discontinuation of fluoxetine. *Clinical Neurology and Neurosurgery,* Vol.110, No.1, (January 2008), pp. 69-70. ISSN 0303-8467

Bond, S.M.; Dietrich, M.S.; Shuster, J.L. Jr. & Murphy, B.A. (2011). Delirium in patients with head and neck cancer in the outpatient treatment setting. *Supportive Care in Cancer,* (May 2011), pp. ISSN 0941-4355.

Branco, B.C.; Inaba, K.; Bukur, M.; Talving, P.; Oliver, M.; David, J.S.; Lam, L. & Demetriades, D. (2011). Risk factors for delirium in trauma patients: the impact of ethanol use and lack of insurance. *The American Surgeon,* Vol.77, No.5, (May 2011), pp. 621-626. ISSN 0003-1348.

Brauer, C.; Morrison, R.S.; Silberzweig, S.B. & Siu, A.L. (2000). The cause of delirium in patients with hip fracture. *Archives of Internal Medicine*, Vol. 160, No. 12, (June 2000), pp. 1856-1860. ISSN 0003-9926.

Brouquet, A.; Cudennec, T.; Benoist, S.; Moulias, S.; Beauchet, A.; Penna, C.; Teillet, L. & Nordlinger, B. (2010). Impaired mobility, ASA status and administration of tramadol are risk factors for postoperative delirium in patients aged 75 years or more after major abdominal surgery. *Annals of Surgery*, Vol.251, No.4, (April 2010), pp. 759-765. ISSN 0003-4932.

Burkhart, C.S.; Dell-Kuster, S.; Gamberini, M.; Moeckli, A.; Grapow M.; Filipovic, M.; Seeberger, M.D.; Monsch, A.U.; Strebel, S.P. & Steiner, L.A. (2010). Modifiable and nonmodifiable risk factors for postoperative delirium after cardiac surgery with cardiopulmonary bypass. *Journal of Cardiothoracic and Vascular Anesthesia*, Vol.24, No.4, (August 2010), pp. 555-559. ISSN 1053-0770.

Burns, A.; Gallagley, A. & Byrne, J. (2004). Delirium. *Journal of Neurology, Neurosurgery and Psychiatry*, Vol.75, No. 3, (March 2004), pp. 362-367. ISSN 0022-3050.

Camus, V., Gonthier, R., Dubos, G., Schwed, P., & Simeone, I. (2000). Etiologic and outcome profiles in hypoactive and hyperactive subtypes of delirium. *Journal of Geriatric Psychiatry and Neurology*, Vol.13, No.1, (April, 2000), pp. 38–42. ISSN 0891-9887.

Cassem, N.H.; Murray, G.B.; Lafayette, J.M. & Stern, T.A. (2004). Delirious Patients. In: *Massachusetts General Hospital Psychiatry*, T.A. Stern ; G.L. Fricchione; N.H. Cassem; M.S. Jellinek & J.F. Rosenbaum, (Ed.) pp. 119-134, Mosby, ISBN-13: 978-0-323-02767-0. ISBN-10: 0-323-02767-9, Philedelphia.

Centorrino, F.; Albert, M.J.; Drago-Ferrante, G.; Koukopoulos, A.E.; Berry, J.M. & Baldessarini, R.J. (2003). Delirium during clozapine treatment: incidence and associated risk factors. *Pharmacopsychiatry* Vol.36, No.4, (July 2003), pp. 156-160. ISSN 0176-3679

Chan, C.H.; Liu, H.C. & Huang, M.C. (2006). Delirium associated with concomitant use of low-dose bupropion sustained release and fluoxetine. *Journal of Clinical Psychopharmacology*, Vol.26, No.6, (December 2006), pp. 677–679. ISSN 0271-0749.

Chistyakova, Y. & Amos J (2008). Delirium associated with lamotrigine and fluoxetine treatment. *The American Journal of Psychiatry* Vol.165, No.7, (July 2008), pp. 918-919. ISSN 0002-953X.

Clegg, A. & Young, J.B. (2011). Which medications to avoid in people at risk of delirium: a systematic review. Age and ageing, Vol.40, No.1, (January 2011), pp.23-29. ISSN 0002-0729.

Cole, M.G. (2004). Delirium in elderly patients. *The American journal of geriatric Psychiatry*, Vol.12, No.1, pp. 7-21. ISSN 1064-7481.

Courtenay, W.H. (2002). Behavioural factors associated with disease: injury and death among men: evidence and implications for prevention. *International Journal of Men's Health*, Vol.1, No.3, (September 2002), pp. 81-142. ISSN 1933-0278 (Online).

Dasgupta, M. & Dumbrell, A.C. (2006). Preoperative risk assessment for delirium after noncardiac surgery: a systematic review. *Journal of the American Geriatrics Society,* Vol. 54, No. 10, (October 2006), pp. 1578–1589. ISSN 0002-8614.

Deiner, S. & Silverstein, J.H. (2009). Postoperative delirium and cognitive dysfunction. *British Journal of Anaesthesia,* Vol.103, No. Suppl, (December 2009), pp. i41-46. ISSN 0007-0912.

Delmas, G.; Rothmann. C. & Flesch F. (2008). Acute overdose with controlled-release levodopa-carbidopa. *Clinical Toxicology,* Vol.46, No.3, (March 2008), pp. 274-277. ISSN 1556-3650.

Dilger, R.N. & Johnson, R.W. (2008). Aging, microglial cell priming, and the discordant central inflammatory response to signals from the peripheral immune system. *Journal of Leukocyte Biology,* Vol.84, No.4, (June 2008), pp. 932–939. ISSN 0741-5400.

Dunn, A.J. (2006). Effects of cytokines and infections on brain neurochemistry. *Clinical Neuroscience Research,* Vol.6, No.1-2, pp. 52–68. ISSN 1566-2772.

Edlund, A.; Lundström, M.; Brännström, B.; Bucht, G. & Gustafson, Y. (2001). Delirium before and after operation for femoral neck fracture. *Journal of the American Geriatrics Society.* Vol.49, No.10 (October 2001), pp. 1335-1340. ISSN 0002-8614

Eikelenboom, P. & Hoogendijk, W.J. (1999). Do delirium and Alzheimer's dementia share specific pathogenetic mechanisms? *Dementia and geriatric cognitive disorders,* Vol.10, No.5, (September-October 1999), pp. 319–324. ISSN 1420-8008.

Eikelenboom, P., Hoogendijk, W. J., Jonker, C., & van Tilburg, W. (2002). Immunological mechanisms and the spectrum of psychiatric syndromes in Alzheimer's disease. *Journal of Psychiatric Research,* Vol.36, No.5, pp. 269–280. ISSN 0022-3956.

Elie, M.; Cole, M.G.; Primeau, F.J. & Bellavance, F. (1998). Delirium risk factors in elderly hospitalized patients. *Journal of General Internal Medicine,* Vol.13, No.3, (March 1998), pp. 204-212. ISSN 0884-8734.

Ely, EW.; Shintani, A.; Truman, B.; Speroff, T.; Gordon, SM.; Harrell, F.E. Jr.; Inouye, S.K.; Bernard, G.R. & Dittus RS. (2004). Delirium as a predictor of mortality in mechanically ventilated patients in the intensive care unit. *JAMA : the journal of the American Medical Association,* Vol.291, No.14, (April 2004), pp. 1753-1762. ISSN 0098-7484.

Fick, D.M.; Agostini, J.V. & Inouye, S.K. (2002). Delirium superimposed on dementia: a systematic review. *Journal of the American Geriatrics Society,* Vol.50, No.10, (October 2002), pp. 1723–1732. ISSN 0002-8614.

Fisher, B.W. & Flowerdew, G. (1995). A simple model for predicting postoperative delirium in older patients undergoing elective orthopedic surgery. *Journal of the American Geriatrics Society,* Vol.43, No.2, (February 1995), pp. 175–178. ISSN 0002-8614.

Flacker, J.M. & Lipsitz, L.A. (1999). Neural mechanisms of delirium: Current hypotheses and evolving concepts. *The Journals of Gerontology. Series A, Biological Sciences and Medical Sciences,* Vol.54, No.6, (June 1999), pp.B239-246. ISSN 1079-5006.

Fong, T.G.; Bogardus, S.T. Jr.; Daftary, A.; Auerbach, E.; Blumenfeld, H.; Modur, S.; Leo-Summers, L.; Seibyl, J. & Inouye, S.K. (2006). Cerebral perfusion changes in older delirious patients using 99mTc HMPAO SPECT. *The Journals of Gerontology. Series A, Biological Sciences and Medical Sciences,* Vol.61, No.12, (December 2006), pp. 1294-1299. ISSN 1079-5006.

Fong, T.G.; Tulebaev, S.R. & Inouye, S.K. (2009). Delirium in elderly adults: diagnosis, prevention and treatment. *Nature reviews. Neurology,* Vol.5, No.4, (April 2009), pp. 210-220. ISSN 1759-4758.

Freter, S. H.; George, J.; Dunbar, M. J.; Morrison, M.; Macknight, C. & Rockwood, K. (2005). Prediction of delirium in fractured neck of femur as part of routine preoperative nursing care. *Age and Ageing,* Vol.34, No.4, (July 2005), pp. 387–388. ISSN 0002-0729.

Gaudreau, J.D. & Gagnon, P. (2005). Psychotogenic drugs and delirium pathogenesis: the central role of the thalamus. *Medical hypothese,* Vol.64, No.3, pp.471–475. ISSN. 0306-9877

Gray, S.L.; Lai, K.V. & Larson, E.B. (1999). Drug-induced cognition disorders in the elderly: incidence, prevention and management. *Drug Safety.* Vol.21, No.2, (August 1999), pp.101-122. ISSN 0114-5916.

Gerretsen, P. & Pollock, B.G. (2011). Drugs with anticholinergic properties: a current perspective on use and safety. *Expert Opinion on Drug Safety,* Vol.10, No.5, (September 2011), pp. 751-765. ISSN 1474-0338.

Gustafson, Y.; Brannstrom, B.; Norberg, A.; Bucht, G. & Winblad, B. (1991). Underdiagnosis and poor documentation of acute confusional states in elderly hip fracture patients. *Journal of the American Geriatrics Society,* Vol.39, No.8, (August 1991), pp. 760–765. ISSN 0002-8614.

Hshieh, T.T.; Fong, T.G.; Marcantonio, E.R. & Inouye, S.K. (2008). Cholinergic deficiency hypothesis in delirium: a synthesis of current evidence. *The Journals of Gerontology. Series A, Biological Sciences and Medical Sciences,* Vol.63, No.7, (July 2008), pp. 764-772. ISSN 1079-5006.

Inouye, S.; Viscili, C.; Horwitz, R.; Hurst, L. & Tinetti M. (1993). A predictive model for delirium in hospitalised elderly medical patients based on admission characteristics. *Annals of Internal Medicine,* Vol.119, No.6, (September 1993), pp. 474-480. ISSN 0003-4819

Inouye, S.K. & Charpentier, P.A. (1996). Precipitating factors for delirium in hospitalized elderly persons. Predictive model and interrelationship with baseline vulnerability. *JAMA : The Journal of the American Medical Association,* Vol.275, No.11, (March 1996), pp. 852-857. ISSN 0098-7484.

Inouye, S. K. (1999). Predisposing and precipitating factors for delirium in hospitalized older patients. *Dementia and Geriatric Cognitive Disorders,* Vol. 10, No.5, (September-October 1999), pp. 393–400. ISSN 1420-8008.

Inouye, S.K. (2006). Delirium in older persons. *The New England Journal of Medicine,* Vol.354, No.11, (March 2006), pp. 1157- 1165. ISSN 0028-4793.

Inouye, S.K. & Ferrucci, L. (2006). Elucidating the pathophysiology of delirium and the interrelationship of delirium and dementia. *The Journals of Gerontology. Series A, Biological Sciences and Medical Sciences,* Vol.61, No.12, (December 2006), pp. 1277-1280. ISSN 1079-5006.

Joosten, E.; Lemiengre, J.; Nelis, T.; Verbeke, G. & Milisen, K. (2006). Is anaemia a risk factor for delirium in an acute geriatric population? *Gerontology,* Vol.52, No.6, (August 2006), pp. 382-385. ISSN 0304-324X 2006.

Kazmierski, J.; Kowman, M.; Banach, M.; Fendler, W.; Okonski, P.; Banys, A.; Jaszewski, R.; Rysz, J.; Mikhailidis, D.P.; Sobow, T.; Kloszewska, I. & IPDACS Study. (2010).

Incidence and predictors of delirium after cardiac surgery: Results from The IPDACS Study. *Journal of Psychosomatic Research*, Vol.69, No.2, (August 2010), pp. 179-85. ISSN 0022-3999.

Kolbeinsson, H. & Jonsson, A. (1993). Delirium and dementia in acute Medical admissions of elderly patients in Iceland. *Acta Psychiatrica Scandinavica*, Vol.87, No.2, (February 1993), pp. 123–127. ISSN 0001-690X.

Kopelman, M.D. (1986). The cholinergic neurotransmitter system in human memory and dementia: A review. *Quarterly Journal of Experimental Psychology*, Vol.38, No.4, (November 1986), pp. 535-573. ISSN 1747-0218.

Korevaar, J.C.; van Munster, B.C. & de Rooij, S.E. (2005). Risk factors for delirium in acutely admitted elderly patients: a prospective cohort study. *BMC geriatrics*, Vol.5, No.1, (April 2005), pp.6. ISSN 1471-2318.

Lee, K.H.; Ha, Y.C.; Lee, Y.K.; Kang, H. & Koo, K.H. (2011). Frequency, risk factors, and prognosis of prolonged delirium in elderly patients after hip fracture surgery. *Clinical Orthopaedics and Related Research*, Vol.469, No.9, (September 2011), pp. 2612-2620. ISSN 0009-921X.

Leigh, H. (2008) Delirium, Dementia, Alcohol Intoxication, and Withdrawal Syndromes, In: *Handbook of Consultation-Liaison Psychiatry*, H. Leigh; J. Streltzer, pp. 74-89, Springer, ISBN 987-0-387-78128-0, New York.

Lindesay, J.; Rockwood, K. & Rolfson, D.B. (2002). The epidemiology of delirium. In: *Delirium in old age*, J. Lindesay, K. Rockwood & A.J. Macdonald, (Eds.), pp. 27–50, Oxford University Press, ISBN 0192632752, 9780192632753 New York.

Leentjens, A.F.; Schieveld, J.N.; Leonard, M.; Lousberg, R.; Verhey, F.R. & Meagher, D.J. (2008). A comparison of the phenomenology of pediatric, adult, and geriatric delirium. *Journal of Psychosomatic Research*, Vol.64, No.2, (February 2008), pp. 219-23. ISSN 0022-3999.

Maclullich, A.M.; Ferguson, K.J.; Miller, T.; de Rooij, S.E. & Cunningham, C. (2008). Unravelling the pathophysiology of delirium: a focus on the role of aberrant stress responses. *Journal of Psychosomatic Research*, Vol.65, No.3, (September 2008), pp. 229-238. ISSN 0022-3999.

Magaziner, J.; Simonsick, E.M.; Kashner, M.; Hebel, J.R. & Kenzora, J.E. (1989). Survival experience of aged hip fracture patients. *American Journal of Public Health*, Vol.79, No.3, (March 1989), pp. 274–278. ISSN 0090-0036.

Maldonado, J.R. (2008). Pathoetiological model of delirium: comprehensive understanding of the neurobiology of delirium and an evidence- based approach to prevention and treatment. *Critical Care Clinics*, Vol.24, No.4, (October 2008), pp. 789-856. ISSN 0749-0704.

Marcantonio, E.; Ta, T.; Duthie, E. & Resnick, N.M. (2002). Delirium severity and psychomotor types: their relationship with outcomes after hip fracture repair. *Journal of the American Geriatrics Society*, Vol.50, No.5, (May 2002), pp. 850-857. ISSN 0002-8614.

Martini, D.R. (2010). Psychiatric Emergencies, In: *Dulcan's Textbook of Child and Adolescent Psychiatry*, M. Dulcan, (Ed.), 588-589, American Psychiatric Publishing, Inc. ISBN: 978-1-58562-323-5, Washington, DC.

Michaud, L.; Büla, C.; Berney, A.; Camus, V.; Voellinger, R.; Stiefel, F. & Burnand, B. (2007). Delirium: guidelines for general hospitals. *Journal of Psychosomatic Research,* Vol.62, No.3, (March 2007), pp. 371-383. ISSN 0022-3999

Milbrandt, E.B.; Deppen, S.; Harrison, P.L.; Shintani, A.K.; Speroff, T.; Stiles, R.A.; Truman, B.; Bernard, G.R.; Dittus, R.S. & Ely, E.W. (2004). Costs associated with delirium in mechanically ventilated patients. Critical care medicine Vol.32, No.4, (April 2004), pp. 955-962. ISSN 0090-3493.

Mittal, V.; Muralee, S.; Williamson, D.; McEnerney, N.; Thomas, J.; Cash, M. & Tampi, R.R. (2011). Review: delirium in the elderly: a comprehensive review. *American Journal of Alzheimer's Disease and Other Dementias,* Vol.26, No.2 (March 2011), pp. 97-109. ISSN 1533-3175.

Morrison, R.S.; Magaziner, J.; Gilbert, M.; Koval, K.J.; McLaughlin, M.A.; Orosz, G.; Strauss, E. & Siu, A.L. (2003). Relationship between pain and opioid analgesics on the development of delirium following hip fracture. *The Journals of Gerontology. Series A, Biological Sciences and Medical Sciences,* Vol.58, No.1, (January 2003), pp. 76–81. ISSN 1079-5006.

Moyer, D.D. (2011). Review article: terminal delirium in geriatric patients with cancer at end of life. *American Journal of Hospice & Palliative Medicine,* Vol.28, No.1, (February 2011), pp. 44-51. ISSN 1049-9091.

Moore, A.R. & O'Keeffe, S.T. (1999). Drug-induced cognitive impairment in the elderly. *Drugs & Aging,* Vol.15, No.1, (July 1999), pp. 15-28. ISSN 1170-229X.

Mussi, C.; Ferrari, R.; Ascari, S. & Salvioli, G. (1999). Importance of serum anticholinergic activity in the assessment of elderly patients with delirium. *Journal of Geriatric Psychiatry and Neurology,* Vol.12, No.2, (Summer 1999), pp. 82-86. ISSN 0891-9887.

National Clinical Guideline Center: delirium: diagnosis, prevention and management. http://guidance.nice.org.uk/CG103/NICEGuidance/pdf/English

Nayeem, K. & O'Keeffe, S. (2003). Delirium. *Clinical Medicine,* Vol.3, No.5, (September-October 2003), pp. 412-415. ISSN 1470-2118.

Norkiene, I.; Ringaitiene, D.; Misiuriene, I.; Samalavicius, R.; Bubulis, R.; Baublys, A. & Uzdavinys, G. (2007). Incidence and precipitating factors of delirium after coronary artery bypass grafting. *Scandinavian Cardiovascular Journal,* Vol.41, No.3, (June 2007), pp. 180-185. ISSN 1401-7431.

Nunez, P.L.; Wingeier, B.M. & Silberstein R.B. (2001). Spatial-temporal structures of human alpha rhythms: theory, microcurrentm sources, multiscale measurements, and global binding of local networks. *Human Brain Mapping* Vol.13, No.3, (July 2001), pp. 125-164. ISSN 1065-9471.

Ouimet, S.; Kavanagh, B.P.; Gottfried, S.B. & Skrobik, Y (2007). Incidence, risk factors and consequences of ICU delirium. *Intensive Care Medicine,* Vol.33, No.1, (January 2007), pp. 66-73. ISSN 0342-4642.

Palmu, R.; Suominen, K.; Vuola, J. & Isometsä, E. (2011). Mental disorders after burn injury: a prospective study. *Burns: journal of the International Society for Burn Injuries,* Vol.37, No.4, (November 2011), pp.601-619. ISSN 0305-4179.

Pandharipande, P.; Shintani, A.; Peterson, J.; Pun, B. T.; Wilkinson, G. R.; Dittus, R. S.; Bernard, G. R. & Ely, E. W. (2006). Lorazepam is an independent risk factor for transitioning to delirium in intensive care unit patients. *Anesthesiology,* Vol.104, No.1, (January 2006), pp. 21-26. ISSN 0003-3022.

Pandharipande, P.; Cotton, B.A.; Shintani, A.; Thompson, J.; Costabile, S.; Truman, Pun B.; Dittus, R. & Ely, E.W. (2007). Motoric subtypes of delirium in mechanically ventilated surgical and trauma intensive care unit patients. *Intensive Care medicine,* Vol.33, No.10, (), pp. 1726-1731. ISSN 0342-4642.

Pisani, M.A.; Murphy, T.E.; Van Ness, P.H.; Araujo, K.L. & Inouye, S.K. (2007). Characteristics associated with delirium in older patients in a medical intensive care unit. *Archives of Internal Medicine,* Vol.167, No.15, (August 2007), pp. 1629-1634. ISSN 0003-9926.

Pisani, M.A.; Murphy, T.E.; Araujo, K.L. & Van Ness, P.H. (2010). Factors associated with persistent delirium after intensive care unit admission in an older medical patient population. *Journal of Critical Care* Vol.25, No.3, (September 2010), pp. 540.e1-7. ISSN 0883-9441.

Pompei, P.; Foreman, M.; Rudberg, M.A.; Inouye, S.K.; Braund, V. & Cassel, C.K. (1994). Delirium in hospitalized older persons: outcomes and predictors. *Journal of the American Geriatrics Society,* Vol.42, No.8, (August 1994), pp. 809-815. ISSN 0002-8614.

Renner, U.D.; Oertel, R. & Kirch, W. (2005). Pharmacokinetics and pharmacodynamics in clinical use of scopolamine. *Therapeutic Drug Monitoring,* Vol.27, No.5, (October 2005), pp. 655-665. ISSN 0163-4356.

Robbins, T.W. & Arnsten, A.F. (2009). The neuropsychopharmacology of fronto-executive function: monoaminergic modulation. *Annual Review of Neuroscience,* Vol.32, No.1, (June 2009), pp. 267-287. ISSN 0147-006X.

Rudolph, J.L.; Ramlawi, B.; Kuchel, G.A.; McElhaney, J.E.; Xie, D.; Sellke, F.W.; Khabbaz, K.; Levkoff, S.E. & Marcantonio, E.R. (2008). Chemokines are associated with delirium after cardiac surgery. *The Journals of Gerontology. Series A, Biological Sciences and Medical Sciences,* Vol.63, No.2, (February 2008), pp. 184–189. ISSN 1079-5006.

Samuels, S.C. & Neugroschl, J.A. (2005). Delirium. In: *Kaplan & Sadock's Comprehensive Textbook of Psychiatry, 8th Edition.* Sadock, Benjamin J.& Sadock, Virginia A, pp. 1055-1068, Lippincott Williams & Wilkins, ISBN: 0781734347, New York.

Sanders, R.D. (2011). Hypothesis for the pathophysiology of delirium: role of baseline brain network connectivity and changes in inhibitory tone. *Medical hypotheses,* Vol.77, No.1, (July 2011), pp. 140-143. ISSN 0306-9877.

Saxena, S. & Lawley, D. (2009). Delirium in the elderly: a clinical review. *Postgraduate Medical Journal,* Vol. 85, No. 1006, (August 2009), pp. 405-413. ISSN 0032-5473.

Scheife, R. & Takeda, M. (2005). Central nervous system safety of anticholinergic drugs for the treatment of overactive bladder in the elderly. *Clinical Therapeutics,* Vol.27, No.2, (February 2005), pp.144-153. ISSN 0149-2918

Schor, J.D.; Levkoff, S.E.; Lipsitz, L.A.; Reilly, C.H.; Cleary, P.D.; Rowe, J.W. & Evans, D.A. (1992). Risk factors for delirium in hospitalized elderly. *JAMA : the journal of the American Medical Association,* Vol.267, No.6, (February 1992), pp. 827-831. ISSN 0098-7484.

Sloan, E.P.; Fenton, G.W. & Standage, K.P. (1992). Anticholinergic drug effects on quantitative electroencephalogram, visual evoked potential, and verbal memory. Biological psychiatry, Vol.31, No.6, (March 1992), pp.600-606. ISSN 0006-3223.

Stanford, B.J. & Stanford S.C. (1999). Postoperative delirium indicating an adverse drug interaction involving the selective serotonin reuptake inhibitor, paroxetine? *Journal of Psychopharmacology*. Vol.13, No.3, (May, 1999), pp. 313-317. ISSN 0269-8811.

Staus, R. (2011). Delirium in the older adult orthopaedic patient: predisposing, precipitating, and organic factors. *Orthopaedic Nursing,* Vol.30, No.4, (Jul-Aug 2011), pp. 231-238. ISSN 0744-6020.

Steiner, L.A. (2011). Postoperative delirium. Part 1: pathophysiology and risk factors. *European Journal of Anaesthesiology,* Vol.28, No.9, (September 2011), pp. 628-636. ISSN 0265-0215.

Thomas, C.; Hestermann, U.; Kopitz, J.; Plaschke, K.; Oster, P.; Driessen, M.; Mundt, C. & Weisbrod, M. (2008). Serum anticholinergic activity and cerebral cholinergic dysfunction: an EEG study in frail elderly with and without delirium. *BMC neuroscience,* Vol.9, No.1, (September 2008), pp.86. ISSN 1471-2202.

Thomason, J.W.W.; Shintani, A.; Peterson, J.F.; Pun, B.T.; Jackson, J.C. & Ely, E.W. (2005). Intensive care unit delirium is an independent predictor of longer hospital stay: a prospective analysis of 261 nonventilated patients. *Critical care,* Vol.9, No.4, (August 2005), pp. R375-381. ISSN 1364-8535.

Trzepacz, P.T. (1999). Update on the neuropathogenesis of delirium. *Dementia and Geriatric Cognitive Disorders,* Vol.10, No.5, (September-october 1999), pp.330-334. ISSN 1420-8008.

Trzepacz, P. & van der Mast, R. (2002). The neuropathophysiology of delirium. In: *Delirium in old age,* J. Lindesay, K. Rockwood & A.J. Macdonald, (Eds.), pp. 27–50, Oxford University Press, ISBN 0192632752, 9780192632753 New York.

Tune, L.E. & Egeli, S. (1999). Acetylcholine and delirium. *Dementia and Geriatric Cognitive Disorders,* Vol.10, No.5, (September-october, 1999), pp. 342–344. ISSN 1420-8008.

Uusvaara, J.; Pitkala, K.H.; Kautiainen, H.; Tilvis, R.S. & Strandberg, T.E. (2011). Association of anticholinergic drugs with hospitalization and mortality among older cardiovascular patients: A prospective study. *Drugs & aging,* Vol.28, No.2, (February 2011), pp.131-138. ISSN1170-229X.

Weinhouse, G.L.; Schwab, R.J.; Watson, P.L.; Patil, N.; Vaccaro, B.; Pandharipande, P. & Ely, E.W. (2009). Bench-to-bedside review: delirium in ICU patients - importance of sleep deprivation. *Critical Care,* Vol.13, No.6, (December 2009), pp.234. ISSN. 1364-8535.

White, C.; McCann, M.A. & Jackson, N. (2007). First do no harm... Terminal restlessness or drug-induced delirium. *Journal of Palliative Medicine,* Vol.10, No.2, (April, 2007), pp.345-351. ISSN 1096-6218.

Williams, D.T. (2007). Delirium and Catatonia, In: *Lewis's Child and Adolescent Psychiatry: A Comprehensive Texbook,* A. Martin, F.R. Volkmar, (Ed.), 647-655, Lippincott Williams & Wilkins, ISBN-13: 978-0-7817-6214-4. ISBN-10: 0-7817-6214-6.

Williams MA, Campbell EB, Raynor WJ, Mlynarczyk SM, Ward SE. Reducing acute confusional states in elderly patients with hip fractures. *Research in Nursing & Health,* Vol.8, No.4, (December 1985), pp. 329–337. ISSN 0160-6891.

Williams-Russo, P.; Urquhart, B.L.; Sharrock, N.E. & Charlson, M.E. (1992). Postoperative delirium: predictors and prognosis in elderly orthopedic patients. *Journal of the*

American Geriatrics Society, Vol.40, No.8, (August 1992), pp. 759–767. ISSN 0002-8614.

Yokota, H.; Ogawa, S.; Kurokawa, A. & Yamamoto, Y. (2003). Regional cerebral blood flow in delirium patients. *Psychiatry and Clinical Neurosciences*, Vol.57, No.3, (June 2003), pp. 337–339. ISSN 1323-1316.

Section 4

Virology and Epidemiology

11

Epidemiology of Simian Polyomavirus SV40 in Different Areas of Russian Federation (RF)

B. Lapin and M. Chikobava
Research Institute of Medical Primatology of the Russian Academy of Medical Sciences, Sochi
Russia

1. Introduction

DNA-containing polyomavirus SV40 was isolated in 1961 from poliovaccine prepared on kidney cell culture of M.mulatta naturally infected with this virus. Main part of poliovaccines (IPV and OPV) was contaminated with SV40. From 1955 till 1963 hundred millions of people in USA, Russia (USSR), and in some other countries were immunized with contaminated SV40 Salk and Sabin vaccine and a lot of people became carriers of SV40. This virus was detected also in some human tumors. Epidemiological researches were not carried out in Russia before 2009. By present time possibility and ways of SV40 excretion into environment and possibility of its horizontal spreading is established. From the beginning of 60s (in Russia a little bit later) vaccines were free from SV40 contamination. In this article the data about SV40 infection of population in Moscow, St. Petersburg, in some cities of the Black Sea coast of Caucasus, in Novosibirsk and in one area of Krasnoyarsk region are presented., Analysis of the source of SV40 people infection is performed.

Small size DNA virus was isolated from mice in 1953. The virus was called "polyomavirus" SV40 (Gross, 1951; Gross, 1953). because it was able to produce multiple malignant tumors in newborn rodents.

Simian SV40 was the second discovered polyomavirus. It was isolated in 1961 from poliovaccine propagated on M.mulatta kidney cell cultures naturally infected with SV40 as it was established later (Eddy et al., 1961; Sweet & Hilleman, 1960).

SV 40 is a small DNA virus which does not have envelope; its capsid consisted of 72 capsomers. The size of virion is 45 nm; the viral genome is represented by two-stranded DNA aprox. 5000 bp long. On character of the changes caused in cell cultures, the virus also has received the name "vacuolating virus"(Sweet & Hilleman, 1960; Butel et al., 1999).

During next years polyomaviruses were isolated from different animals including different monkey species and from humans with different pathology as well (Simon,2008; Gjoerup, 2010; Voevodin, 2009).).

In 1957 baboon polyomavirus was discovered (Gardner et al., 1989); polyovavirus of African green monkeys was discovered in 1979 (zur Hausen & Giosmann, 1979), after that polyomaviruses of M.fascicularis and chimpanzee were discovered (but not isolated). Two human polyomaviruses BKV and JCV were firstly isolated in 1971: JCV from a patient with Progressive multifocal leukoencephalopathy (Padgett et al., 1971), BKV from patient with nephropathy (Gardner et al., 1971; Padgett et al., 1971).

Later 3 more polyomaviruses were isolated: KI, Wu from respiratory tract and MCV from rare malignant skin tumor - Merkel carcinoma (Feng et al., 2008)

Among human viruses such ubiquitous viruses as JCV and BKV are widely known and are determined from 60 to 90% of cases in humans according to data of different authors (Knowles et al., 2006; Maginnis & Atwood, 2009).

However many publications often contradictory were associated with simian polyomavirus SV40. The virus was unintentionally introduced into human populations together with poliovaccine contaminated with SV40 as it turned out later (Shah, 2007).

The middle 50s of the last century was marked by epoch-making event - creating of 2 types of poliovaccines: Salk formolvaccine (IPV) and live attenuated Sabin vaccine (OPV). More than 100 million people were immunized in USA beginning from 1956 till 1963 using the above mentioned 2 types of vaccines; more than 70 million people were immunized in Russia (USSR) in 1960 using Sabin vaccine (Fisher, 1999. Rizzo, 1999, Peden, 2008, Drozdov, 2005, Mironova et al., 2006). Significant amount of predominantly young people were immunized in different European countries (Shah & Nathanson, 1976).

It is necessary to look back to the history of poliovaccine creation by Salk and Sabin. Both vaccines (Salk inactivated formolvaccine and Sabin live attenuated vaccine) were poliovirus propagated on M. mulatta kidney cell culture. Soon it was shown that in high percent of cases M.mulatta had been already infected with SV40 in natural conditions (Sweet &Hilleman, 1960; Lapin et al., 1965). That is why many poliovaccine lots were contaminated with this virus. As it was found out later Salk method of vaccine preparation did not provide full inactivation of the vaccine (Carbone et al., 1997). As to the Sabin vaccine - it was initially contaminated with polyomavirus (Peden, 2008).

Zoonotic SV40 origin perhaps is beyond doubt but some authors advance an opinion in their publications about preexisting of this virus in humans (Levine, 1998; Geissler, 1985; Paracchini, 2005). This assumption could be supported if SV40 (or DNA sequences of this virus or antibodies to it) could be reliably detected in human materials obtained before mass poliovaccination. Some publications contain information about detection the antibodies to SV40 before beginning the vaccination against poliomyelitis (Geissler, 1985). It can be supposed that the virus could be introduced into human population from the countries of monkey natural habitat (Southeast Asia and India). Serological investigations revealed SV40 infection of Zoo workers and in workers of India companies exporting monkeys and contacting with animals. SV40 footprints were detected in their blood (Horvath, 1965; Engels et al., 2004; Shah, 1966). All this testifies the possibility of contact infection humans from animals carriers of the virus.(citation from: Vastad, JAMA, 2002, 288, 1337-1338). However the quantity of people infected with SV40 greatly increased particularly after beginning of mass poliovaccination which testifies this supposition.

Thus mass vaccination of millions of people with poliovaccine which made it possible to eradicate poliomyelitis as an epidemic disease simultaneously led to infection of people with simian polyomavirus SV40.

In 1961 as it was mentioned above USA investigators revealed contamination of poliovaccine with simian (M.mulatta) virus SV40.

Serological investigation and PCR revealed antibodies to SV40 and virus DNA sequences in polio immunized people. To the researcher's surprise the antibodies to SV40 were also detected in not vaccinated people. In connection with this fact the researchers came out with a suggestion that in human populations virus can spread horizontally (Knowles et al., 2006) It has been shown that virus can excrete into surrounding with excrements, breast milk, sperm, that supports the assumption about the possibility of horizontal spreading of the virus (David, 2001; Martini, 1996; Vastag, 2002).

Some investigators described discovery of polyomaviruses in sewage and in sea and river waters which undoubtedly could be the source of horizontal spreading of infection in regions with high SV40 prevalence (Vastag, 2002; Bofill-Mas et al., 2009).

Appearance of people infected with SV40 after immunization with polio vaccine caused anxiety of physicians due to virus ability to induce malignant tumors in laboratory rodents. However absence of apparent increase of tumors in polio vaccinated people reduced the interest to SV40 in people. A new wave of anxiety and long lasting discussions continuing up to now was caused by discovery of DNA sequencing of SV40 in some human tumors. As a result great many contradictory publications appeared describing infection of people with this virus, its origin, ways of spreading and possible connection with human pathology (Carbone, 1994, 1997,1999; De Rizzo, 1998, 2001; Arrington, 2000; Tognon, 2001; Lednicky,2001; Bergsagel, 1992; Vilchez, 2002; Klein, 2002; Bocchetta, 2001; Lapin & Chikobava, 2011; Cutrone et al., 2005; Carter et al., 2003; Hübner R. & Van Marck E.2002; Martini et al., 1998; Barbanti-Brodane et al., 2004).

Some researchers considered discovery of SV40 in human blood and in tumors as artifact (Shah, 1976; Lopez-Rios, 2004; Manfredi, 2005; Mayall, 2003, and many others). Disagreement was caused mainly by high homology of SV40 with ubiquitous human polyomaviruses JCV and BKV and consequently with their immunologic and molecular-biological reactivity (Testa, 1998; Lopez-Rios, 2004; Heinsohn, 2005; Shah & Nathanson, 1976; Shah, 2007; Carter et al., 2003). Some researchers denied infection people with SV40 and believed that discovered antibodies and DNA sequencing belong to human polyomaviruses JCV and BKV.

Because M.mulatta are carriers of polyomavirus SV40 in natural conditions WHO recommended to replace in manufacture poliovaccines kidneys of rhesus monkeys with kidneys of green monkeys not containing this virus. At the same time methods of vaccine decontamination were improved. It is possible to assert that in the period from 1960 till 1962 poliovaccine produced by USA, Great Britain, and some other European countries was free from SV40 contamination. However by that period of time hundred millions of people had been already immunized with contaminated SV40 vaccine in USA, Russia (USSR) and many other countries. In Russia (USSR) that produced vaccine for own needs and also for export to east European countries and countries of southeast Asia clearing vaccine from contamination happened some years later Chumakov et al., 1961;Chumarjvet al., 1963; Scovranek, 1961)

Vaccine produced in east countries was contaminated with SV40 till 1978 according to data of USA and English researchers who investigated SV40 contamination in poliovaccine samples produced in different time in different countries. Authors of the publication note that method of heat inactivation of the vaccine in the presence of $MgCl_2$ inactivated SV40 not completely (Cutrone et al., 2005).

Epidemiological investigations carried out in different countries revealed infection of population with SV40. K. Leithner et al (2005) in Fig 4 of their article published a schematic map demonstrating data on infection of population with SV40 in European countries where contaminated SV40 vaccine was used and afterwards SV40 infection of population was revealed and also those countries where contaminated vaccine was also used but the population was not examined for SV40 infection. Such countries were Russia, Ukraine, Byelorussia, and some East European countries in which vaccination was carried out with OPV Sabin vaccine perhaps produced in Russia (USSR).

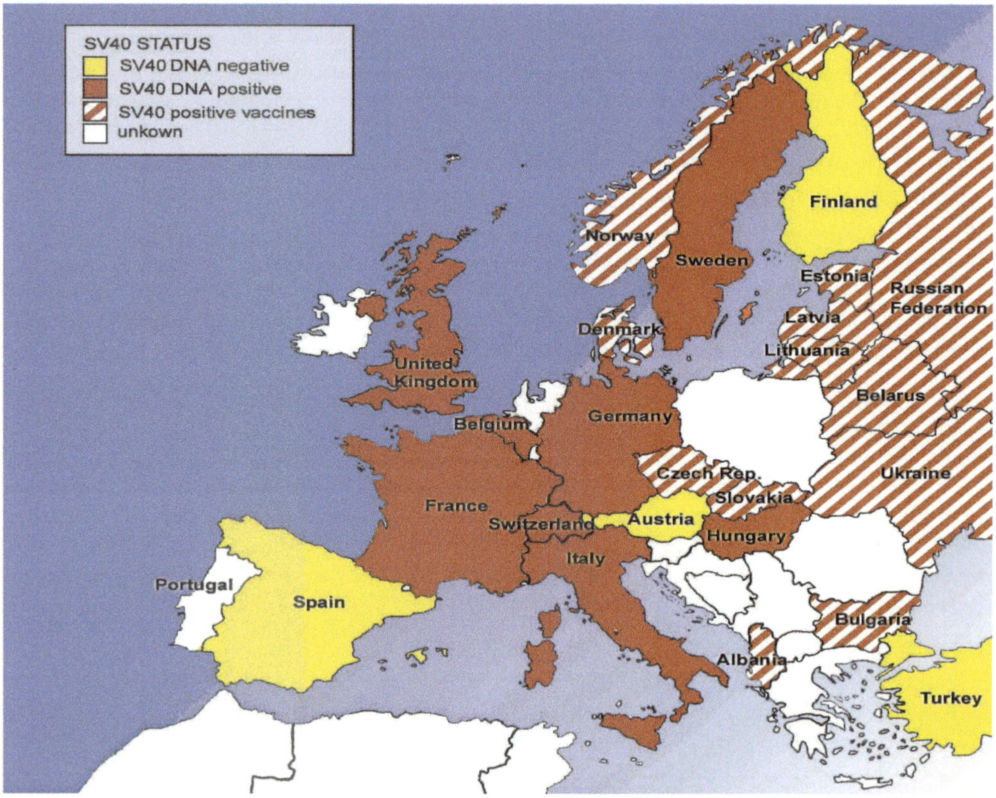

Fig. 1. Red color designates countries where contaminated SV40 vaccine was used and SV40 carriers were discovered (continuous coloring does not mean degree of prevalence). Shaded area designates countries where contaminated vaccine was also used but people were not tested for SV40 carriers. (Leithner 2005). See also Table 1.

Authors of this publication prepared a Table on the basis of literary data which helps to understand where the source of SV40 infection was.

Country	Rating of contamination of polio vaccines with SV40	Vaccines, vaccination programs and origin of vaccines
Albania	Positive	Contaminated Russian vaccine (OPV) used since 1960 (Chumakov et al, 1961;Chumakov et al, 1963; Shah & Nathanson, 1990; Levine et al, 1998).
Austria	Negative	Mass vaccinations with SV40-free British vaccine (OPV) since winter 1961/62 (Kundratitz, 1962; Friza, 1962)
Bulgaria	Positive	Contaminated Russian vaccine (OPV) used since 1960 (Chumakov et al, 1961; Chumakov et al, 1963; Shah & Nathanson, 1990; Levine et al, 1998).
CSSR	Positive	Since 1960: limited use of IPV, mass vaccinations with OPV, partly with contaminated Russian vaccine (Chumakov et al, 1961; Chumakov et al, 1963; Shah & Nathanson, 1990; Levine et al, 1998; Skovranek,1961; Chron Wld Hlth Org, 1960)
Denmark	Positive	Vaccinations from 1955 with widely contaminated Danish vaccine (IPV), SV40-free from 1963 (Engels, 2003). A combined schedule was introduced in 1968 (Murdin et al, 1996).
Finland	Negative	Mass vaccinations since 1957 with SV40-free Belgium vaccine (IPV) (Hirvonen, 1999). Finland has never used OPV on a routine basis (Murdin et al, 1996)
Germany East	Positive	Contaminated Russian vaccine (OPV) used since 1960 (Geissler, 1983; Chumakov et al, 1963; Shah & Nathanson ,1976; Prog Med Virol, 1990; Levine et al,1998, Belian & Rademacher, 1961).
Hungary	Positive	Since 1957: limited use of IPV, mass vaccinations with vaccines from the US, Canada, Hungary and Russia (also OPV) (Chumakov et al, 1963; Shah & Nathanson, 1976; Geissler, 1990; Levine et al, 1998)

Norway	Positive	Vaccinations started 1956 with Danish vaccine (IPV); since 1957 potentially contaminated U.S.vaccine (IPV) (Thu et al, 2006), change to OPV from 1967 to 1979, then back to IPV from 1979 onwards (Murdin et al, 1996).
Poland	Unclear	Mass vaccinations (OPV) since 1958 with Koprowski strain live vaccine [94]; vaccine was claimed to be Russian made (Minor et al, 2003), but Russian vaccines were derived from Sabin's strain (Chumakov et al, 1961)
Russia (USSR)	Positive	Mass vaccinations since 1959 with contaminated Russian vaccine (OPV). A small proportion of persons were vaccinated with IPV at the beginning of the mass vaccinations (Chumakov et al, 1961; Chumakov et al, 1963; Shah & Nathanson , 1976; Levine et al, 1998;Chron Wld Hlth Org 1960).
Spain	Unclear	Mass vaccinations since 1963 with British vaccine (OPV) [101]; British vaccines were SV40-free since 1962 (Sangar et al, 1999); in contrast some vaccines were later claimed to have been contaminated (De Sanjose et al, 2003).
Sweden	Positive	In 1957 potentially contaminated U.S. vaccine (IPV), from 1958 SV40-free Swedish vaccine (IPV). Sweden has never used OPV (Murdin et al, 1996)
Turkey	Negative	Vaccination was not started before 1970, at a time where polio vaccines were required to be SV40-free (De Rienzo et al, 2002). The type of the vaccine is unclear. In a global poliomyelitis eradication initiative starting in 1989, OPV was used.
United Kingdom	Positive	Vaccination started in 1956 with OPV (Chron Wld Hlth Org, 1958; Chron Wld Hlth Org, 1960). SV40-free since 1962 (Rev Sanid Hi Publica, 1965)

Table 1. (Leithner, 2005)

We were aimed at carrying out epidemiological investigation and determining infection of population with polyomavirus SV40 in different regions of Russia and also determine intensity and source of infection. Investigation was carried out mainly anonymously. Each sample was accompanied with information about the place from where the sample was delivered, sex and age of the person.

To determine SV40 infection of population in Russia we decided to determine virus DNA sequences in blood samples of persons of different sex and age delivered to us by different medical institutions from different regions of Russia. Investigation of biological samples for SV40 is rather difficult because standard PCR and immunological tests (IFA, western blotting) do not allow differentiation of SV40 from widely spread ubiquitous human polyomaviruses JCV and BKV which have cross-immunological and cross molecular-biological-reactivity with SV40 (Viscidi, 2003). That is why for SV40 detection we chose the recommended method Real Time PCR (RQ-PCR) with TaqMan probe addressed to the area with 9-nucleotid deletion distinguishing SV40 from JVC and BKV.

2. Methods

For PCR analysis 100 ul of blood was put into a test tube containing EDTA and kept at 4° C until it was delivered to the laboratory for DNA extraction. After extraction DNA samples were kept at -20° C.

Genome of SV40 can be present in the cell in 2 forms: episomal or integrated into genome of host cell. Because of few SV40 copies in the sample the best method allowing detecting episomal forms of SV40 DNA in RQ-PCR are methods based on DNA sorption by SiO_2. That is why we used modified GuSCN protocol (Boom et al., 1992, Testa et al., 1998) for extraction of DNA from whole blood.

Three hundreds microliters of solution containing 5 M GuSCN,1% Triton X-100(v/v), 20 mM EDTA, 50 mM Tris-HCl (pH 6,4), 10 ul SiO_2 was added to the blood sample (100 ul) and incubated 15 min, centrifugated and the sediment was washed once in 5 M GuSCN, 50 mM Tris-HCl (pH 6,4) and twice in 10 mM Tris-HCl (pH 7,3), 50 mM NaCl, 50% ethanol. The sample was desiccated in thermostat and DNA was eluted by TE-buffer (10 mM Tris-HCl (pH 8,0), 1Mm EDTA). For PCR amplification 5 ul were used. Rest was kept at -20° C.

As it was mentioned above SV40 detection was carried out by RQ-PCR method with internal probe directed to SV40 genome region in 4517 position, characterized by deletion of 9 nucleotides distinguishing SV40 from viruses JCV and BKV. PCR was carried out on BioRad Thermocycler according to the following program: 5 min initial denaturation, then 8 sec at 94°C, 23 sec at 60°C, 30 sec at 72°C, during 50 cycles. DNA extracted from M.mulatta blood was used as positive control. Water 5 ul from opened test tube kept together with extracted DNA samples was used as negative control.

3. Results

In total 768 blood samples obtained from different cities and regions of Russian Federation (St. Petersburg - 56, Moscow - 50, Krasnodar region - 352, Novosibirsk - 108, Krasnoyarsk region - 202) have been investigated by RQ-PCR. Results of these investigations are presented in Table 2.

Region	Number of samples	Number of SV40 positive	
		Absolute number	%
Krasnodar region	100	49	49
Moscow	50	8	16
St. Petersburg	56	8	14
Novosibirsk	108	32	29.6
Krasnoyarsk region	202	64	26.7

Table 2.

Because this investigation revealed a rather high number of SV40 carriers in Krasnodar region we decided to check the situation in Sochi and Adler (Table 3).

Region	Number of samples	Number of SV40 positive	
		Absolute number	%
Sochi	102	44	43
Adler	150	48	32

Table 3.

To confirm the results of RQ PCR, and prepare amplicons for sequencing another sets (SV5/SV6) of primers directed to conservative region 173-bp length of SV40 T-ag were used. These PCR primers amplify a region of SV40 that could be distinguished from BK and JC viral DNA. (Testa *et al.* 1998).

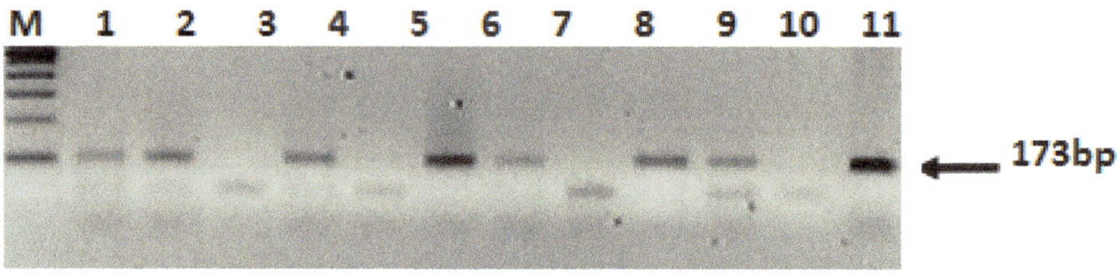

Fig. 2.

The ethidium bromide-stained 2.5% agarose gel shows the PCR products of 9 blood samples, some of which are SV40 positive. N10(-) control (water), 11 (+) control (DNA extracted from blood of SV40+ positive M. mulatta).

The obtained samples were sequenced on a ABI Prism 377 sequenator. Result of sequencing confirmed belonging of amplified regions to SV40.

We believe that the results can be corrected both towards the increase and towards reduction on the basis of age, sex and other factor analyzes of representative groups.

Nevertheless obtained material allows drawing some conclusions. High percent of SV40 infected children in Sochi and Krasnodar region at the age of 10 years who were immunized with poliovaccine reliably free from contamination with this virus definitely testifies horizontal way of contamination.

Numerous publications are devoted to polyomavirus problem and a great part of them to SV40 problem: reliability or unauthenticity of SV40 detection in healthy people, in human neoplasm, SV40 role in tumor emergence, SV40 origin and ways of spreading are discussed. In a great degree a lot of publications are connected with scandalous character of the problem - SV40 introduction into human population during immunization against poliomyelitis.

Despite the fact that preparing vaccines on rhesus kidney cell cultures was stopped about 30 years ago SV40 carrying is still determined in high percent of cases in healthy persons and also in some malignant human neoplasm (brain tumors, mesotheliomas, osteosarcomas etc.).

Polyomavirus SV40 has been detected practically on all continents (Fig. 2). After introduction it into human population it should be considered as human virus - man has become its reservoir. The virus circulates among people, spreading horizontally, excretes into surrounding, pollutes it and this is perhaps a very important factor of its epidemiology.

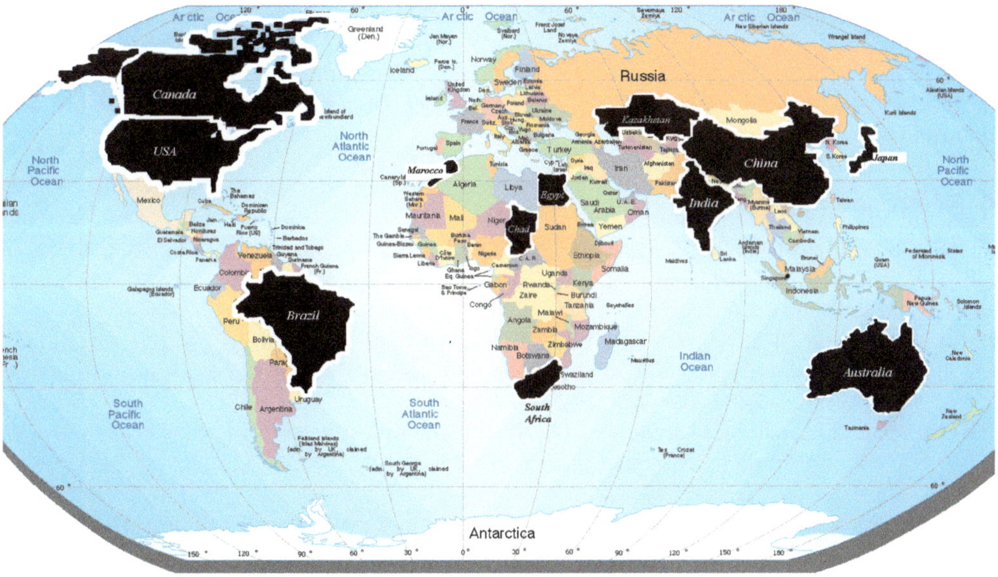

Fig. 3. SV40 infection of population was discovered on all Continents. Black color designates countries where SV40 carriers were discovered. However it does not mean the prevalence of SV40 infection.

4. Conclusion

In this article data on analysis of SV40 polyomavirus contamination of population in some regions of Russia are presented. Infection was detected by PCR in real time (RQ-PCR) with TaqMan probe directed to the site of 9 nucleotide deletion distinguishing SV40 from ubiquitous human viruses JCV and BKV, The source of infection was mainly vaccination with Sabin OPV vaccine contaminated with SV40. Virus SV40 was detected in archive vaccine samples produced in East European countries before 1978 because heating with $MgCl_2$ did not free the vaccine from SV40 contamination. Infection rate was investigated in 5 Russian regions: Russia (Moscow, St. Petersburg, cities of the Black Sea coast, Novosibirsk and Krasnoyarsk region).

The highest values were detected on the Black Sea and the lowest in St. Petersburg. Presence of SV40 in children vaccinated with reliably decontaminated vaccine confirms possibility of horizontal spreading of the virus. According to reference data contamination of population was revealed on all Continents.

Despite the fact that preparing polio vaccine on culture of M.mulatta kidney cells was stopped 30 years ago SV40 carriage still exists in healthy people in rather high percent and also in human malignant neoplasms practically in all countries, on all Continents (Basetse, 2002; Leithner et al., 2006; Minor et al., 2003; Zekri et al., 2007; Dang-Tan et al., 2004). Polyomavirus SV40 was introduced into human population and should be considered as human virus. Man has become its reservoir. The virus circulates among people, spreads horizontally, excretes into environment and pollutes it and this is an important factor in its epidemiology.

Perhaps true value of SV40 prevalence in different regions can be established at examination of randomized groups generated on age, sex, place of residing, conditions of life and cultural skills.

5. References

Arrington AS, Lednicky JA, & Butel JS (2000): Molecular characterization of SV40 DNA in multiple samples from a human mesothelioma. Anticancer Res. 20: 879 - 884, ISSN 0250-7005

Barbanti-Brodano G, & Tognon M (1996): SV40 early region and large T antigen in human brain tumors, peripheral blood cells, and sperm fluids from healthy individuals. Cancer Res. 56: 4820 - 4825, ISSN 0008-5472

Basetse HR, Lecatsas G, &Gerber LJ.(2002) An investigation of the occurrence of SV40 antibodies in South Africa. S Afr Med J. Oct;92(10):825-8, ISSN 0256-9574

Belian W & Rademacher I (1961): Vaccination with live poliovirus vaccine in the German Democratic Republic. In The control of poliomyelitis by live poliovirus vaccine Edited by: Weissfeiler J. Budapest, Akademiai Kiado; 53-56.

Bergsagel DJ, Finegold MJ, Butel JS, Kupsky WJ, & Garcea RL(1992): DNA sequences similar to those of simian virus 40 in ependymomas and choroid plexus tumors of childhood. N. Engl. J. Med. 326: 988 -993, ISSN 0028-4793

Bocchetta M, Di Resta I, Powers A, Fresco R, Tosolini A, Testa JR, Pass HI, Rizzo P, & Carbone M (2000) : Human mesothelial cells are unusually susceptible to simian virus 40-mediated transformation and asbestos cocarcinogenicity. Proc. Natl. Acad. Sci. 97: 10214 -10219.

Boom R, Sol CJ, Salimans MM, Jansen CL, Wertheim-van Dillen PM, & van der Noordaa J (1990): Rapid and simple method for purification of nucleic acids. J.Clin. Microbiol. 28, 495- 50, ISSN 0095-1137

Brown F, Lewis AM (eds) (1998): Simian virus 40 (SV40): A possible human polyomavirus. Dev Biol Stand. Basel, Karger, vol 94, ISSN 0301-5149

Butel JS, Lednicky JA. (1999): Cell and molecular biology of simian virus 40: implications for human infections and disease. J. Natl. Cancer .Inst. 91: 119- 134, ISSN1052-6773

Carbone M, Pass HI, Rizzo P, Marinetti M, Di Muzio M, Mew DJ, Levine AS, & Procopio A. (1994) Simian virus 40-like DNA sequences in human pleural mesothelioma. Oncogene 9: 1781-1790, ISSN 0950-9232

Carbone M, Rizzo P, & Pass HI (1997): Simian virus 40, poliovaccines and human tumors: A review of recent developments. Oncogene 15: 1877- 1888, ISSN 0950-9232

Carbone M. (1999)Simian virus 40 and human tumors: It is time to study mechanisms. J. Cellular Biochemistry 76: 189- 193, ISSN 0733-1959

Carter JJ, Madeleine MM, Wipf GC, Garcea RL, Pipkin PA, Minor PD & Galloway DA (2003)Lack of serologic evidence for prevalent simian virus 40 infection in humans. J Natl Cancer Inst. Oct 15;95(20):1522-30, ISSN 1052-6773,

Chron Wld Hlth Org 1958, 12:163-166. Four years of poliomye,litis research, ISSN 1010-3090,

Chron Wld Hlth Org 1960, 14:137-142. Live poliovirus vaccine, ISSN 10103090,

Chron Wld Hlth Org, 1960, 14:142-144. Live poliovirus vaccination in the USSR, Poland and Czechsolovakia, ISSN 1010-3090,

Chron Wld Hlth Org 1960, 14:462-468. Poliomyelitis prevention, ISSN 1010-3090

Chumakov MP, Voroshilova MK, Drozdov SG, Dzagurov SG,Lashkevich VA, Mironova LL, Ralph NM, Gagarina AV, Dobrova IN, Ashmarina EE, Shirman GA, Fleer GP, Tolskaya EA, Sokolova IS, Elbert LB & Sinyak KM (1961): Some results of the work on mass immunization of the population in the soviet union with live poliovirus vaccine from Albert S. Sabin's strains. In The control of poliomyelitis by live poliovirus vaccine Edited by: Weissfeiler J. Budapest,Akademiai Kiado, p.19-39.

Chumakov MP. (1961a)Some results of mass immunization of the population of the Soviet Union against poliomyelitis with live vaccine from Sabin strains.Vestn Akad Med Nauk SSSR. 16(4):30-43. Russian, ISSN 0869-6047

Chumakov MP.(1961b) Some results of the work on mass immunization in the Soviet Union with live poliovirus vaccine prepared from Sabin strains.Bull World Health Organ. 25:79-91, ISSN 0042-9686

Chumakov MP, Dzagurov SG, Lashkevich VA, Grachev VP, Mironova LL, Ralf NM & Elbert LB (1963): Methods and results of preparing live poliovirus vaccine without SV40 impurities. In: Poliomyelitis and other enterovirus infections : . Proc.of the 2nd scientific session of the Moscow, Institute of Poliomyelitis and Viral Encephalitides; p.201-202, Moscow.

Cicala C, Pompetti, & Carbone M (1993). SV40 induces mesotheliomas in hamsters. Am. J. Pathology 142: 1524- 1533, ISSN 0002-9440

Cutrone R, Lednicky J, Dunn G, Rizzo P, Bocchetta M, Chumakov K, Minor P, & Carbone M.(2005) Some Oral Poliovirus Vaccines Were Contaminated with Infectious SV40 after 1961. Cancer Res 65(22): 10273-10279, ISSN 0008-5472

Dang-Tan T, Mahmud SM, Puntoni R & Franco EL. (2004) Polio vaccines, Simian Virus 40, and human cancer: the epidemiologic evidence for a causal association. Oncogene. Aug 23;23(38):6535-40, ISSN 0950-9232

David H, Mendoza S, Konishi T, & Miller CW (2001): Simian virus 40 is present in human lymphomas and normal blood. Cancer Lett 162: 57- 64, ISSN 0304-3835

De Rienzo A, Tor M, Sterman DH, Aksoy F, Alblda SM, & Testa JR. (2002)Detection of SV40 DNA sequences in malignant mesothelioma specimens from the United States, but not from Turkey. J. Cell. Biochem. 84(3):455- 459, ISSN 0733-1959

De Sanjose S, Shah KV, Domingo-Domenech E, Engels EA, Fernandez DS, Alvaro T, Garcia-Villanueva M, Romagosa V, Gonzalez-Barca E & Viscidi RP (2003): Lack of serological evidence for an association between simian virus 40 and lymphoma. Int J Cancer 104:522-524, ISSN 0020-7136

David H, Mendoza S, Konishi T & Miller CW (2001). Simian virus 40 is present in human lymphomas and normal blood. Cancer Lett. Jan 10;162(1):57-64, ISSN 0304-3835

Drozdov SG, Lashkevich VA. (2005) [The fiftieth anniversary of the M. P. Chumakov Institute of Poliomyelitis and Viral Encephalitides, Russian Academy of Medical Sciences]. vopr Virusol. May-Jun;50(3):4-7, ISSN 0507-4088

Eddy BE, Borman GS, Berkeley W, & Young RD. (1961)Tumors induced in hamsters by injection of rhesus monkey kidney cell extracts. Proc. Soc. Exp. Biol. (NY) 107: 191-197, ISSN 0037-0727

Engels EA, Katki HA, Nielsen NM, Winther JF, Hjalgrim H, Gjerris F,Rosenberg PS & Frisch M (2003): Cancer incidence in Denmark following exposure to poliovirus vaccine contaminated with simian virus 40. J Natl Cancer Inst 95:532-539, ISSN 1052-6773

Feng H, Shuda M, Chang Y & Moore PS (2008) Clonal integration of a polyomavirus in human Merkel cell carcinoma. Science. Feb 22;319(5866):1096-100. Epub 2008 Jan 17, ISSN 0036-8075

Fisher SG, Weber L, & Carbone M (1999) Cancer risk associated with simian virus 40 contaminated polio vaccine. Anticancer Res. 19(3B): 2173- 2180, ISSN 0250-7005

Friza F (1961): Organisation und Durchfuhrung der ersten Schutzimpfung gegen Kinderlahmung mit Lebendvakzine nach Sabin in Osterreich im Winter 1961-1962. Mitt d osterr Sanitatsverw , 63:359-362.

Gallardo P.F, Clavel VL & Galan GJ (1965): Resultados de la Campana nacional de vacunacion antipoliomielitica por via oral en Espana. Rev Sanid Hi Publica, 39:537-561.

Gardner SD, Field AM, Coleman DV & Hulme B(1971)New human papovavirus (B.K.) isolated from urine after renal transplantation. Lancet. Jun 19;1(7712):1253-7, ISSN 0099-5355

Gardner SD, Knowles WA, Hand JF & Porter AA(1989) Characterization of a new polyomavirus (Polyomavirus papionis-2) isolated from baboon kidney cell cultures. Arch Virol. 105(3-4):223-33, ISSN 0304-8608

Geissler E, Konzer P, Scherneck S, & Zimmermann W(1985) Sera collected before introduction of contaminated polio vaccine contain antibodies against SV40. Acta Virologica 29: 420- 423, ISSN 0001-723X

Geissler E, Staneczek. W (1988) SV40 and human brain tumors. Archive fur Geschwulstforschung 58: 129- 134.

Geissler E (1990) SV40 and human brain tumors. Prog Med Virol 37:211–222, ISSN 0079-645X

Gjoerup O, Chang Y (2010), Update on Human Polyomaviruses and Cancer. Adv Cancer Res. 106:1- 51, ISSN 0065-230X

Gross L (1951) "Spontaneous" leukemia developing in C3H mice following inoculation in infancy, with AK-leukemic extracts, or AK-embrvos. Proc. Soc. Exp. Biol. Med. 76: 27–32, ISSN 0037-9727

Gross L (1953) A filterable agent, recovered from Ak leukemic extracts, causing salivary gland carcinomas in C3H mice. Proc. Soc. Exp. Biol. Med. Jun; 83(2):414-21, ISSN 0037-9727

zur Hausen H, Gissmann L (1979) Lymphotropic papovaviruses isolated from African green monkey and human cells. Med Microbiol Immunol. Aug;167(3):137-53, ISSN 0300-8584

Heinsohn S., Golta S., Abisch H., & zur Stadt U (2005), Standardized detection of Simian virus 40 by real-time quantitative polymerase chain reaction in pediatric malignancies. Haematologica 90: 94- 99, ISSN 0390-6078

Hirvonen A, Mattson K, Karjalainen A, Ollikainen T, Tammilehto L,Hovi T, Vainio H, Pass HI, Di Resta I, Carbone M & Linnainmaa K (1999): Simian virus 40 (SV40)-like DNA sequences not detectable in finnish mesothelioma patients not exposed to SV40-contaminated polio vaccines. Mol Carcinog 26:93-99, ISSN 0899-1987

Horvath LB (1965), Incidence of SV40 virus neutralizing antibodies in sera of laboratory workers. Acta Microbiol. Acad. Sci. Hung 12(2):201-205, ISSN 0001-6187

Hübner R,Van Marck E. Reappraisal of the strong association between simian virus 40 and human malignant mesothelioma of the pleura (Belgium) (2002) Cancer Causes Control Mar 13 (2):121-9, 11936818.

Jasani B, Cristaudo A, Emri SA, Gazdar AF, Gibbs A, Krynska B, Miller C, Mutti L, Radu C, Tognon M, Procopio A. Association of SV40 with human tumors. Semin Cancer Biol. 2001; 11:49- 61, ISSN 1044-578X

Klein G, Powers A, & Croce C (2002): Association of SV40 with human tumors. Oncogene 21: 1141–1149, ISSN 0950-9232

Knowles WA (2006) Discovery and epidemiology of the human polyomaviruses BK virus (BKV) and JC virus (JCV). Adv. Exp, Med, Biol. 577:19- 45, ISSN 0065-2598

Kundratitz K (1962): Akutelle Impfprobleme. Mitt d osterr Sanitatsverw 63:192-198.

Martini F, Iaccheri L, Lazzarin L, Carinci P, Corallini A, Gerosa M, Iuzzolino P, Barbanti-Brodano G & Tognon M (1996) SV40 early region and large T antigen in human brain tumors, peripheral blood cells, and sperm fluids from healthy individuals. Cancer Res. Oct 15;56(20):4820-5, ISSN 0008-5472

Lapin BA, Dzhikidze EK, Iakovleva LA, Chumakova MK & Adzhigitov FI (1965) SV-40 virus infection of monkeys in North Vietnamese jungle Vopr Virusol. Mar-Apr;10(2):226-8. Russia, ISSN 0507-4088

Lapin BA. Chikobava MG (2009a)Detection of SV40 in blood samples from healthy subjects in the Russian Federation by RT-PCR. Vestn Ross Akad Med Nauk. (4):7-10, ISSN 0869-6047

Lapin B A, Chikobava MG (2009b) Epidemiology of SV-40 simian virus in different regions of the Russian federation. Bull Exp Biol Med. Dec;148(6):924-6, ISSN 0007-4888

Lednicky JA, Butel JS (2001): Simian virus 40 regulatory region struc-tural diversity and the association of viral archetypal regulatory regions with human brain tumors. Semin Cancer. Biol. 11: 39 - 47, ISSN 1044-579X

Leithner A, Weinhaeusel A, Windhager R, Schlegl R, Waldner P, Lang S, Dominkus M, Zoubek A, Popper HH & Haas OA (2002): Absence of SV40 in Austrian tumors correlates with low incidence of mesotheliomas. Cancer Biol Ther 1:375-379, ISSN 1538-4047

Leithner K, Leithner A, Clar H, Weinhaeusel A, Radl R, Krippl P, Rehak P, Windhager R, Haas OA, & Olschewski H. (2006) Mesothelioma mortality in Europe: impact of asbestos consumption and simian virus 40. Orphanet J Rare Dis. Nov 7;1:44, ISSN 1750-1172

Levine A, Butel J, Dorries K, Goedert J, Frisque R, Garcea R, Morris A, O'Neill F, & Shah K. (1998) SV40 as a putative human commensal. Developments in Biological Standardization 94: 245 269, ISSN 0301-5149

López-Rios F, Illei PB, Rusch V, & Ladanyi M. (2004) Evidence against a role for SV40 infection in human mesotheliomas and high risk of false-positive PCR results owing to presence of SV40 sequences in common laboratory plasmids Lancet, 364 (9440), 1157- 1166, ISSN 0099-3090

Maginnis MS, Atwood WJ. (2009) JC virus : an oncogenic virus in animals and humans? Semin Cancer Biol. Aug;19(4):261-9. Epub 2009 Feb 24. Review, ISSN 1044-579X

Manfredi, J.J, Jianli Dong, Wen-jun Liu, Lois Resnick-Silverman, Rui Qiao, Philippe Chahinian, Marko Saric, Allen R. Gibbs, James I. Phillips, J. Murray, Charles W. Axt en, Robe rt P. Nolan, & Stuart A. Aaronson (2005) Evidence against a Role for SV40 in Human Mesothelioma. Cancer Res. 65(7): 2602- 2609, ISSN 0008-5472

Mayall F, Barratt K, & Shanks J (2003) The detection of Simian virus 40 in mesotheliomas from New Zealand and England using real time FRET probe PCR protocols. J. Clin. Pathol. Oct;56(10):728-730, ISSN 0021-9746

Minor P, Pipkin P, Jarzebek Z & Knowles W (2003) Studies of neutralising antibodies to SV40 in human sera. J Med Virol. Jul;70(3):490-5, ISSN 0146-6615

Murdin AD, Barreto L, Plotkin S (1996): Inactivated poliovirus vaccine: past and present experience. Vaccine 14:735-746.

Padgett BL, Walker DL, ZuRhein GM, Eckroade RJ, Dessel BH (1971) Cultivation of papova-like virus from human brain with progressive multifocal leucoencephalopathy. Lancet. Jun 19;1(7712):1257-60, ISSN 0099-5355

Paracchini V, Garte S, Pedotti P, Poli F, Frison S, Taioli E (2005) Molecular identification of simian virus 40 infection in healthy Italian subjects by birth cohort. Mol Med. Jan-Dec;11(1-12):48-51.

Peden, K. (2008) Recovery of strains of the polyomavirus SV40 from rhesus monkey kidney cells dating from the 1950s to the early 1960s Virology, 370 (1), 63-76

Rizzo P, Bocchetta M, Powers A, Foddis R, Stekala E, Pass HI, & Carbone M (2001): SV40 and the pathogenesis of mesothelioma. Semin Cancer Biol. 11: 63–71, ISSN 1044-579X

Rizzo P, Di Resta I, Stach R, Mutti L, Picci P, Kast WM, Pass HI, & Carbone M (1998): Evidence for and implications of SV40-like sequences in human mesotheliomas and osteosarcomas. Dev. Biol. Stand. 94: 33– 40, ISSN 0301-5149

Rizzo P, Resta ID, Powers A, Ratner H, & Carbone M (1999) Unique strains of SV40 in commercial poliovaccines from 1955 not readily identifiable with current testing for SV40 infection. Cancer Research 59: 6103- 6108, ISSN 0008-5472

Sangar D, Pipkin PA, Wood DJ & Minor PD (1999): Examination of poliovirus vaccine preparations for SV40 sequences. Biologicals ,27:1-10.

Shah KV (2007) SV40 and human cancer: a review of recent data. Int J Cancer. Jan 15;120(2):215-23. Review, ISSN 0020-7136

Shah K, Nathanson N (1976) Human exposure to SV40: Reviews and Comment.. Am. J. Epidemiol. 103:11-12.

Simon M (2008), Polyomaviruses of Nonhuman Primates: implications for research. Comp. Med. Feb. 58(1): 51- 56, ISSN 1532-0820

Skovranek V (1961): The organization and results of mass vaccination against poliomyelitis in CSSR. In The control of poliomyelitis by live poliovirus vaccine Edited by: Weissfeiler J. Budapest, Akademiai Kiado :41-51.

Sweet BH, Hilleman MR (1960): The vacuolating virus SV40. Proc. Soc.Exper. Biol .Med. 105: 420 - 427,

Schuler F (2006) No evidence for simian virus 40 DNA sequences in malignant non-Hodgkin lymphomas. Int. J. Cancer 118, 498–504, ISSN 0020-7136

Testa JR, Carbone M, Hirvonen A, Khalili K, Krynska B, Linnainmaa K, Pooley FD, Rizzo P, Rusch V & Xiao, GH (1998) A multi-institutional study confirms the presence and expression of simian virus 40 in human malignant mesothelioma. Cancer Res., 58: 4505–4509, ISSN 0008-5472

Thu GO, Hem LY, Hansen S, Moller B, Norstein J, Nokleby H & Grotmol T (2006): Is there an association between SV40 contaminated polio vaccine and lymphoproliferative disorders? An age period-cohort analysis on Norwegian data from 1953 to 1997. Int J Cancer 118(8):2035-9, ISSN 0020-7136

Tognon M, Martini F, Iaccheri L, Cultrera R, & Contini C (2001): Inves-tigation of the simian polyomavirus SV40 as a potential causative agent of human neurological disorders in AIDS patients. J. Med. Microbiol. 50: 165–172, ISSN 0022-2615

Vastag B (2002) Sewage Yields Clues to SV40 Transmission *JAMA* 288 (11): 1337- 1338, ISSN 0098-7484

Vilchez RA, Madden CR, Kozinetz CA, Halvorson SJ, White ZS, Jorgenson JL, Finch CJ & Butel JS (2002): Association between simian virus 40 and non-Hodgkin lymphoma. Lancet 359: 817- 823, ISSN 0099-5355

Viscidi RP, Rollison DE, Viscidi E, Clayman B, Rubalcaba E, Daniel R, Major EO & Shah KV (2003) Serological cross-reactivities between antibodies to simian virus 40, BK virus, and JC virus assessed by virus-like-particle-based enzyme immunoassays. Clin Diagn Lab Immunol. Mar;10(2):278-85

Voevodin A. & Marx PA Simian Virology,2009, Wiley-Blackwell, ISBN-13: 978-0-8138-2432-1, UK

Zekri AR, Bahnassy AA, Mohamed WS, Hassan N, Abdel-Rahman AR, El-Kassem FA & Gaafar R (2007) Evaluation of simian virus-40 as a biological prognostic factor in Egyptian patients with malignant pleural mesothelioma. Pathol Int. Aug;57(8):493-501, ISSN 1320-5463

12

Modeling Infectious Diseases Dynamics: Dengue Fever, a Case Study

Maíra Aguiar[1], Nico Stollenwerk[1] and Bob W. Kooi[2]
[1]*Centro de Matemática e Aplicações Fundamentais, Lisbon University*
[2]*Faculty of Earth and Life Sciences, Department of Theoretical Biology, Vrije Universiteit*
[1]*Portugal*
[2]*The Netherlands*

1. Introduction

Throughout human history, infectious diseases have caused debilitation and premature death to large portions of the human population, leading to serious social-economic concerns. Many factors have contributed to the persistence and increase in the occurrence of infectious disease (demographic factors, political, social and economic changes, environmental change, public health care and infrastructure, microbial adaptation, etc.), which according to the World Health Organization (WHO), are the second leading cause of death globally ($\approx$ 23 % of deaths) after cardiovascular diseases (WHO, 2010).

Research on basic and applied aspects of host, pathogen, and environmental factors that influence disease emergence, transmission and spread have been supported so far, and the development of diagnostics, vaccines, and therapeutics has been greatly increased. In recent years, mathematical modeling became an interesting tool for the understanding of infectious diseases epidemiology and dynamics, leading to great advances in providing tools for identifying possible approaches to control, including vaccination programs, and for assessing the potential impact of different intervention measures.

Epidemiological models are a formal framework to convey ideas about the components of a host-parasite interaction and can act as a tool to predict, understand and develop strategies to control the spread of infectious diseases by helping to understand the behaviour of the system under various conditions. They can also aid data collection, data and interpretation and parameter estimation. The purpose of epidemiological models is to take different aspects of the disease as inputs and to make predictions about the numbers of infected and susceptible people over time as output.

In the early 20th century, mathematical models were introduced into infectious disease epidemiology, and a series of deterministic compartment models such as SI (susceptible-infected), SIS (susceptible-infected-susceptible), and e.g SIR (susceptible-infected-recovered) have been proposed based on the flow patterns between compartments of hosts. In our days, most of the models developed try to incorporate other factors focusing on several different aspects of the disease, which can imply rich dynamic behaviour even in the most basic dynamical models. Factors that can go into the models include the duration of disease, the duration of infectivity, the infection rate, the waning immunity, and so forth. In such a way, differential equation models are a simplified representation of reality, which are designed to facilitate prediction and calculation of rates of change as functions of the conditions or the components of the system.

There are two common approaches in modeling, the deterministic and the stochastic one. In the first case, the model is one in which the variable states are uniquely determined by parameters in the model and by sets of previous states of these variables. In mathematics, a deterministic system is a system in which no randomness is involved in the development of future states of the system. In a stochastic model, randomness is present, and variable states are not described by unique values, but rather by probability distributions. Stochastic epidemic models are appropriate stochastic processes that can be used to model disease propagation. Disease propagation is an inherently stochastic phenomenon and there are a number of reasons why one should use stochastic models to capture the transmission process. Real life epidemics, in the absence of intervention from outside, can either go extinct with a limited number of individuals getting ultimately infected, or end up with a significant proportion of the population having contracted the disease in question. It is only stochastic, as opposed to deterministic, models that can capture this behavior and the probability of each event taking place.

Only few stochastic processes can be solved explicitly. The simplest and most thoroughly studied stochastic model of epidemics are based on the assumption of homogeneous mixing, i.e. individuals interact randomly at a certain rate. The mean field approximation is a good approximation to be used in order to understand better the behavior of the stochastic systems in certain parameter regions, where the dynamics of the mean quantities are approximated by neglecting correlations, giving closed ordinary differential equations (ODE) systems, hence mathematically deterministic systems which are easier to analyze.

In the following section of this chapter we present the properties of the basic SIR epidemic model for infectious diseases with a summary of the analysis of the dynamics, identifying the thresholds and equilibrium points. The goal is to introduce notation, terminology, and results that will be generalized in later sections on more advanced models motivated by dengue fever epidemiology as an example of multi-strain systems.

2. The SIR epidemic model

The SIR epidemic model divides the population into three classes: susceptible (S), Infected (I) and Recovered (R). It can be applied to infectious diseases where waning immunity can happen, and assuming that the transmission of the disease is contagious from person to person, the susceptibles become infected and infectious, are cured and become recovered. After a waning immunity period, the recovered individual can become susceptible again. This model was for the first time proposed by William Ogilvy Kermack and Anderson Gray McKendrick in 1927 (Weisstein, 2010). The model was brought back to prominence after decades of neglect by Anderson and May (Anderson & May, 1979).

In the simple SIR epidemics without strain structure of the pathogens we have the following reaction scheme for the possible transitions from one to another disease related state, susceptibles S, infected I and recovered R,

$$S + I \xrightarrow{\beta} I + I$$
$$I \xrightarrow{\gamma} R$$
$$R \xrightarrow{\alpha} S$$

for a host population of N individuals, with contact and infection rate β, recovery rate γ and waning immunity rate α. The dynamic model in terms of ordinary differential equations (ODE) reads,

$$\dot{S} = -\frac{\beta}{N} IS + \alpha(N - S - I) \quad (1)$$

$$\dot{I} = \frac{\beta}{N} IS - \gamma I \quad , \quad (2)$$

where we use the time derivative $\dot{S} = dS/dt$ with time t for a constant population size of $N = S + I + R$ individuals. The solution of $R(t)$ is given by $R(t) = N - I(t) - S(t)$ which can be calculated using the solution of the ODEs. The susceptible individuals become infected with infection rate β, recover from the infection with recovery rate γ and become susceptible again after waning immunity rate α.

In Fig. 1 we show the dynamical behavior of the susceptible, infected and recovered individuals in a given population N, when solving the above ODE system.

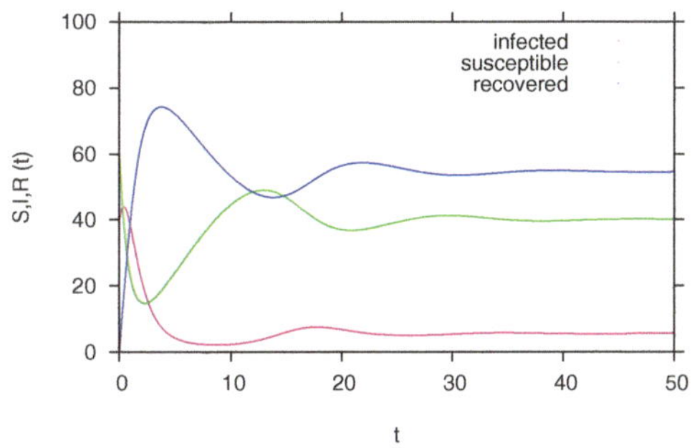

Fig. 1. Time dependent solution simulation for the SIR epidemic model. With a population $N = 100$, and starting values $I = 40$, $S = 60$ and $R = 0$, we fixed $\beta = 2.5$, $\alpha = 0.1$, and $\gamma = 1$. In green the dynamics for the susceptibles $S(t)$, in pink the dynamics for the infected $I(t)$ and in blue the dynamics of the recovered $R(t)$. Note that $N = 100$ allows for the interpretation for the class abundances in percentages.

The basic SIR model has only fixed points as possible stationary solutions, that can be calculated setting the rates of change $\dot{S}$ and $\dot{I}$ to zero. For the disease free equilibrium state, the solution is given by

$$I_1^* = 0 \quad (3)$$
$$S_1^* = N \quad (4)$$

and for the disease endemic equilibrium state, the solution is

$$I_2^* = N\left(1-\frac{\gamma}{\beta}\right)\frac{\alpha}{(\alpha+\gamma)} \tag{5}$$

$$S_2^* = N\frac{\gamma}{\beta} \quad . \tag{6}$$

The epidemic dynamic as a function of the parameter β shows the spread of the epidemic when $\beta > \gamma$ (see Fig. 2 a)), and its extinction when $\beta < \gamma$ (see Fig. 2 b)).

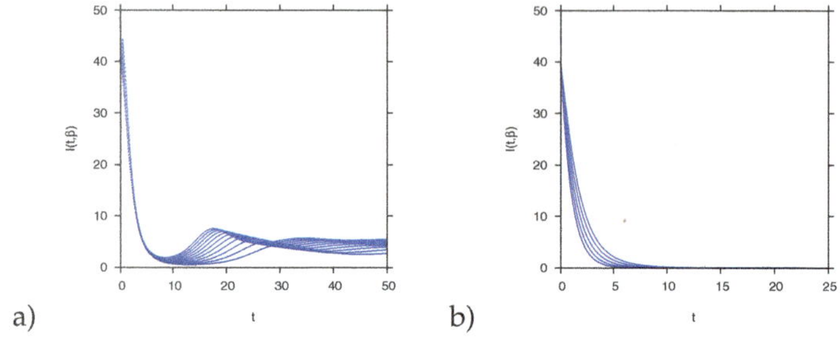

Fig. 2. Epidemic dynamics as a function of β. With the same initial values as used in Fig. 1, we plot time dependent solutions $I(t)$ for several β values. In a)$\beta \in [1.5, 2.5]$, with a resolution $\Delta\beta = 0.1$ and in b) $\beta \in [0, 0.9]$ where $\Delta\beta = 0.2$.

In order to analyze the stability of the equilibrium states, we look at the Jacobian matrix and its eigenvalues. Let the dynamics for the state $\underline{x} := (S, I)$ be $\underline{f}(\underline{x})$, hence $\frac{d}{dt}\underline{x} = \underline{f}(\underline{x})$ which explicitly gives $\Delta\underline{x} := \underline{x}(t) - \underline{x}^*$ as a small perturbation around the fixed point $\underline{x}^*$. We linearize the dynamic $\frac{d}{dt}\Delta\underline{x} = \frac{d}{dt}(\underline{x}(t) - x^*)$ applying Taylor's expansion

$$\underline{f}(\underline{x}^* + \Delta\underline{x}) = \underline{f}(\underline{x}^*) + \left.\frac{d\underline{f}}{d\underline{x}}\right|_{x^*} \cdot (\Delta\underline{x}) + \mathcal{O}((\Delta x)^2) \tag{7}$$

with $\underline{f}(\underline{x}^*) = 0$ for the fixed point and neglecting higher order terms. For our system we have the following linear differential equation system

$$\frac{d}{dt}\begin{pmatrix} S(t) - S^* \\ I(t) - I^* \end{pmatrix} = \left.\begin{pmatrix} \frac{\partial f}{\partial S} & \frac{\partial f}{\partial I} \\ \frac{\partial g}{\partial S} & \frac{\partial g}{\partial I} \end{pmatrix}\right|_{\begin{pmatrix} S \\ I \end{pmatrix} = \begin{pmatrix} S^* \\ I^* \end{pmatrix}} \cdot \begin{pmatrix} S - S^* \\ I - I^* \end{pmatrix} \tag{8}$$

where $\underline{f} := (f, g)$ and the Jacobian matrix is explicitly given by

$$\begin{pmatrix} -\frac{\beta}{N}I^* - \alpha & -\frac{\beta}{N}S^* - \alpha \\ \frac{\beta}{N}I^* & \frac{\beta}{N}S^* - \gamma \end{pmatrix} =: A \tag{9}$$

where we have to insert for S^* and I^*, the respective steady states. In order to decoupled the linear differential equation system, we diagonalize the matrix A, (9), with the eigenvalue decomposition $A\ \underline{u} = \lambda\ \underline{u}$, $\underline{u}$ is an eigenvector of A, and λ is an eigenvalue of A corresponding to the eigenvector $\underline{u}$.

The eigenvalues can be calculated setting the determinant of $[A - \lambda\ \mathbb{1}]$ equal zero.

2.1 The disease free equilibrium state

For the disease free equilibrium state (I_1^* and S_1^*), Eq.(3) and Eq. (4), the eigenvalues are given by

$$\lambda_1 = \beta - \gamma \tag{10}$$

$$\lambda_2 = -\alpha \quad . \tag{11}$$

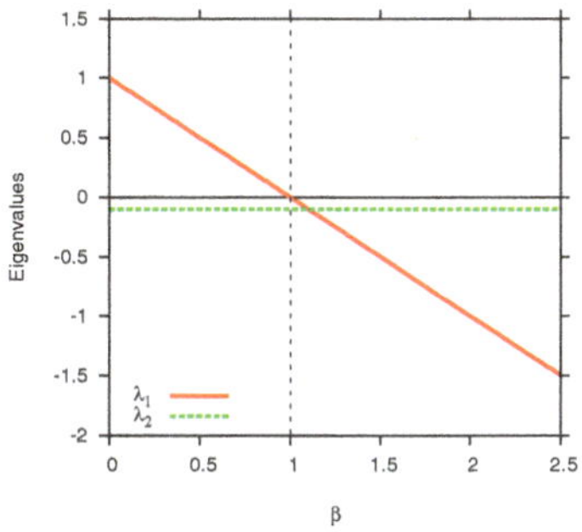

Fig. 3. Eigenvalues for the disease free equilibrium state as functions of β when fixing $\alpha = 0.1$ and $\gamma = 1.0$.

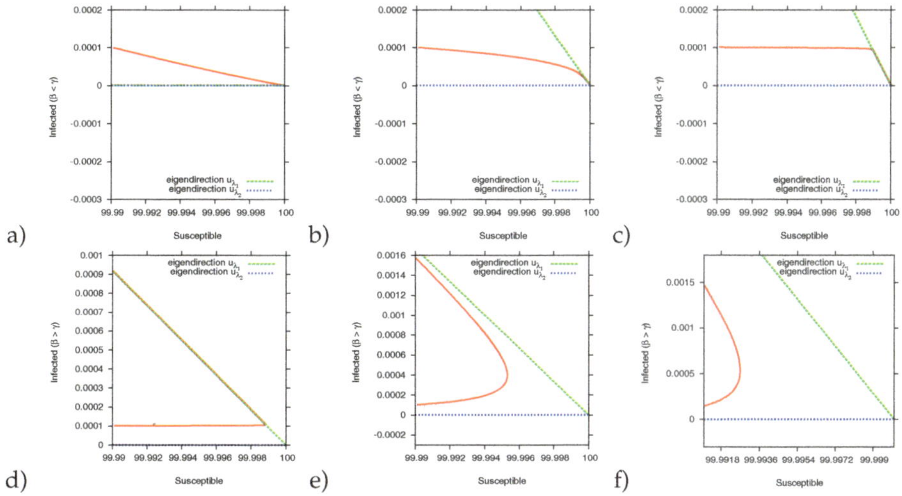

Fig. 4. eigenvectors for the disease free equilibrium state in function of β. For a population $N = 100$, where $I = 0.0001$, $S = 99.99$, and $R = N - I - S$, in a) $\beta = 0.9$, in b) $\beta = 0.97$, in c) $\beta = 0.999$, in d) $\beta = 1.001$, in e) $\beta = 1.1$, and in f) $\beta = 1.3$.

When looking at Eq. (10) and Eq. (11) we see that for $\beta < \gamma$ both eigenvalues are negative, i.e. the fixed point I_1^* is stable. The eigenvalues λ_1 and λ_2 are equal at the point $\beta = \gamma - \alpha$ and for $\beta > \gamma$, λ_1 is positive and λ_2 is negative, therefore the fixed point $I_1^* = 0$ is unstable. The stability of the system changes when one of the eigenvalues of the system becomes zero. At this point, $\beta_c = \gamma$, when I_1^* becomes unstable and I_2^* stable. Fig. 3 shows the eigenvalues for the disease free equilibrium state as functions of β.

To calculate the corresponding eigenvectors we use $(A - \lambda \mathbb{1})\,\underline{u} = 0$, with λ_i and $\underline{u}_i =: \begin{pmatrix} u_{1i} \\ u_{2i} \end{pmatrix}$. For the first eigenvalue, λ_1, the correspondent eigenvector $\underline{u}_1$ is giving by

$$\underline{u}_1 = \frac{1}{\sqrt{1 + \left(\frac{\gamma-\beta-\alpha}{\beta+\alpha}\right)^2}} \cdot \left(\begin{matrix} 1 \\ \left(\frac{\gamma-\beta-\alpha}{\beta+\alpha}\right) \end{matrix} \right) \quad ,$$

and for λ_2, the correspondent eigenvector $\underline{u}_2$ is is giving by

$$\underline{u}_2 = \begin{pmatrix} 1 \\ 0 \end{pmatrix} \quad .$$

In Fig. 4 we show the eigenvectors for the disease free equilibrium state as functions of β, when fixing $\alpha = 0.1$, and $\gamma = 1$. We plot the eigenvectors, $\underline{u}_1$ (blue line) and $\underline{u}_2$ (green line) on top of the trajectory of the infected individuals (red line). Note that $\lambda_1 = \lambda_2$ at $\beta = (\gamma - \alpha)$, i.e. the eigenvectors $\underline{u}_1 = \underline{u}_2$ (see Fig. 4a)). By increasing β toward the critical value $\beta_c = \gamma$ the trajectory needs longer time to hit the fixed point (see Fig. 4b) and 4c)). For $\beta > \gamma$, the trajectory goes toward the other fixed point I_2^* (see Fig. 4d) and 4e)).

2.2 The disease endemic equilibrium state

For the disease endemic equilibrium state (I_2^* and S_2^*), Eq. (5) and Eq. (6), the eigenvalues are giving by

$$\lambda_1 = -\frac{\alpha}{2}\left(1 + \frac{\beta-\gamma}{\alpha+\gamma}\right) + \sqrt{\left[\frac{\alpha}{2}\left(1 + \frac{\beta-\gamma}{\alpha+\gamma}\right)\right]^2 - (\beta-\gamma)\alpha} \tag{12}$$

$$\lambda_2 = -\frac{\alpha}{2}\left(1 + \frac{\beta-\gamma}{\alpha+\gamma}\right) - \sqrt{\left[\frac{\alpha}{2}\left(1 + \frac{\beta-\gamma}{\alpha+\gamma}\right)\right]^2 - (\beta-\gamma)\alpha} \quad . \tag{13}$$

In order to simplify the notation, let $-\frac{\alpha}{2}\left(1 + \frac{\beta-\gamma}{\alpha+\gamma}\right) =: a$ and $\left[\frac{\alpha}{2}\left(1 + \frac{\beta-\gamma}{\alpha+\gamma}\right)\right]^2 - (\beta-\gamma)\alpha =: b$. If $b > 0$ the eigenvalues are real numbers, giving the contraction or expansion of the trajectories near to the considered fixed point, and can be written as

$$\lambda_1 = a + \sqrt{b} \tag{14}$$

$$\lambda_2 = a - \sqrt{b} \quad . \tag{15}$$

If $b < 0$, the eigenvalues

$$\lambda_1 = a + i\sqrt{|b|} \tag{16}$$

$$\lambda_2 = a - i\sqrt{|b|} \tag{17}$$

become complex, where the real part a gives the contraction or expansion, and the imaginary part $i\sqrt{|b|}$ gives the frequency of oscillations of the trajectories spiraling into the fixed point as is shown in Fig. 5. The parabola curve shows the contraction and expansion of the eigenvalues. For $\beta < \gamma$ the fixed I_2^* point is unstable, with one positive eigenvalue.

For $\beta > \gamma$, the fixed point I_2^* becomes stable with both eigenvalues negative. The system changes stability when $\beta_c = \gamma$ and becomes complex when $\lambda_1 = \lambda_2$ (see Fig. 5).

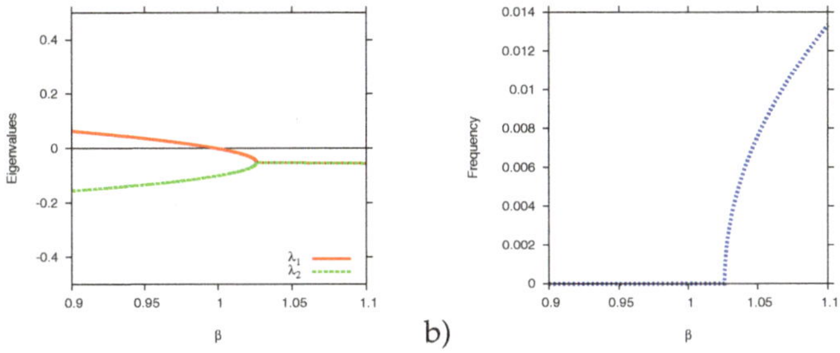

a) b)

Fig. 5. Plot of the eigenvalues as functions of β when fixing $\alpha = 0.1$ and $\gamma = 1.0$. In a) the real part a of the eigenvalues gives the contraction and expansion of the trajectories. For $\beta < \gamma$ the fixed point is unstable ($\lambda_1 > 0$). The system changes stability when $\beta_c = \gamma$ and becomes complex when $\lambda_1 = \lambda_2$. Here, the straight green line represents only the real parts of the complex eigenvalues obtained putting $\sqrt{-b} = 0$. In b) the imaginary part of the eigenvalues gives the frequency of the oscillatory behavior on the trajectory toward at the fixed point.

The correspondent eigenvectors of the disease endemic equilibrium state can be calculated for the eigenvalues in the same manner as it was shown above. For the first eigenvalue λ_1, the correspondent eigenvector $\underline{u}_1$ is given by

$$\underline{u}_1 = \frac{1}{\sqrt{1+\left(\frac{a-\sqrt{b}}{\gamma+\alpha}\right)^2}} \cdot \begin{pmatrix} 1 \\ \frac{a-\sqrt{b}}{\gamma+\alpha} \cdot \frac{1}{\sqrt{1+\left(\frac{a-\sqrt{b}}{\gamma+\alpha}\right)^2}} \end{pmatrix} \quad . \tag{18}$$

and for the second eigenvalue λ_2, the correspondent eigenvector $\underline{u}_2$ is given by

$$\underline{u}_2 = \frac{1}{\sqrt{1+\left(\frac{a+\sqrt{b}}{\gamma+\alpha}\right)}} \cdot \begin{pmatrix} 1 \\ \frac{a+\sqrt{b}}{\gamma+\alpha} \end{pmatrix} \quad . \tag{19}$$

In Fig. 6 we show the eigenvectors for the disease endemic equilibrium state in function of β.

For the real eigenvalue the general solution of the linearized system is given by

$$\underline{x}(t) = C_1 e^{\lambda_1 t} \underline{u_1} + C_2 e^{\lambda_2 t} \underline{u_2}$$

when $\lambda_1 \neq \lambda_2$. By including the respective eigenvalues, Eq. (10) and Eq.(11), we get as a solution

$$\underline{x}(t) = C_1 e^{(\beta-\gamma)t} \underline{u_1} + C_2 e^{-\alpha t} \underline{u_2} \tag{20}$$

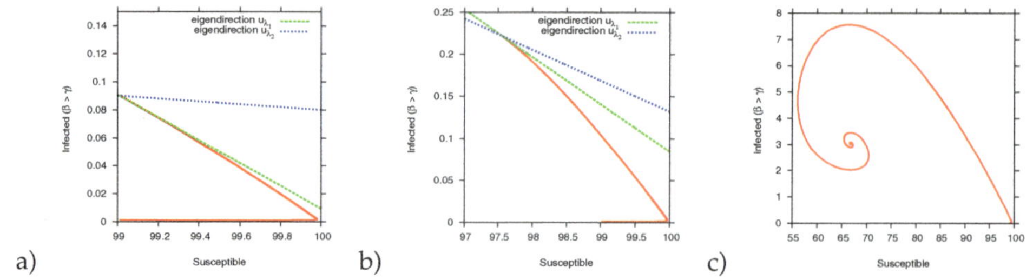

Fig. 6. eigenvectors for the disease endemic equilibrium state in function of β. For a population $N = 100$, where $I = 0.001$ and $S = 99$, we fixed $\alpha = 0.1$, $\gamma = 1$ and vary β. We plot the eigenvectors, $\underline{u}_1$ (blue line) and $\underline{u}_2$ (greenline), on top of the trajectory of the infected individuals toward the second fixed point I_2^*. In a) $\beta = 1.01$, and in b) $\beta = 1.025$. In c) we show the oscillatory trajectory toward the fixed point when $\beta = 2.5$

where the eigenvector $\underline{u_1}$ is the driving force for $t \to \infty$, since $\lambda_1 > \lambda_2$ (see Fig. 4b) to 4f)). When $\lambda_1 < \lambda_2$ the eigenvector $\underline{u_2}$ is the driving force for $t \to \infty$.

For the special case where $\lambda_1 = \lambda_2 =: \lambda$ and therefore the eigenvectors $\underline{u_1} = \underline{u_2} =: \underline{u}$ the general solution is then given by

$$\underline{x}(t) = C_1 e^{\lambda t} \underline{u} + C_2 (t e^{\lambda t} \underline{u} + e^{\lambda t} \underline{w})$$

where $\underline{w}$ is the so called generalized eigenvector, satisfying $(A - \lambda \mathbb{1})\, \underline{w} = \underline{u}$. In this case, for $t \to \infty$, the eigenvector $\underline{u}$ is again the driving force (see Fig. 4a)).

For the complex eigenvalues, where the real part a gives the contraction or expansion, and the imaginary part $i\sqrt{|b|}$ gives the frequency of oscillations of the trajectories spiraling into the fixed point, the general solution of the linearized system is given by

$$\underline{x}(t) = 2e^{at}\left(\left[C_1 \cos\left(\sqrt{b}t\right) - C_2 \sin\left(\sqrt{b}t\right)\right] \underline{u_1} - \left[C_1 \sin\left(\sqrt{b}t\right) + C_2 \cos\left(\sqrt{b}t\right)\right] \underline{u_2}\right) \quad ,$$

where C_1 and C_2 depend on the initial conditions and $\underline{u_i}$, respectively the real and imaginary parts of the complex eigenvector. This expression shows that the stability of the fixed point depends on the sign of a. For detailed information on the solution of a linear two dimensional ODE system, see (Mattheij & Molenaar, 1996).

The stochastic SIR epidemic is modeled as a time-continuous Markov process to capture population noise. The dynamics of the probability of integer infected and integer susceptibles, while the recovered follow from this due to constant population size, can be give as a master equation (van Kampen, 1992) in the following form

$$\begin{aligned} \frac{dp(S,I,t)}{dt} &= \frac{\beta}{N}(S+1)(I-1) \quad p(S+1, I-1, t) + \gamma(I+1) \quad p(S, I+1, t) \\ &+ \alpha(N-(S-1)-I) \quad p(S-1, I, t) - \left(\frac{\beta}{N} + \gamma I + \alpha(N-S-I)\right) \quad p(S,I,t) \quad . \end{aligned} \tag{21}$$

This process can be simulated by the Gillespie algorithm giving stochastic realizations of infected and susceptibles in time (Gillespie, 1976, 1978).

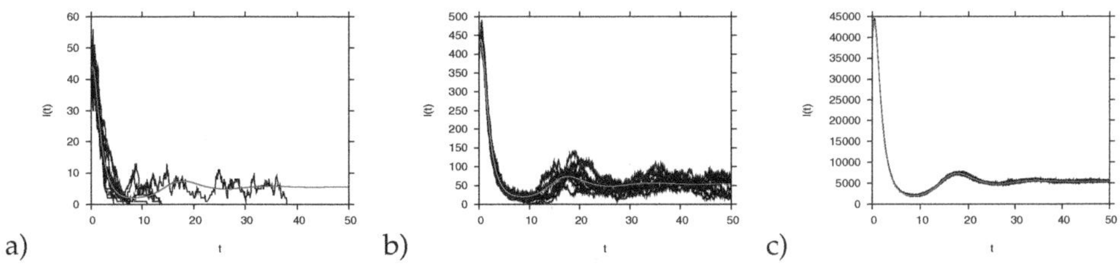

Fig. 7. Stochastic simulations for the basic SIR epidemic model. Here 10 realizations are plotted. We fixed $\alpha = 0.1$, $\gamma = 1$ and $\beta = 2.5$. The deterministic trajectory is shown (pink line) top of the stochastic realizations for different population size N a. In a) $N = 100$, in b) $N = 1000$ and in c) $N = 100000$.

For mean values of infected $\langle I \rangle$ and susceptibles $\langle S \rangle$, defined as e.g.

$$\langle I \rangle(t) := \sum_{S=0}^{N} \sum_{I=0}^{N} I \, p(S,I,t) \quad . \tag{22}$$

one can calculate the dynamics by inserting the master equation into the definition of the mean values obtaining

$$\begin{aligned} \frac{d}{dt}\langle S \rangle &= \alpha \langle R \rangle - \frac{\beta}{N} \langle SI \rangle \\ \frac{d}{dt}\langle I \rangle &= \frac{\beta}{N} \langle SI \rangle - \gamma \langle I \rangle \end{aligned} \tag{23}$$

with $\langle R \rangle = N - \langle S \rangle - \langle I \rangle$. For more details on the calculations see e.g. (Stollenwerk & Jansen, 2010). These equations for the mean dynamics include now due to the nonlinear transition rates in the master equation also higher moments $\langle S \cdot I \rangle$. The simplest approximation to obtain a closed ODE system is to neglect cross-correlations $\langle S \cdot I \rangle - \langle S \rangle \cdot \langle I \rangle \approx 0$, the so-called mean field approximation (originally introduced for spatially extended systems in statistical physics (Stollenwerk et al., 2010)). Hence, the equation system (23) gives with identifying the higher moment $\langle S \cdot I \rangle = \langle S \rangle \cdot \langle I \rangle$ by a product of simple moments gives again the ODE system for SIR system, as it was just presented above. For certain parameter regions the mean field approximation describes the system well in terms of its mean dynamics and only small fluctuations around it. Then the previously shown analysis of the system is appropriate. However, noise can stabilize transients, a feature which becomes important in parameter regions where in the deterministic description a fixed point is reached via decreasing oscillations, as we have observed them in the SIR system. The noisy system would show here continued oscillations (Alonso et al., 2006).

In Fig. 7 we compare the deterministic and stochastic dynamics and we see that the magnitude of stochastic fluctuations decreases when the population size increases. However, the good approximation (see Fig. 7c)) is only achieved when the population size is large enough (see Fig. 7a) where most simulations die out very quickly for small population size).

Almost all mathematical models of diseases start from the same basic premise: that the population can be subdivided into a set of distinct classes. The most commonly used framework for epidemiological systems, is still the SIR type model, a good and simple model for many infectious diseases. However, different extensions of the classical single-strain SIR model show a rich dynamic behavior, e.g. (Stone et al., 2007) in measles, or in generalized multi-strain SIR type models to describe the epidemiology of dengue fever (Aguiar et al., 2008).

3. Dengue fever epidemiology

Dengue is a viral mosquito-borne infection which in recent years has become a major international public health concern. According to the estimates given by (PDVI, 2011), 3.6 billion (55% of world population) are at risk of acquiring dengue infection (see Fig. 8a)). It is estimated that every year, there are 70 – 500 million dengue infections, 36 million cases of dengue fever (DF) and 2.1 million cases of dengue hemorragic fever (DHF), with more than 20.000 deaths per year (CDC, 2011; PDVI, 2011; WHO, 2009). In many countries in Asia and South America DF and DHF has become a substantial public health concern leading to serious social-economic costs.

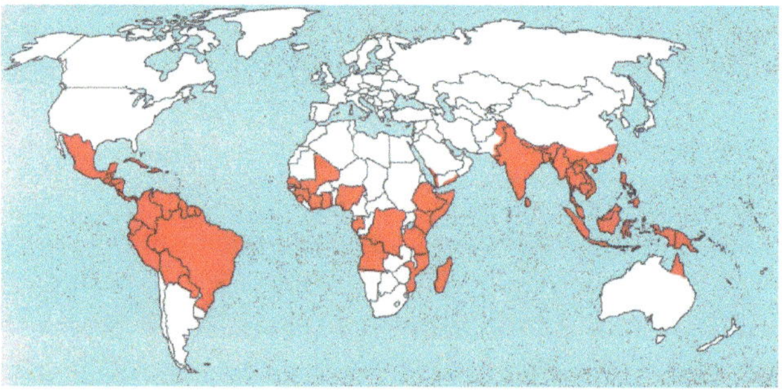

Fig. 8. Worldwide Dengue distribution 2010. In red Countries and areas where dengue has been reported Data source: World Health Organization (WHO) & Centers for Disease Control and Prevention (CDC). Adapted from (Gubler, 2002; Mackenzie et al., 2004).

Dengue fever is transmitted by the female domestic mosquito Aedes aegypti, although Ae. albopictus and Ae. polynesiensis can also act as transmission vector (Favier et al., 2005). Virus transmission in its simplest form involves the ingestion of viremic blood by mosquitoes and passage to a second susceptible human host. The mosquito becomes infected when taking a blood meal from a viremic person. After an extrinsic incubation period, the mosquito becomes infective and remains so during its entire life span (Rigau-Pérez et al., 1998). As the blood meal stimulates ovoposition, which undergoes at least one, often more, reproductive cycles there is an opportunity of vertical transmission to the eggs, passing the virus to the next generation of mosquitoes (CDC, 2011; Monath, 1994; Rosen et al., 1983).

There are four antigenically distinct dengue viruses, designated DEN-1, DEN-2, DEN-3, and DEN-4 (Guzmán et al., 2010; Halstead, 1994; SES, 2010; WHO, 2009). Infection by one serotype confers life-long immunity to only that serotype and a short temporary cross-immunity period to other serotypes exists. It lasts from three to nine months, when the antibody levels created during the response to that infection would be enough to protect against infection by a different but related serotype (Dejnirattisai et al., 2010; Halstead, 1994; Matheus et al., 2005; SES, 2010; WHO, 2009). Two variants of the disease exist: dengue fever (DF), a non-fatal form of illness, and dengue hemorrhagic fever (DHF), which may evolve toward a severe form known as dengue shock syndrome (DSS).

Epidemiological studies support the association of DHF with secondary dengue infection (Guzmán et al., 2000; Halstead, 1982, 2003; Nisalak et al., 2003; Vaughn, 2000), and there is good evidence that sequential infection increases the risk of developing DHF, due to a process described as antibody-dependent enhancement (ADE), where the pre-existing antibodies to previous dengue infection cannot neutralize but rather enhance the new infection.

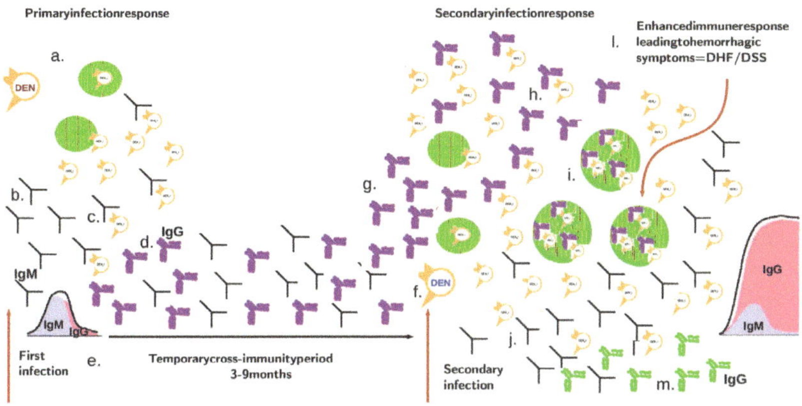

Fig. 9. Scheme of the immunological response on recurrent dengue infections. In (a.) the first infection with a given dengue virus serotype, in (b.) production of antibodies (Immunoglobulin M (IgM)), in (c.) inactivation of the virus and in (d.) production of antibodies (IgG class, the so called memory antibodies). In (e.) the temporary cross immunity period, that lasts between 3-9 months. After that period, the individual can get infected again with another dengue virus serotype (f.). In (g.) the IgG from the previous dengue infection binds to the new virus but do not inactivate them. In (h.) the complex antibody-virus enhances the new infection (i.). In (j.) the production of antibodies (IgM class) which is then able to inactivate the new viruses, leading to (l.), an enhanced immune response, such that hemorrhagic symptoms are observed. In (m.) production of IgG antibodies.

In the first dengue infection virus particles will be captured and processed by so-called antigen presenting cells. These viruses will be presented to T-cells causing them to become activated. And likewise B-cells will encounter their antigen free floating and become activated. B-cells produce antibodies that are used to tag the viruses to encourage their uptake by macrophages and inactivate them. In a secondary infection the antibodies from the first infection will attach to the virus particles but will not inactivate them. The antibody-virus complex suppresses innate immune responses, increasing intracellular infection and generating inflammatory citokines and chemokines that, collectively, result in enhanced disease (Dejnirattisai et al., 2010; Guzmán et al., 2010; Halstead, 1982, 1994, 2003; Mackenzie et al., 2004; WHO, 2009). Fig.9 is an scheme to illustrate the immunological response on recurrent dengue infections.

DF is characterized by headache, retro-orbital pain, myalgia, arthralgia, rash, leukopenia, and mild thrombocytopenia. The symptoms resolve after 27 days. DHF is a potentially deadly complication that is characterized by high fever and hemorrhagic phenomenae. DHF develops rapidly, usually over a period of hours, and resolves within 12 days in patients who receive appropriate fluid resuscitation. Otherwise, it can quickly progress to shock (CDC, 2011; WHO, 2009).

Treatment of uncomplicated dengue cases is only supportive, and severe dengue cases requires careful attention to fluid management and proactive treatment of hemorrhagic symptoms (CDC, 2011; WHO, 2009). A vaccine against dengue is not yet available, since it would have to simulate a protective immune response to all four serotypes (Stephenson, 2005), although several candidates of tetravalent vaccines are at various stages of development (WHO, 2011).

Mathematical models describing the transmission of dengue viruses appeared in the literature early as 1970 (Fischer & Halstead, 1970). More recently, mathematical models describing the transmission of dengue viruses have focused on the ADE effect and temporary cross immunity trying to explain the irregular behavior of dengue epidemics. Such models ultimately aim to be used as a predictive tool with the objective to guide the policies of prevention and control of the dengue virus transmission, including the implementation of vaccination programs when the candidate dengue fever vaccines will be accessible. In the literature the multi-strain interaction leading to deterministic chaos via ADE has been described previously, e.g. (Billings et al., 2007; Ferguson et al., 1999; Schwartz et al, 2005) but neglecting temporary cross immunity. Consideration of temporary cross immunity is rather complicated and up to now not in detail analyzed. Models formulated in (Loureço & Recker, 2010; Nagao & Koelle, 2008; Recker et al., 2009; Wearing & Rohani, 2006), did not investigate closer the possible dynamical structures. In (Aguiar & Stollenwerk, 2007; Aguiar et al., 2008, 2009, 2011 a) by including temporary cross immunity into dengue models with ADE, a rich dynamic structure including deterministic chaos was found in wider and more biologically realistic parameter regions.

4. Multi-strain models motivated by dengue fever epidemiology: a review

Multi-strain dynamics are generally modelled with SIR-type models and have demonstrated to show critical fluctuations with power law distributions of disease cases, exemplified in meningitis and dengue epidemiology (Massad et al., 2008; Stollenwerk & Jansen, 2003; Stollenwerk et al., 2004). Dengue models including multi-strain interactions via ADE but without temporary cross immunity period e.g. (Billings et al., 2007; Ferguson et al., 1999; Schwartz et al, 2005) have shown deterministic chaos when strong infectivity on secondary infection was assumed. The addition of the temporary cross immunity period in such models shows a new chaotic attractor in an unexpected parameter region of reduced infectivity on secondary infection (Aguiar & Stollenwerk, 2007; Aguiar et al., 2008, 2009, 2011 a), i.e. deterministic chaos was found in a wider parameter regions. This indicates that deterministic chaos is much more important in multi-strain models than previously thought, and opens new ways to data analysis of existing dengue time series, as will be shown below. It offers a promising perspective on parameter values inference from dengue cases notifications.

The basic multi-strain model divides the population into ten classes: susceptible to both strains, 1 and 2 (S), primarily infected with strain one (I_1) or strain two (I_2), recovered from the first infection with strain one (R_1) or strain two (R_2), susceptible with a previous infection with strain one (S_1) or strain two (S_2), secondarily infected with strain one when the first infection was caused by strain two (I_{21}) or for second time infected with strain two when the first infection was caused by strain one (I_{12}). Notice that infection by one serotype confers life-long immunity to that serotype. Then the individuals recover from the secondary infection (R).

To capture differences in primary infection by one strain and secondary infection by another strain we consider a basic two-strain SIR-type model for the host population, which is only slightly refined as opposed to previously suggested models for dengue fever (Billings et al., 2007; Ferguson et al., 1999; Schwartz et al, 2005).

The stochastic version of the multi-strain dengue model is now in complete analogy to the previously described SIR model, and the mean field ODE system for the multi-strain dengue model can be read from the following reaction scheme (24), describing the transitions for first infection with strain 1 and secondary infection with strain 2, and for the reverse process, where the first infection is caused by strain 2 and the secondary infection is caused by strain 1, the same reaction scheme can be used to describe the transitions by just changing labels.

$$\begin{aligned} S + I_1 &\xrightarrow{\beta} I_1 + I_1 \\ S + I_{21} &\xrightarrow{\phi\beta} I_1 + I_{21} \\ I_1 &\xrightarrow{\gamma} R_1 \\ R_1 &\xrightarrow{\alpha} S_1 \\ S_1 + I_2 &\xrightarrow{\beta} I_{12} + I_2 \\ S_1 + I_{12} &\xrightarrow{\phi\beta} I_{12} + I_{12} \\ I_{12} &\xrightarrow{\gamma} R \end{aligned} \tag{24}$$

The demographic transitions are $S, I_1, I_2, R_1, R_2, S_1, S_2, I_{12}, I_{21}, R \xrightarrow{\mu} S$ defining the system of two strains completely (for more information on the deterministic ODE system and its parametrization, see (Aguiar et al., 2011 a)).

The complete system of ordinary differential equations for the two strain epidemiological system is given by Eq. system (25) and the dynamics are described as follows. Susceptibles to both strains can get the first infection with strain one or strain two with force of infection $\frac{\beta I}{N}$ when the infection is acquired via an individual in his first infection or $\frac{\phi\beta I}{N}$ when the infection is acquired via an individual in his second infection. They recover from the first infection with a recovery rate γ, conferring full and life-long immunity against the strain that they were exposed to, and also a short period of temporary cross-immunity α against the other strain, becoming susceptible to a second infection with a different strain. The susceptible with a previous infection gets the secondary infection with force of infection $\frac{\beta I}{N}$ or $\frac{\phi\beta I}{N}$ depending on whom (individual on his primary or secondary infection) is transmitting the infection. Then, with recovery rate γ, the individuals recover and become immune against all strains. We assume no epidemiological asymmetry between strains, i.e. infections with strain one or strain two contribute in the same way to the force of infection. Here, the only relevant difference concerning disease transmissibility is that the force of infection varies accordingly to the number of previous infections the hosts have experienced. The parameter ϕ in our model, is the ratio of secondary infection contribution to the force of infection. For more information on the parametrization of ADE and secondary dengue infection by ϕ, see (Aguiar et al., 2008; Ferguson et al., 1999). The parameter values are given in Table 1, if not otherwise explicitly stated.

$$\begin{aligned}
\dot{S} &= -\frac{\beta}{N} S(I_1 + \phi I_{21}) - \frac{\beta}{N} S(I_2 + \phi I_{12}) + \mu(N - S) \\
\dot{I_1} &= \frac{\beta}{N} S(I_1 + \phi I_{21}) - (\gamma + \mu) I_1 \\
\dot{I_2} &= \frac{\beta}{N} S(I_2 + \phi I_{12}) - (\gamma + \mu) I_2 \\
\dot{R_1} &= \gamma I_1 - (\alpha + \mu) R_1 \\
\dot{R_2} &= \gamma I_2 - (\alpha + \mu) R_2 \\
\dot{S_1} &= -\frac{\beta}{N} S_1(I_2 + \phi I_{12}) + \alpha R_1 - \mu S_1 \\
\dot{S_2} &= -\frac{\beta}{N} S_2(I_1 + \phi I_{21}) + \alpha R_2 - \mu S_2 \\
\dot{I_{12}} &= \frac{\beta}{N} S_1(I_2 + \phi I_{12}) - (\gamma + \mu) I_{12} \\
\dot{I_{21}} &= \frac{\beta}{N} S_2(I_1 + \phi I_{21}) - (\gamma + \mu) I_{21} \\
\dot{R} &= \gamma(I_{12} + I_{21}) - \mu R \quad ,
\end{aligned} \tag{25}$$

Par.	Description	Values	Ref
N	population size	100	—
μ	new born susceptible rate	$1/65y$	(UNWPP, 2008)
γ	recovery rate	$52y^{-1}$	(Gubler et al., 1981; WHO, 2009)
β	infection rate	2γ	(Ferguson et al., 1999)
α	temporary cross-immunity rate	$2y^{-1}$	(Matheus et al., 2005; SES, 2010)
ϕ	ratio of contrib. to force of inf.	variable	—

Table 1. Parameter set, rates given in units per year, ratio without unit

The stationary states can be calculated analytically by setting the time derivatives in Eq. system (25) to zero,

$$
\begin{aligned}
S^* &= \frac{\mu N - (\gamma+\mu)(I_1^* + I_2^*)}{\mu} \\
I_{21}^* &= \frac{1}{\phi_1}\left(\frac{N}{\beta_1 S^*}(\gamma+\mu) - 1\right) I_1^* \\
I_{12}^* &= \frac{1}{\phi_2}\left(\frac{N}{\beta_2 S^*}(\gamma+\mu) - 1\right) I_2^* \\
S_1^* &= \frac{(\gamma+\mu) I_{12}^*}{(I_2^* + \phi_2 I_{12}^*)} \frac{N}{\beta_2} \\
S_2^* &= \frac{(\gamma+\mu) I_{21}^*}{(I_1^* + \phi_1 I_{21}^*)} \frac{N}{\beta_1} \\
R_1^* &= \frac{\gamma}{\alpha+\mu} I_1^* \\
R_2^* &= \frac{\gamma}{\alpha+\mu} I_2^* \quad ,
\end{aligned}
\tag{26}
$$

where still the stationary values of I_1^* and I_2^* have to be determined.

The solution of coexistence of both strains for $I_1 = I_2 = I^*$ is given by the following expression

$$
I_1^* = I_2^* = -\left[\frac{\frac{\alpha\gamma}{(\alpha+\mu)(\gamma+\mu)}\phi + \left(\frac{(\gamma+\mu)}{\beta} - 3\right)}{4\frac{(\gamma+\mu)}{\mu}\left(1 - \frac{\alpha\gamma}{(\alpha+\mu)(\gamma+\mu)}\phi\right)}\right] N \tag{27}
$$

$$
- \sqrt{\frac{N^2}{4}\left[\frac{\frac{\alpha\gamma}{(\alpha+\mu)(\gamma+\mu)}\phi + \left(\frac{(\gamma+\mu)}{\beta} - 3\right)}{2\frac{(\gamma+\mu)}{\mu}\left(1 - \frac{\alpha\gamma}{(\alpha+\mu)(\gamma+\mu)}\phi\right)}\right]^2 + \left[\frac{N^2\mu\left(\frac{(\gamma+\mu)}{\beta} - 1\right)}{2\frac{(\gamma+\mu)^2}{\mu}\left(1 - \frac{\alpha\gamma}{(\alpha+\mu)(\gamma+\mu)}\phi\right)}\right]} \quad ,
$$

and the solution of the extinction of one of the strains is as follows

$$
\begin{aligned}
I_1^* &= \frac{\mu N(\beta - (\gamma+\mu))}{(\gamma+\mu)\beta} \\
I_2^* &= 0 \quad .
\end{aligned}
\tag{28}
$$

Finally, the stationary value of R^*, when hosts have been recovered from both strains, is given by the balance equation for the total population size N, explicitly

$$
R^* = N - (S^* + I_1^* + I_2^* + R_1^* + R_2^* + S_1^* + S_2^* + I_{12}^* + I_{21}^*) \quad . \tag{29}
$$

The time series for $\phi < 1$ shows that the total number of infected $I := I_1 + I_2 + I_{12} + I_{21}$ stays quite away from zero, avoiding the chance of extinction in stochastic systems with reasonable system size (see Fig. 10 a)). The parameter region previously considered to model ADE effects on dengue epidemiology, i.e. $\phi > 1$, leads to rather low troughs for the total number of infected giving unrealistically low numbers of infected. In Fig. 10 b) the logarithm of total number of infected goes as low as -70 for $\phi = 2.7$ in the chaotic region of $\phi > 1$. Population fluctuations would in this case drive almost surely the system to extinction.

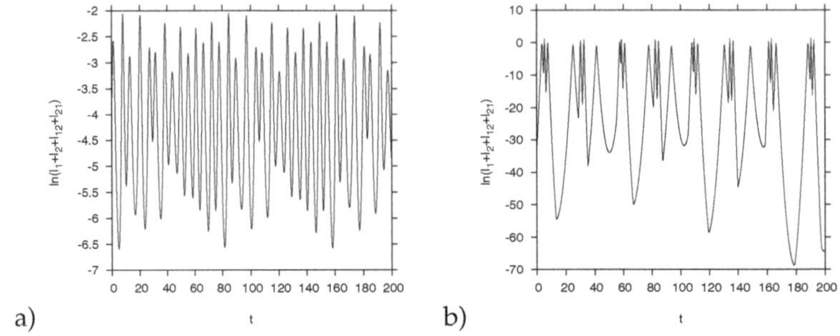

Fig. 10. Time series of the logarithm of the overall infected ($\ln(I)$) comparison: a) simulation for $\phi = 2.7$ and b) simulation for $\phi = 0.6$ for the same time interval.

The state space plots in terms of the variables S and the logarithm of the total number of infected I show a rich dynamical behavior with bifurcations from fixed point to limit cycles, till completely irregular behavior (see Fig. 11).

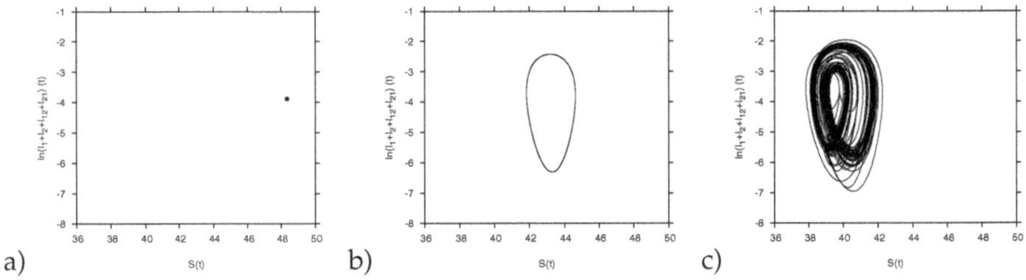

Fig. 11. Attractors for various values of $\phi < 1$: a) fixed point for $\phi = 0.1$, and b) limit cycle for $\phi = 0.4$, and c) chaotic attractor for $\phi = 0.6$.

Looking for higher values of ϕ, the chaotic attractor becomes unstable, just leaving simple limit cycles as attractors for large parameter regions beyond $\phi = 1$ (Aguiar & Stollenwerk, 2007; Aguiar et al., 2008). Only for much higher values of $\phi >> 1$, another chaotic attractor appears, the classical "ADE chaotic attractor" (Aguiar & Stollenwerk, 2007; Aguiar et al., 2008; Ferguson et al., 1999).

The bifurcation diagram was obtained plotting the local extrema of $ln(I)$ over the varying parameter ϕ (see Fig. 12). Fixed points appear as one dot per parameter value, limit cycles appear as two dots, double-limit cycles as four dots, more complicated limit cycles as more dots, and chaotic attractors as continuously distributed dots for a single ϕ value (Ruelle, 1989). We observe two chaotic windows, one for $\phi < 1$, where this dynamical behavior has never been described before, and also another one for $\phi > 1$ (see Fig. 12a)) where the minimal values go to very low numbers of infected, which already has been described (see Fig. 12b)) in previous publications (Billings et al., 2007; Ferguson et al., 1999; Schwartz et al, 2005). In Fig. 12b) the dynamical behavior was obtained when neglecting the temporary cross-immunity

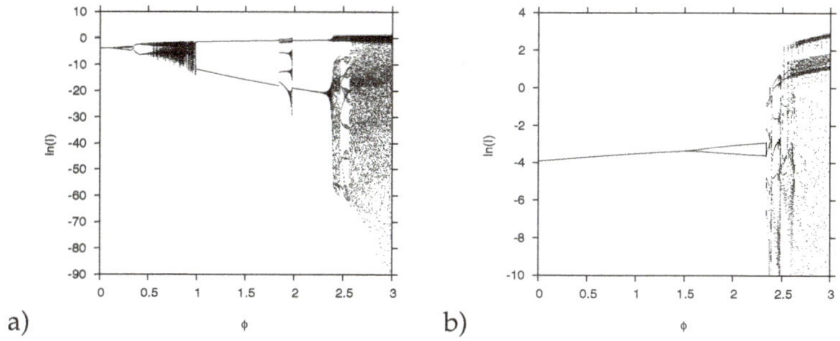

Fig. 12. Bifurcation diagram for the local extrema of the overall infected with changing parameter ϕ. In a) $\alpha = 2$ (six month) and in b) $\alpha = 52$ (one week).

period, i.e. by putting $\alpha \to \infty$. The recovered individuals can be immediately infected with another strain, whereas consideration of temporary cross-immunity brings a new chaotic attractor found first by Aguiar et al. (Aguiar & Stollenwerk, 2007; Aguiar et al., 2008).

This finding encourages to look closer to the parameter region of $\phi < 1$, when dengue patients in a secondary infection evolving to severe disease because of the ADE phenomenon contribute less to the force of infection, and not more, as previous models suggested. This assumption is likely to be more realistic for dengue fever since the possible severity of a secondary infection may hospitalize people, not contributing to the force of infections as much as people with first infection.

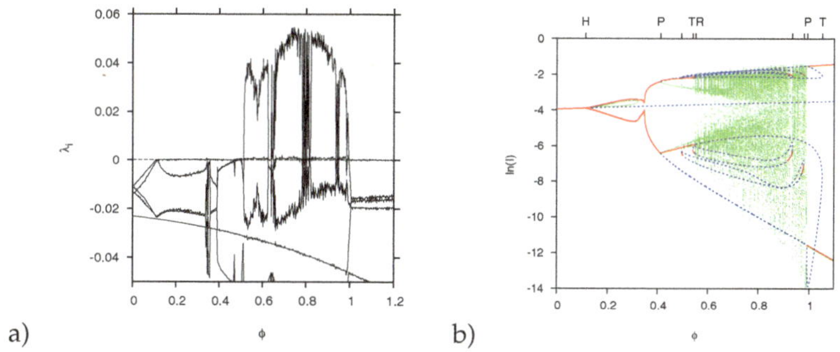

Fig. 13. In a) spectrum of the four largest Lyapunov exponents with changing parameter ϕ and fixed $\alpha = 2$. In b) we show the one-parameter bifurcation diagram with temporary cross-immunity rate $\alpha = 2$ and varying the ratio of secondary infection contribution to the force of infection ϕ. Solid lines denote stable equilibria or limit cycles, and dashed lines unstable equilibria or limit cycles.

We quantify the attractor structure, fixed point, limit cycle or chaotic attractor etc., by calculating Lyapunov exponents (Ott, 1993; Ruelle, 1989), which were calculated using an iterated technique along a trajectory using the QR decomposition algorithm via Householder matrices (see (Aguiar et al., 2008; Holzfuss & Lauterborn, 1989; Holzfuss & Parlitz, 1991)). Lyapunov exponents are essentially a generalization of eigenvalues determining stability versus instability along trajectories. A negative largest Lyapunov exponent indicates a stable fixed point as attractor, a zero largest Lyapunov exponent indicates a stable limit cycle and a positive largest Lyapunov exponent indicates a chaotic attractor. Fig. 13a) shows the largest four Lyapunov exponents as a function of ϕ. We observe that for small ϕ up to 0.1 all four Lyapunov exponents are negative, indicating the stable fixed point solution. Then follows a region up to $\phi = 0.5$ where the largest Lyapunov exponent is zero, characteristic for stable limit cycles. Above $\phi = 0.5$ a positive Lyapunov exponent, clearly separated from the second largest Lyapunov exponent being zero, indicates deterministically chaotic attractors. In the chaotic window between $\phi = 0.5$ and $\phi = 1$ also periodic windows appear, giving a zero largest Lyapunov exponent. These findings are in good agreement with the numerical bifurcation diagram, Fig. 13b).

A further analysis of the bifurcation structure, in the region of interest of $\phi < 1$, was performed using the numerical software AUTO (AUTO, 2009). Various bifurcations were found: Hopf bifurcation $H(\phi = 0.11326)$, pitchfork bifurcations $P(\phi = 0.41145, 0.99214)$, torus bifurcation $TR(\phi = 0.55069)$ and tangent bifurcations $T(\phi = 0.4.9406, 0.53874, 0.93103, 0.97825, 1.05242)$. In addition to this main bifurcation pattern we found two isolas, consisting of isolated limit cycles existing between two tangent bifurcations (see Fig. 13b), for more information on the isolas see (Aguiar et al., 2008, 2009). These results agree very well with the simulation results shown in the bifurcation diagram for the maxima and minima of the overall infected in Fig. 12a).

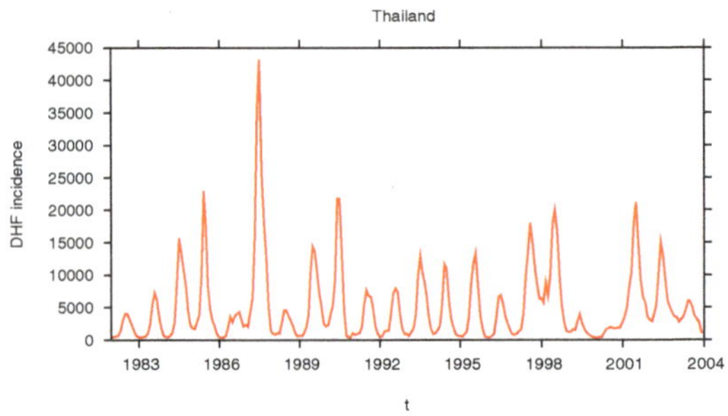

Fig. 14. Time series of DHF incidence in Thailand.

Dengue fever epidemiology is characterized as a yearly cycle of incidences (see Fig. **??**), therefore in order to be able to reproduce the yearly cycle in dengue incidence seasonal forcing and a low import of infected have to be included in the models. The first recorded epidemic of DHF in Thailand (population of approximately 66 million people (Wikipedia, 2011)) was in 1958 (WHO, 2009). The co-circulation of all four dengue serotypes and their capacity to produce severe dengue disease was demonstrated as early as 1960 in Bangkok, Thailand (Halstead et al., 1969). DHF occurred first only in Bangkok, but was disseminated to the whole region during the 1970s (Chareonsook et al., 1999; Gubler, 2002; Halstead et al., 1969). Physicians in Thailand are trained to recognize and treat dengue fever and practically all cases of DHF and DSS are hospitalized. A system for reporting communicable diseases including DHF/DSS was considered fully installed in 1974 and the data bank of DHF and DSS is available at the Ministry of Public Health, Bangkok (Chareonsook et al., 1999).

We extend the previously studied non-seasonal model by adding seasonal forcing, mimicking the vectorial dynamics, and a low import of infected individuals, which is realistic in the dynamics of infectious diseases, in order to get a more realistic pattern of dengue fever epidemics, with irregular, yearly and smooth outbreaks.

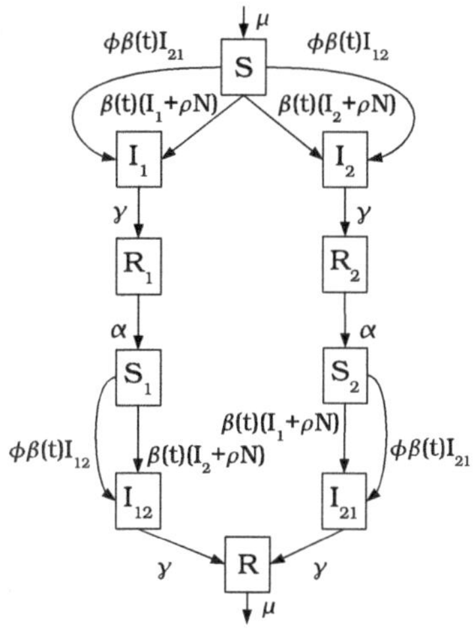

Fig. 15. The state flow diagram for the seasonal multi-strain model. The transition rate μ coming out of the class R represents the death rates of all classes, $S, I_1, I_2, R_1, R_2, S_1, S_2, I_{12}, I_{21}, R$, getting into the class S as a birth rate.

The seasonal multi-strain model is represented in Fig. 15 by using a state flow diagram where the boxes represent the disease related stages and the arrows indicate the transition rates. In the same manner as described for the non-seasonal, the population is divided into ten classes, with constant size $N = S + I_1 + I_2 + R_1 + R_2 + S_1 + S_2 + I_{12} + I_{21} + R$. The complete system of ordinary differential equations for the seasonal multi-strain epidemiological can be written as shown in system (25), with the difference that now the parameter β takes the seasonal forcing into account as a cosine function given explicitly by

$$\beta(t) = \beta_0 \cdot (1 + \eta \cdot \cos(\omega \cdot t)) \quad , \tag{30}$$

where β_0 is the infection rate, and η is the degree of seasonality. In this model, a susceptible individual can become infected also by meeting an infected individual from an external population (hence $(\beta/N \cdot S \cdot I)$ goes to $(\beta/N \cdot S \cdot (I + \rho \cdot N)))$ contributing to the force of infection with an import parameter ρ.

The parameters are fixed, temporary cross immunity rate $\alpha = 2y^{-1}$, recovery rate $\gamma = 52y^{-1}$, infection rate $\beta_0 = 2 \cdot \gamma$, seasonality $\eta = 0.35$, import factor $\rho = 10^{-10}$, birth and death rate $\mu = 1/65y$ and the ratio of secondary infection contribution to the force of infection $\phi = 0.9$.

In Fig. 16a) the time series simulation results for the total number of infected $(I_1 + I_2 + I_{12} + I_{21})$ in the non-seasonal system, previously studied in (Aguiar et al., 2008), is shown. Besides showing an irregular pattern of outbreaks that happens every 5 years, the non-seasonal system and its time series are not able to represent dengue fever epidemiology that is characterized as a yearly cycle of incidences. By adding low seasonality into the system, the epidemic outbreaks appear every year (see (Aguiar et al., 2011 a)). However, between two large outbreaks there is a very low number of cases in subsequent years, which is also not data alike. In Fig. 7c), the time series simulation in the high seasonal system with a low import of infected contributing to the force of infection is shown. The addition of import into the

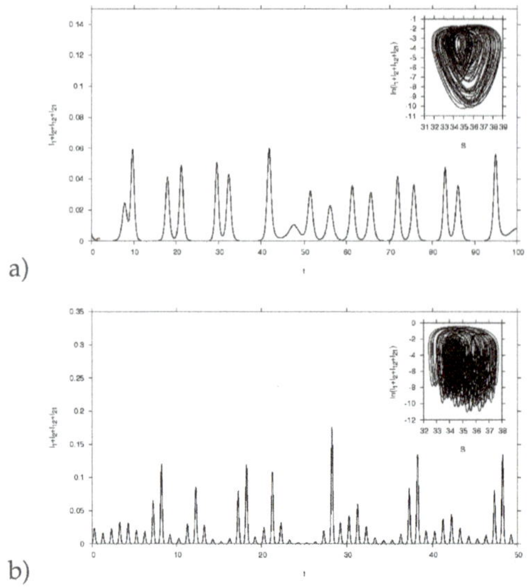

Fig. 16. Time series simulations. In a) time series simulation for the non-seasonal model ($\eta = 0$). In b) time series simulation for the seasonal model with a low import of infected. Here, the degree of seasonality is $\eta = 0.35$ and the import of infected $\rho = 10^{-10}$.

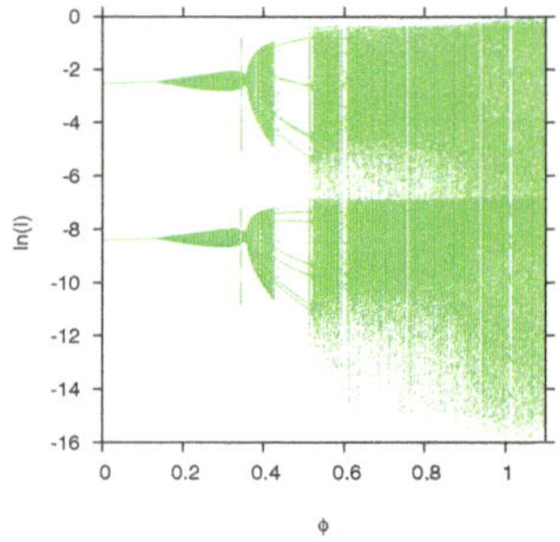

Fig. 17. Bifurcation diagram for the seasonal model with import. Here, the degree of seasonality $\eta = 0.35$ and the import factor $\rho = 10^{-10}$.

seasonal system gives a much more realistic pattern of dengue fever epidemics, with irregular, yearly and smooth outbreaks. The system has a reasonable size (the number of infected stays quite away from zero), avoiding the chance of extinction in stochastic systems. For detailed analysis on the attractors in state space for the seasonal model, see (Aguiar et al., 2011 a). The bifurcation diagram for the seasonal model with import is shown in Fig. 17.

For the seasonal model with import AUTO predicted a torus bifurcation TR at $\phi = 0.13$, and at $\phi = 0.522$ which are also predicted very well when comparing with the results given by the Lyapunov exponent calculation. In the limiting case where the amplitude of the seasonal forcing is zero, the torus bifurcation TR of the seasonally forced system coincides with the Hopf bifurcation H of the non-seasonal system, as was shown in (Aguiar et al., 2011 a).

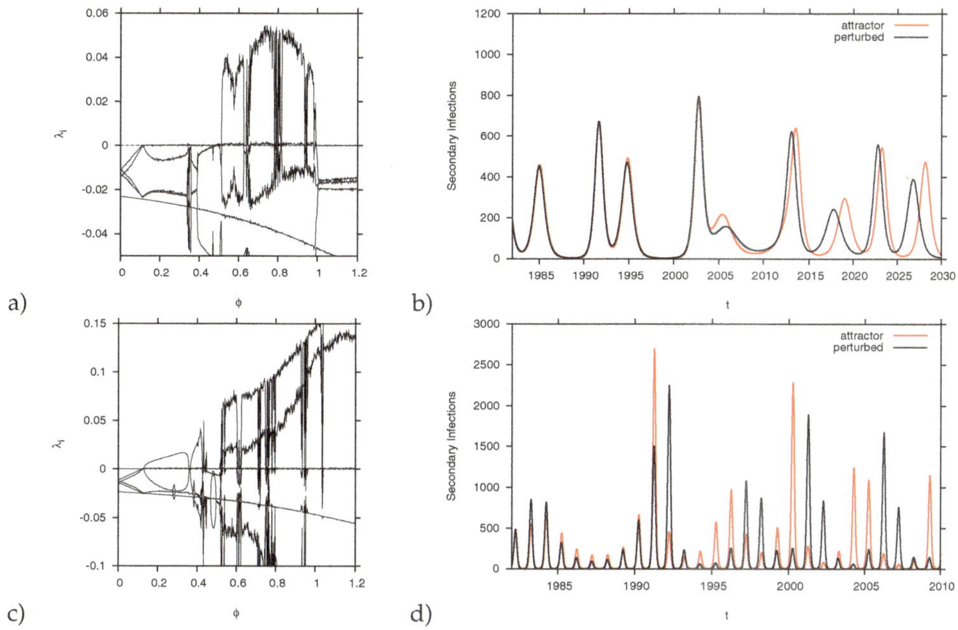

Fig. 18. Qualitative insight into the predictability in the monthly time series. In a) the Lyapunov spectrum and in b) the time series for the non-seasonal model. In c) the Lyapunov spectrum and in d) the time series for the seasonal model with import.

In Fig. 18 the Lyapunov spectrum for both non-seasonal model and the seasonal model with import are shown and compared concerning the prediction horizon of the monthly peaks in the multi-strain dengue model time series. We take as an example the Dominant Lyapunov Exponent (DLE) for $\phi = 0.9$ in the region where the system is chaotic (positive DLE). For the non-seasonal system, the DLE $= 0.04$ giving around 25 years of prediction horizon in the monthly time series (see Fig. 18b)), whereas for the seasonal system with import,the DLE$=$ 0.118 giving around 8.5 years of prediction horizon in the monthly time series. It is clear that the addition of seasonal forcing into the system by itself decreases the practical predictability, however, the addition of a low import into the seasonally forced system helps to get a more complex dynamics and a better prediction horizon in the monthly time series. In order to get a qualitative insight into the predictability in the monthly sampled time series, i.e. to show how the original system behaves under a small perturbation we plot two different trajectories of the same system (for the non-seasonal model in Fig. 18b), and for the seasonal model with import of infected in Fig. 18d)), where the perturbed system (black line) is compared with the original model simulation (red line). To get the trajectory of the perturbed system, we keep the last point of the transient of the original system and use those values as starting values to compute the new and perturbed trajectory. The perturbation is given by $S_p = S + R \cdot \epsilon$ and $R_p = R \cdot (1.0 - \epsilon)$, where S_p is the susceptibles perturbed and R_p is the recovered perturbed with $\epsilon = 0.001$. (for details on the perturbed system see (Aguiar et al., 2011 a)).

The inspection of the available DHF incidence data in Thailand shows a smooth behavior with a well defined maximum each year of irregular hight for the Northern Provinces.

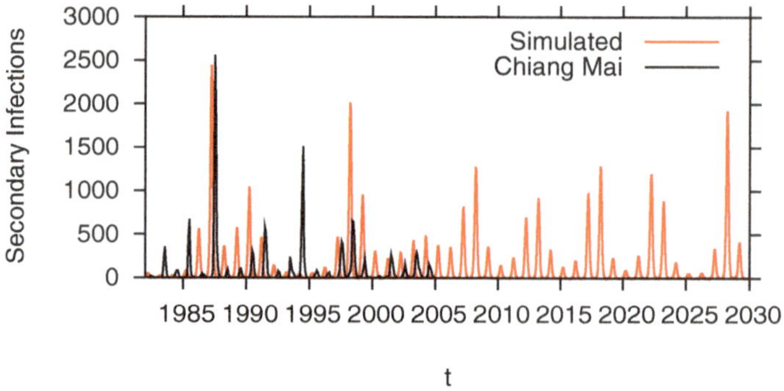

Fig. 19. Empirical DHF incidence data matched with the model simulation.

We take the Province of Chiang Mai as a case study where the empirical DHF incidence data and the time series simulation for the seasonal model with import are compared (see Fig. 19)). The seasonal model with import shows complex dynamics and qualitatively a very good result when comparing empirical DHF and simulations. However, the extended model needs to be parametrized on data referring to incidence of severe disease.

5. Discussions

In this chapter we presented the properties of the basic SIR epidemic model for infectious diseases with a summary of the analysis of the dynamics, identifying the thresholds and equilibrium points in order to introduce notation, terminology. The results that were generalized to more advanced models motivated by dengue fever epidemiology.

The epidemiology of dengue fever was described presenting the relevant biological features that are taken into the modeling process. Then, multi-strain models previously described in the literature were presented. We focused in a minimal model motivated by dengue fever epidemiology, formulated first by Aguiar et al. (Aguiar & Stollenwerk, 2007), where the notion of at least two different strains is needed to describe differences between primary infections, often asymptomatic, and secondary infection, associated with the severe form of the disease. We discussed the role of seasonal forcing and the import of infected individuals in such systems, the biological relevance and its implications for the analysis of the available dengue data. The extended model (Aguiar et al., 2011 a) shows complex dynamics and qualitatively a good agreement between empirical DHF monitoring data and the obtained model simulation. This suggests that the used parameter set can be the starting set for a more detailed parameter estimation procedure. Such a technical parameter estimation is notoriously difficult for chaotic time series but temporally local approaches are possible (He et al., 2010; Ionides et al., 2006). At the moment only such minimalistic models have a chance to be qualitatively understood well and eventually tested against existing data.

The introduction of stochasticity is needed to explain the fluctuations observed in some of the available data sets, revealing a scenario where noise and complex deterministic skeleton strongly interact (Aguiar et al., 2011 b). For large enough population size, the stochastic system can be well described by the deterministic skeleton gaining insight into the relevant parameter values purely on topological information of the dynamics, rather than classical parameter estimation of which application is in general restricted to fairly simple dynamical scenarios.

6. Conclusions

Being able to predict future outbreaks of dengue in the absence of human interventions is a major goal if one wants to understand the effects of control measures. Even after a dengue virus vaccine has become accessible, this holds true for the implementation of a vaccination program. For example, to perform a vaccine trial in a year with normally low numbers of cases would make statistical tests of vaccine efficacy much more difficult than when it was performed in a year with naturally high numbers of cases. Thus predictability of the next season's hight of the dengue peak on the basis of deterministic balance of infected and susceptible would be of major practical use.

7. Acknowledgments

The research presented in this book chapter has been supported by the Fundação para a Ciência e a Tecnologia, FCT grant SFRH/BD/43236/2008, and has been further supported by the Portuguese FCT project PTDC/MAT/115168/2009 and by the EU project EPIWORK under Framework Program 7. The work was carried out at Centro de Matemática e Aplicações Fundamentais, Science Faculty, Lisbon University, Portugal.

8. References

Aguiar, M. & Stollenwerk, N. (2007). A new chaotic attractor in a basic multi-strain epidemiological model with temporary cross-immunity. *arXiv:0704.3174v1 [nlin.CD].*

Aguiar, M., Kooi, B. W. & Stollenwerk, N. (2008). Epidemiology of Dengue Fever: A Model with Temporary Cross-Immunity and Possible Secondary Infection Shows Bifurcations and Chaotic Behaviour in Wide Parameter Regions. *Math. Model. Nat. Phenom.,* 4, 48–70, ISSN 0973-5348.

Aguiar, M., Stollenwerk, N. & Kooi, B. W. (2009). Torus bifurcations, isolas and chaotic attractors in a simple dengue model with ADE and temporary cross immunity. *International Journal of Computer Mathematics,* 86, 1867–1877, ISSN 0020-7160.

Aguiar, M., et al. (2011 a). The role of seasonality and import in a minimalistic multi-strain dengue model capturing differences between primary and secondary infections: complex dynamics and its implications for data analysis. *Journal of Theoretical Biology,* 289, 181–196, ISSN 0022-5193.

Aguiar, M., Kooi B. W., & Stollenwerk N. (2011 b). Scaling of stochasticity in DHF epidemics. *Under review.*

Alonso, D., McKane, A. & Pascual, M. (2006). Stochastic Amplification in Epidemics. *Journal of the Royal Society Interface,* 4, 575–582, ISSN 1742-5689.

Anderson, R. M. & May, R. M. (1979). Population biology of infectious diseases: Part I. *Nature,* 280, 361–67, ISSN 0028-0836.

Doedel J. E. and Oldeman, B. (2009). AUTO 07P âĂŞ Continuation and bifurcation software for ordinary differential equations. *Technical Report: Concordia University, Montreal, Canada,* Retrieved from http://indy.cs.concordia.ca/auto/

Billings, L., et al. (2007). Instabilities in multiserotype disease models with antibody-dependent enhancement. *Journal of Theoretical Biology,* 246, 18–27, ISSN 0022-5193.

Centers for Disease Control and Prevention. (2011). *Dengue.* Retrieved from http://www.cdc.gov/dengue/

Chareonsook, O.et al. (1999). Changing epidemiology of dengue hemorrhagic fever in Thailand. *Epidemiol. Infect.,* 122, 161–166, ISSN 0950-2688.

Dejnirattisai, W. et al. (2010). Cross-Reacting Antibodies Enhance Dengue Virus Infection in Humans. *Science,* 328, 745–748, ISSN 0036-8075.

Favier, C., et al. (2005). Influence of spatial heterogeneity on an emerging infectious disease: the case of dengue epidemics. *Proc. Biol. Sci.,* 272, 1171–7, ISSN 0962-8452.

Ferguson, N., Anderson, R. and Gupta, S. (1999). The effect of antibody-dependent enhancement on the transmission dynamics and persistence of multiple-strain pathogens. *Proc. Natl. Acad. Sci. USA,* 96, 790–94, ISSN 0027-8424.

Fischer, D. B. & Halstead, S. B. (1970). Observations related to pathogenesis of dengue hemorrhagic fever. V. Examination of age specific sequential infection rates using a mathematical model. *J. Biol. Med.,* 42, 329–49.

Gillespie, D.T. (1976). A general method for numerically simulating the stochastic time evolution of coupled chemical reactions. *Journal of Computational Physics,* 22, 403–434, ISSN 0021-9991.

Gillespie, D.T. (1978). Monte Carlo simulation of random walks with residence time dependent transition probability rates. *Journal of Computational Physics,* 28, 395–407, ISSN 0021-9991.

Gubler, J. D., Suharyono, W., Tan, R., Abidin, M. and Sie, A. (1981). Viraemia in patients with naturally acquired dengue infection. *Bull. World Health Organ.,* 59, 623–630, ISSN 0042-9686.

Gubler D. J., (2002). Epidemic dengue/dengue hemorrhagic fever as a public health, social and economic problem in the 21st century. *Trends in Microbiology,* 10, 100–103, ISSN: 0966-842X.

Guzmán, M.G. et al. (2000). Epidemiologic Studies on Dengue in Santiago de Cuba, 1997. *Am. J. Epidemiol.,* 152, 793–799, ISSN 0002-9262.

Guzmán, M.G. et al. (2010). Dengue: a continuing global threat. *Nature Reviews Microbiology,* 8, S7–S16, ISSN : 1740-1526.

Halstead S. B., et al. (1969). Dengue and chikungunya virus infection in man in Thailand, 1962–1964. V. Epidemiologic observations outside Bangkok. *Am. J. Trop. Med. Hyg.* 18, 1022–33, ISSN: 0002-9637.

Halstead, S.B. (1982). Immune enhancement of viral infection. *Progress in Allergy,* 31, 301–364,ISSN 0079-6034.

Halstead, S. B. (1994). Antibody-dependent Enhancement of Infection: A Mechanism for Indirect Virus Entry into Cells. *Cellular Receptors for Animal Viruses,* 28, Chapter 25, 493–516, ISBN 0-87969-429-7. (Cold Spring Harbor Laboratory Press).

Halstead, S.B. (2003). Neutralization and antibody-dependent enhancement of dengue viruses. *Advances in Virus Research,* 60, 421–467, ISSN 0065-3527.

He, D., Ionides, E. L., King, A. A. (2010). Plug-and-play inference for disease dynamics: measles in large and small populations as a case study. *J. R. Soc. Interface,* 7, 271–283, ISSN 1742-5689.

Holzfuss, J. & Lauterborn, W. (1989). Liapunov exponents from a time series of acoustic chaos. *Physical Review A,* 39, 2146–2152, ISSN 1943-2879.

Holzfuss, J. & Parlitz, U. (1991). Lyapunov exponents from time series. *Lecture Notes in Mathematics,* 1486, 263–270, ISSN: 0075-8434.

Ionides, E., Breto, C., & King, A. A. (2006). Inference for nonlinear dynamical systems. *Proc. Natl. Acad. Sci. USA,* 103, 18438–18443, ISSN 0027-8424.

Lourenço, J. & Recker, M. (2010). Viral and Epidemiological Determinants of the Invasion Dynamics of Novel Dengue Genotypes. *PLoS Negl. Trop. Dis.,* 4, e894, ISSN 1935-2735.

Mackenzie, J. S., Gubler, D. J. & Petersen, L. R. (2004). Emerging flaviviruses: the spread and resurgence of Japanese encephalitis, West Nile and dengue viruses. *Nature Medicine Review,* 12, S98–S109, ISSN : 1078-8956.

Massad, E.,et al. (2008). Scale-free network of a dengue epidemic. *Applied Mathematics and Computation,* 195, 376–381, ISSN: 0096-3003.

Matheus, S. et al. (2005). Discrimination between Primary and Secondary Dengue Virus Infection by an Immunoglobulin G Aviditnoy Test Using a Single Acute-Phase Serum Sample. *Journal of Clinical Microbiology,* 43, 2793–2797, ISSN: 0095-1137.

Mattheij, R. M. M. and Molenaar, J. (1996). *Ordinary differential equations in theory and practice.,* ISBN 0-89871-531-8, (Wiley, Chichester and New York).

Monath T. P., (1994). Dengue: The risk to developed and developing countries. *Proc. Natl. Acad. Sci. U.S.A.,* 91, 2395–2400, ISSN 0027-8424.

Nagao, Y. & Koelle, K.(2008). Decreases in dengue transmission may act to increase the incidence of dengue hemorrhagic fever. *Proc. Natl. Acad. Sci. USA,* 105, 2238–2243, ISSN 0027-8424.

Nisalak, A. et al. (2003). Serotype-specific dengue virus circulation and dengue disease in Bangkok, Thailand from 1973 to 1999. *Am. J. Trop. Med. Hyg.,* 68, 191–202, ISSN: 0002-9637.

Ott, E. (1993). *Chaos in Dynamical Systems,* ISBN 0-52143-799-7. (Cambridge University Press, Cambridge, 2nd edition).

Pediatric Dengue Vaccine Initiative. International Vaccine Institute (IVI). *Global Burden of Dengue.* Retrieved from http://www.pdvi.org/about_dengue/GBD.asp

Recker, M. et al. (2009). Immunological serotype interactions and their effect on the epidemiological pattern of dengue. *Proc. R. Soc. B.,* 276, 2541–2548, ISSN: 1471-2954.

Rigau-Pérez, J. G., et al. (1998). Dengue and dengue haemorrhagic fever. *The Lancet,* 352, 971–77, ISSN: 0140-6736.

Rosen, L. et al. (1983). Transovarial transmission of dengue viruses by mosquitoes: A. albopictus and A. aegypti. *Am. J. Trop. Med. Hyg.,* 32, 1108–19, ISSN: 0002-9637.

D. Ruelle. (1989). *Chaotic Evolution and Strange Attractors,* ISBN 978-0-52136-272-6 (Cambridge University Press, Cambridge).

Pers comm.: Francisco Lemos, Secretaria de Estado de Saúde de Minas Gerais, Brazil; Sônia Diniz, Fundação Ezequiel Dias, Minas Gerais, Brazil and Scott Halstead, Pedriatic Dengue Vaccine Initiative, Maryland, USA.

Schwartz, I. B., et al. (2005). Chaotic desynchronization of multi-strain diseases. *Physical Review,* E 72, 066201–6, ISSN 1943-2879.

Stephenson, J. R., (2005). Understanding dengue pathogenesis: implications for vaccine design. *Bull. World Health Organ.,* 83, 308–14, ISSN 0042-9686.

Stollenwerk, N., & Jansen, V. A. A. (2003). Meningitis, pathogenicity near criticality: the epidemiology of meningococcal disease as a model for accidental pathogens. *J. Theor. Biol.*, 222, 347–359, ISSN 0022-5193.

Stollenwerk, N., Maiden, M.C.J. & Jansen, V.A.A. (2004). Diversity in pathogenicity can cause outbreaks of menigococcal disease. *Proc. Natl. Acad. Sci. USA*, 101, 10229–10234, ISSN 0027-8424.

Stollenwerk, N., & Jansen, V. (2010). *Population biology and criticality*, ISBN 978-1-84816-401-7. (Imperial College Press, London).

Stollenwerk, N., van Noort, S., Martins, J., Aguiar, M., Hilker, F., Pinto, A. & Gomes G. (2010). A spatially stochastic epidemic model with partial immunization shows in mean field approximation the reinfection threshold. *Journal Of Biological Dynamics*, 4, 634–649, ISSN: 1751-3758.

Stone, L., Olinky, R., & Amit Huppert, A. (2007). Seasonal dynamics of recurrent epidemics. *Nature*, 446, 533–36, ISSN 0028-0836.

World Population Prospects: The 2008 Revision. *Population Database*. Retrieved from http://esa.un.org/unpp/index.asp?panel=2

van Kampen, N. G. (1992). *Stochastic Processes in Physics and Chemistry*, ISBN 978-0-44452-965-7. (North-Holland, Amsterdam).

Vaughn, D. W. (2000). Invited Commentary: Dengue Lessons from Cuba. *Am. J. Epidemiol.*, 152, 800–803, ISSN 0950-2688.

Wearing, H.J. & Rohani, P. (2006). Ecological and immunological determinants of dengue epidemics *Proc. Natl. Acad. Sci. USA* , 103, 11802–11807, ISSN 0027-8424.

Weisstein, E. W. (2010). *"Kermack-McKendrick Model." From MathWorld – A Wolfram Web Resource.* Retrieved from http://mathworld.wolfram.com/Kermack-McKendrickModel.html

Wikipedia contributors. Wikipedia, The Free Encyclopedia. *Provinces of Thailand*. Retrieved from http://en.wikipedia.org/wiki/Provinces_of_Thailand

World Health Organization. (2009). *Dengue and Dengue Hemorrhagic Fever, Fact sheet 117*. Retrieved from http://www.who.int/mediacentre/factsheets/fs117/en/

World Health Organization: Health statistics and health information systems (2010). *The global burden of disease: 2004 update*, ISBN 978-9-24156-371-0. Retrieved from http://www.who.int/healthinfo/global_burden_disease/GBD_report__2004update_AnnexA.pdf

World Health Organization – Programs and Projects: Initiative for Vaccine Research (2011). *Vector borne infections*. Retrieved from http://www.who.int/vaccine_research/diseases/vector/en/index1.html#virology

13

The SIALON Project: Report on HIV Prevalence and Risk Behaviour Among MSM in Six European Cities

Massimo Mirandola et al.*
Azienda Ospedaliera Universitaria Integrata Verona (The Hospital Trust of Verona), Coordinamento Regionale per il Management e la Progettazione Europea (Regional Coordination Centre for European Project Management), Veneto Region, Verona, Italy

1. Introduction

The following chapter describes the process and results of a survey conducted in six cities in Southern and Eastern Europe to obtain data on (i) the prevalence of HIV and Syphilis among Men who have Sex with Men (MSM), (ii) sexual behaviour risk patterns of MSM and (iii) the determinants of access to Voluntary Counselling and Testing (VCT) by MSM.

The chapter describes how the survey was undertaken against a backdrop of evidence indicating a rising incidence of HIV infection in Europe and in the context of a gap in information on HIV incidence and prevalence amongst the MSM community which has been identified as an at risk population for HIV infection.

In this context, the methodology used for obtaining reliable information and data, represents a key factor in the process. The Time-Location Sampling (TLS) method has proven to be an effective means for gathering both behavioural and biological data in hidden or hard to reach populations, such as MSM.

The chapter provides a description of the implementation of TLS for epidemiological purposes and a summary of the main results of the survey which reveal (i) a high unawareness of HIV positive serostatus, (ii) a higher risk among younger people of obtaining the HIV infection due to their risk behaviour (e.g. unprotected anal intercourse)

* Jean-Pierre Foschia[2], Michele Breveglieri[2], Martina Furegato[2], Enrica Castellani[2], Ruth Joanna Davis[1], Lorenzo Gios[1], Dunia Ramarli[3] and Paola Coato[4]
[1]*Azienda Ospedaliera Universitaria Integrata Verona (The Hospital Trust of Verona), Coordinamento Regionale per il Management e la Progettazione Europea (Regional Coordination Centre for European Project Management), Veneto Region, Verona, Italy*
[2]*ULSS20, Veneto Region, Verona, Italy*
[3]*UO immunologia (Department of Pathology, Immunology), Azienda Ospedaliera Universitaria Integrata Verona (The Hospital Trust of Verona), Verona, Italy*
[4]*UO immunologia (Department of Pathology, Microbiology), Azienda Ospedaliera Universitaria Integrata Verona (The Hospital Trust of Verona), Verona, Italy*

and a more limited access to HIV screening services and prevention programmes, (iii) the correlation between HIV infection and STIs and Syphilis and (iv) the association between HIV risk and alcohol and drug use.

This chapter also discusses the use of UNGASS indicators and the Second Generation Surveillance System (SGSS) approach in the survey and in general as key features to be considered as part of a comprehensive surveillance system.

Finally, a number of conclusions are drawn with regard to the need for repeated epidemiological studies focusing on hard to reach populations as well as to the need for targeted health promotion and prevention campaigns.

2. Background

HIV infection remains a relevant issue in Europe in the field of public health. Moreover, scientific literature suggests an increasing HIV transmission in several European countries. MSM represent one of the most at risk populations for acquiring HIV. In 2009, 9,023 newly diagnosed HIV infections were reported among this population in Europe, which accounts for 35% of all HIV diagnoses in that year (European Centre for Disease Prevention and Control ECDC/World Health Organisation WHO - Regional Office for Europe, 2010; Likatavičius et al., 2008). Moreover, in this specific population, a high level of risk behaviours associated with an increasing incidence of other Sexually Transmitted Infections (STI) clearly show the need for specific and targeted prevention campaigns (Dodds et al., 2005; Van de Laar et al., 2009).

Due to a lack of risk perception and also to perceived social stigma, MSM tend to refer a low level of VCT and active health seeking behaviours (MacKellar et al., 2005). In addition, social and cultural obstacles to testing can be perceived by MSM also in health facilities. From a methodological point of view, since the introduction of Highly Active Anti-Retroviral Therapy (HAART), AIDS has become less indicative of the underlying trends in HIV infection, for this population in particular. Data based on the clinical records, at the same time, seems to not realistically reflect the HIV trends for two reasons. On the one hand, clinical records often do not include information regarding hard-to-reach MSM, who are less likely to ask for VCT and regular testing. On the other hand, a low level of knowledge about the real serostatus is reported among MSM (Williamson & Hart, 2007; Mirandola et al., 2009). Therefore, specific surveillance and outreach research targeting MSM who cannot attend the clinical facilities, is strongly required in order to obtain a more realistic estimation of the HIV epidemic.

In this context, a need for reliable and comparable data across different countries is also a key issue in monitoring the spread of HIV and in providing meaningful prevention. Unfortunately, data are often collected across a number of countries or in the same country using different sampling methods, or different testing methods, or different testing algorithms. In addition, questionnaire items used in various studies are often based on different assumptions and they can vary greatly in terms of time frame of the questions (last 12 or 3 months, last intercourse), definition of risk sexual practice, etc. Finally, specific HIV surveys focusing on MSM are rarely repeated on a regular basis. For that reason, a lack of reliable data and trends on HIV epidemic is available for this at risk population.

In this framework, a specific Declaration of Commitment on HIV/AIDS and a Political Declaration on HIV/AIDS were proposed and adopted by the UN General Assembly in 2001. In these documents, a specific set of epidemiological and surveillance activities are suggested, as well as the adoption of the so-called UNGASS indicators. UNGASS indicators are a set of measures to be used among different countries in order to effectively monitor the HIV epidemic (Joint United Nations Programme on HIV/AIDS UNAIDS & World Health Organization WHO, 2009). The Declaration provides a comprehensive framework to achieve the Millennium Development Goal in order to reverse the HIV epidemic by 2015.

In addition, specific indications for developing and implementing a more effective surveillance system are provided in UNAIDS and WHO publications (UNAIDS & WHO, 2002, 2005). These documents suggest the adoption of the so-called Second Generation Surveillance System (SGSS), which foresees a set of detailed managerial and epidemiological procedures, as well as standardized processes and actions for managing surveillance studies . The SGSS foresees the implementation of surveys repeated on a regular basis according to different indicators, which require the collection of both behavioural and biological data. The SGSS provides a meaningful tool for developing prevention initiatives according to reliable data on HIV epidemics and behavioural patterns, which represent the major challenge for the coming years.

The "Capacity building in HIV/Syphilis prevalence estimation using non-invasive methods among MSM in Southern and Eastern Europe" - SIALON project was developed and implemented according to the main procedures and processes foreseen in the UNGASS declaration and in the SGSS approach. The SIALON project was funded in the framework of the 2003-2008 Public Health Programme (Work Plan 2007) and implemented by a team of European Public Institutions under the leadership of the Veneto Region in close collaboration with local partners ranging from Universities, teaching hospitals, epidemiological centres and Gay NGOs. In particular, the SIALON study was carried out in six cities of Southern and Eastern European countries: Barcelona (Spain), Bratislava (Slovakia), Bucharest (Romania), Ljubljana (Slovenia), Prague (Czech Republic), Verona (Italy).

3. Methods

3.1 Study design

The study conducted during the SIALON project was a cross-sectional study targeting MSM who have had sex with another man during the last 12 months. The data collection was conducted according to the Time-Location (or Time-Space) Sampling (TLS) procedure. This method was used to recruit men visiting the selected gay settings in each participating city, allowing to construe a representative sample with known properties. The cross-sectional study was conducted using a self-administered pen-and-paper questionnaire and an oral fluid collector to gather both behavioural and biological data for each participant.

The study design was planned and implemented in line with the Second Generation Surveillance System (SGSS) criteria (UNAIDS & WHO, 2002, 2005) and the United Nations General Assembly Special Session (UNGASS) Indicators (UNAIDS & WHO, 2009).

3.1.1 Study population

According to data and the results of some seroprevalence studies, levels of HIV prevalence are between 10 and 20% among MSM. As mentioned in section 2, this specific sub-population continues to be at high risk of HIV infection, especially in Europe, and according to the available data a hidden HIV epidemic seems currently underway (ECDC, 2010; Likatavičius et al., 2008). Because of a high level of risk sexual practices, MSM become a key population for HIV surveillance. In addition, especially because of stigma, a low level of VCT is reported, particularly among hard-to-reach MSM who do not attend health services regularly. Moreover, since the introduction of HAART, AIDS has become less indicative of the underlying trends in HIV infection, for this population in particular. For these reasons, field research and surveillance activities targeting this specific population seem to be essential in monitoring the HIV epidemic and in developing preventive action in Europe.

3.1.2 Sampling

The sample size estimation for a prevalence study was calculated on the basis of previous prevalence estimation studies, where available (Folch et al., 2005). According to this calculation, a total of 2,800 persons (400 per city) were planned to be included in the data collection process.

Time-Location (or Time-Space) Sampling (TLS) was used to recruit representative samples of men visiting the gay scene in each city. This specific approach was used in previous studies (Williamson & Hart, 2007; Stueve et al., 2001; MacKellar et al., 2007; Gallagher et al., 2007; Muhib et al., 2001), and has proven to be a good and reliable method for gathering both behavioural and biological data in hidden or hard to reach populations. According to the TLS method, spaces (locations) are venues attended by the target population, in this case MSM, while times refer to specific days and time periods when the target population attends each identified space or setting. This sampling approach allows to construe a sample with known properties, enabling statistical inferences to be made to the larger population of venue visitors (ideally, all MSM attending the gay scene in each city).

In order to identify timing and settings, a specific formative research was conducted in each city. The first step in the formative research was the identification and selection of all gay venues in the given city. Bars, discos, saunas, cruising venues, sex-shops, sex-clubs were therefore identified. All venues were mapped and visited when information was not sufficient. This process allowed to identify the potential TLS units (the attendance time frame, opening days and hours) and to create a specific data collection calendar. The spaces and their associated days were divided into standardised time segments (four-hour periods). MSM were then enrolled over the entire TLS unit time period. During the data collection sessions, information regarding the number of refusals per unit was registered. In order to include all possible time and location units that did not occur frequently but that may attract members of the target population, also settings or special gay events were identified and mapped, creating a "special events" category. A list of TLS units was created according to this sampling approach, where the TLS units were the "primary sampling units" (PSU). In addition, in creating the final list of TLS units, safety and feasibility of data collection in different settings and at different times (especially in cruising venues) was taken into account. At this stage, the PSU were randomly selected from complete list of eligible TLS list in each participating city.

3.2 Data collection and analysis

3.2.1 Questionnaire

The SIALON questionnaire was specifically designed according to the international literature and according both to the study design and the data collection procedures. The self-administered pen-and-paper questionnaire was developed to obtain information on a range of different aspects and taking into account both UNGASS and ECDC indicators. The first part refers to background data. The second part lists items on sexual practices, risk-reducing strategies, condom use, STI history and self-reported/perceived serostatus.

Moreover, questions regarding number of both steady and casual partners were foreseen, as well as frequency and type of sexual practices in both cases. In construing the different questions, specific attention was paid to the social/cultural/environmental and contextual variables, as well as to access and barriers to VCT.

From a structural point of view, the questionnaire contained items referring to different time-spans: last 12 months, last 6 months, and last time (last sexual intercourse). This structure allowed to include all items needed for the construction of the UNGASS and ECDC indicators.

In terms of the UNGASS and ECDC indicators themselves, according to the WHO-UNAIDS documents, questions referring to UNGASS 8 (testing), 9 (prevention campaigns), 19 (condom use) and 23 (HIV prevalence) were included.

Finally, specific attention was paid to the time span required to fulfill the questionnaire: a maximum of 20 minutes was required for completing the questionnaire. For this purpose, specific piloting was conducted.

3.2.2 Enrolment

With regard to the enrolment of subjects, a specific easy-to-use and practical manual was provided to all data collectors, in order to standardise all procedures and to guarantee the safety and reliability of data collected. Following the data collection calendar created through the TLS method, trained field workers from gay associations attended the different gay venues in specific time-location units. The self-administered pen-and-paper questionnaires were distributed, as well as the Oracol devices for oral fluid collection (Malvern Medical Developments, Worcester, UK). Both self-completed questionnaires (behavioural data) and oral fluid samples (biological data) were collected for each subject. A unique barcode for each subject was used to link behavioural and biological information.

Finally, regarding the enrolment period, this varied between the different participating cities, according to the different situations and calendars (from 2 months to 9 months), starting in November 2008 and ending in October 2009.

3.2.3 Statistical analysis

Mean, median, standard deviation, quartiles and inter-quartiles were calculated and proportions with 95% confidence intervals (CI) were adopted for all variables and indicators. With regard to the UNGASS indicators calculation, specific reference to the UNGASS-WHO publications was made. Finally, STATA 11 survey commands suite was used.

3.3 Laboratory testing

3.3.1 Oral fluid sampling and testing

To collect oral fluids, Oracol oral fluid collection kits (Malvern Medical Developments, Worcester, UK) were used. The main advantages for replacing serum with oral fluid were easy access and non-invasive collection. After collection, oral fluid samples were kept refrigerated and sent to the national reference laboratory for HIV/AIDS in the respective countries no more than 72 hours after collection.

3.3.2 HIV testing

The oral fluid samples were sent for the analysis by each national reference laboratory to the Teaching Hospital-University of Verona, Immunology Unit, Verona, Italy. EIA testing GENSCREEN HIV 1/2 version 2, BIO-RAD on oral fluid sample was performed according to the manufacturer's instructions. All positive samples were confirmed with a Western Blot test. In terms of quality control, for each oral fluid sample, a total IgG antibodies ELISA test was performed in order to assess the sample suitability for testing. Samples below 3.5 titre (cut-off) were excluded from the study as invalid (see Fig. 1: Survey testing algorithm). A validation

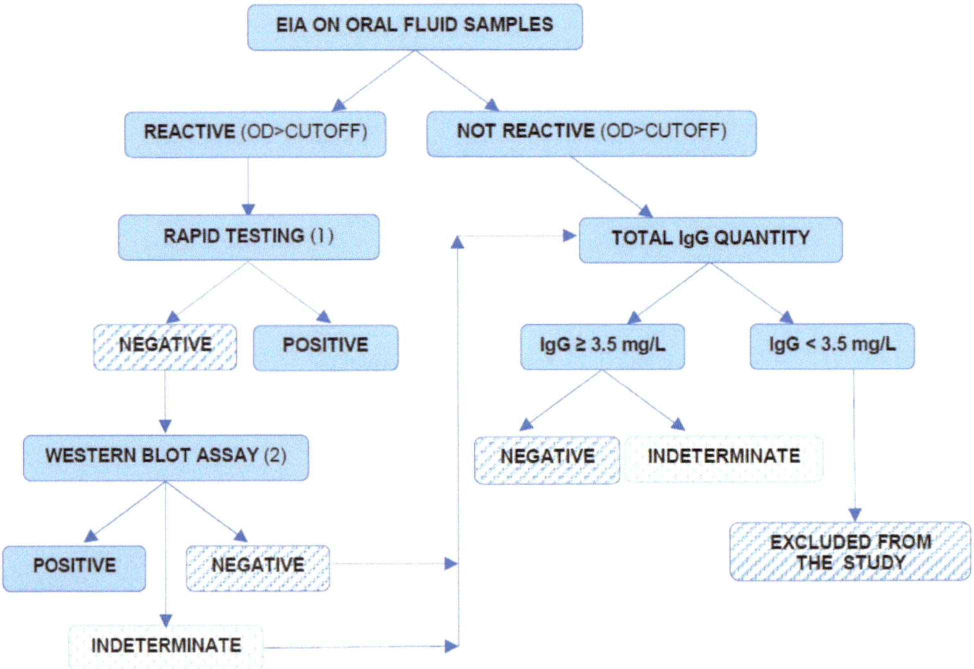

(1) Rapid Immunocromatograpy Determine HIV 1/2 (Unipath Ltd, Bedford UK) CE marked for serum were used
(2) HIV 1/2 BLOT 2.2 (MP Biomedical, China) CE marked for serum

Fig. 1. HIV testing algorithm on oral fluid samples

study of Bio-Rad OF testing comparing serological testing involving 37 HIV positive patients and 35 controls per country was carried out according to Commission decision of 7 May 2002 on common technical specifications for in vitro medical devices. EIA on oral fluid samples from 259 of the 263 HIV positive subjects were positive, giving a sensitivity of 98.5% (CI 96.2-99.6). All 233 controls were found negative for HIV in oral fluid and no false positives were detected (100% specificity; CI 98.4-100). The positive and negative predictive values of the OF test according to HIV prevalence are presented in Table 1.

Prevalence	5 %	15 %
PPV	100 %	100 %
NPV	99.9 %	99.7 %

Table 1. PPV and NPV according to prevalence

4. Results

4.1 General description of the sample

In this section, the description of the sample is provided in terms of number of MSM recruited, questionnaires and oral fluid samples collected, and characteristics of the sample.

4.1.1 Numbers of subjects recruited

A total of 2,592 subjects were recruited as follows: 408 MSM in Prague, 185 in Athens, 405 in Verona, 398 in Bucharest, 394 in Bratislava, 401 in Ljubljana and 401 in Barcelona. This study does not include the analysis of data from Athens as the Greek partner did not achieve the data collection.

4.1.2 Questionnaires and oral fluid samples collected

Table 2 shows the number of questionnaires and the number of oral fluid samples gathered during the data collection period for each country. Both the number of valid and invalid questionnaires and OF samples are given. From a general point of view, the percentage of invalid questionnaires is low, with the highest percentage in Ljubljana (0.7%). In three cases the percentage is 0% (Athens, Bucharest and Bratislava). With regards to the OF samples, in

	Prague	Athens	Verona	Bucharest	Bratislava	Ljubljana	Barcelona
Questionnaires	408	185	405	398	394	401	401
Valid	407	185	404	398	394	398	400
% invalid	0.2	0.0	0.2	0.0	0.0	0.7	0.2
OF samples	418	178	400	398	396	399	399
Invalid	31	28	9	53	10	10	10
% invalid	7.4	15.7	2.3	13.3	2.5	2.5	2.5

Table 2. Number of questionnaires and OF samples collected and percentage of valid samples

two cities the percentage of invalid samples is higher than 10% (Athens 15.7%; Bucharest 13.3%). In the other cities the percentage is low, ranging from 2.3% (Verona) to 2.5% (Ljubljana, Barcelona and Bratislava).

4.1.3 Venue types

The proportion of subjects recruited by venue type is shown in Fig. 2. 47.1% of the respondents were recruited in a disco (1,128 MSM). With the exception of Verona, discos were the main location where questionnaires and oral fluid were collected (36.7% in Prague, 71.3% in Bratislava, 65.2% in Bucharest, 64.0% in Ljubljana). Bars represented the second location in each city, in terms of number of participants (22.6% of the total, 540 subjects). The percentage of subjects recruited in this location ranged from 3.0% in Bratislava to 32.2% in Verona. With regard to saunas, 39.1% of the sample was recruited in this setting in Verona, 26.3% in Barcelona, 15.5% in Prague, 15.3% in Ljubljana and 13.7% in Bratislava. In Bucharest there is no sauna. Taking into account the total of the sample, the percentage of MSM recruited in a sauna was 18.4%. Low percentages of participants were recruited in cruising settings. Naked sex party and sex clubs were not present in Bucharest and Ljubljana, and the percentages of MSM recruited in this type of venue ranged from 6.4% in Verona up to 15.5% in Prague.

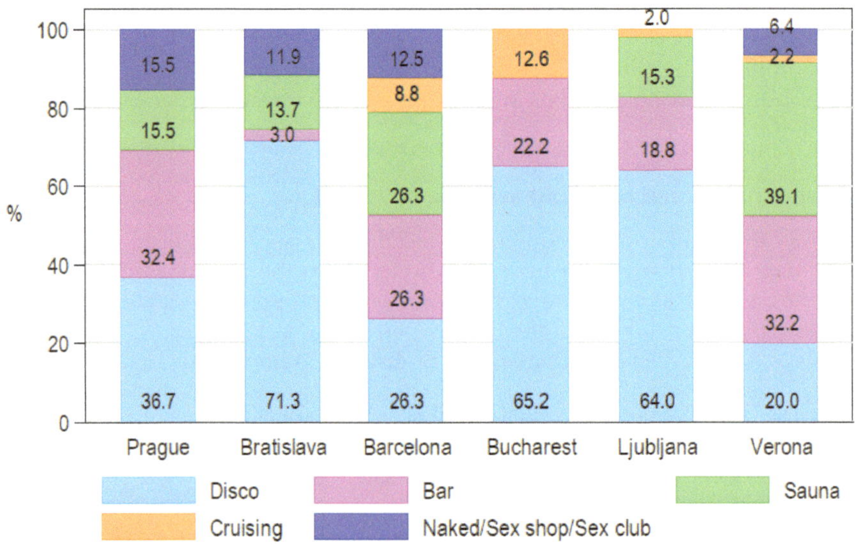

Fig. 2. Subjects recruited by venue type

4.1.4 Age of subjects

Median age and age distribution by city are presented in Figure 3. Respondents in Barcelona and Verona had a similar age distribution and were older (38 and 35 years respectively) than those in Eastern European cities.

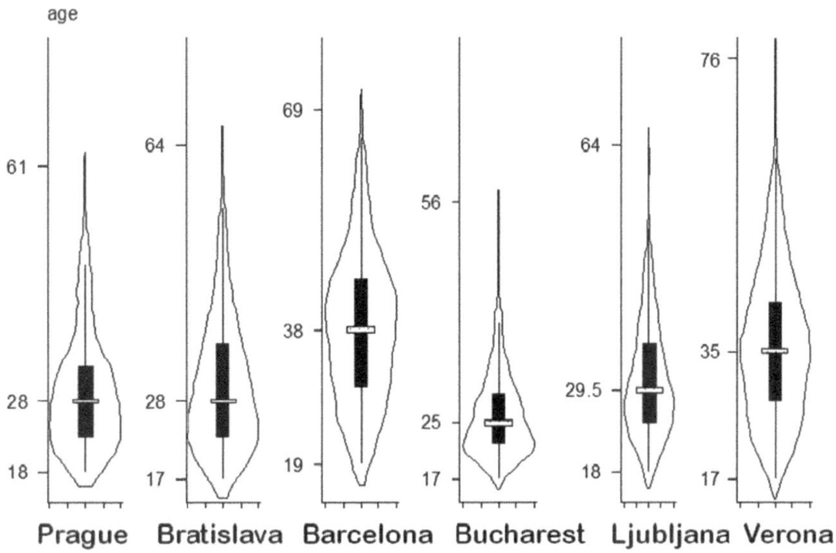

Fig. 3. Age distribution of MSM recruited by city

4.2 UNGASS indicators

In this section, the main data referring to the UNGASS indicators are provided. As mentioned in section 2, a specific Declaration of Commitment on HIV/AIDS and a Political Declaration on HIV/AIDS were proposed and adopted by the UN General Assembly in 2001. In these documents, a specific set of epidemiological and surveillance activities are proposed, as well as the adoption of the so-called UNGASS indicators. UNGASS indicators are a set of measures to be used among different countries in order to effectively monitor the HIV epidemic (UNAIDS & WHO, 2009). The idea which is behind the UNGASS indicators is that all data provided by the different countries can represent a reliable picture of the status of the epidemic and on the different prevention activities implemented against the spread of HIV in specific and general population.

The national-level UNGASS indicators are basically divided into three categories. The first one refers to the National commitment and action, taking into account topics as policy decisions, financial plan and activities for the HIV prevention, testing and treatment, drugs and care as well. The second category refers to knowledge and behaviour in different population, while the third category refers to the national level programme impact. For all these three areas, specific guidelines and procedures on how these indicators have to be calculated are provided (for instance, they provide specific numerators and denominators to calculate the different percentages and levels of the indicators).

Despite the relevance and importance of the UNGASS Declaration and the number of countries involved in this process, it should be mentioned that to date, a number of limitations in the UNGASS reporting have emerged. For instance, in 2008 less than half of those countries that stated the indicators and procedures referring to the most-at-risk populations (MSM included) were able to provide data based on these very indicators.

In this regard, one of the added values of the SIALON project is to provide reliable data on behaviours and HIV infection levels based on the UNGASS procedures and indicators. In some of the participating countries, the results of the SIALON project represent the first time in which UNGASS indicators were put into practice at the National level through a cross-sectional survey. In designing the SIALON questionnaire, four indicators were taken into account, focusing on high risk population, namely MSM. UNGASS indicators have proven to be effective measures to be considered in surveillance systems and in a comprehensive national monitoring and in an evidence-based evaluation approach.

4.2.1 UNGASS indicator N°8

In order to measure the HIV testing level, a specific UNGASS indicator was set, namely the UNGASS 8. This indicator refers to the percentage of MSM tested for HIV in the last 12 months and who know/collected the result, with the purpose of monitoring advancement in promoting HIV VCT among most-at-risk populations, in this case MSM. The indicator foresees as a numerator the number of most-at-risk population respondents who have been tested for HIV during the last 12 months and who know the results and as denominators the number of most-at-risk population included in the sample (Fig. 4).

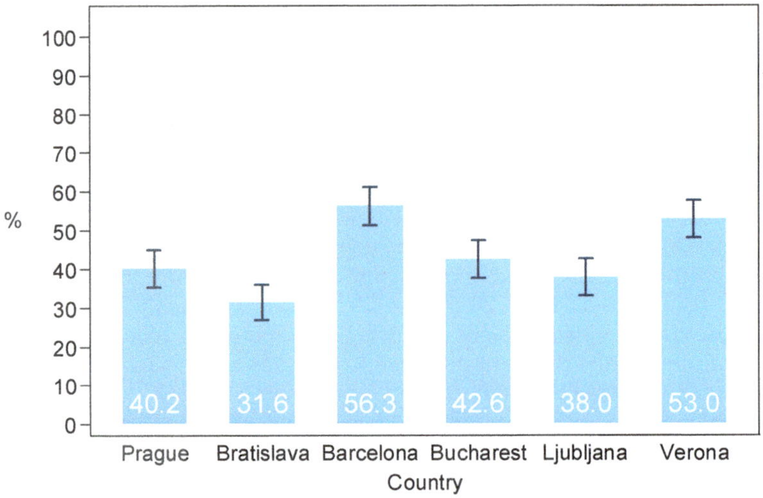

Fig. 4. UNGASS indicator N. 8: MSM who were tested in the last 12 month and knew the result

The Southern European cities had a high percentage of tested people who collected the test result (56.3% in Barcelona and 53.0% in Verona). In the other cities, low percentages are reported: 31.6% in Bratislava, 42.6% in Bucharest, 38.0% in Ljubljana and 40.2% in Prague.

4.2.2 UNGASS indicator N°9

This indicator refers to the percentage of most-at-risk populations reached with HIV prevention programmes. With regard to the construction of the indicator, the numerator is the number of respondents who replied that they have been given condoms for free in the last 12 months and knew where to go if they wished to be given an HIV test. The denominator is the number of MSM involved in the survey (Fig. 5).

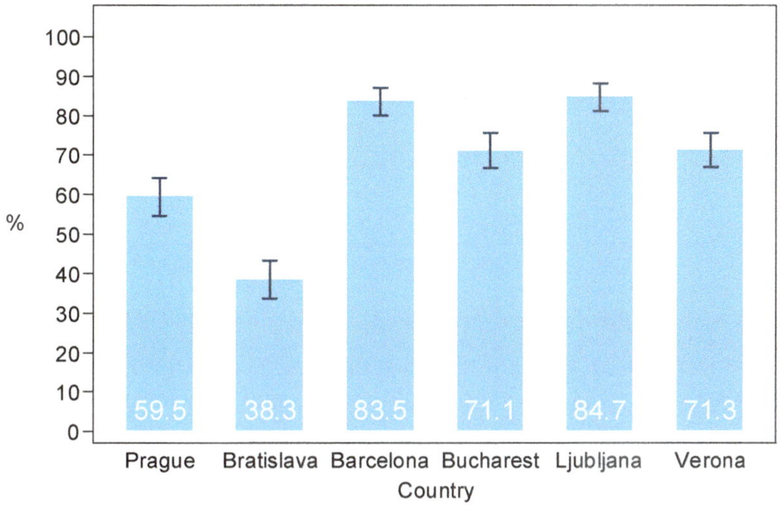

Fig. 5. UNGASS indicator N. 9: MSM reached by prevention programmes

The highest percentages of participants reached by prevention programmes are reported in Ljubljana (84.7%) and Barcelona (83.5%), while the lowest are in Prague (59.5%) and Bratislava (38.3%). In Verona, the percentage is 71.3%, while in Bucharest it is 71.1%. According to the UNGASS request of disaggregating the data according to the age group (<25/25+), young people (< 25 years old) were less reached by prevention programmes than older people (61.4% and 72.0% respectively).

4.2.3 UNGASS indicator N°19

This indicator describes the percentage of men reporting the use of a condom during their last anal sex intercourse with a male partner. The goal is to monitor the condom use among MSM, as it represents the main means for risk reduction. In this case, the numerator is the number of respondents who reported that a condom was used the last time they had anal sex, while the denominator is the number of respondents who reported having had anal sex with a male partner in the last six months (Fig. 6).

UNGASS 19 with steady and casual partner was calculated. As shown in Fig. 6, the percentage of participants who reported the use of a condom the last time they had anal sex with a male partner in the last 6 months with their steady partner was highest in Barcelona (35.1%) and lowest in Prague (19.1%). The percentage with occasional partner was highest in Barcelona (64.3%) and lowest in Bratislava (39.7%).

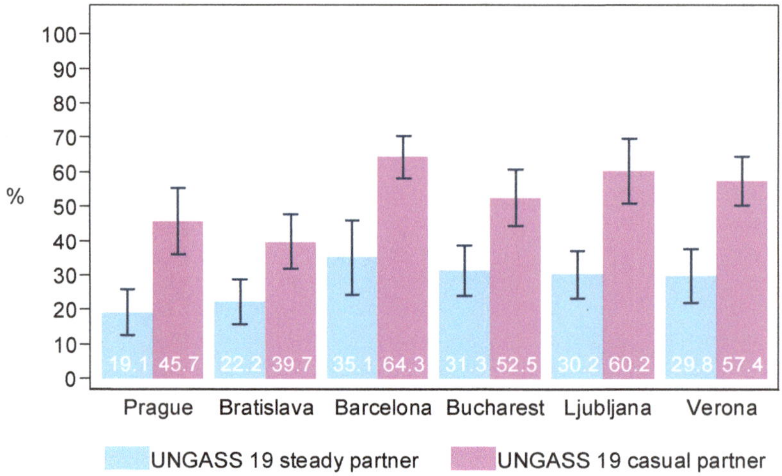

Fig. 6. UNGASS indicator N. 19: MSM reporting the use of a condom the last time they had anal sex with a male partner in the last 6 months: steady and occasional partners.

4.2.4 UNGASS indicator N°23

The UNGASS 23 refers to the HIV prevalence in a specific population, representing therefore the main indicator. This indicator allows to directly assess improvement in containing HIV levels among most-at-risk, namely MSM. In this case, the prevalence was calculated from the oral fluid tests performed in the central laboratory (Fig. 7).

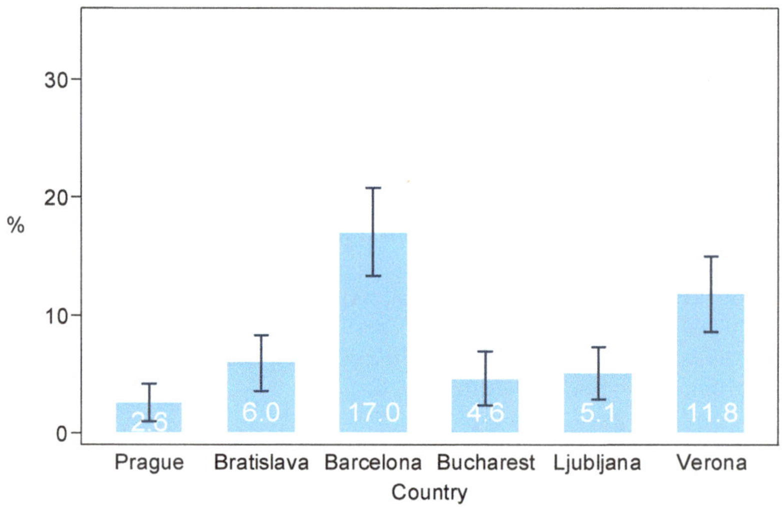

Fig. 7. UNGASS indicator N. 23 HIV prevalence

HIV percentages are 17.0% in Barcelona and 11.8% in Verona. Lower percentages were calculated in Bratislava (6.0%), Bucharest (4.6%) and Ljubljana (5.1%). In Prague, HIV level was 2.6%.

4.3 HIV prevalence

As reported in the UNGASS 23, data regarding HIV prevalence levels were calculated through the oral fluid samples tests. As mentioned before, the cities with the highest HIV prevalence were Barcelona (17.0%) and Verona (11.8%). Lower percentages were reported in Bratislava (6.0%), Bucharest (4.6%) and Ljubljana (5.1%). Prague had the lowest HIV prevalence (2.6%). The overall prevalence of HIV positive oral fluid samples was 7.9%. Previous studies carried out in some of the participating cities, came to quite different prevalence estimates. For instance, in Barcelona HIV prevalence found in previous studies using a convenience sample was slightly higher than the prevalence found in the SIALON study. The lower levels reported in Ljubljana and Bratislava in previous studies may be partly due to the different sampling method adopted and lower number of MSM recruited in the study.

4.3.1 HIV prevalence by age

The prevalence according to age group is represented in Table 3. In the overall sample, prevalence of HIV among young people (less than 25 years old) was significantly lower than among people of over 25 years of age (3.5% vs 9.6%). This difference in prevalence according to age group was also significant in Ljubljana where no HIV positive cases were found among younger MSM, and in Bratislava where 1.7% of younger MSM were HIV positive compared to 7.6% of older ones.

	Negative				Positive				Total	
Age group	No.	%	95% Conf. Interval		No.	%	95% Conf. Interval		No.	%
< 25	553	96.5	95.0	98.0	20	3.5	2.0	5.0	573	100.0
>= 25	1447	90.4	88.9	91.8	154	9.6	8.2	11.1	1601	100.0
Total	2000	92.0	91.0	93.2	174	8.0	6.8	9.0	2174	100.0

Table 3. HIV result according to age group

The mean age of HIV positive MSM was 36, significantly higher than the mean for HIV negative people (31.6 years). Table 4 shows the mean age of HIV positive people by country. This figure was lowest in Bucharest (27.1 years old) and the highest in Verona (38.9 years old).

Age group	Mean	95% Conf. Interval	
Prague	32.3	28.2	36.3
Bratislava	34.8	30.9	38.8
Barcelona	37.5	35.1	39.8
Bucharest	27.1	23.5	30.8
Ljubljana	35.1	32.2	38.0
Verona	38.9	36.3	41.5
Total	36.0	34.7	37.4

Table 4. Mean of age of HIV positive people by country

4.3.2 HIV prevalence by venue type

As shown in Fig. 8, HIV prevalence, based on oral fluid samples, was higher in subjects recruited in sex-focused venues like saunas (14.3%), cruising venues (15.2%) sex shops and naked parties (11.5%) than in other venues such as discos and bars (4.6% and 6.7% respectively).

At city level, HIV prevalence by type of venue (sex focused versus non-sex focused) was significantly higher in sex focused venues in Verona, Bratislava and Ljubljana.

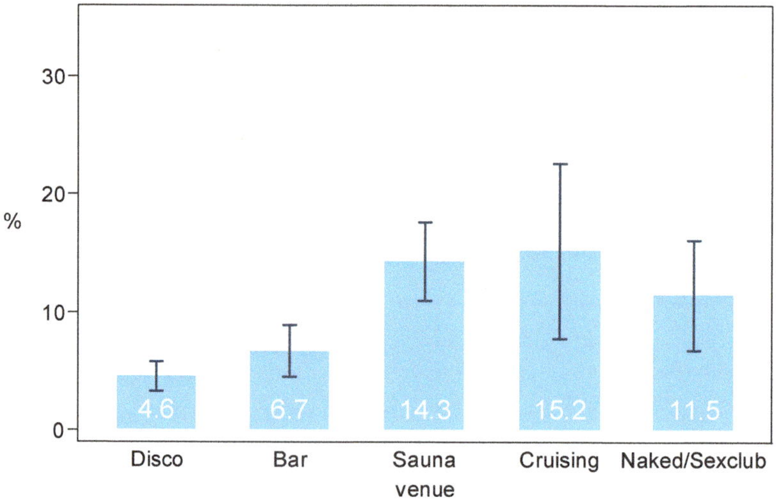

Fig. 8. HIV Prevalence by venue type

4.3.3 Knowledge of actual HIV status and undiagnosed infection

56% of HIV positive people were not aware of their HIV serostatus, that is, they declared they had never been tested (7.8%), were found to be HIV negative at their last HIV test (47.6%) or didn't collect their result (0.6%). As shown in Fig. 9, the rates of people unaware of their HIV positive status were almost 80% in Bucharest and Ljubljana and lower than 50% only in Barcelona.

Moreover, the average age of people unaware of their HIV positive status was 33.9 y/o lower than that of subjects that knew their seropositivity that was 37.9 y/o, based on their reported last HIV test. Another important fact is that among oral fluid HIV positive subjects, nearly one third (30.9%) reported a negative HIV test over the last 12 months. This data seems to indicate that quite a number of infections were acquired over the last 12 months. At city level this percentage was higher than 50% in Ljubljana while the lowest figure was in Bratislava (less than 20%). All other cities had intermediate values (nearly 30%).

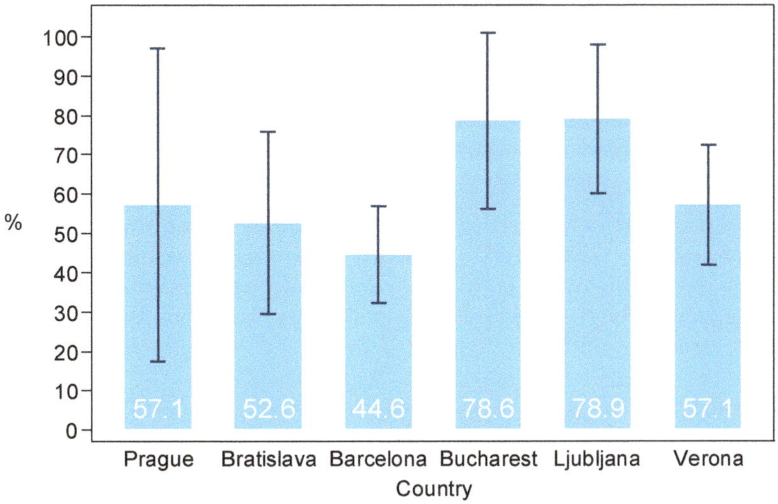

Fig. 9. Percentage of HIV positive MSM unaware of their HIV status

4.4 Other STI infections

4.4.1 STI history

Of the overall sample, 11.7% of respondents declared that they had at least one STI during the last 12 months. The highest proportion of people with a declared STI history was in Barcelona (15.3%) and the lowest in Bucharest (6.5%). For the details from all participating cities, see Fig. 10.

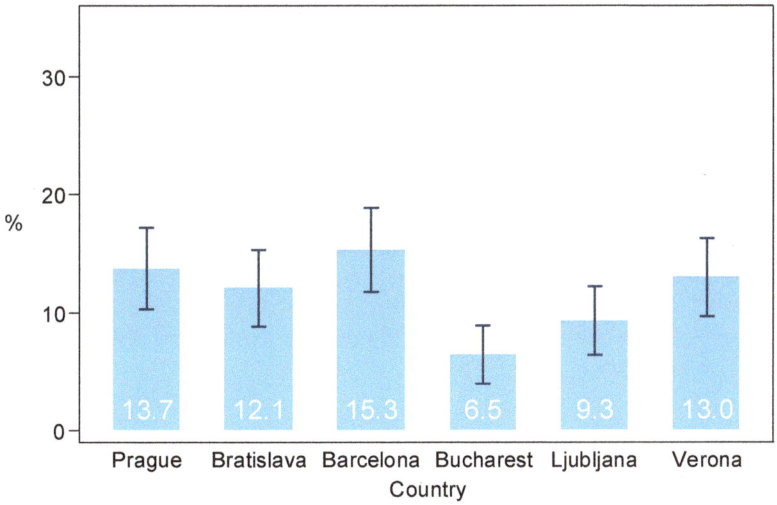

Fig. 10. STI during the last 12 months

4.4.2 Self reported history of Syphilis

2.5% of the overall sample had had Syphilis during the last year. The highest percentage was in Barcelona (5.6%) followed by Verona and Prague (3.7% and 3.4% respectively) while Bratislava, Bucharest and Ljubljana had the lowest figures (less than 1%).

4.4.3 Other STIs

The most frequent STI was Urethritis (6.2% including Gonorrhoea and Chlamydia), followed by anogenital warts (2.5%), Hepatitis B (1.2%) and genital herpes (1.0%). The distribution by city is shown in Fig. 11. The Urethritis category, including Gonorrhoea and Chlamydia, appears to be the most frequent in all cities. The second most frequent STI was anogenital warts in all the cities.

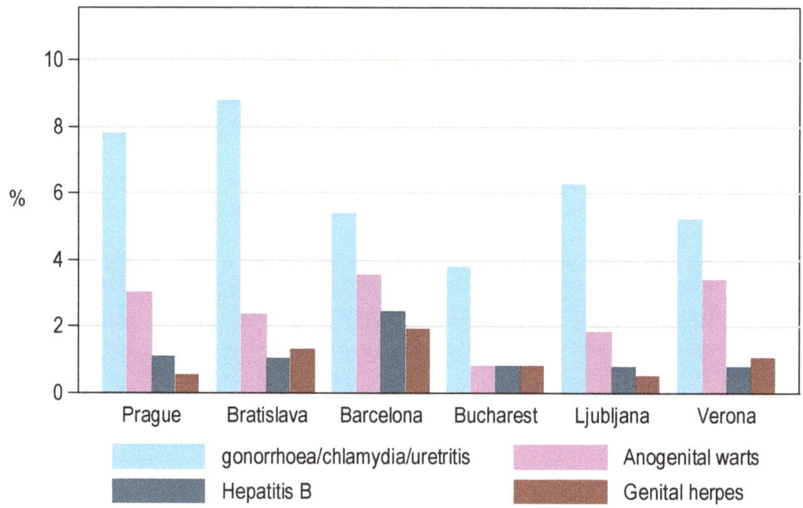

Fig. 11. Other STIs during the last 12 months by city

4.5 Risk behaviour

As mentioned in section 3.2.1, when designing the questionnaire, a number of questions were included to collect information on risk behaviours, which are proven to be widely adopted in the MSM community. This section provides data collected regarding the most at risk behaviours, namely unprotected anal intercourse (UAI) and the use of alcohol and drugs before or while having sex.

4.5.1 UAI

Unprotected anal intercourse during the last 6 months with steady and casual partners was calculated. As shown in Fig. 12, the percentage of participants who reported UAI over the last 6 months with their steady partner was highest in Prague (74.2%) and Bratislava (72.5%)

and lowest in Verona (58.1%). With regard to UAI with an occasional partner, this behaviour was reported in Bucharest in almost 60% of respondents, while in Prague the percentage reaches 46.5%, in Bratislava 45.7%, and similar percentages in Barcelona, Ljubljana and Verona (33.7%, 32.0%, 33.0% in this order). The percentage of MSM reporting UAI was significantly higher among young people (<25 years of age, according to the UNGASS disaggregation cut-off) with a steady (70.8%) and occasional (51.2%) partner (P<0.05 and P<0.001 respectively) compared to older people (64.9% and 37.8% in that order).

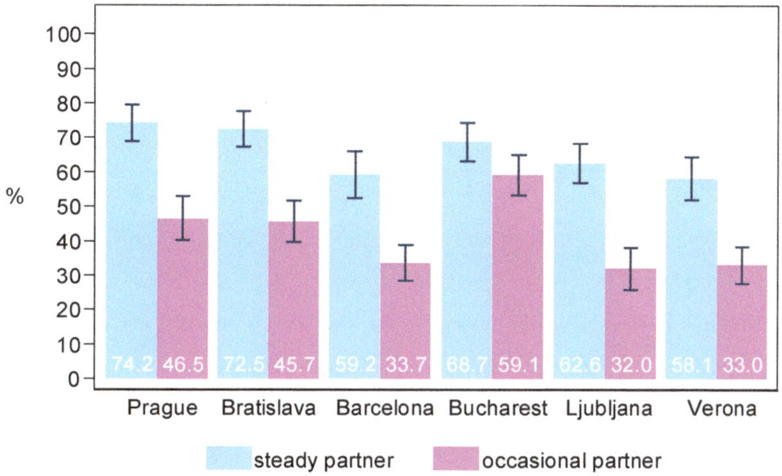

Fig. 12. UAI in the last 6 months with steady and occasional partner

4.5.2 Alcohol and drug use

As the alcohol and recreational drug use seems to be connected to an increase in unprotected sexual practices, the use of alcohol and drug before or during sex was included in the questionnaire.

With regard to alcohol use is concerned (Fig. 13), a significant percentage of respondents in the overall sample stated that they had used alcohol before or during sex in the last 6 months. The percentage of subjects reach 82.9% in Bratislava, 54.2% in Verona, 85.0% in Prague, 66.0% in Barcelona, 64.3% in Bucharest, while the level is of 72.3% in Ljubljana. With regards to the alcohol use before or during their last sexual encounter, percentages are lower compared with the last 6 months. The levels of alcohol use are in this case high in Prague (56.0%), Bucharest (46.3%), Bratislava (45.2%), Barcelona (43.0%), while rates lower than 40% were found only in Ljubljana and Verona (32.2% and 23.2% respectively).

With regard to drug use (see Fig. 14), drug use before or during sex in the last 6 months seems to be widely present in the sample. In Ljubljana the percentage reaches 58.8%, in Barcelona 57.1%, in Prague 52.7%. Low percentages are reported in Bucharest (33.2%), Verona (34.3%) and Bratislava (44.5%). Here again the proportion of people using drugs during sex was significantly higher among HIV positive (68.5%) than negative (44.9%) people (P<0.001).

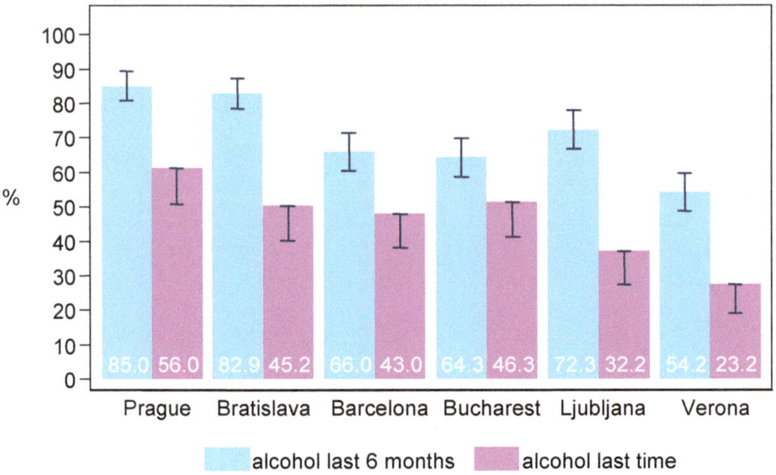

Fig. 13. Alcohol use before or while having sex in the last six months and in the last sexual intercourse

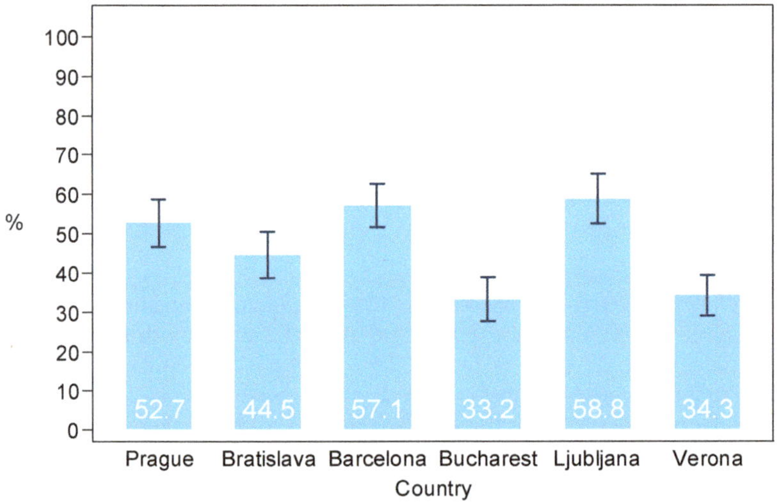

Fig. 14. Drug use before or while having sex in the last six months

5. Conclusions

In terms of the methodology, the use of TLS as a sampling method proved to be efficient and easily applicable especially in cities where gay scenes are highly developed and, in line with the scientific literature, it increases the possibility of involving a variety of participants from the target population.

In implementing this method, the formative research is a crucial step of the process. The initial identification and selection of all gay venues (bars, discos, saunas, cruising venues, sex-shops, sex-clubs, special events) is a key factor for including all possible places and events and creating a list of all possible time-space units.

Moreover, it should be pointed out that in this project different ways of recruiting MSM, such as internet, chat rooms and so on, were excluded. In actual fact, these virtual settings seem to play a very important role in the process of socialising and finding potential sexual partners among MSM. Nevertheless, the selection of "real" gay venues allowed to collect both behavioural data (questionnaire) and biological data (oral fluid sample). In this way, it was possible to triangulate behavioural data, risk factors, and HIV prevalence and to obtain reliable information on epidemic patterns.

With regard to oral fluid sample collection, this procedure has clear advantages in terms of simplifying both the data collection and the diagnostic processes in community settings, compared to venopuncture. Oral fluid testing proved to be an ideal tool for surveillance and epidemiological purposes in outreach settings among high-risk and hard to reach populations, namely MSM. The acceptability of this biological data collection procedure in gay settings is proven by the number of samples collected in all sites confirmed.

Furthermore, the SIALON project methodology included several epidemiological approaches: first of all, the Second Generation Surveillance System philosophy, which strongly suggests the combination of both behavioural and biological data and the regular replication of surveillance survey. Secondly, the implementation of UNGASS indicators, which proved to be very useful in focusing on specific topics such as access to prevention (testing and prevention programmes), high risk behaviours and HIV prevalence. Indicators related to HIV testing, prevention programs, condom use, and understanding of how to protect against HIV infection, revealed how many MSM are unaware of their HIV status and fail to practice behaviour that could protect them from infection.

This very approach seems to be a crucial activity in order to develop, pilot and validate multi-faceted epidemiological approaches in monitoring HIV epidemic.

In terms of the data collected, the highest rates of HIV seroprevalence were found in Southern European cities, namely Barcelona and Verona. This could be partly attributed to the older samples and therefore to longer exposure to risk, since HIV prevalence was higher among MSM of over 25.

The highest rates of syphilis prevalence were also found in Barcelona and Verona. In general, data confirms that a correlation exists between STI, previous syphilis, IgG anti-Treponema seroprevalence and HIV infection.

Alarming findings included undiagnosed HIV infections. Over half the respondents were unaware of their HIV positive status. This proportion was slightly lower only in Barcelona, but very high (nearly 80%) in Ljubljana and Bucharest. Moreover, nearly one third of MSM found to be HIV-positive through oral fluid samples reported a negative HIV test result over the last 12 months, so the undiagnosed infections were recent. This figure was highest in Bucharest (over 50%) and lowest in Bratislava (less than 20%).

The risk of HIV infection was assessed with a major focus on unprotected anal intercourse (UAI). Two respondents out of ten reported having had UAI with an occasional partner the last time they had sex, while four out of ten reported having had UAI in the last 6 months with this kind of partner or partners. The percentages of UAI with an occasional partner were highest in Bucharest, Prague and Bratislava both for the last sexual encounter and for encounters over the previous 6 months. In line with this finding, in these cities MSM reported less use of a condom for anal intercourse the last time they had anal sex. Young MSM exhibited the riskiest behaviour, as the highest rates of UAI with occasional partners, both last time and in the last 6 months, were found amongst young people under 25 years old. As expected, UAI with a steady partner was more frequent than with an occasional partner, in the overall sample and in all the cities.

Finally, the association between HIV risk and alcohol and drug use was confirmed. At least one third of respondents had used drugs before or during sex over the last six months and half the respondents had used alcohol. This proportion was above half in Ljubljana, Barcelona and Prague for drugs, and higher than 80% in Prague and Bratislava.

This data suggests the (i) the need for health promotion and prevention messages particularly focused on sexual behaviour and alcohol and drug use (ii) the need for prevention and information programmes for STIs given that the presence of an STIs increases the risk of HIV infection (iii) the need for policies and strategies promoting VCT among hard to reach populations such as MSM, especially young MSM.

6. Acknowledgements

Financial support:
The Capacity building in HIV/Syphilis prevalence estimation using non-invasive methods among MSM in Southern and Eastern Europe - SIALON project was funded by the European Commission under the European Commission Public Health Programme 2003-2008.

The sole responsibility for this article lies with the authors and the European Commission is not responsible for any use that might be made of the information contained therein.

The SIALON Network is composed by:
Yuri Amirkhanian (CAIR - Medical College of Wisconsin, USA) Eva Baldassari (Mental Health Department, ULSS20, Verona) Luigi Bertinato (Service for International Social and Health Relations, ULSS20, Veneto Region, Verona) Chrisoula Botsi (HCDCP, Athens) Michele Breveglieri (Regional Centre for Health Promotion, Verona) Enrica Castellani (Regional Centre for Health Promotion, Verona) Paola Coato (Azienda Ospedaliera Universitaria Integrata Verona, Department of Pathology, Section of Microbiology) Jonathan Elford (City University London) Cinta Folch (CEEISCAT Badalona Barcelona) Roberta Fontana (Microbiology - Verona University Hospital) Mauro Fornasiero (University of Bristol, England, UK) Jean-Pierre Foschia (Regional Centre for Health Promotion, Verona) Martina Furegato (Regional Centre for Health Promotion, Verona) Lorenzo Gios (Azienda Ospedaliera Universitaria Integrata Verona, Verona) Jaroslav Gyurik (Association of AIDS Help, Bratislava) Victoria Gonzalez (CEEISCAT Hospital Universitari Germans Trias i PUjol, Badalona) Valentina Guarnieri (Microbiology - Azienda Ospedaliera Universitaria

Integrata Verona) Monika Habekova (NRC HIV/AIDS Slovak Univeristy, Bratislava) Alex Horky (Czech Youth Queer Organisation) Jaroslav Jedlicka (NIPH, Prague) Kostantinos Kampourakis (Act-up Hellas, Athens) Igor Krampac (Regional Public Health Institute Maribor, Slovenia) Massimiliano Lanzafame (Azienda Ospedaliera Universitaria Integrata Verona, Infectious Diseases Unit) Emanuela Lattuada (Azienda Ospedaliera Universitaria Integrata Verona) Roberta Martini (International Health and Social Affairs, Veneto Region) Massimo Mirandola (Azienda Ospedaliera Universitaria Integrata Verona, Verona) Zeno Menegazzi (Arcigay Pianeta Urano, Verona) Silvana Menichelli (Regional Centre for Health Promotion, Verona) Gianmichele Moise (STD Centre, Gorizia) Sabrina Montante (Veneto Region) Rafael Muñoz Castro (STOP SIDA, Barcelona) Daniela Negri (Veneto Region) Georgios Nikolopoulos (HCDCP, Athens) Irina Nita (ACCEPT, Bucharest) Paolo Patanè (Arcigay, Italy) Daniela Pitigoi (Matei Bals Institute, Bucharest) Peter Porubsky (Czech Aids Help Society) Ivo Prochazka (Czech Aids Help Society, Prague) Alexandru Rafila (Matei Bals Institute, Bucharest) Dunia Ramarli (Azienda Ospedaliera Universitaria Integrata Verona, Department of Pathology, Section of Immunology) David Rivett (independent consultant specialising in Health Promotion and Education) Miran Solinc (SKUC Magnus, Ljubljana) Danica Staneková (NRC HIV/AIDS Slovak University, Bratislava) Dzamila Stehlikova (NIPH, Prague) Barbara Suligoi (ISS, Rome) Igor Toskin (Department of Reproductive Health & Research WHO, Geneva) Lev Zohrabyan (Regional Support Team, Europe and Central Asia UNAIDS, Moscow) Elisabetta Tonolli (Azienda Ospedaliera Universitaria Integrata Verona, Department of Pathology, Section of Microbiology) Ruggero Ughetti (Regional Centre for Health Promotion, Verona) (Hana Zakoucka (NIPH, Prague) Alessandro Zan (Arcigay Veneto) Alin Robert Zoltan (ACCEPT, Bucharest)

7. References

Dodds, J.D.; Mercey, D.E.; Parry, J.V.; Johnson, A.M. (2004). Increasing risk behaviour and high levels of undiagnosed HIV infection in a community sample of homosexual men. *Sexually Transmitted Infections*, vol. 80, 2004, pp. 236-240, ISSN 1472-3263

European Centre for Disease Prevention and Control (ECDC) & World Health Organization (WHO) - Regional Office for Europe. *HIV/AIDS surveillance in Europe 2009.* Stockholm: European Centre for Disease Prevention and Control, 2010

Folch, C.; Casabona, J.; Munoz, R.; Zaragoza, K. (2005). [Trends in the prevalence of HIV infection and risk behaviours in homo- and bisexual men]. *Gaceta Sanitaria,* vol. 19(4), 2005, pp. 294-301, ISSN 0213-9111, Spanish

Gallagher, K.M.; Finlayson, T.; Sanchez, T.; Lansky, A.; Sullivan, P.S. (2007). Surveillance of HIV risk and prevention behaviors of men who have sex with men-a national application of venue-based, time-space sampling. *Public Health Reports,* vol. 122 Suppl. 1, 2007, pp. 39-47, ISSN 0033-3549

Joint United Nations Programme on HIV/AIDS (UNAIDS) and World Health Organization (WHO) (2009). *Monitoring the Declaration of Commitment on HIV/AIDS: guidelines on construction of core indicators: 2010 reporting*. Geneva: UNAIDS 2009, available from: http://www.unaids.org

Joint United Nations Programme on HIV/AIDS (UNAIDS) and World Health Organization (WHO) (2002). *Initiating second generation HIV surveillance systems: practical guidelines.* UNAIDS-WHO, retrieved from: http://www.who.int/hiv/pub/surveillance/guidelines/en/index.html

Joint United Nations Programme on HIV/AIDS (UNAIDS) and World Health Organization (WHO) (2005). *The pre-surveillance assessment. Guidelines for planning serosurveillance of HIV, prevalence of sexually transmitted infections and behavioural components of second generation surveillance of HIV*. UNAIDS-WHO, retrieved from: http://www.who.int/hiv/pub/surveillance/sti/en/index.html

Likatavičius, G.; Klavs, I.; Devaux, I.; Alix, J.; Nardone, A. (2008). An increase in newly diagnosed HIV cases reported among men who have sex with men in Europe, 2000–6: implications for a European public health strategy, *Sexually Transmitted Infections*, vol. 84, 2008, pp. 499-505, ISSN 1472-3263

MacKellar, D.A.; Gallagher, K.M.; Finlayson, T.; Sanchez, T.; Lansky, A.; Sullivan, P.S. (2007). Surveillance of HIV risk and prevention behaviors of men who have sex with men: a national application of venue-based, time-space sampling. *Public Health Reports*, vol. 122 Suppl. 1, 2007, pp.39-47, ISSN 0033-3549

MacKellar, D.A.; Valleroy, L.A.; Secura, G.M.; Behel, S.; Bingham, T.; Celentano, D.D.; Koblin, B.A.; Lalota, M.; McFarland, W.; Shehan, D.; Thiede, H.; Torian, L.V.; Janssen, R.S.; Young Men's Survey Study Group. (2005). Unrecognized HIV infection, risk behaviors, and perceptions of risk among young men who have sex with men: opportunities for advancing HIV prevention in the third decade of HIV/AIDS. *Journal of Acquired Immune Deficiency Syndromes*, vol. 38(5), 2005, pp. 603-14, ISSN 1525-4135

Mirandola, M.; Folch Toda, C.; Krampac, I.; Nita, I.; Stanekova, D.; Stehlikova, D.; Toskin, I.; Gios, L.; Foschia, J.P.; Breveglieri, M.; Furegato, M.; Castellani, E.; Bonavina, M.G.; the SIALON network. (2009). HIV bio-behavioural survey among men who have sex with men in Barcelona, Bratislava, Bucharest, Ljubljana, Prague and Verona, 2008-2009. *Euro Surveillance*, vol. 14(48), ISSN 1560-7917, retrieved from: http://www.eurosurveillance.org/ViewArticle.aspx?ArticleId=19427

Muhib, FB.; Lin, LS.; Stueve, A.; Miller, R.L.; Ford, W.L.; Johnson, W.D. (2001). A venue-based method for sampling hard-to-reach populations. *Public Health Reports*, vol. 116 Suppl. 1, 2001, pp. 216-22, ISSN 0033-3549

Stueve, A. ; O'Donnell L.N.; Duran, R.; San Doval, A.; Blome, J. (2001). Time-space sampling in minority communities: results with young Latino men who have sex with men. *American Journal of Public Health*, vol. 91(6), 2001, pp. 922-6, ISSN 1541-0048

Van de Laar, M.J. (2009). HIV/AIDS and other STI in men who have sex with men - a continuous challenge for public health. *Euro Surveillance*, vol. 14(47), ISSN 1560-7917

Williamson, L.M. & Hart, G.J. (2007). HIV prevalence and undiagnosed infection among a community sample of gay men in Scotland. *Journal of Acquired Immune Deficiency Syndromes*, vol. 45(2), 2007, pp. 224-30, ISSN 1525-4135

Section 5

Epidemiology of Wildlife Tuberculosis

14

Wildlife Tuberculosis: A Systematic Review of the Epidemiology in Iberian Peninsula

Nuno Santos[1], Margarida Correia-Neves[1], Virgílio Almeida[2] and Christian Gortázar[3]
[1]*Life and Health Sciences Research Institute (ICVS) School of Health Sciences, University of Minho, Campus de Gualtar, Braga*
[2]*Centro de Investigação Interdisciplinar em Sanidade Animal – Faculdade de Medicina Veterinária (CIISA/FMV), TULisbon, Pólo Universitário do Alto da Ajuda, Lisbon*
[3]*IREC National Wildlife Research Institute (CSIC-UCLM-JCCM), Ciudad Real*
[1,2]*Portugal*
[3]*Spain*

1. Introduction

Mycobacterium bovis is the main etiological agent of bovine tuberculosis, infecting many species of wild and domestic mammals and also man. Bovine tuberculosis is a chronic and contagious infectious disease that has been reported to infect wild ungulates, carnivores, marsupials and primates (de Lisle *et al.*, 2002). Bovine tuberculosis (bTB) also occurs worldwide in livestock (Humblet *et al.*, 2009), causing annual economic losses estimated at 3 billion USD in 1995 (Steele, 1995). It remains a serious risk for animal health, and a threat for human health in many developing countries (Etter *et al.*, 2006). Several countries successfully eradicated bovine tuberculosis in livestock through test-and-slaughter and/or abattoir surveillance programs. Yet other countries, using similar strategies, did not achieve eradication and some even face the re-emergence of the disease (Schiller *et al.*, 2010). In Europe for instance, the prevalence of bTB in cattle is increasing in several countries (Gordejo & Vermeersch, 2006). Moreover current eradication and control programs in livestock in Europe are facing a range of challenges as stamping out is becoming a less attractive option for economic and environmental reasons and due to animal welfare concerns (Whiting, 2003).

Some of the abovementioned difficulties in eradicating bTB in cattle may relate with the occurrence of the disease in wildlife (Schiller *et al.*, 2010). In fact it has been demonstrated that the complete elimination of bTB can be extremely complicated by persistent infection of wild hosts, such as badgers in the United Kingdom, white tailed deer in the United States and brushtail possum in New Zealand (Corner, 2006). The single successful example of bTB eradication in a wildlife host is the Australian case, where it was accomplished through stamping out, which eliminated introduced water buffalo *Bubalus arnee*, the only maintenance host in that ecosystem, (Corner, 2006). This is not an option when autochthonous, protected or economic and socially valuable species are involved (Artois *et al.*, 2001). In most cases, an integrated control program is needed (Horan *et al.*,

2008), but this is often hampered by the lack of epidemiological data (Artois *et al.*, 2001; Corner, 2006).

Bovine tuberculosis control programs in cattle are in place for several decades in Iberian Peninsula and consequently incidence has been decreasing (Allepuz *et al.*, 2011; Cunha *et al.*, 2011). However in the last few years incidence has stabilized, or even slightly increased in both Portugal and Spain (Allepuz *et al.*, 2011; Cunha *et al.*, 2011). The role of wildlife hosts in this scenario remains speculative; nevertheless the existence of wildlife reservoirs may compromise the goal of eradication in cattle. Besides livestock, attention should be given to spill-over from wildlife to other domestic animals (e.g. goats and free-ranging pigs) and even to humans, namely hunters and others that handle wild ungulate carcasses (Gortazar *et al.*, 2011b, in press). Wildlife-to-human transmission of *M. bovis* is hard to prove and no single case has been documented in Iberian Peninsula, but it is known to occur elsewhere (e.g. USA - Wilkins *et al.*, 2008). Bovine tuberculosis is also one of the main infectious diseases affecting the critically endangered Iberian lynx *Lynx pardinus*, with several free-ranging and captive lynx killed by this infection (Millán *et al.*, 2009). Iberian lynx is subject to an intensive multinational conservation program in Iberian Peninsula, which includes releasing captive-bred animals to former range. The persistence of *M. bovis* on the environment and in prey species poses a threat to this conservation action (Millán *et al.*, 2009).

Iberian Peninsula ecosystems display a high degree of human intervention and have experienced some profound changes in the last decades. The most important alterations were a shift from domestic ungulate to wild ungulate production for hunting purposes (Miguel *et al.* 1999) and an increasing intensification of the later (Vargas *et al.* 1995). This management of wild ungulate populations aims to increase profits by increasing harvest, translating into increased densities of hunted species. This has been accomplished through introduction/restocking, provision of food and water (mostly during the summer shortage), fencing and sometimes even medication (Miguel *et al.* 1999, Gortázar *et al.*, 2006). All these changes have potential implications on bTB epidemiology (Gortázar *et al.*, 2006).

In the Iberian Peninsula, ungulates such as the wild boar *Sus scrofa* and the red deer *Cervus elaphus* have been recognized as the most important maintenance hosts for wildlife tuberculosis (Gortázar *et al.*, 2011b). Nevertheless other species have also been identified as locally non-negligible hosts, such as the fallow deer *Dama dama* and the badger *Meles meles* (Gortázar *et al.*, 2011b; Balseiro *et al.*, 2011). Several other species of ungulates and carnivores were also found infected (Rodriguez *et al.*, 2010). This situation fits the definition of a multi-host pathogen within a multi-species ecosystem (Renwick *et al.*, 2007; Gortázar *et al.*, in press), in which pathogen persistence and spread is dependent on the density of each maintenance host species and also on the effective interspecies contact rate (dependent on the ecology of each species).

Research on host-pathogen interaction usually deals with single-host single-pathogen systems, where disease persistence depends solely on the intra-species transmission rate (Tompkins *et al.*, 2001). If transmission is density-dependent, then population thresholds for disease invasion and persistence are expected and have been described (Swinton *et al.*, 2001). By contrast, in multi-host pathogens systems, disease persistence is dependent on both intra and inter-species transmission rates and densities of several host species (Renwick *et al.*, 2007). Moreover, these rates depend on pathological, epidemiological, ecological and behavioural factors (Corner, 2006).

In such a complex epidemiological setting, it is imperative to determine the precise role of each host species in pathogen maintenance before comprehensive control measures are undertaken. Much has been investigated in the last decade regarding wildlife tuberculosis epidemiology in Iberian Peninsula. In order to contribute to understanding the mechanisms underlying wildlife tuberculosis persistence in the multi-host ecosystems of this region, under widely different ecological and management pressures, we report a systematic bibliographic review on this subject. The aim of this review was to survey the peer-reviewed literature for evidence of the: *i*) epidemiological status of each host species; *ii*) determinants of wildlife tuberculosis occurrence; *iii*) geographical structuring of wildlife tuberculosis in the Iberian Peninsula; *iv*) time trends in wildlife tuberculosis occurrence.

2. Methods

We conducted a systematic bibliographic review for epidemiological studies on tuberculosis in wildlife in Iberian Peninsula by searching MEDLINE/PubMed, up to the 31st of August 2011, using MeSH and keywords: "*Mycobacterium bovis*", "*Mycobacterium caprae*", "wild boar", "deer", "epidemiology", "Iberian Peninsula", "Portugal" and "Spain". Combinations used were: ("Portugal" OR "Spain") AND ("*Mycobacterium bovis*" OR "*Mycobacterium caprae*"), ("*Mycobacterium bovis*" OR "*Mycobacterium caprae*") AND "wild boar" AND "epidemiology" and ("*Mycobacterium bovis*" OR "*Mycobacterium caprae*") AND "deer" AND "epidemiology". Abstracts were selected according to their relevancy and excluded if dealing exclusively with laboratory or pathology investigations, domestic species or humans or other geographical regions. Articles were reviewed in full text.

For each article, information about the type of epidemiological study and study design, sample size and sampling methodology, screening and diagnostic tests used, prevalence rate, time frame of the study, study areas, characteristics of the populations studied, risk factors identified and host epidemiological status was summarized and presented in table format for easy comparison. Due to their idiosyncrasies, molecular epidemiology articles were characterized differently according to the number of isolates studied, genotyping technique, mycobacterial species reported, number of genotypes found, host and geographical clustering of genotypes and study areas. Due to differing methodologies and sometimes incomplete reporting of results, meta-analysis was not applicable except for a small number of studies.

For the purpose of this review, wildlife tuberculosis was defined according to the OIE definition of bovine tuberculosis, but *Mycobacterium caprae* was also considered etiological agent, besides *M. bovis*.

3. Results

The bibliographic search yielded 286 articles. Initially, title and abstracts were reviewed and 247 articles excluded because they deal only with laboratory/pathology investigations (n=74), domestic animals (n=41), humans (n=50), other geographical regions (n=79), or were review/model articles (n=3). Full text papers were then reviewed and further 6 papers were excluded because they focused exclusively on laboratory/pathology investigations. Therefore 33 articles were selected as of interest to the present review.

Reference	Type	Sampling strategy	Sample n	Screening test	Diagnostic test	Time frame & tendency	Prevalence (rate)	Fencing	Study areas
Aranaz *et al.* (2004)	SU	Targeted (hunted)	96		BC		51 (53,1%)	MX	7 area SW Spain
Acevedo-Whitehouse *et al.* (2005)	CS	Targeted (hunted)	175		BC	2000-2003	82 (47%)	MX	7 areas SW Spain
Parra *et al.* (2005)	CS	Scanning (hunted)	112	MI	BC		112	FE	1 region W Spain
de Mendoza *et al.* (2006)	CS	Scanning (hunted)	8.478	MI	BC	1992-2004 increasing	333 (3,92%)	MX	1 area W Spain
Parra *et al.* (2006)	CS	Scanning (hunted)	34.582	MI	BC	1997-2002 increasing	625 (1,81%)	MX	1 region W Spain
Vicente *et al.* (2006a)	CS	Targeted (hunted)	1.060		GP BC (not all)	1999-2004	(42,51%, mean estate rate)	MX	57 areas SW Spain
Vicente *et al.* (2006b)	CS	Targeted (hunted)	412		GP BC (not all)	1999-2004	(18,2%-100%)	FE	19 area SW Spain
Gortázar *et al.* (2008)	CS	Targeted (culled)	124		BC	2006-2007	65 (52,4%)	FR	1 area SW Spain
Romero *et al.* (2008)	SU	Targeted (culled)	214		BC	1998-2003	60 (28,0%)	FR	1 area SW Spain
Santos *et al.* (2009)	CS	Targeted (hunted)	162		BC	2005-2007	18 (11,1%)	FR	8 areas South-central Portugal
Cunha *et al.* (2011)	SU	Scanning (hunted)	343	MI	BC	2002-2010	(63%)	MX	Several areas across Portugal
Gortázar *et al.* (2011a)	CS	Targeted (culled)	124		BC	2006-2007	62 (50%)	FR	1 area SW Spain
Pinto *et al.* (2011)	CS	Targeted (hunted)	132	GP	BC	2008-2009	21 (15,9%)	MX	1 area Central Portugal

Table 1. Studies dealing with wild boar included in the analysis. Classification: SU – survey; CS - cross sectional study; CC – case-control study; Screening/diagnostic test: MI – official meat inspection scheme; GP – gross pathology; BC – bacteriological culture; SE – serology; Fencing: FR – free-ranging populations; FE – fenced populations; MX – mixed free-ranging and fenced populations.

3.1 Characterization of published articles

Investigation of bTB epidemiology in wild boar and red deer (most often studied hosts) are mostly cross-sectional (11/14), the rest being surveys (Tables 1-2). Most studies opt for targeted surveillance on hunted (6/14) or culled (3/14) animals, the rest relying on scanning surveillance in routine meat inspection schemes for detection of macroscopic lesions-like lesions (Table 1-2). The mean number of animals studied in targeted-design studies is 278 for wild boar (n=9, range 96-1.060) and 401 for red deer (n=6, range 95-1.368). Thirteen out of fourteen studies use bacteriological culture as the diagnostic test. Nevertheless most of them (9/14) also include a previous screening test (usually gross pathology or routine meat inspection schemes), followed by bacteriological culture when macroscopic lesions were observed (Table 1-2).

As regards studies on other host species (ungulates and carnivores), 5/14 are case reports, 6/14 surveys while 3/14 are cross sectional studies (Table 3). Five out of twelve studies rely on passive surveillance of haphazardly found carcasses and 3/12 on targeted surveillance of purposefully trapped animals. Most of these studies deal with carnivore species. As expected regarding novel host species, 3/12 studies are case reports (Table 3). Mean number of animals studied in survey studies is 105 for fallow deer (n=4, range 89-134), 63 for badger (n=3, range 2-157) and 15 for Iberian lynx (n=5, range 1-39). Most other species (Table 5) are dealt in single studies, usually as case reports. Serologic tests were used in 3/9 studies investigating other host species, such as Barbary sheep and carnivores (Table 3).

3.2 Prevalence rates

For the wild boar populations surveyed by targeted-design studies using bacteriological culture as diagnostic test on all animals (n=6), prevalence rates ranged 0,11-0,53, with a meta prevalence rate of 0,36 (Table 5). Including all studies, regardless of design, prevalence rates ranged 0,18-1 (Table 1). For the red deer populations surveyed by targeted-design studies using bacteriological culture as diagnostic test on all animals samples (n=3), prevalence rates ranged 0,02-0,27, with a meta prevalence rate of 0,21 (Table 5). Including all studies, regardless of design, prevalence rates ranged 0,01-0,44 (Table 2). For the fallow deer populations surveyed by targeted-design studies using bacteriological culture as diagnostic test on all animals samples (n=4), prevalence rates ranged 0,13-0,67, with a meta prevalence rate of 0,28 (Table 5). For other host species, the sample size and/or the study design do not allow meta analysis.

3.3 Trends

Few studies address or allow addressing the time trend of bTB prevalence rates. In Doñana, bTB was not detected in targeted wildlife health surveillance until 1990's, when the population of cattle greatly increased, while in 2000's high prevalence rates were found in all ungulate species (Gortázar *et al.*, 2008). In fact, prevalence rates in this area increased from 1998-2003 to 2006-2007 by 100% in wild boar and 50% in red deer (Gortázar *et al.*, 2011b). In Extremadura region, West-central Spain, prevalence rates detected in routine meat inspection schemes steadily raised from 1994-2004, while not detected in 1992-1993 (de Mendonza *et al.*, 2006). One study area in South-eastern Portugal showed an increase in *M. bovis* infection rates in wild boar from 0,46 in 2005/06 (Santos *et al.*, 2009) to 0,78 in 2009/11 (Santos *et al.*, unpublished data).

Reference	Type	Sampling strategy	Sample n	Screening test	Diagnostic test	Time frame & tendency	Prevalence (rate)	Fencing	Study areas
Aranaz *et al.* (2004)	SU	Targeted (hunted)	108		BC		26 (24,1%)	MX	5 areas SW Spain
Parra *et al.* (2005)	CS	Scanning (hunted)	59	MI	BC		59	FE	1 region W Spain
de Mendoza *et al.* (2006)	CS	Scanning (hunted)	36.144	MI	BC	1992-2004 increasing	394 (1,09%)	MX	1 area W Spain
Parra *et al.* (2006)	CS	Scanning (hunted)	50.009	MI	BC	1997-2002 increasing	591 (1,18%)	MX	1 region W Spain
Vicente *et al.* (2006a)	CS	Targeted (hunted)	1.368		GP BC (not all)	1999-2004	(13,71% mean rate)	MX	21 areas SW Spain
Vicente *et al.* (2006b)	CS	Targeted (hunted)	574		GP BC (not all)	1999-2004	(0-44,0%)	FE	19 areas SW Spain
Gortázar *et al.* (2008)	CS	Targeted (culled)	95		BC	2006-2007	26 (27,4%)	FR	1 area SW Spain
Romero *et al.* (2008)	SU	Targeted (culled)	168		BC	1998-2003	26 (15,5%)	FR	1 area SW Spain
Castillo *et al.* (2010)	CS	Scanning (hunted)	551	MI	BC	2007-2009	28 (5,1%)	MX	2 areas SW Spain
Cunha *et al.* (2011)	SU	Scanning (hunted)	544 samples with lesion	MI	BC	2002-2010	(51%)	MX	Several areas across Portugal
Gortázar *et al.* (2011a)	CS	Targeted (culled)	95		BC	2006-2007	24 (25,3%)	FR	1 study area SW Spain
Pinto *et al.* (2011)	CS	Targeted (hunted)	339	GP	BC	2008-2009	35 (10,3%)	MX	1 area Central Portugal

Table 2. Studies dealing with red deer included in the analysis. Classification: SU – survey; CS - cross sectional study; CC – case-control study; Screening/diagnostic test: MI – official meat inspection scheme; GP – gross pathology; BC – bacteriological culture; SE – serology; Fencing: FR – free-ranging populations; FE – fenced populations; MX – mixed free-ranging and fenced populations.

Reference	Type	Sampling strategy	Sample n	Diagnostic test	Time frame	Prevalence (rate)	Fencing	Study areas
Briones *et al.* (2000)	CR		1 Iberian lynx	BC		1	FR	1 - SW Spain
Pérez *et al.* (2001)	CR		1 Iberian lynx	BC		1	FR	1 - SW Spain
Aranaz *et al.* (2004)	SU	Targeted (hunted)	89 fallow deer	BC		60 fallow deer (67,4%)	MX	2 area SW Spain
		Scanning (carcasses)	4 Iberian lynx			3 Iberian lynx		
Atance *et al.* (2005)	SU	Scanning (carcasses)	7 red fox 2 mongoose 2 genets 1 Iberian lynx 4 mustelids	BC		1 red fox	FR	1 area SW Spain
Atance *et al.* (2006)	SU	Targeted (trapped)	118 red fox 5 mongoose 4 genets 39 Iberian lynx 32 mustelids	SE (ELISA MPB70)		5 red fox (4%) 1 Iberian lynx (3%) 7 badger (23%)	FR	1 area SW Spain
Gortázar *et al.* (2008)	CS	Targeted (culled)	97 fallow deer	BC	2006-2007	18 (18,5%)	FR	1 area SW Spain
Millán *et al.* (2008)	CR		1 red fox	BC		1	FR	1 area SW Spain
Romero *et al.* (2008)	SU	Targeted (culled)	134 fallow deer	BC	1998-2003	17 (12,7%)	FR	1 area SW Spain
		Scanning (carcasses)	10 Iberian lynx			4 (40%)		
			5 red fox			2 (40%)		
Sobrino *et al.* (2008)	CR		1 badger	BC		1	FR	1 area SW Spain
Candela *et al.* (2009)	CS	Targeted (hunted)	61 Barbary sheep	SE (icELISA MPB70)	1999	(50%)	FR	1 area SE Spain
Millán *et al.* (2009)	SU	Targeted (trapped) Scanning (carcasses)	26 Iberian lynx 33 red fox 24 mongoose 10 gennet 2 badger	BC PCR SE (cELISA MPB70)	2004-2006	SE: 1 red fox 1 mongoose 2 badger BC: 2 red fox 2 Iberian lynx	FR	2 area SW Spain
Balseiro *et al.* (2009)	CR		1 roe deer	PCR IHC		1	FR	1 area N Spain
Gortázar *et al.* (2011a)	CS	Targeted (culled)	100 fallow deer	BC	2006-2007	21 (21%)	FR	1 area SW Spain
Balseiro *et al.* (2011)	SU	Targeted (trapped) Passive (carcasses)	157 badger (121 found dead, 36 trapped)	BC	2006-2010	8 found dead (6,6%) 0 trapped	FR	Several areas across Spain

Table 3. Studies dealing with other host species included in the analysis. Classification: SU - survey; CS - cross sectional study; CC - case-control study; Screening/diagnostic test: MI - official meat inspection scheme; GP - gross pathology; BC - bacteriological culture; SE - serology; IHC - immunohistochemistry; ELISA - enzyme-linked immune serum assay; Fencing: FR - free-ranging populations; FE - fenced populations; MX - mixed free-ranging and fenced populations.

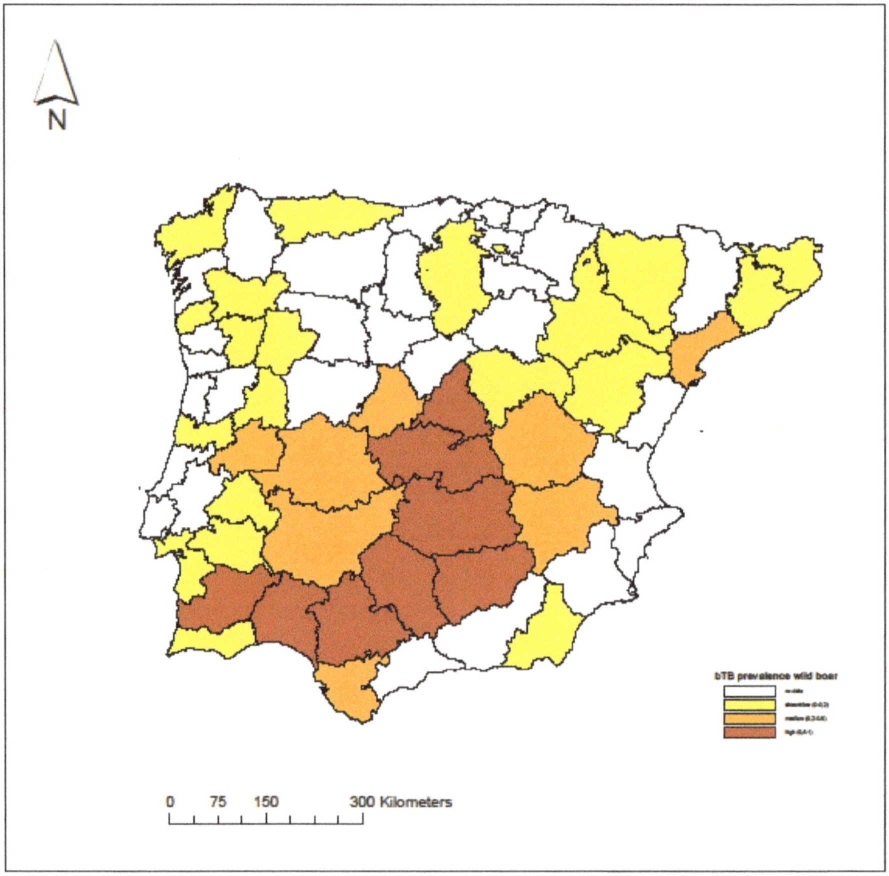

Fig. 1. Map displaying reported prevalence rates for bTB in the wild boar by administrative divisions of Iberian Peninsula (provinces in Spain, districts in Portugal). Bacteriological culture data (Aranaz *et al.*, 2004; de Mendoza *et al.*, 2006; Vicente *et al.*, 2006a; Gortázar *et al.*, 2008; Santos *et al.*, 2009; Pinto *et al.*, 2011) and serology data (Boadella *et al.*, 2011; Santos *et al.*, unpublished data) combined. The highest recorded prevalence for each administrative division is shown.

Again, few published articles address or allow addressing the geographical trend in bTB prevalence rates. In South-central Spain, an area roughly corresponding to Sierra Morena and Montes de Toledo was shown to have high prevalence rates, which declined towards the periphery of the area (Vicente *et al.*, 2006a). In Doñana, wild boar and red deer show an increasing South-North gradient in prevalence rates (Gortázar *et al.*, 2008). In Portugal, bTB was not detected in western regions, while present in the eastern portion of the country (Santos *et al.*, 2009). Also in Eastern-central Portugal, wild boar and red deer populations show an increasing North-South gradient in prevalence rates (Pinto *et al.*, 2011). In South-central Spain, lack of geographical autocorrelation in prevalence rates was reported (Vicente *et al.*, 2006b).

3.4 Determinant factors of disease

Several risk and protective factors for bTB in both wild boar and red deer have been identified (Table 4). Most of the identified risk factors relate to host and other sympatric host's population factors, but also to environmental, management and historical factors. On the other hand, protective factors are mainly associated with environmental variables (Table 4). Notably, only one study has identified fencing, feeding and watering of wild ungulate populations as risk factors.

Determinants of disease		Wild boar	Red deer
	Type of risk factor		
Risk factors	Host population	Reproductive season Age Sex bTB prevalence rate in sympatric wild boar Wild boar abundance	Reproductive season Age Sex bTB prevalence rate in sympatric red deer
	Other hosts	Red deer presence Red deer abundance bTb prevalence rate in sympatric red deer	bTb prevalence rate in sympatric wild boar
	Environmental	Agro forestry land cover	
	Management	Aggregation at watering sites	Aggregation of wild boar at watering and feeding sites Fencing Supplementary feeding Presence water ponds Presence of livestock
	Historical	Past cattle density Distance to historical refuges	Past cattle density
Protective factors	All	Shrub land cover Distance to freshwater Sparse forestry land cover Genetic variability	Distance to freshwater

Table 4. Determinant factors of bTB occurrence identified in wild boar and red deer epidemiological studies in the Iberian Peninsula.

3.5 Host epidemiological status

Wild boar and red deer are usually considered maintenance hosts in Iberian Peninsula and epidemiological evidence has been gathered to support this view (Table 5) based on the characterization of populations maintaining high bTB prevalence rates despite long-term lack of contacts with cattle. Fallow deer, Barbary sheep and badger are also discussed as possible maintenance hosts, while all other reported hosts are considered spillover. Wild boar, red and fallow deer have been suggested as possible reservoirs of infection for livestock.

3.6 Molecular epidemiology

The most commonly identified causative agent of bTB in Iberian Peninsula has been *M. bovis*, although a small proportion (0,05, n=829) of *Mycobacterium caprae* was reported in 6/15 studies. *M. caprae* is much more frequent among isolates from wild boar (0,08, n=502) than from red deer (0,01, n=327). *Mycobacterium avium*-complex mycobacteria and other mycobacteria have also been isolated from wild hosts, but they fall out of the scope of the present review. Molecular epidemiology studies rely mostly on spoligotyping (14/15), usually coupled with MIRU-VNTR typing (9/15) (Table 6).

4. Discussion

4.1 Characterization of published articles

Most epidemiological studies on wild boar or red deer are cross-sectional, allowing for the estimation of prevalence rates and simultaneously the identification of risk or protective factors. A few of the earliest studies were surveys; also classified as such were some molecular epidemiology articles that allow calculating prevalence rates. As knowledge of bTB on other species is more recent, a larger proportion of these studies are case reports and surveys. A comparatively large number of studies address molecular epidemiology.

Notably absent from the literature are case-control studies, which could shed light on the importance of specific determinants of disease, such as fencing and provision of feed and water. The same should be mentioned for experimental studies, were exposure to a certain determinant of disease is manipulated and the effect on disease occurrence is then measured. This design could be of great help to ascertain the role of each species in the persistence of bTB, trough manipulation of host density. The same can be said for epidemiological modelling, which could provide a theoretical framework for understanding bTB persistence in Iberian Peninsula and test the effect of different control measures (Thrushfield *et al.*, 1995) and also to identify key data on host populations and wildlife tuberculosis that is missing or that is not feasible or up to date.

Most articles resort to targeted surveillance of hunted or culled animals, which allows prevalence estimation. Culling is expected to be less sex and age-biased than recreational hunting, which focuses on specific age (adults) and sex (males) classes. The hunting method used for harvesting the animals (drive hunts) is less selective than trophy hunting, allowing access also to females and juvenile/subadult animals (Fernández-Llario & Mateos-Quesada, 2003; Martínez *et al.*, 2005). Hunted animals are usually considered a representative sample of the population for health monitoring, at least for non neurological or debilitating diseases (Conner *et al.*, 2000). Nevertheless it should be kept in mind that some sampling biases can be present (Wilson *et al.*, 2001).

Taxonomic Order	Species	Diagnostic technique	Mycobacterial species	Meta prevalence	Epidemiological status	References
Artiodactyla	Wild boar *Sus scrofa*	Bacteriology culture other	*M. bovis* *M. caprae*	276/771 (35,8%)	Maintenance host Reservoir?	Aranaz *et al.* (2004) Acevedo-Whitehouse *et al.* (2005) Gortázar *et al.* (2008) Romero *et al.* (2008) Santos *et al.* (2009) Pinto *et al.* (2011) others
	Red deer *Cervus elaphus*	Bacteriology culture other	*M. bovis* *M. caprae*	78/371 (21,0%)	Maintenance host Reservoir?	Aranaz *et al.* (2004) Gortázar *et al.* (2008) Romero *et al.* (2008) Pinto *et al.* (2011) others
	Fallow deer *Dama dama*	Bacteriology culture other	*M. bovis*	116/420 (27,6%)	Maintenance host? Spillover host? Reservoir host?	Aranaz *et al.* (2004) Gortázar *et al.* (2008, 2011) Romero *et al.* (2008) others
	Chamois *Rupicapra pyrenaica*	Bacteriology culture	*M. bovis*		Spillover host	Rodríguez *et al.* (2010)
	Mouflon *Ovis orientalis*	Bacteriology culture	*M. bovis*		Spillover host	Rodríguez *et al.* (2010)
	Barbary sheep *Ammotragus lervia*	Bacteriology culture other	*M. bovis*		Spillover host? Maintenance host?	Candela *et al.* (2009) Rodríguez *et al.* (2010)
	Roe deer *Capreolus capreolus*	IHC PCR	*M. bovis*		Spillover host	Balseiro *et al.* (2009)
Carnivora	Iberian lynx *Lynx pardina*	Bacteriology culture other	*M. bovis*	9/40	Spillover host	Briones *et al.* (2000) Pérez *et al.* (2001) Aranaz *et al.* (2004) Atance *et al.* (2006) Romero *et al.* (2008) Millán *et al.* (2009) Rodríguez *et al.* (2010)
	Red fox *Vulpes vulpes*	Bacteriology culture other	*M. bovis* *M. caprae*	5/45	Spillover host	Atance *et al.* (2005, 2006) Millán *et al.* (2008, 2009) Romero *et al.* (2008) Rodríguez *et al.* (2010)
	Badger *Meles meles*	Bacteriology culture other	*M. bovis*	8/121	Maintenance host	Atance *et al.* (2006) Sobrino *et al.* (2008) Rodríguez *et al.* (2010) Balseiro *et al.* (2011)

Table 5. Bovine tuberculosis host species described in the Iberian Peninsula. For references and meta prevalence rate calculations for wild boar, red and fallow deer only targeted-design studies using bacteriological culture as diagnostic test on all animals samples are used. Meta prevalence in carnivores is exclusively based on passive-design studies.

Reference	Sample n (Isolates)	Technique	Time frame	Genotypes n	Host clustering	Study areas
Aranaz *et al*. (1996)	4 wild boar 2 red deer (129 cattle, 44 goat, 1 sheep, 2 cat)	SP		24 spoligotypes (2 clusters)	Sheep/goat isolates clustered apart from other species	
Parra *et al*. (2003)	37 wild boar (25 Iberian pig)	SP MV	1998-2001	8 spoligotypes 43 combined (14 clusters, 21 unique profiles)	4 Iberian pig-only clusters 7 wild boar-only clusters 2 common clusters (14 genotypes)	1 area W Spain
Aranaz *et al*. (2004)	33 red deer 62 fallow deer 58 wild boar 3 Iberian lynx (50 cattle)	SP	1996-2002	21 spoligotypes	17 genotypes in wild boar (4 exclusive) 8 genotypes red deer (none exclusive) 6 fallow deer (1 exclusive) 10 cattle (3 exclusive)	7 areas SW Spain
Gortázar *et al*. (2005)	58 wild boar 19 red deer	SP MV	1999-2002	11 spoligotypes 19 combined	10 spoligotypes wild boar (5 exclusive) 6 spoligotypes red deer (1 exclusive)	24 areas SW Spain
Parra *et al*. (2005)	112 wild boar 59 red deer (6 cattle, 28 Iberian pig, 2 goat)	SP MV	1998-2003	14 spoligotypes 131 combined (28 clusters, 76 unique profiles)	22 clusters wild boar (8 exclusive) 13 clusters red deer (3 exclusive) 7 clusters pig (2 exclusive) 3 clusters cattle (1 exclusive) 1 cluster goat	1 area W Spain
de Mendoza *et al*. (2006)	11 wild boar 8 red deer (5 cattle)	SP MV	1992-2004	(4 clusters, 10 unique profiles)		1 area W Spain
Duarte *et al*. (2008)	21 red deer 6 wild boar (258 cattle, 8 goat)	SP	2002-2007	29 spoligotypes	11 spoligotypes red deer (2 exclusive) 5 spoligotypes wild boar (none exclusive) 27 spoligotypes cattle (15 exclusive)	Portugal
Romero *et al*. (2008)	60 wild boar 26 red deer 17 fallow deer 4 Iberian lynx 2 red fox (54 cattle)	SP MV	1998-2003	9 spoligotypes	3 spoligotypes wild boar (none exclusive) 2 spoligotypes red & fallow deer & red fox (none exclusive) 2 spoligotypes Iberian lynx (1 exclusive) 11 spoligotypes cattle (8 exclusive)	1 area SW Spain
Duarte *et al*. (2009)	13 red deer 4 wild boar (157 cattle, 7 goat)	MV	2002-2007	87 genotypes	12 genotypes red deer (8 exclusive) 4 genotypes wild boar (1 exclusive) 78 genotypes cattle (71 exclusive)	Portugal
Santos *et al*. (2009)	14 wild boar	SP	2005-2006	4 spoligotypes		3 areas Portugal
Rodríguez *et al*. (2010)	204 wild boar 141 red deer 229 fallow deer 2 chamois 1 mouflon 6 Iberian lynx 2 red fox 1 badger	SP	1992-2007	252 spoligotypes	26 spoligotypes wild boar (6 exclusive) 22 spoligotypes red deer (2 exclusive) 13 spoligotypes fallow deer (1 exclusive) 1 spoligotype chamois (none exclusive) 1 spoligotype mouflon (1 exclusive) 3 spoligotypes lynx (none exclusive)	Spain

	(5585 cattle, 33 goat, 7 pig, 3 cat, 1 dog)				2 spoligotypes red fox (none exclusive) 1 spoligotype badger (none exclusive) 239 spoligotypes cattle (207 exclusive) 3 spoligotypes goat (1 exclusive) 2 spoligotypes pig (none exclusive) 3 spoligotypes cat (1 exclusive) 1 spoligotype dog (none exclusive)	
Cunha *et al.* (2012)	74 red deer 36 wild boar	SP MV	2008-2009	27 spoligotypes	21 spoligotypes red deer (11 exclusive) 15 spoligotypes wild boar (5 exclusive) 6 spoligotypes exclusive of wildlife vs 23 spoligotypes exclusive of domestic species	4 regions South-Central Portugal
Gortázar *et al.* (2011)	24 red deer 21 fallow deer 62 wild boar	SP MV	2006-2007	9 spoligotypes 13 genotypes combined	8 genotypes red deer (2 exclusive) 6 genotypes fallow deer (none exclusive) 5 genotypes wild boar (none exclusive)	1 area SW Spain
Pinto *et al.* (2011)	27 red deer 21 wild boar	SP	2008-2009	8 spoligotypes	8 spoligotypes red deer (4 exclusive) 4 spoligotypes wild boar (none exclusive)	1 area Central Portugal
Rodriguez *et al.* (2011)	14 wild boar 1 red deer 1 red fox (542 goat, 229 cattle, 2 sheep, 2 pig)	SP MV	1992-2009	15 spoligotypes	4 spoligotypes wild boar (none exclusive) 1 spoligotype red (none exclusive) 1 spoligotype red fox (none exclusive) 12 spoligotypes goat (6 exclusive) 9 spoligotypes cattle (2 exclusive) 2 spoligotypes sheep, pig (none)	Spain

Table 6. Molecular biology studies included in the analysis. SP: spoligotyping, MV: MIRU-VNTR mycobacterial interspersed repetitive units-variable number of tandem repeats.

On the other hand, studies of wild ungulates relying on routine meat inspection for detection of macroscopic tuberculosis-like lesions, do not allow for a reliable estimation of prevalence, which is underestimated in this situation (de Mendonza *et al.*, 2006). Nevertheless this type of design allows increasing sample size, which makes them suited for long-term surveillance rather than detailed epidemiological studies (de Mendonza *et al.*, 2006) and were mostly used in the first surveys and cross-sectional studies after bTB was detected in wildlife in Iberian Peninsula. The investigations on carnivore species, most of which are not hunted, tend to rely on passive surveillance schemes based on haphazardly found carcasses. This sampling design does not allow to estimate prevalence rates due to extensive sampling bias (e.g. Taylor *et al.*, 2002). Targeted sampling in these species has been attempted using serological tests but results should be interpreted with caution since these techniques have not yet been validated in these species.

The number of animals studied is usually adequate to determine prevalence rates with relatively small confidence intervals, at least in the easily available hunted species. The same cannot be said for most studies on protected carnivore species, where the collection of biological samples from a large number of animals is inherently difficult.

Bacteriological culture is the reference test for diagnosing bTB although it is expensive and time-consuming (de Lisle *et al.*, 2002). As the financial resources needed to perform bacteriological culture on a large number of samples are scarcely available, most surveys use other methods (usually gross pathology) as screening tests and only perform bacteriological culture for lesion-positive animals, sometimes as pooled samples. This introduces a bias and it was shown that the sensitivity of gross pathology was 72,2% of that obtained from bacteriology in the wild boar (Santos *et al.*, 2010). The same trend has been reported elsewhere for deer (Rohonczy *et al.*, 1996; O'Brien *et al.*, 2004).

4.2 Prevalence rates

Overall prevalence rates reported for bTB in wild boar, red deer and fallow deer in Iberian Peninsula are among the highest recorded for these species worldwide (Corner, 2006; Nishi *et al.*; 2006, Wilson *et al.*, 2008). Interestingly, prevalence rates in wild boar are invariably higher than in sympatric red or fallow deer (Gortázar *et al.*, in press).

Most studies report no sex differences in infection rates, but Santos *et al.* (2009) reported a significantly higher infection rate in female wild boar, presumably linked to more frequent social behaviour of females compared to males. Several studies report age differences in infection rates in wild boar, but data is conflicting since some authors reported increasing prevalence rates with age (e.g. Vicente *et al.*, 2006a,b), while others found higher prevalence rate in juveniles (e.g. Gortázar *et al.*, 2008; Santos *et al.*, 2009). Age and sex differences in prevalence rates were also reported in red deer (Vicente *et al.*, 2006a), which were higher for males and increased with age. This gender difference was already reported for cervids in North America (O'Brien *et al.*, 2006).

4.3 Trends

The few published data about the temporal dynamics of bTB prevalence rates are unanimous in showing an increasing trend across Iberian Peninsula in both wild boar and red deer (de Mendonza *et al.*, 2006; Gortázar *et al.*, 2008, 2011b, in press; Santos *et al.*, 2009, unpublished data). Gortázar *et al.*, (2011b) recently reported that 11/14 wild ungulate populations from central Spain show increasing bTB prevalence rates as assessed by gross pathology. This strongly supports previous interpretations that bTB is an emerging disease in wildlife in Iberian Peninsula.

The highest prevalence rates for bTB reported in wild ungulates in Iberian Peninsula lie in the central-south-western mountain chains of Montes de Toledo-Sierra Morena-Contenda (e.g. Vicente *et al.*, 2006a; Santos *et al.*, 2009) and Doñana (Gortázar *et al.*, 2008). Prevalence rates decline to the periphery of this region; the detected limits of this bTB core area are the provinces of Cáceres/Ávila to the north, eastern Portugal to the West, the Mediterranean coast to the South and Teruel to the East. bTB has not been detected or only sporadically in the northern, western and eastern periphery of Iberian Peninsula, despite locally intense surveillance (Gortázar *et al.*, 2011b). This pattern, coupled with the abovementioned increase in prevalence over time, strongly suggests that the disease is expanding from the central core area.

Interestingly, this core region of high bTB prevalence rates coincides with the main historical refuge of the wild boar in Spain (Tellería & Saez-Royuela, 1985) and, to some extent, in Portugal (Lopes & Borges, 2004). In the beginning of the XXth century, Iberian populations of wild ungulates were at their lowest level due to intense direct persecution and were largely restricted to a few mountain regions. Starting in 1960's, wild boar populations expanded from these refuges (Tellería & Saez-Royuela, 1985; Acevedo *et al.*, 2011) to a point they nowadays occupy almost all Iberian Peninsula (Rosell, 2001). Natural expansion of red deer also occurred but not to such a great extent as in the wild boar case and was much dependent upon translocations (Soriguer, 1998; Acevedo *et al.*, 2011).

As suggested by Santos *et al.* (2009) for Portugal, wildlife bTB could be similarly expanding from the historical refuges with a lag comparative to its host's expansion. This lag could be explained by the threshold theory for disease persistence, as reported for other bTB hosts such as the possum *Trichosurus vulpecula* in New Zealand - Lloyd-Smith *et al.*, 2005). As wild ungulate populations expanded, densities at the front of the expansion wave were too low (Holland *et al.*, 2007) to allow for the persistence of bTB, even if presumably some infected hosts were involved in that expansion event. As a consequence, wildlife bTB initially remained confined to the historical refuges, despite dispersion of infected hosts. As ungulate distribution continued to expand, densities increased in a gradient centred at the historical refuges and eventually reached the threshold level. At that point, bTB, introduced by infected immigrants from the historical refuges, could persist and spread its distribution, a process seemingly still taking place.

This hypothesis could be tested by comprehensive geographical spatial analysis of the distribution of bTB in Iberian Peninsula, but the proposed natural expansion pattern has probably been much obscured by translocation and intensive management of ungulates for hunting purposes (Vargas *et al.* 1995; Miguel *et al.* 1999; Castillo *et al.*, 2010). In fact, in South-central Spain lack of geographical autocorrelation in prevalence rates was suggested to be due to extensive fencing of intensively-managed big game hunting estates, which impair animal movements (Vicente *et al.*, 2006b). On the other hand, wild ungulate translocations for hunting purposes occur frequently and may spread *M. bovis* to areas where it is absent today. Interestingly, *M. bovis* was isolated from wild boar in Portugal in two areas widely out of the known distribution of the disease (Santos *et al.*, 2009; Cunha *et al.*, 2012), one of which coincides with the release site of red deer originating from a population harbouring the same genotype of *M. bovis*. This provides circumstantial evidence for the role of translocations on bTB geographical spread.

More spatial data of bTb occurrence in Iberian Peninsula is urgently needed. The advent of sensitive, specific, reproducible and cheap serologic tests allows such large-scale research to be conducted, at least for wild boar (Boadella *et al.*, 2011). This should improve the understanding of bTB occurrence across Iberian Peninsula.

4.4 Disease determinant factors

Most risk factors for bTB in wild boar and red deer identified in Iberian Peninsula are host population factors, most of them abundance-related. It is interesting to note that in the wild boar-red deer system, the abundance of each species influences bTB occurrence in the other species, further supporting the multi-host pathogen status of bTB in Iberian Peninsula ecosystems.

The number of risk factors related to management is greater for the red deer (n=5) than for the wild boar (n=1). This suggests that bTB occurrence in red deer populations is more dependent on management practices, while wild boar is competent to act as maintenance host under low-intensity management. This hypothesis could be tested by a case-control study of bTB occurrence in both species across a gradient of intensity of management.

Interestingly, among the protective risk factors described for bTB in Doñana, distance to freshwater sources is highlighted. Much remains to be known on the conditions necessary for the survival of mycobacteria in the environment, but humidity seems to favour it (Humblet *et al.*, 2009), particularly in the arid summer conditions of southern Iberian Peninsula. This suggests that environmental contamination with mycobacteria, particularly at watering sites, and indirect routes could play a role in disease transmission among wild ungulate species.

4.5 Host status

Wild boar and red deer are usually referred as maintenance hosts in Iberian Peninsula and evidence is available as populations maintaining high prevalence rates for several years, even decades, in the absence of domestic cattle which could theoretically serve as reservoirs for wildlife (e.g. Vicente *et al.*, 2006a; Gortázar *et al.*, 2008). It seems consensual that high-density sympatric populations of wild boar and red deer can maintain bTB at a high prevalence independent of the existence of other hosts (e.g. de Mendonza *et al.*, 2006; Vicente *et al.*, 2006a; Gortázar *et al.*, in press). This seems also to be independent of intensity of management for hunting purposes, favouring high density of animals through habitat management, feeding and watering (Miguel *et al.*, 1999), as even non-intensively managed but high-density populations of wild boar show high bTB prevalence rates (Santos *et al.*, 2009).

It should be noted that in most of Iberian Peninsula densities far above the natural carrying capacity of wild boar and red deer occur, even in the absence of intensive management, because natural predators of these species (essentially wolf *Canis lupus*) have been eliminated during the last 50 years (Rico & Torrente, 2000). Packer *et al.* (2003) have shown through modelling that removal of predators can lead to an increase on pathogens' prevalence. Furthermore, Barber-Meyer *et al.* (2007) have shown that wolf restoration in Yellowstone had significant impacts on the seroprevalence of several pathogens of deer, even though those populations were previously subject to predation by other species.

It could be hypothesized that the current bTB high prevalence rates in wildlife in Iberian Peninsula derives from severe changes on the ecosystems caused by intensive management for hunting purposes (Gortázar *et al.*, 2006) and eventually also predator eradication (Rico & Torrente, 2000). Experimental studies where host density is manipulated through large-scale culling are absent from the literature and could help to understand the role of artificialization of the ecosystems in the persistence and expansion of bTB. The picture is further complicated by the difficulty in separating the effect of each host species, as they usually occur in sympatry in the core area. Nevertheless, wild boar populations have been reported to show high bTB prevalence rates even in the absence of sympatric deer (Vicente *et al.*, 2006a).

Fallow deer and badger are most likely local maintenance hosts where they occur at high density, notably in scattered populations of fallow deer and in Atlantic Iberian Peninsula for the badger. On the other hand, other carnivore and ungulate species infected in Iberian Peninsula are most likely spillover hosts, with the possible exception of exotic Barbary sheep.

4.6 Molecular epidemiology

Studies reviewed are rather concordant in concluding that genotypes seem to be geographically clustered as each location has a few predominant genotypes, responsible for the majority of the infections. Concurrently, there is also a wide variety of locally rare genotypes. Local genotypes tend to be the same in different sympatric species, both domestic and wild, supporting the local interspecies transmission of *M. bovis*.

5. Conclusion

In summary, published evidence suggests that bTB is a natural pathogen of autochthonous wild ungulates in Iberian Peninsula, where wild boar and red deer act as maintenance hosts. Bovine tuberculosis is an emergent disease in these hosts, the expansion from the core high prevalence area in south-western Iberian Peninsula being fuelled by high densities of these species due to intensive management for hunting purposes. Several other species of ungulates and carnivores are affected by bTB, most probably as spillover hosts, but fallow deer and badger could serve as maintenance host in some locations. Although shown to be an important emerging infection, large gaps remain in the knowledge of the epidemiology of bTB in wildlife, such as intra and inter-species transmission routes, geographical distribution and effectiveness of control methods. Applying different epidemiological study designs, such as case-control and experimental studies, spatial analysis and modelling could shed light on this subject.

6. References

Acevedo, P., Farfán, M., Márquez, A., Delibes-Mateos, M., Real, R. & Vargas, J. (2011) Past, present and future of wild ungulates in relation to changes in land use. *Landscape Ecology*, 26:19–31, ISSN 0921-2973

Acevedo-Whitehouse, K., Vicente, J., Gortázar, C., Höfle, U., Fernández-de-Mera, I. & Amos, W. (2005) Genetic resistance to bovine tuberculosis in the Iberian wild boar. *Molecular Ecology*, 14: 3209–3217, ISSN 0962-1083

Allepuz, A., Casals, J., Nappa, S., Saez, M., Alba, A., Vilar, M., Domingo, M., González, M., DuranFerrer, M., Vicente, J., Álvarez, J., Muñoz, M. & Saez, J. (2011) Analysis of the spatial variation of bovine tuberculosis disease risk in Spain (2006–2009). *Preventive Veterinary Medicine*, 100(1): 44-52, ISSN 0167-5877

Aranaz, A., Liébana, E., Mateos, A., Domínguez, L., Vidal, D., Domingo, M., González, O., Rodriguez-Ferri, E., bunschoten, A., van Embden, J. & Cousins, D. (1996) Spacer oligonucleotide typing of *Mycobacterium bovis* strains from cattle and other animals: a tool for studying epidemiology of tuberculosis. *Journal of Clinical Microbiology*, 34(11): 2734–2740

Aranaz, A., de Juan, L., Montero, N., Sánchez, C., Galka, M., Delso, C., Álvarez, J., Romero, B., Bezos, J., Vela, A., Briones, V., Mateos, A. & Domínguez, L. (2004) Bovine tuberculosis (*Mycobacterium bovis*) in wildlife in Spain. *Journal of Clinical Microbiology*, 42(6): 2602–2608

Artois, M., Delahay, R., Guberti, V. & Cheeseman, C. (2001) Control of infectious diseases of wildlife in Europe. *Veterinary Journal*, 162: 141–152, ISSN 1090-0233

Atance, P., Palomares, F., Candela, M., Revilla, E., Cubero, M., Calzada, J. & Vizcaíno, L. (2005) Bovine tuberculosis in a free ranging red fox (*Vulpes vulpes*) from Doñana National Park (Spain). *Journal of Wildlife Diseases*, 41(2): 435–436, ISSN 0090-3558

Atance, P., Vizcaíno, L., Palomares, F., Revilla, E., Candela, M., Calzada, Cubero-Pablo, J. & Delibes, M. (2006) Antibodies to *Mycobacterium bovis* in Wild Carnivores from

Doñana National Park (Spain). *Journal of Wildlife Diseases*, 42(3): 704–708, ISSN 0090-3558

Balseiro, A., Oleaga, A., Orusa, R., Robetto, S., Domenis, L., Zoppi, S., Dondo, A., Goria, M., Gortázar, C. & Marín, J. (2009) Tuberculosis in roe deer from Spain and Italy. *Veterinary Record*, 164: 468-470, ISSN 0042-4900

Balseiro, A., Rodríguez, O., González-Quirós, P., Merediz, I., Sevilla, I., Davé, D., Dalley, D., Lesellier, D., Chambers, M., Bezos, J., Muñoz, M., Delahay, R., Gortázar, C. & Prieto, J. (2011) Infection of Eurasian badgers (*Meles meles*) with *Mycobacterium bovis* and *Mycobacterium avium* complex in Spain. *Veterinary Journal*, 190(2): 21-25, ISSN 1090-0233

Barber-Meyer, S., Whit, P. & Mech, L. (2007) Survey of Selected Pathogens and Blood Parameters of Northern Yellowstone Elk: Wolf Sanitation Effect Implications. *American Midland Naturalist*, 158: 369–381, ISSN 0003-0031

Boadella, M., Lyashchenko, K., Greenwald, R., Esfandiari, J., Jaroso, R., Carta, T., Garrido, J., Vicente, J., de la Fuente, J. & Gortázar, C. (2011) Serologic tests for detecting antibodies against *Mycobacterium bovis* and *Mycobacterium avium* subspecies *paratuberculosis* in Eurasian wild boar (*Sus scrofa scrofa*). *Journal Veterinary Diagnostic Investigations*, 23: 77-83, ISSN 1040-6387

Boadella, M., Acevedo, P., Vicente, J., Mentaberre, G., Balseiro, A., Arnal, M., Martínez, D., García-Bocanegra, I., Casal, C., Álvarez, J., Oleaga, A., Lavín, S., Muñoz, M., Sáez-Llorente, J., de la Fuente, J. & Gortázar, C. (2011) Spatio-temporal trends of Iberian wild boar contact with *Mycobacterium tuberculosis* complex detected by ELISA. *EcoHealth*, doi: 10.1007/s10393-011-0713-y, ISSN 1612-9210

Briones, V., de Juan, L., Sánchez, C., Vela, A., Galka, M., Montero, N., Goyache, J., Aranaz, A., Mateos, A. & Domínguez, L. (2000) Bovine tuberculosis and the endangered Iberian Lynx. *Emerging Infectious Diseases*, 6(2): 189-191, ISSN 1080-6040

Candela, M., Serrano, E., Martinez-Carrasco, C., Martín-Atance, C., Cubero, M., Alonso, F. & Leon, L. (2009) Coinfection is an important factor in epidemiological studies: the first serosurvey of the aoudad (*Ammotragus lervia*). *European Journal of Clinical Microbiology Infectious Diseases*, 28:481–489, ISSN 0934-9723

Castillo, L., Fernández-Llario, p., Mateos, C., Carranza, J., Benítez-Medina, J., García-Jiménez, W., Bermejo-Martín, F. & de Mendoza, J. (2010) Management practices and their association with *Mycobacterium tuberculosis* complex prevalence in red deer populations in Southwestern Spain. *Preventive Veterinary Medicine*, 98(1): 58-63, ISSN 0167-5877

Clifton-Hadley, R., Sauter-Louis, C., Lugton, I., Jackson, R., Durr, P. & Wilesmith, J. (2001) *Mycobacterium bovis* infections, In: *Infectious diseases of wild mammals*. E. Williams & I. Barker, pp. 340-361, 3rd edition, Manson Publishing/The Veterinary Press, ISBN 9781840760057, London

Conner, M., McCarty, C. & Miller, M. (2000) Detection of bias in harvest-based estimates of Chronic Wasting Disease prevalence in Mule deer. *Journal of Wildlife Diseases*, 36(4): 691-699, ISSN 0090-3558

Corner, L. (2006) The role of wild animal populations in the epidemiology of tuberculosis in domestic animals: how to assess the risk. *Veterinary Microbiology*, 112: 303–312, ISSN 0378-1135

Cunha, M., Monteiro, M., Carvalho, P., Mendonça, P., Albuquerque, T. & Botelho, A. (2011) Multihost tuberculosis: insights from the Portuguese control program. *Veterinary Medicine International*, 2011: doi:10.4061/2011/795165, ISSN 2042-0048

Cunha, M., Matos, F., Canto, A., Albuquerque, T., Alberto, J., Aranha, J., Pinto, M. & Botelho, A. (2012) Implications and challenges of tuberculosis in wildlife ungulates in Portugal: A molecular epidemiology perspective. *Research in Veterinary Science*, 92(2): 225-235, ISSN 0034-5288

Etter, E., Donado, P., Jori, F., Caron, A., Goutard, F. & Roger, F. (2006) Risk analysis and bovine tuberculosis, a re-emerging zoonosis, *Annals New York Academy Sciences*, 1081:61–73, ISSN 0077-8923

Fernández-Llario, P. & Mateos-Quesada, P. (2003) Population structure of the wild boar (*Sus scrofa*) in two Mediterranean habitats in the western Iberian Peninsula. *Folia Zoologica*, 52(2): 143–148, ISSN 1573-1189

Gordejo, F. & Vermeersch, J. (2006) Towards eradication of bovine tuberculosis in the European Union. *Veterinary Microbiology*, 112: 101–109, ISSN 0378-1135

Gortázar, C., Acevedo, P., Ruiz-Fons, F. & Vicente, J. (2006) Disease risks and overabundance of game species. *European Journal Wildlife Research*, 52: 81–87, ISSN 1439-0574

Gortázar, C., Torres, M., Vicente, J., Acevedo, P., Reglero, M., de la Fuente, J., Negro, J. & Aznar-Martín, J. (2008) Bovine tuberculosis in Doñana Biosphere Reserve: the role of wild ungulates as disease reservoirs in the last Iberian Lynx strongholds. *PLoS ONE*, 3(7): e2776. doi:10.1371/journal.pone.0002776, ISSN 1932-6203

Gortázar, C., Torres, M., Acevedo, P., Aznar, J., Negro, J., de la Fuente, J. & Vicente, J. (2011a) Fine-tuning the space, time, and host distribution of mycobacteria in wildlife. *BMC Microbiology*, 2011, 11:27, ISSN 1471-2180

Gortázar, C., Vicente, J., Boadella, M., Ballesteros, C., Galindo, R., Garrido, J., Aranaz, A. & de la Fuente, J. (2011b) Progress in the control of bovine tuberculosis in Spanish wildlife. *Veterinary Microbiology*, 151(1-2): 170-178, ISSN 0378-1135

Gortázar, C., Delahay, R., McDonal, R., Boadella, M., Gavier-Widen, D., Acevedo, P. (in press) The status of tuberculosis in European wild mammals. *Mammal Review*, ISSN 1365-2907

Holland, E., Aegerter, J. & Smith, G. (2007) Spatial sensitivity of a generic population model, using wild boar (*Sus scrofa*) as a test case. *Ecological Modelling*, 205: 146–158, ISSN 0304-3800

Horan, R., Wolf, C., Fenichel, E. & Mathews, K. (2008) Joint management of wildlife and livestock disease. *Environmental & Resources Economics*, 41:47–70 doi: 10.1007/s10640-007-9180-x, ISSN 1573-1502

Humblet, M., Boschiroli, M. & Saegerman, C. (2009) Classification of worldwide bovine tuberculosis risk factors in cattle: a stratified approach. *Veterinary Research*, 40:50 doi: 10.1051/vetres/20090 , ISSN 0928-4249

de Lisle, G., Bengis, R., Schmitt, S. & O'Brien, D. (2002) Tuberculosis in free-ranging wildlife: detection, diagnosis and management. *Revue Scientific et Technique Office International des Epizooties*, 21: 317–334, ISSN 0253-1933

Lloyd-smith, J., Cross, P., Briggs, C., Daugherty, M., Getz, W., Latto, J., Sanchez, M., Smith, A. & Swei, A. (2005) Should we expect population thresholds for wildlife disease? *Trends in Ecology and Evolution*, 20: 511–520, ISSN 0169-5347

Lopes, F. & Borges, J. (2004) Wild boar in Portugal. *Galemys*, 16: 243–251, ISSN 1137-8700

Lyashchenko, K., Greenwald, R., Esfandiari, J., Chambers, A., Vicente, J., Gortazar, C., Santos, N., Correia-Neves, M., Buddle, B., Jackson, R., O'Brien, D., Schmitt, S., Palmer, M., Delahay, R. & Waters, R. (2008) Animal-side serologic assay for rapid detection of *Mycobacterium bovis* infection in multiple species of free-ranging wildlife. *Veterinary Microbiology*, 132: 283-292, ISSN 0378-1135

Martínez, M., Rodríguez-Vigal, C., Jones, O., Coulson, T. & San Miguel, A. (2005) Different hunting strategies select for different weights in red deer. *Biology Letters*, 1: 353–356, ISSN 1744-9561

Matos, F., Cunha, M., Canto, A., Albuquerque, T., Amado, A. & Botelho, A. (2010) Snapshot of *Mycobacterium bovis* and *Mycobacterium caprae* infections in livestock in a bovine tuberculosis low incidence scenario. *Journal of Clinical Microbiology*, 48: 4337–4339, ISSN 0095-1137

de Mendoza, J., Parra, A., Tato, A., Alonso, J., Rey, J., Peña, J., García-Sánchez, A., Larrasa, J., Teixidó, J., Manzano, G., Cerrato, R., Pereira, G., Fernández-Llario, P. & de Mendoza, M. (2006) Bovine tuberculosis in wild boar (*Sus scrofa*), red deer (*Cervus elaphus*) and cattle (*Bos taurus*) in a Mediterranean ecosystem (1992–2004). *Preventive Veterinary Medicine*, 74: 239–247, ISSN 0167-5877

Miguel, A., Pérez-Carral, C. & Roig, S. (1999) Deer and traditional agrosilvopastoral systems of Mediterranean Spain. A new problem of sustainability for a new concept of land use. *Options Méditerranéennes*, 39: 261-264, ISSN 1016-1228.

Millán, J., Jiménez, M., Viota, M., Candela, M., Peña, L. & Vizcaíno, L. (2008) Disseminated bovine tuberculosis in a wild red fox (*Vulpes vulpes*) in Southern Spain. *Journal of Wildlife Diseases*, 44(3): 701–706, ISSN 0090-3558

Millán, J., Candela, M., Palomares, F., Cubero, M., Rodríguez, A., Barral, M., de la Fuente, J., Almería, S. & Vizcaíno, L. (2009) Disease threats to the endangered Iberian lynx (*Lynx pardinus*). *Veterinary Journal*, 182: 114–124, ISSN 1090-0233

Nishi, J., Shury, T. &, Elkin, B. (2006) Wildlife reservoirs for bovine tuberculosis (*Mycobacterium bovis*) in Canada: strategies for management and research. *Veterinary Microbiology*, 112: 325–338, ISSN 0378-1135

O'Brien, D., Schmitt, S., Berry, D., Fitzgerald, S., Vanneste, J., Lyon, T., Magsig, D., Fierke, J., Cooley, T., Zwick, L. & Thomsen, B. (2004) Estimating the true prevalence of *Mycobacterium bovis* in hunter-harvested white-tailed deer in Michigan. *Journal of Wildlife Diseases*, 40(1): 42–52, ISSN 0090-3558

O'Brien, D., Fitzgerald, S., Berry, D. & Hickling, G. (2006) Managing the wildlife reservoir of *Mycobacterium bovis*: the Michigan, USA, experience. *Veterinary Microbiology*, 112: 313- 323, ISSN 0378-1135

Packer, C., Holt, R., Hudson, P., Lafferty, K. & Dobson, A. (2003) Keeping the herds healthy and alert: implications of predator control for infectious disease. *Ecology Letters*, 6: 797–802, ISSN 1461-023X

Parra, A., Larrasa, J., García, A., Alonso, J. & de Mendoza, J. (2005) Molecular epidemiology of bovine tuberculosis in wild animals in Spain: A first approach to risk factor analysis. *Veterinary Microbiology*, 110 (3-4): 293-300, ISSN 0378-1135

Parra, A., Inglis, N., Tato, A., Alonso, J., de Mendoza, M., de Mendoza, J. & Larrasa, J. (2006) An epidemiological evaluation of *Mycobacterium bovis* infections in wild game animals of the Spanish Mediterranean ecosystem. *Research in Veterinary Science*, 80: 140–146, ISSN 0034-5288

Pérez, J., Calzada, J., Vizcaíno, L., Cubero, M., Velarde, J. & Mozos, E. (2001) Tuberculosis in an Iberian lynx (*Lynx pardina*). *Veterinary Record*, 148: 414-415, ISSN 0042-4900

Pinto, M., Alberto, J., Aranha, J., Serejo, J., Canto, A., Cunha, M. & Botelho, A. (2011) Combined evaluation of bovine tuberculosis in wild boar (*Sus scrofa*) and red deer (*Cervus elaphus*) from Central-East Portugal. *European Journal of Wildlife Research*, doi 10.1007/s10344-011-0532-z, ISSN 1612-4642

Renwick, A., White, P. & Bengis, R. (2007) Bovine tuberculosis in southern African wildlife : a multi-species host-pathogen system. *Epidemiology and Infection*, 135: 529-540, ISSN 0950-2688

Rico, M. & Torrente, J. (2000) Caza y rarificación del lobo en españa: investigación histórica y conclusiones biológicas. *Galemys*, 12:163-179, ISSN 1137-8700

Rodríguez, S., Romero, B., Bezos, J., de Juan, L., Álvarez, J., Castellanos, E., Moya, N., Lozano, F., González, S., Sáez-Llorente, J., Mateos, A., Domínguez, L., Aranaz, A. (2010) High spoligotype diversity within a *Mycobacterium bovis* population: clues to understanding the demography of the pathogen in Europe. *Veterinary Microbiology*, 141: 89-95, ISSN 0378-1135

Rodríguez, S., Bezos, J., Romero, B., de Juan, L., Álvarez, J., Castellanos, E., Moya, N., Lozano, F., Javed, M., Sáez-Llorente, J., Liébana, E., Mateos, A., Domínguez, L., Aranaz, A. (2011) *Mycobacterium caprae* infection in livestock and wildlife, Spain. Emerging Infectious Diseases, 17(3): 532-535, ISSN 1080-6059

Rohonczy, E., Balachandran, A., Dukes, T., Payeur, J., Rhyan, J., Saari, D., Whiting, T., Wilson, S. & Jarnagin, J. (1996) A comparison of gross pathology, histopathology, and mycobacterial culture for the diagnosis of tuberculosis in elk (*Cervus elaphus*). *Canadian Journal of Veterinary Research*, 60: 108–114, ISSN 0830-9000

Romero, B., Aranaz, A., Sandoval, A., Álvarez, J., de Juan, L., Bezos, J., Sánchez, C., Galka, M., Fernández, P., Mateos, A. & Domínguez, L. (2008) Persistence and molecular evolution of *Mycobacterium bovis* population from cattle and wildlife in Doñana National Park revealed by genotype variation. *Veterinary Microbiology*, 132: 87–95, ISSN 0378-1135

Rosell, C., Fernández-Llario, P. & Herrero, J. (2001) El jabalí (*Sus scrofa* Linnaeus, 1758). *Galemys*, 13(2): 1-25, ISSN 1137-8700

Santos, N., Correia-Neves, M., Ghebremichael, S., Källenius, G., Svenson, S. & Almeida, V. (2009) Epidemiology of *Mycobacterium bovis* infection in wild boar *Sus scrofa* from Portugal. *Journal of Wildlife Diseases*, 45(4): 1048-1061, ISSN 0090-3558

Santos, N., Geraldes, M., Afonso, A., Almeida, V. & Correia-Neves, M. (2010) Diagnosis of tuberculosis in the wild boar (*Sus scrofa*): a comparison of methods applicable to hunter-harvested animals. *PLoS-ONE*, 5(9): e12663, ISSN 1932-6203

Schiller, I., Oesch, B., Vordermeier, M., Palmer, M., Harris, B., Orloski, K., Buddle, B., Thacker, T., Lyashchenko, K. & Waters, W. (2010) Bovine tuberculosis: a review of current and emerging diagnostic techniques in view of their relevance for disease control and eradication. *Transboundary and Emerging Diseases* doi:10.1111/j.1865-1682.2010.01148.x, ISSN 1865-1674

Sobrino, R., Martín-Hernando, M., Vicente, J., Aurtenetxe, O., Garrido, J. & Gortázar, C. (2008) Bovine tuberculosis in a badger (*Meles meles*) from Spain. *Veterinary Record*, 163(5): 159-160, ISSN 0042-4900

Soriguer, R., Márquez, F. & Pérez, J. (1998) Las translocaciones (introducciones y reintroducciones) de espécies cinegéticas y sus effectos medioambientales. *Galemys*, 10(2): 19-35, ISSN 1137-8700

Steele, J. (1995) Regional and Country Status Report, In: *Mycobacterium bovis infection in animals and humans*, Thoen, C.O. & J.H. Steele, pp. 169–172, Iowa Press, ISBN 9780470344538, Ames

Swinton, J., Woolhouse, M., Begon, M., Dobson, A., Ferroglio, E., Grenfell, B., Guberti, V., Hails, R., Heesterbeek, J., Lavazza, A., Roberts, M., White, P. & Wilson, K. (2001) Microparasite transmission and persistence, In: *The Ecology of Wildlife Diseases*, P. Hudson, A. Rizzoli, B. Grenfell, H. Heesterbeek, A. Dobson, pp. 83-101, Oxford University Press, ISBN 0198506198, Oxford

Taylor, S., Buergelt, C., Roelke-Parker, M., Homer, B. & Rotstein, D. (2002) Causes of mortality of free-ranging Florida panthers. *Journal of Wildlife Diseases*, 38(1): 107-114, ISSN 0090-3558

Tellería, J. & Saez-Royuela, Y. (1985) L'évolution démographique du sanglier (*Sus scrofa*) en Espagne. *Mammalia* 49: 195–202, ISSN 0025-1461

Thrushfield, M. (1995) *Veterinary epidemiology*. 2nd edition, Blackwell Science, ISBN 0632048514, Oxford

Tompkins, D., Dobson, A., Arneberg, P., Begon, M., Cattadori, I., Greenman, J., Heesterbeek, J., Hudson, P., Newborn, D., Pugliese, A., Rizzoli, A., Rosa, R., Rosso, F. & Wilson, K. (2001) Parasites and host population dynamics, In: *The Ecology of Wildlife Disease,*. P. Hudson, A. Rizzoli, B. Grenfell, H. Heesterbeek, A. Dobson, pp. 45-62, Oxford University Press, ISBN 0198506198, Oxford

Vargas, J. Calvo, J. & Aparicio, M, (1995) Red deer *(Cervus elaphus hispanicus)* management in the dehesa system in Central Extremadura, Spain. *Agroforestry Systems*, 29: 77-89, ISSN 0167-4366.

Vicente, J., Höfle, U., Garrido, J., Fernández-de-Mera, I., Juste, R., Barral, M. & Gortazar, C. (2006a) Wild boar and red deer display high prevalences of tuberculosis-like lesions in Spain. *Veterinary Research*, 37: 107–119, ISSN 0928-4249

Vicente, J., Höfle, U., Garrido, J., Fernández-de-Mera, I., acevedo, P., Juste, R., Barral, M. & Gortazar, C. (2006b) Risk factors associated with the prevalence of tuberculosis-like lesions in fenced wild boar and red deer in south central Spain. *Veterinary Research*, 38: 1-15, ISSN 0928-4249

Whiting, T. (2003) Foreign animal disease outbreaks, the animal welfare implications for Canada: risks apparent from international experience. *Canadian Veterinary Journal*: 44: 805–815, ISSN 0008-5286

Wilkins, M., Meyerson, J., Bartlett, P., Spieldenner, S., Berry, D., Mosher, L., Kaneene, J., Robinson-Dunn, B., Stobierski, M. & Boulton, M. (2008) Human *Mycobacterium bovis* infection and bovine tuberculosis outbreak, Michigan, 1994–2007. *Emerging Infectious Diseases*, 14(4):657-660, ISSN 1080-6040

Wilson, K., Bjornstad, O., Dobson, A., Merler, S., Poglayen, G., Randolph, S., Read, A. & Skorping, A. (2001) Heterogenities in macroparasite infections: patterns and processes, In *The Ecology of Wildlife Diseases*, P. Hudson, A. Rizzoli, B. Grenfell, H. Heesterbeek, A. Dobson, pp. 6-44, Oxford University Press, ISBN 0198506198, Oxford

Wilson, G., Broughan, J., Chambers, M., Clifton-Hadley, R., Crawshaw, T., de la Fuente, J., Delahay, R., Gavier-Widen, D., Gortazar, C., Hewinson, G., Jackson, V., Martín-Hernando, M., Neimanis, A., Salguero, F., Vicente, J., Ward, A. & McDonald, R. (2008) Scientific review on Tuberculosis in wildlife in the European Union. *Technical Report submitted to EFSA*, 117 pp.

Section 6

Microbial Quality of Milk and Milk Products: Epidemiological Aspects

15

Microbial Properties of Ethiopian Marketed Milk and Milk Products and Associated Critical Points of Contamination: An Epidemiological Perspective

Zelalem Yilma
East Africa Dairy Development (EADD) Program, Addis Ababa Ethiopia

1. Introduction

In Ethiopia, milk production systems can be categorized into urban, peri-urban and rural, based on location (Reda, 2001). Located around Addis Ababa and regional towns, urban and peri-urban systems are market oriented and make use of the high demand in urban areas. The rural system is part of the subsistence farming system and includes pastoralists, agro-pastoralists, and mixed crop-livestock producers mainly in the highlands. As this system is not market oriented, most of the milk produced is retained for home consumption. The surplus is mainly processed using traditional technologies into more shelf stable products such as *Ergo* (Ethiopian naturally fermented milk), butter, ghee and *Ayib* (Ethiopian cottage cheese) that are marketed through the informal channel (Reda, 2001).

In Sub Saharan countries the traditional sector, which is characterized by small herd size dominated by indigenous zebu breeds of low milk production with very little or no specialized inputs, is the dominant type of production system accounting to 70 - 80% of Africa's cattle population (Ibrahim and Olaloku, 2000). In Ethiopia, around 97% of the annual milk production is accounted by the traditional milk production system (Felleke, 2003), which is likewise dominated by indigenous breeds. Most of the milk produced in the country is accordingly processed on-farm using traditional technologies that are generally not well understood. Most of the very few enterprises currently operating in and around the capital entirely depend on the traditional sector for their milk intake, while others depend on it for the majority of their intake. These underscore the importance of understanding the traditional sector in order to make improvement interventions.

Cows contribute to about 95% of the total annual milk produced by cows and camels at national level (CSA, 2010). In 2010, the cattle population was estimated at about 50.9 million (99.19% indigenous, 0.72% hybrid and 0.09% pure exotic breeds). The female cattle population accounted for about 55% of the total. The large livestock population; the favorable climate for improved, high-yielding animal breeds; and the relatively animal disease-free environment make Ethiopia to hold a substantial potential for dairy development. In 2010, a total of 2940 million liters of milk was produced from about 9.6 million cows at national level. During the same year, dairying has created an estimated

588,000 full-time on-farm jobs. However, Ethiopia is a net importer of dairy products with import values significantly exceeding export values. In five reference years, for instance, export values increased from about 73000 USD in 2005 to 123000 USD in 2009, while import values increased from about 5,6 million USD in 2005 to about 10,3 million USD in 2009 (a 4,7 million USD increment).

The importance of milk in the Ethiopian diet differs according to the farming system and the socio-cultural set-ups. Generally, in the lowlands especially where livestock keeping is the main occupation, milk is consumed by all groups of the society. In the highlands, the rural people are sedentary farmers raising both livestock and crops. The main part of their diet consists of cereals and legumes. Milk is used for rearing calves and children, and the surplus is soured for making different fermented milk products. The major ones include: *Ergo, Ayib,* butter (three types of butter can be distinguished namely *Lega, Mekakelegna* and *Besal,* which refer to fresh, semi-rancid and rancid), *Nitir kibie* (melted butter or ghee), *Arrera* (defatted sour milk, a by-product of butter-making and a raw material for *Ayib*-making) and *Aguat* (whey). The demand for milk and milk products is a function of several factors that include: population growth, seasonality of demand and supply, low per capita consumption and high transaction costs. The per capita milk consumption (about 17kg) for Ethiopia is much lower as compared to that for Africa (about 25kg), that recommended by World Health Organization (WHO) (200 liters), the 62.5 kg recommended by FAO (1990) as a minimum level to be kept for a balanced diet and the world's per capita average of about 100 liters/year (FAO, 2010).

In Ethiopia, milk marketing system is not well developed and for the majority of smallholder producers, access to market is limited. In year 2010, for instance, only less that 7 percent of the annual milk production is estimated to be marketed at national level. In 2009, there were 180 cooperatives involved in milk production and marketing in the entire nation, accounting for only 2% of the total number of agro-based cooperatives. In most of the cases, existing dairy cooperatives are operating in areas that are accessible to transportation and market. This means that a substantial amount of milk does not reach the market and a number of producers keep on producing at a subsistence level.

Post harvest losses of up to 40% of milk and its derivatives have been reported from milking to consumption (Felleke, 2003). Such loses are mainly attributed to mishandling in the dairy value chain from farm to fork. These include: contamination during milking and further handling coupled with long storage time at high tropical ambient temperature before consumption; deliberate adulteration of milk; substandard handling, transportation and distribution systems; inefficient processing technologies; inadequate fresh milk outlet; and spillage losses during milking. According to FAO (cited by ENA, 2004), the value of annual milk and dairy product losses due mainly to mishandling across five African and the Middle East countries (Kenya, Tanzania, Uganda, Ethiopia and Syria) is over 90 million USD. Reducing such losses and improving quality are effective ways of making more and safer milk available that benefits both producers and consumers.

Provision of milk and milk products of good hygienic quality is desirable from consumer health point of view. This is one reason why milk testing and quality control include hygiene as well as microbial qualities in addition to testing for fat content and heat stability (Giangiacomo, 2000). The consumption of raw milk and its derivatives is common in Ethiopia (Yilma, 2003), which is not safe from consumer health point of view as it may lead to the transmission of various diseases. Prior to the discovery and widespread adoption of pasteurization for instance, raw milk and its products were responsible for serious bacterial infections such as diphtheria, scarlet fever and tuberculosis (Spreer, 1998). The consumption of unpasteurized, incorrectly pasteurized or post pasteurization contaminated milk and its derivatives have been reported to cause illnesses (Duffy, Garvey & Sheridan, 2002; Desenclos *et al.*, 1996; Cody *et al.*, 1999).

Consumers all over the world are increasingly concerned about the safety of their food in general and milk and milk products in particular. Therefore, quality should not be ignored at all stages of the dairy value chain from farm to table. As the bacterial quality of raw milk is important to product shelf-life, flavor and product yield, it is important that dairy enterprises should strive to obtain the highest quality raw material possible from their own farm as well as their suppliers. It is therefore essential to produce best quality raw milk in the dairy barn in order to manufacture milk products of not only acceptable quality but of high standard premium throughout the year.

Putting a functional quality control system in place is an important tool to bring about improvement in the dairy sector. However, in Ethiopia there is no a properly operational formal marketing and grading system that is geared towards relating quality of products to market price. Establishing a formal marketing system that relates quality to market price has a potential to enhance commercialization of the smallholder dairy sector. Such an approach provides an incentive for producers to supply products of good quality from nutritional as well as consumer health perspective.

2. Study approach

This chapter is essentially based on primary data collection using questionnaire, key informants, group discussions, personal observation and review of available literature. Data were generated from ten dairy potential areas in the Ethiopian highlands (Addis Ababa, Asella, Debre Birhan, Debre Zeit, Holetta, Sululta, Selale, Adama, Sheno, Jimma). A semi-structured questionnaire was used to collect information on hygienic practices at different stages of the dairy value chain from a total of 765 smallholder producers and 22 primary dairy cooperatives.

The milk quality assessment includes preliminary quality tests (specific gravity or milk density, clot-on-boiling and alcohol tests), while the microbial analysis include Aerobic Mesophilic Bacteria, *Enterobacteriaceae*, Coliform, and Yeast and mould counts.

3. Hygienic conditions during production, processing, storage and marketing of milk and milk products

3.1 Milk production

3.1.1 Milking environment

In Ethiopia, there is no standard hygienic condition followed by producers during milk production. The hygienic conditions are different according to the production system, adapted practices, level of awareness, and availability of resources. In most of the cases under smallholder condition, the common hygienic measures taken during milk production especially during milking are limited to letting the calf to suckle for few minutes and/or washing the udder before milking. The quality of the water used for cleaning purpose (to wash the udder, milk equipment, hands), however, is not secured (Yilma, 2003).

Maintaining the sanitary condition of milking area is important for the production of good quality milk. The drainage condition of the milking area, in this regard, is one of the most determinant factors. As observed during the current study, about 71% of the respondents had well drained and easy to clean barns. This is mainly attributed to the large proportion (80.4%) of the respondents from all the study areas that used housed type of barn for their crossbred cows. Since housed and well built barns can drain easily, it has positive correlation with overall hygienic conditions of a given milking environment rendering the production of better quality milk. However, the barns owned by about 29% of the respondents were observed to be not well drained and difficult to clean, which leads to poor quality milk production. It is therefore important that producers consider appropriate drainage conditions of the milking environment as an integral part of production hygiene to ensure the supply of safe and good quality milk and its derivatives. It is also essential to implement a regular barn cleaning scheme. Although, about 87% of the respondents cleaned their barn on daily basis, about 9% of them cleaned only once or twice a week, and the remaining 4% did not clean at all.

3.1.2 The cow and the milker

Cleaning the udder of cows before milking is important since it could have direct contact with the ground, urine, dung and feed refusals while resting. Not washing udder before milking can impart possible contaminants into the milk. Milk is highly nutritious; therefore spoilage as well as pathogenic microorganisms present in the dust, urine, dung and feed refusals, once get access, can easily multiply and deteriorate the quality of milk making it unsafe for consumption and unfit for further processing. As observed during the present study, over 31 and 14% of the respondents owning local and crossbred dairy cows, respectively, do not wash the cow's udder before milking. They rather let calves to suckle before milking. Such practice, however, cannot replace washing. Producers should therefore make udder washing a regular practice in order to minimize contamination and produce good quality milk.

About 39 and 36% of the respondents owning local and crossbred milking cows, respectively, reported to not use towel at all, while about 10 and 20% of local and crossbred cow owners, respectively, responded to use collective towel to clean the udder of two or more milking cows. Such practice, in addition to its effect on milk quality, can lead to cross contamination of udder health problems of milking cows and related complications. In the current study about 27% of the respondents reported to have encountered udder health problems and over 18% of them reported the problem to have occurred more than twice a year. To reverse the situation, producers spent 650 birr per crossbred and 242 birr per local milking cows per year as treatment cost. The reported milk disposal from infected udders was estimated to amount to 1056 birr per crossbred and 560 birr per local cows. The use of individual towel and following essential cleaning practices during milking is important for the production of good quality milk and need be practiced by all producers.

Milkers, in addition to keeping good personal hygiene, should be in good health during milk operation. In this study, about 94 and 96% of the respondents reported to wash their hands before milking their local and crossbred cows, respectively. Covering hair and dressing gown during milking and handling of milk and milk products are important practices milkers need to obey, which weren't observed in any of the farms visited.

3.1.3 Milking utensils

About 81 and 3.4% of the respondents used plastic and stainless equipment, respectively, while 6.6% of them used clay pot. Equipment used for milking, processing and storage determine the quality of milk and milk products. Producers need therefore pay particular attention for the type as well as cleanliness of milk equipment. Milking equipment should be easy to clean. Aluminum and stainless steel equipment are mostly preferred.

3.1.4 Source of water used for cleaning

Although, about 45% of the respondents reported to use tap water for cleaning purpose (udder, milk equipment and hand), about 19 and 16% of them reported to use river and ground water, respectively, while the remaining about 20% reported to use water from either of the aforementioned sources (Fig. 1). Moreover, about 60% of the respondents that reported to use water from non tap sources neither boil nor filter it before use (Fig. 2). When water from non tap sources is used for cleaning purpose, it is important that producers should at least filter and heat treat it before use.

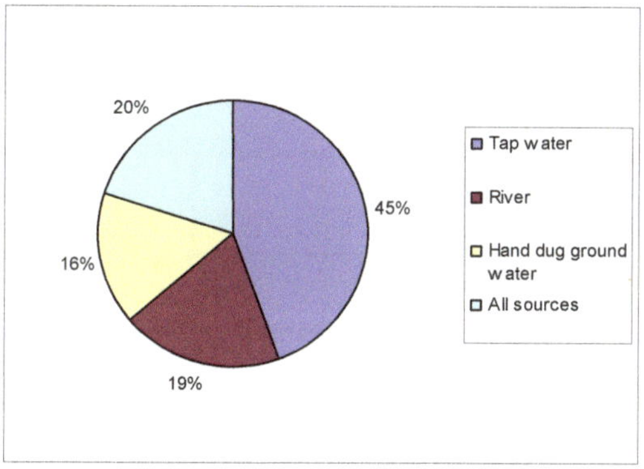

Fig. 1. Source of water used for cleaning purpose (cleaning udder, hands and milk equipment)

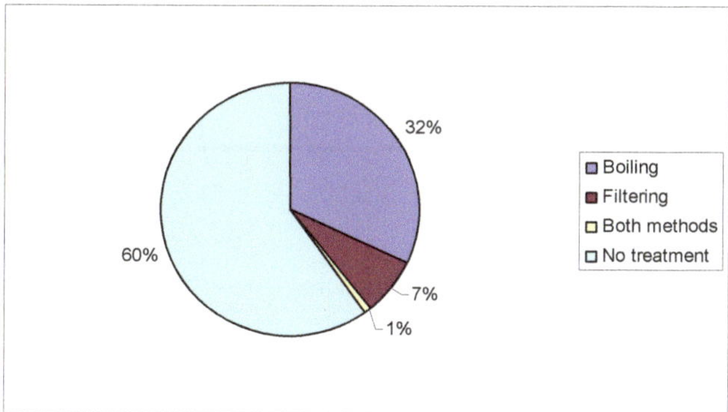

Fig. 2. Treatment of water from non tap sources before use (cleaning udder, hand, milk equipment)

3.2 Milk processing

Although various traditional milk processing and storage equipment are used in different parts of Ethiopia, clay pot is the most commonly available and used. Though not regularly practiced, 74.4% of the producers process milk in to different products. Butter, *Ergo* and *Ayib* are the major fermented milk products, while clay pot is the most commonly used equipment under smallholder condition. Flow diagram of smallholder milk processing is presented in Fig. 3 and Fig. 4 depicts utilization of milk and milk products under smallholder condition. In Ethiopia, heating milk to sterilization temperature of above 100°C for 15 to 40 minutes followed by cooling and inoculation with known bacteria culture (starter) to achieve a controlled fermentation (O'Connor, 1994) is not practiced by smallholders.

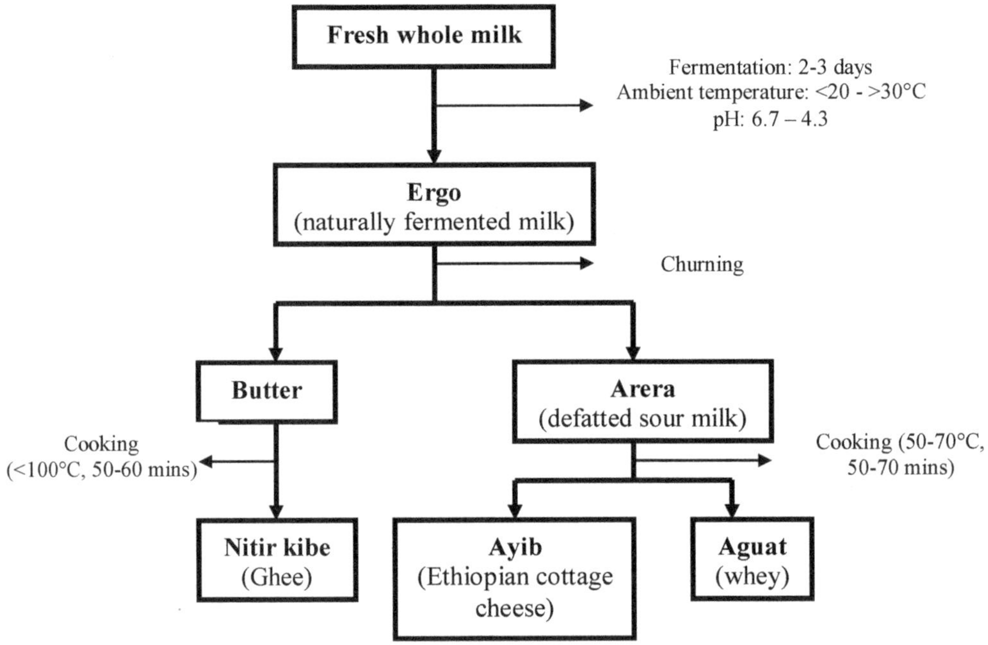

Fig. 3. Flow diagram of smallholder milk processing in the highlands of Ethiopia

Fermented milk is reported to have a storage stability of 15 to 20 days at a temperature of about 16 to 18°C (O'Connor, 1994). About 48% of the interviewees use clay pot for milk souring and/or churning for butter-making. In smallholder butter-making, microbial contamination can come from unclean surfaces, the butter maker and wash water. Packaging materials such as cups and leaves can also represent important sources of contamination. Although washing and smoking the churn reduce bacterial numbers, traditional equipments are often porous and difficult to clean, therefore can serve as a reservoir for many organisms (O'Connor, 1994). Over 61% of the respondents in the study areas reported to use clay pot as a churn and for storage. *Ayib* is made by heating *Arera* or sour skim milk in a clay pot or another material on a low fire to about 40-50°C (FAO, 1990; O'Connor, 1993). In the current study, over 59% of the respondents reported to use clay pot for *Ayib*-making and storage.

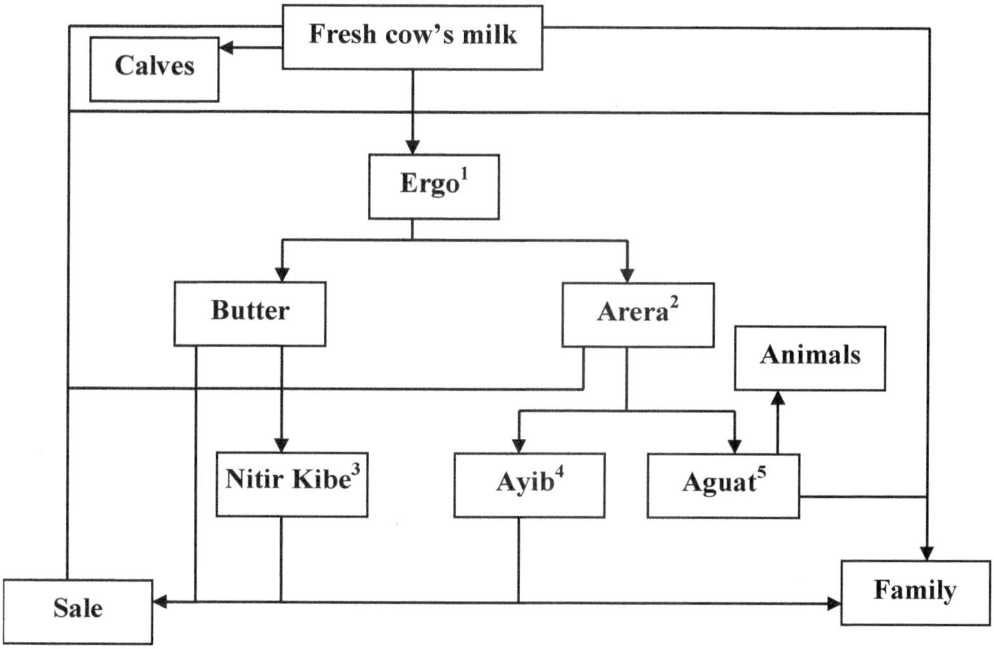

[1]Naturally fermented cow's milk, [2]Defatted sour milk, [3]Ghee, [4]Ethiopian cottage cheese, [5]whey

Fig. 4. Flow scheme of smallholder utilization of milk and milk products

Milk cooperatives sell fresh whole milk directly without further processing as well as process into more shelf stable products whenever there is no market for fresh whole milk. Unlike smallholder producers, cooperatives use hand operated cream separator and therefore, milk makes the basis of processing in cooperative settings (Fig. 5). Although, smallholder and cooperative milk processing differs, both produce similar major marketable products: butter and Ayib. Cooperatives also use manual churn for butter-making.

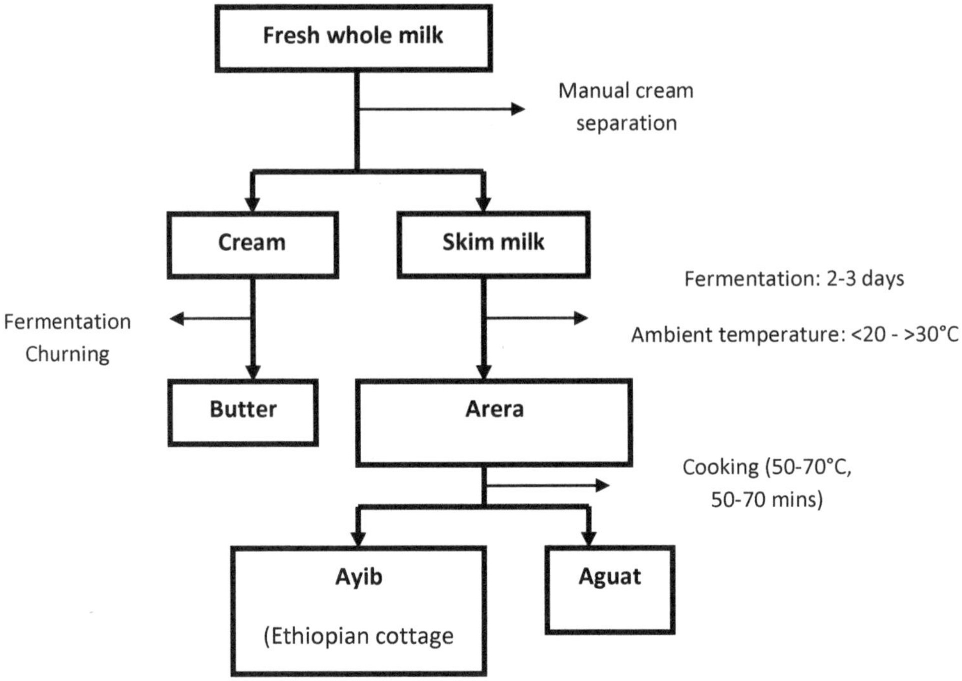

Fig. 5. Flow diagram of milk processing in cooperative centers in the highlands of Ethiopia

3.3 Storage

Milk products are generally more stable than fresh milk because they are more acidic and/or contain less moisture. Salt may also be added to milk products to prolong their shelf life. Applying principles of acidification, moisture reduction and salting (O'Mahony and Peters, 1987) can thus make milk products of good storage stability. All of the smallholder producers interviewed and about 82% of cooperatives stored their products at ambient temperatures. However, about 9% of the cooperatives have a refrigerator and the rest used cold water to store their products in cool conditions. Type of equipment used for different milk operations in the cooperative settings is presented in Table 1.

Purpose	N	Equipment used (frequencies, %)		
		Aluminum/Stainless steel	Plastic containers	Wooden containers
Milk collection	22	65.9	34.0	-
Milk storage	22	76.2	23.8	-
Cream storage	22	77.5	22.5	-
Butter storage	22	55.0	15.0	30.0
Cheese storage	22	88.2	11.8	-

Table 1. Equipment used for different milk operations in cooperative settings

3.4 Marketing of milk and milk products

There are basically two marketing systems in the central highlands of Ethiopia: formal and informal. In the formal system milk is collected at cooperative or private milk collection centers and transported to processing plants. In this system, there are somehow milk quality tests (alcohol and clot-on-boiling tests and density) up on delivery, and therefore the quality of milk is fairly secured. Producers supplying milk in this system pay a due emphasis in the production, storage and transportation of milk if their milk has to be accepted. In the informal system producers supply their surplus production to their neighbors and/or in local markets, either as liquid milk or in the form of butter and/or *Ayib* (O'Connor, 1992). In this system, the quality of milk and milk products is very poor mainly due to the prevailing situation where producers have limited knowledge of dairy product handling coupled with the inadequacy of dairy infrastructure such as electricity and clean water in the production areas.

In Ethiopia, there is no an operational hygienic regulation set for smallholder marketed dairy products. This indicates that the health of the dairy consuming community is not secured. This particularly holds true for *Ayib,* which is consumed with *Enjera* without farther treatment (Duteurtre, 1998). On open markets buyers of milk products practice organoleptic tests. The transaction of *Ayib* is particularly subject to such tests and it is uncommon that a buyer of *Ayib* is not tongue-testing the *Ayib* before buying it. This type of test is only partly associated with the effects of putrefactive microorganisms that can be detected by a simple tongue test. The presence of pathogenic microorganisms, however, cannot be detected by such tests.

There are reports that depict experiences of certain cooperatives around the Selale area (about 14%) (Yilma, 1999) that had a rewarding mechanism through better payment for good quality milk supplied. Such an approach encourages cooperative member and non-member farmers to be concerned about sanitary conditions during milk production and subsequent handling.

3.5 Major milk quality related constraints

Milk quality related constraints ranked during group discussions with dairy cooperatives are presented in Table 2. The major milk quality related constrains include: limited

Constraints	Rank
Limited awareness on hygienic handling	1st
Shortage of capital	1st
Lack of clean water	3rd
Poor type of barn	3rd
Hygiene of the milker	5th
Lack of transport facilities	6th
Mastitis (udder health problem)	7th
Inappropriate materials used for milk production and handling	8th

Table 2. Major milk quality related problems ranked using pair-wise comparison during group discussions

awareness on hygienic handling of milk and milk products, which could mainly be attributed to inefficient extension services; shortage of capital to purchase recommended equipment (milk containers, and processing and packaging materials); lack of clean water for sanitation purpose and poor condition of barn or milking area that is directly related to shortage of capital and limited awareness of its implication on milk quality.

4. Quality of milk and milk products

4.1 Density and freshness of products

Milk, at its normal state, has unique physico-chemical properties, which are used as quality indicators. The density of milk, among others, is commonly used for quality test mainly to check for the addition of water to milk or removal of cream. Addition of water to milk reduces milk density, while removal of cream increases it (O'Connor, 1994). The solid constituents of milk make milk an important food item from nutritional as well as processing point of view. Milk fat and protein are most important components of different varieties of most shelf stable milk products. All the 22 milk cooperatives used specific gravity test as an indicator of milk quality. The average specific gravity of 72 milk samples tested was 1.028 and 1.029 for Holetta and Selale areas, respectively (Fig. 6). These values fall within the range between 1.028 and 1.032 given to unadulterated milk (O'Connor, 1994). About 21% of the same samples checked with alcohol test were positive, while only 14% of the samples were positive for clot-on-boiling test. The results indicate that certain farmers deliver milk to collectors that has undergone fermentation that occurred either through long time elapsed between milking and delivery; mixing evening and morning milk; or use of insufficiently cleaned milk containers.

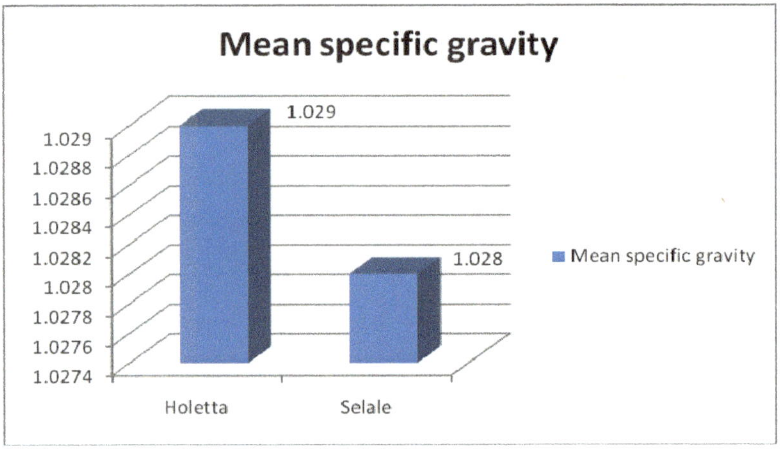

Fig. 6. Specific gravity/density of milk samples in Selale and Holetta areas

The mean pH values of whole milk ranged from 6.29 for Debre Birhan to 6.66 for Selale (data not presented). This variation and low pH may be attributed to the long time elapsed between milking and supply to collection centers. Three of the 24 samples of pasteurized milk checked with alcohol test were positive, while 5 of the samples were positive for clot-on-boiling test. These results are consistent with the results of pH values observed for the same samples that ranged from the lowest 5.46 to the highest 6.14 with an overall mean value of 5.87. The relatively low pH of *Ergo*, ranging from 4.3 to 4.5 retards the growth of undesirable microorganisms, such as pathogens and spoilage bacteria, and enables its further storage (Gonfa *et al.*, 2001).

4.2 Microbial properties of milk and milk products

The microbial content of milk indicates the hygienic levels during milking that include cleanliness of the milking utensils, proper storage and transport as well as the wholesomeness of the udder of the individual cow (Spreer, 1998). The most commonly used microbial quality tests for milk and milk products include determination of total bacterial count (TBC) or standard plate count (SPC) and colifom count (CC). Estimation of yeast and mould counts is also useful for evaluating sanitary practices (O'Connor, 1994). Microorganisms can enter milk via the cow, air, feeds, milk handling equipment and the milker. Once they get into the milk their numbers increase rapidly. It is therefore more effective to exclude microorganisms than trying to control their growth once they get access into the milk.

There are varieties of traditionally fermented dairy products in Ethiopia, for which the exact type of desirable lactic acid bacteria responsible for fermentation is unknown due mainly to uncontrolled and spontaneous fermentation. Most of these products are produced by smallholder producers where access to the required dairy infrastructure is limited. Results of the present study and selected reports of relevant earlier research efforts on the microbial properties of locally produced milk and milk products that have been carried out in different parts of the country are briefly summarized below.

Source	No of Obs.	TBC	*Enterobacteriaceae*	Coliform	YMC
Overall mean	630	8.35	5.10	4.53	8.32
Whole milk	135	9.10	5.49	4.58	-
Ergo	105	9.49	4.95	4.51	8.38
Butter	105	6.67	4.95	4.58	8.32
Arera	75	9.35	4.94	4.65	-
Ayib	105	7.01	4.84	4.42	8.26
Skim milk	105	9.37	5.34	4.44	-

TBC: Total Bacterial Count; YMC: Yeast and Mould Count

Table 3. Overall bacterial and yeast and mould counts (log10) per ml/g of milk and milk product samples collected from different sources (sites and producer groups)

Although there are slight variations between sample sources (locations/producer groups) in microbial counts, the figures observed in the present study are generally much higher than acceptable limits (Table 3). TBC is generally high in samples of whole milk, *Ergo* and skim milk. Counts of *Enterobacteriaceae* and coliform counts are higher than acceptable limits: *Enterobacteriaceae* <1 and coliform <10 cfu/ml for pasteurized milk, and coliform <100 cfu/ml for raw milk intended for direct consumption (Council Directives 92/46/EEC, 1992). The higher count in milk indicates substandard hygienic conditions practiced during production and subsequent handling. The high count in fermented milk products, however, can be partly explained by lactic acid bacteria.

4.2.1 Whole milk

Mean total bacterial counts ranged from 10.12 log cfu/ml of milk collected from Jimma to 8.30 log cfu/ml of milk sampled from Debre Zeit and Adama with the average value being 9.10 log cfu/ml. These values exceed the acceptable value of 10^5 cfu/ml for milk in most European counties (Council Directives 92/46/EEC, 1992; IFCN, 2006). Mean counts of *Enterobacteriaceae* were greater than 5 log cfu/ml and coliform counts greater than 4 log cfu/ml of milk sampled from all study sites.

In Ethiopia, milking animals are kept with the rest of the stock in a shade or enclosure during the night. Milking is done in the shade, grazing field in front of the homestead, or under a tree. However, as these areas are not generally kept clean enough, milking cows usually become soiled with dung and urine. Moreover, cleaning of the udder and hind quarters of the cow is not a common practice. This coupled with the unhygienic cleaning and handling of milk containers result in microbial contamination of milk (Tola, 2002; Gonfa *et al.*, 2001).

According to an earlier report, milk samples collected form smallholder producers in East Wollayta (Southern Ethiopia) had average total microbial count of 7.60 log cfu/ml (Tola, 2002). A total bacterial count ranging from 6.0 to 8.8 log cfu/ml in which 15% of the samples had a count equal or above 7.7 log cfu/ml in raw milk samples in Southern Ethiopia was also reported (Beyene, 1994). In another report, milk sampled from most of the dairy cooperatives operating in the country had total bacterial count of 10^8 cfu/ml (Francesconi, 2006). These values are much higher than the acceptable limits in different countries (10^4 to 10^5 cfu/ml) (IFCN, 2006). This implies that the sanitary conditions in which milk has been produced and handled are substandard subjecting the product to microbial contamination and multiplication. It is indicated that total bacterial count is a good indicator for monitoring the sanitary conditions practiced during production, collection, and handling of raw milk (Chambers, 2002). A good instance worth mentioning is a reduced total bacterial count observed in milk sampled from farmers who received training on hygienic milk production and handling, and who used recommended milk containers as compared to that produced by the traditional milk producers (control) (Tola, 2002; Nebiyu, 2008; Sintayehu *et al.*, 2008). A similar result was also reported for large-scale producers and research centers where there is a better access to dairy facilities as compared to small-scale producers (Yilma and Faye, 2006).

According to a report from Southern Ethiopia, raw cow's milk sampled from smallholder producers contained coliform counts of about 4.46 log cfu/ml (Tola, 2002). Similar counts were also observed in raw milk sampled from smallholder producers in the central highlands of Ethiopia (Yilma and Faye, 2006; Yilma *et al.*, 2007a). Higher counts of different species of *Enterobacteriaceae* were reported with *Escherichia coli* being the most abundantly isolated species (Yilma *et al.*, 2007a), which is a good indicator of recent fecal contamination (Bintsis *et al.*, 2008).

In a study focused on the identification of major bacterial species found in milk as it comes from the udder, it is reported that *Micrococci* represent the largest proportion followed by *Streptococci* and rods (O'Connor, 1994). In a separate study, *Staphylococci* and *Micrococci* are reported to be the most common udder-specific bacteria of environmental origin in milk samples taken directly from the udder (Godefaye and Molla, 2000).

Producer	Whole milk	Ergo*	Butter	Arera	Ayib	Skim milk
Total bacteria						
Smallholder farmers	8.87	9.48	6.86	9.35	7.16	-
Cooperatives	9.49	9.54	6.14	-	6.51	9.25
Overall mean	9.10	9.49	6.67	9.35	7.00	9.25
Enterobacteria						
Smallholder farmers	5.51	4.94	4.97	4.94	4.85	-
Cooperatives	5.45	4.98	4.90	-	4.82	5.30
Overall mean	5.48	4.95	4.95	4.94	4.84	5.30
Coliforms						
Smallholder farmers	5.59	4.48	4.60	4.65	4.44	-
Cooperatives	4.54	4.61	4.53	-	4.37	4.37
Overall mean	4.58	4.51	4.58	4.65	4.42	4.37
Yeast and mould						
Smallholder farmers	-	8.39	8.34	-	8.26	-
Cooperatives	-	8.34	8.27	-	8.27	-
Overall mean	-	8.38	8.32	-	8.26	-

*Ergo refers to fermented whole milk for smallholder farmers, while it refers to fermented skim milk for cooperatives

Table 4. Microbial count (log10) per ml/g of milk and milk products categorized by sample source (producer type)

Total aerobic plate counts were 1.1 x 10^5, 4 x 10^6 and 1.9 x 10^8 cfu/ml respectively for milk samples taken from milking bucket, storage container and processing plant on arrival (Godefaye and Molla, 2000). In the same study, mean coliform counts were reported to range from 1.3 x 10^4 cfu/ml (storage container) to 7.1 x 10^6 cfu/ml (on arrival at the processing plant). The hygienic quality of the milk from a collection center was poor with a mean total bacterial count of 1.3 x 10^7 cfu/ml. In another study, 4 x 10^7 and 1 x 10^9 cfu/ml total microbial counts were reported as lowest and highest values, respectively for raw milk samples at a processing plant in Addis Ababa. Of the total counts in raw milk, psychrophilic, thermoduric and thermophilic organisms made up 98.1, 1.4 and 0.5%, respectively.

4.2.2 Ergo – Naturally fermented milk

Ergo is made by natural fermentation of milk under ambient temperature, without the addition of starter cultures (Assefa *et al.*, 2008). The use of a portion of ergo from a previous batch as a starter in highland areas where ambient temperature is relatively low is reported (Kassa, 2008). This practice is technically adapted to overcome the effect of low ambient temperature, which slows down the growth of lactic acid bacteria (LAB) in the absence of starter culture thus prolongs the fermentation time. The temperature and duration of incubation varies from place to place depending on the prevailing environmental conditions. According to a previous report, five LAB genera were identified from *Ergo* that include *Lactobacillus, Lactococcus, Leuconostoc, Entrococcus* and *Streptococcus* (Assefa *et al.*, 2008). They also indicated the LAB species identified in *Ergo* to be *Streptococcus thermophilus, Strep. acidominus, Enterococcus faecalis* var. *liquefaciens, Strep. bovis, Strep. mitis, Strep. agalactiae, Lactococcus cremoris, Leuconostoc dextranicum, Leuc. lactis, Lactobacillus xylosus* and

Lact. lactis. The isolation of similar genera, and *Micrococci* and coliforms, which are present in low numbers was also reported (Gonfa *et al.*, 2001). An average LAB count of 7.68 log cfu/ml for *Ergo* samples collected from different producers in Addis Ababa and major cities around Addis Ababa was also reported (Yilma and Faye, 2006).

LAB are reported to have antimicrobial activities. The use of different LAB species to create a stationary phase for *Staphylococcus aureus* and a higher density of LAB in modeled starter culture could result in complete inhibition of the bacterium (Le Marc *et al*, (2009). Another report also indicated that 12 LAB isolates from *Ergo* that include *Lactobacillus plantarum, Lactococcus lactic* ssp *cremoris, Lactococcus lactic* ssp *lactic, Lactobacillus acidophyilus, Leuconostoc lactic, Pediococcus pentosace* and *Pediococcus* sp. have antimicrobial activities against different pathogenic microbes including *Shigella flexinery, Salmonella typhi, Escherichia coli* and *Staphylococcus aureus* (Assefa *et al.*, 2008).

TBC of *Ergo* was generally high ranging from 7.71 cfu/ml in samples collected from Sheno to about 10 cfu/ml in samples from Jimma. Average *Enterobacteriaceae* and coliform counts were greater than 4 cfu/ml of *Ergo* sampled from all study sites with differences between the lowest and highest counts ranging from 0.25 to 0.37 cfu/ml.

Mean yeast and mould counts observed in the current study exceeded 8 cfu/ml of *Ergo* sampled from all the sites considered. However, a lower value (2×10^5 cfu/ml) was reported (Gonfa *et al.*, 2001). Yeast and mould count of up to 4.6 log cfu/ml of fermented milk sampled from Southern Ethiopia was also reported (Beyene, 1994). These values are much higher than the acceptable value (<10 cfu/gm for yoghurt) (Mostert and Jooste, 2002). The presence of different species of yeast in milk and its products may result in the spoilage of the product or conversely could contribute to the enhancement of the flavor of fermented milk, since different yeast species are able to assimilate different milk substrates (Gadaga *et al.*, 2000). Bacterial species namely *Klebsiella pneumoniae, Klebsiella oxytoca, Enterobacter cloacae, Citrobacter freundii* and *Enterobacter sakazakii* were isolated from *Ergo* samples collected from smallholder producers in the central Ethiopia (Yilma *et al.*, 2007a). Coliform count averaging at 6.57 log cfu/ml was reported for *Ergo* samples (Yilma and Faye, 2006). Lower values were also observed in which 75% of the samples showed coliform count less than 4.4 log cfu/ml (Beyene, 1994). However, the same author also reported TBC of greater than 8.6 log cfu/ml for 3/4th of fermented milk samples collected from three villages in Southern Ethiopia and coliform counts of higher than 4.4 log cfu/ml in 15% of two fermented milk varieties.

The common traditional milk processing techniques involve smoking of processing utensils using embers of *Olea africana*. This smoking practice is reported to be beneficial to keep better quality of *Ergo* through its inhibitory effect on spoilage and pathogenic organisms. For instance, the inhibitory effect of smoking on *Listeria monocytogenes* was reported (Ashenafi, 1994). The effect of lower pH of *Ergo* in controlling the proliferation of undesirable microorganisms is more effective after 24 hours of incubation. However, at this time, the *ergo* is considered to be too sour for direct consumption since *ergo* coagulates within 24 hours and preferably consumed at this time for its good flavor (Ashenafi, 2006). Accordingly, the same author recommended that milk should be boiled beforehand and a small amount of 3-days-old *Ergo* that is normally free from pathogens but contains enough LAB should be inoculated to initiate fermentation.

4.2.3 Kibe – Traditional butter

Different studies on various aspects of traditional butter-making in Ethiopia have been undertaken in different parts of the country. Traditional butter-making is based on sour milk that has been accumulated over a few days commonly in a clay pot. Once the amount of the accumulated sour milk justifies churning, the sour milk is mixed thoroughly by using a wooden stick with 3 to 5 finger-like projections at one end (*mesbekia* in amahric) then churned using different techniques until butter granules are formed.

Mean total bacterial counts ranged from 6.18 cfu/g in butter samples collected from Selale area to 7.25 cfu/g in samples from Sululta. These values are higher than the acceptable limit of 5×10^4 cfu/g (Mostert and Jooste, 2002). Average *Enterobacteriaceae* and coliform counts were greater than 4 cfu/g of butter sampled from all study sites both of which are higher than the acceptable value of <10 cfu/g (Mostert and Jooste, 2002). Mean yeast and mould counts observed in the current study exceeded 8 cfu/g of butter sampled from all the sites considered.

TBC of 3.15×10^7 and the presence of high variability among samples depending on the sources were reported (Mamo, 2007). Samples collected from open markets and rural producers, for instance, had higher counts as compared to that obtained from dairy farms and urban producers. Coliform counts ranging from 1.92 to 4.5 log cfu/gm of butter are reported (Mamo, 2007; Asfaw, 2008; Yilma *et al.*, 2007a). These differences could be attributed to the wide variation in hygienic handling during milking, processing, storage and transport to market. *Klebsiella pneumoniae, Klebsiella oxytoca, Enterobacter cloacae, Citrobacter freundii,* and *Esherichia coli* were isolated from *ergo* samples collected in the central Ethiopia (Yilma *et al.*, 2007ab), and these microbes are considered to be pathogenic and spoilage (Walstra *et al.*, 2006). On the other hand, yeast and mould counts ranging between 4.3 and 6.86 log cfu/g of butter sampled from Wollayta area are reported (Asfaw, 2008). Average yeast and mould count of 4.5×10^7 cfu/g of butter was also reported (Mamo, 2007). Higher values are observed (Yilma *et al.*, 2005) that varied depending on the type of producer where lower counts were observed for butter sampled from research centers and small-scale producers than that from large-scale producers. TBC of fresh butter sampled from rural and public butter markets in Addis Ababa ranged from 6.2×10^4 to 1.86×10^8 per gram of butter and coliforms were found in all samples that indicate poor hygienic practices (ILCA, 1992). These high deviations from the acceptable value of 10 cfu/gm (Mostert and Jooste, 2002) indicate substandard handling conditions at all stages in the milk chain.

4.2.4 Arera – Defatted sour milk

Average counts of total bacteria, *Enterobacteriaceae* and coliforms were greater than 9, 4.7 and 4.2 cfu/ml, respectively of *Arera* sampled from all study sites both of which are higher than the acceptable value of <10 cfu/gm (Mostert and Jooste, 2002). Traditionally produced *Arera* sampled from Wollayta area had total bacterial count of about 9 log cfu/ml (Nebiyu, 2008). The same author also reported coliform count of 4.86 log cfu/ml. Different species of bacteria were identified in *Arera* samples collected during both dry and wet seasons, which include: *Klebsiella pneumoniae, Klebsiella oxytoca, Enterobacter cloacae, Enterobacter sakazakii, Esherichia coli* and some species of *Salmonella* (Yilma *et al.*, 2007a).

4.2.5 Ayib – Ethiopian cottage cheese

Mean TBC ranged from 6.46 cfu/g in *Ayib* samples collected from Arsi and Selale area to 7.87 cfu/g in samples from Sululta with the overall mean being 7.01 cfu/g. Average *Enterobacteriaceae* and coliform counts were greater than 4 cfu/g of *Ayib* sampled from all study sites. Mean yeast and mould counts observed in the current study exceeded 8 cfu/g of *Ayib* sampled from all the sites considered.

Ayib samples contained high numbers of mesophilic bacteria, *Enterococci*, and yeasts (Ashenafi, 2002). The author also reported aerobic mesophilic bacterial counts of over 10^8 cfu/g for more than 90% of the samples collected in Southern Ethiopia. Works undertaken to identify bacterial species in *ayib* samples reported *Klebsiella pneumoniae, Klebsiella oxytoca, Enterobacter cloacae* (Yilma *et al.*, 2007b), *Staphylococcus aureus* and *Bacillus cereus* (Ashenafi, 2002).

Several earlier works carried out in different parts of the country reported coliform counts of *ayib* samples that ranged between 2 log cfu/gm (Ashenafi, 2002, 2006) and 5.68 log cfu/gm (Yilma *et al.*, 2005) with differences being a function of source of samples and handling conditions. Coliform counts varied among samples collected from different producers where samples from research centers had lower coliform counts (4.85 log cfu/gm) as compared to samples from large-scale (5.68 log cfu/gm) and small-scale (5.48 log cfu/gm) farms showing variations in the hygienic conditions practiced among the different producers (Yilma *et al.*, 2005). However, in all cases values are higher than the acceptable level of <10 cfu/gm (Mostert and Jooste, 2002) indicating the poor hygienic conditions practiced during processing and handling.

Ayib samples collected from an open market in Awassa showed high numbers of mesophilic bacteria, enterococci and yeasts (Table 19). More than 90% of the samples had aerobic mesophilic counts of ≥ 10^8 cfu/g while more than 75% of the samples had yeast counts of ≥ 10^7 cfu/g, and over 85% contained *Enterococci* in numbers of ≥ 10^7 cfu/g. The majority of the samples had mould and lactic acid bacteria counts of 10^5 cfu/g or higher, spore-formers of about 10^4 and psychrotrophs of about 10^6 cfu/g. Over 32% had coliform counts of more than 10^2/g and about 27% contained fecal coliform loads of more than 10^2/g. *Bacillus cereus* and *Staphylococcus aureus* were isolated in 63% and 23% of the samples, respectively, but at low numbers (10^2 to 10^3 cfu/g) (Ashenafi, 1990).

4.2.6 Domestic commercial pasteurized milk

Mean total bacterial counts ranged from 6.60 to 7.54 $\log_{10}$ cfu/ml of domestic pasteurized milk collected from different kiosks and supermarkets in Addis Ababa with the average value being 7.28 $\log_{10}$ cfu/ml (Table 5). Mean counts of coliform bacteria and *Enterobacteriaceae* were 2.87 and 3.69 $\log_{10}$ cfu/ml, respectively. These values are much higher than the acceptable values. As presented in microbiological safety limits for major milk products in community legislation in force by the European Commission, the maximum limit for total bacterial and coliform counts in pasteurized milk intended for drinking is 5×10^5 and 5 cfu/ml, respectively, while *Enterobacteriaceae* count should be <1 cfu/ml and pathogenic microorganisms should not be detected in 25 ml of the product (Council Directives 92/46 EEC, 1992).

The pasteurized milk samples considered in the present study were between 5 to 2 days before the expiry date as indicated on the packaging materials. Although, the high total bacterial count observed in the current study can partly be attributed by lactic acid bacteria, which can be explained by the low mean pH value of 5.87, the higher counts of coliform bacteria and *Enterobacteriaceae* imply that there was a problem either in the pasteurization process or there occurred post pasteurization contamination during packaging. Protection from post-pasteurization contamination before the milk product is packaged is a critical factor in achieving a safe food. Ingredients added after pasteurization of the milk portion of the food can be a source of pathogens. The control of potential sources of contamination can be addressed by following production practices based on Good Manufacturing Practices.

Pasteurized milk had mesophilic aerobic counts of 7 x 10^5 cfu/ml as it left the pasteurizing unit (Mahari and Gashe, 1990). According to the same source, psychrophilic, thermoduric and thermophilic organisms constituted 53.0, 39.5 and 7.5%, respectively and the isolates belonged mostly to the genera *Bacillus, Streptococcus, Lactobacillus, Arthrobacter, Alcaligenes, Aeromonas* and *Pseudomonas*. *Cocci* were more predominant than rod-shaped bacteria and of the rod-shaped bacteria 73% were gram-negative. As indicated by the same authors, utensils holding the raw and pasteurized milk and plastic sheets used for bagging the pasteurized milk were reported to contribute for the high bacterial count, which were either thermoduric or thermophilic.

Pasteurized milk sample*	No. of obs.	Count, Log10 cfu/ml		
		TBC	CC	EntC
A	4	7.28	3.18	3.58
B	4	6.60	3.28	3.94
C	4	7.47	3.26	4.26
D	4	7.37	2.34	3.63
E	4	7.54	2.77	3.68
F	4	7.42	2.40	3.05
Overall mean	24	7.28	2.87	3.69

*Different letters represent different brands of pasteurized milk marketed in Addis Ababa;
TBC: Total Bacterial Count; CC: Coliform Count; EntC: *Enterobacteriaceae* Count; cfu/ml: Colony Forming Units per millilitre

Table 5. Microbial quality of domestic commercial pasteurized milk sampled from different kiosks and supermarkets in Addis Ababa

5. Critical control points in the milk chain

As with hygiene and food safety, the issue of quality has been growing prominently in recent years and the optimum approach to these two areas is remarkably similar. Providing quality assured products to the consumer has traditionally relied on quality control of finished products, that is, a set of procedures to test and analyze the product to ensure it conforms to the required specification. This approach has drawbacks that include incidents of food poisoning in spite of quality control procedures, less effective as microorganisms are not evenly distributed in products, and high cost of rejected products as the quality control is based solely on finished product testing. This is one reason why, developments in quality management have focused on the prevention of defects in the first place (through effective design and hazard elimination) rather than trying to measure defects once the product has been manufactured. Applying this approach to hygiene has led to the development of preventive

Quality Assurance (QA) systems. Hazard Analysis and Critical Control Point (HACCP) in particular is employed in the identification of stages in the food chain where spoilage as well as pathogenic microorganisms can enter, survive and proliferate in the food and managing these as the key control strategy rather than relying on testing end products (IDF, 1994).

In the Ethiopian smallholder context, six Critical Control Points (CCPs) where milk and milk products can be contaminated can be identified (Fig. 7). These include:

i. *During milk production*: During milking, contamination can come from the cow, the milker, utensils used for milking, storage and filtering the milk, and the barn or the milking environment.
ii. *During fermentation*: Milk containers used for fermentation, wash water of poor quality used, ingredients added with the intention of improving the flavor of the final product can represent potential sources of contamination.
iii. *During churning (butter-making)*: Churns and warm water added to facilitate the churning process (speed-up butter recovery) can be possible sources of contamination.
iv. *During Ayib-making*: Low cooking temperatures that may not be enough to kill spoilage as well as pathogenic microorganisms can be considered as an important point for the poor quality of the final product. Other potential sources of microbial contamination include: materials used for *Ayib*-making, other utensils such as that used for draining the whey or ladling out the *Ayib*, and filtration.
v. *Packaging/storage of butter and Nitir Kibe/ghee*: Potential sources of contamination here include: product container/packaging, high keeping temperature, and poor personal hygiene of people handling the product.
vi. *Packaging/storage of Ayib*: Potential sources of contamination here are similar with that under v above.

CCPs at dairy cooperatives are summarized in Fig. 8:

i. *The milk/reception*: The raw material milk can be contaminated via the cow; the milker; the barn; utensils used for milking, filtering, storage (at farm and cooperative center) and transport.
ii. *During cream separation*: Contamination at this point can come from the separator, wash water, personnel, and environment.
iii. *During fermentation of skim milk*: Containers used for fermentation, poor quality wash water, personnel and the environment represent potential sources of contamination.
iv. *During churning (butter-making)*: Contamination at this point can come from the churn (container), personnel, wash water, and environment.
v. *During Ayib-making*: Low cooking temperatures that may not be enough to kill spoilage as well as pathogenic microorganisms can be considered as an important point for the poor quality of the final product. Other potential sources of contamination include: materials used for *Ayib*-making, other utensils such as that used for draining the whey or ladling out the *Ayib*, and filtration.
vi. *Packaging/storage of butter*: Potential sources of contamination here include: product container/packaging, high keeping temperature, poor personal hygiene of people handling the product, and environment.
vii. *Packaging/storage of Ayib*: Potential sources of contamination here are similar with that under vi above.

The aforementioned critical points of contaminations can be considered for making improvement interventions.

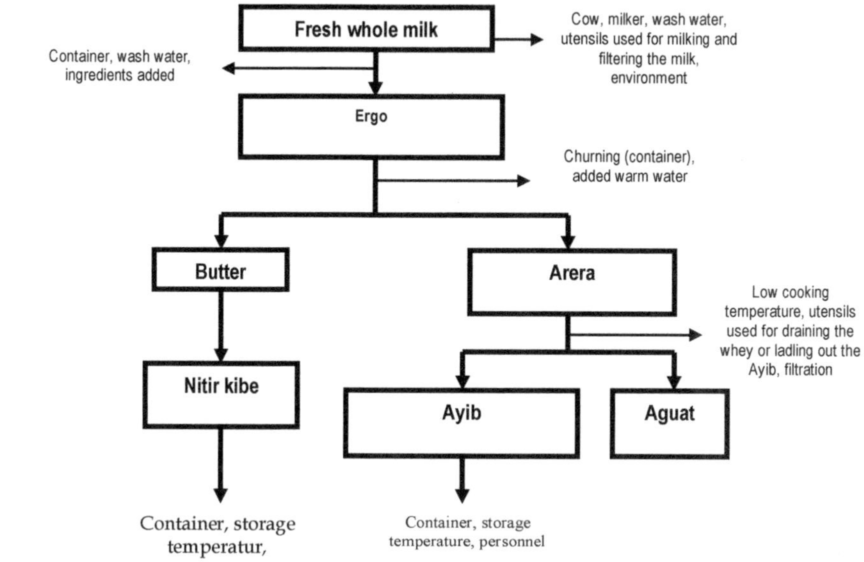

Fig. 7. Flow scheme of critical points of microbial contamination during traditional milk processing in the central Ethiopian highlands

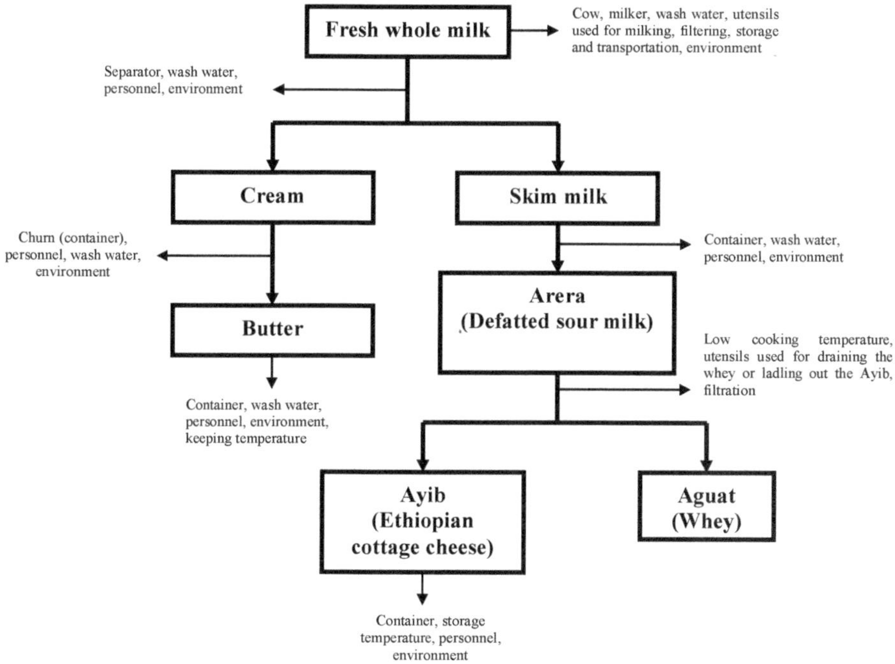

Fig. 8. Flow scheme of critical points of microbial contamination of milk and milk products at cooperative centers in different parts of Ethiopia

6. International quality standards practiced in different countries

As food safety and quality are a growing concern all over the world, different organizations in many countries implement quality control programs and established quality standards for all food items including animal products to ensure the health of the consumer. Health hazards to the consumer are often grouped into microbiological, physical and chemical (FDA, 2004). A microbial criteria stipulate that a type of microorganism, groups of microorganisms, toxin produced by a microorganism must either not be present at all, be present in only a limited number of samples, or be present at less than a specified number or amount in a given quantity of a food ingredient (NRC, 1985).

Different microbiological tests are used to indicate the hygienic condition of manufacturing of a given product. Coliform count provides an indication of unsanitary production practices and/or mastitis infection. A count less than 100 Colony Forming Units (CFU)/ml is considered acceptable for milk intended to be pasteurized before consumption. Counts of 10 CFU/ml or less are achievable and desirable if raw milk will be consumed directly (Jones and Sumner, 1999; Ruegg, 2003). Estimation of the total bacteria count is the procedure used to measure the general sanitary quality of milk. The number of bacteria in aseptically drawn milk varies from animal to animal and even from different quarters of the same animal. On average, aseptically drawn milk from healthy udders contains between 500 and 1000 bacteria ml^{-1}. High initial counts (>10^5 bacteria ml^{-1}) are evidence of poor production hygiene (O'Connor, 1994). Somatic cell count (SCC) is another indirect indicator of the microbial quality of milk. The number of somatic cells increases in response to pus-producing bacteria like *Staphylococcus aureus*, a cause of mastitis (Kleinschmit and Gompert, 2007).

Legal and voluntary bacteriological standards vary widely from country to country and there are different standards for different groups and species of microorganisms specific to specific products. Standard plate count (SPC) values for raw milk can range from <1000ml^{-1}, where contamination during production is minimal, to >1 x $10^5 ml^{-1}$. Consequently, high initial SPC values (>10^5ml-1) are evidence of serious hygienic problem during production, likewise SPC values of <$2x10^4 ml^{-1}$ reflect good sanitary practices (IDF, 1994).

Somatic Cell Count/ml	Drug residue	Country	Source
< 7.5 x 10^5	Absent	USA	IFCN, 2006; CDFA, 2008
< 4.99 x 10^5	Absent	Canada	IFCN, 2006; CDFA, 2008
< 4 x 10^5	Absent	France	IFCN, 2006; CDFA, 2008
< 4 x 10^5	Absent	Sweden	IFCN, 2006; CDFA, 2008
< 10^6	Absent	Russian	IFCN, 2006
< 6 x 10^5	Absent	Israel	IFCN, 2006
< 4 x 10^5	Absent	South Africa	IFCN, 2006
< 7 x 10^5	Absent	Brazil	IFCN, 2006
< 5 x 10^5	Absent	China	IFCN, 2006
< 2.5 x 10^5	Absent	Australia	IFCN, 2006

Table 6. Commonly used safety limits of somatic cell count and drug residue for raw milk employed in selected countries

In many countries, a standard for Grade 'A' raw milk is an SPC of <10 ml^{-1} for milk intended for heat treatment before consumption or further processing. For milk that is to be

Milk product	Microorganism	Maximum limit (cfu/ml or g)
Raw cow's milk intended for processing	Total bacteria	10^5
	Staphylococcus aureus	2×10^3
Raw cow's milk intended for direct human consumption	*Salmonella*	Absent in 25g
	S. aureus	5×10^2
	Total bacteria	5×10^4
Pasteurized drinking milk	Pathogenic microorganisms	Absent in 25g
	Coliforms	5
	Total bacteria	5×10^5
UHT milk and sterilized milk	Total bacteria	100
Cheese made from raw and thermized milk	*Listeria monocytogenes*	Absent in 1g hard cheese or in 25g other cheese varieties
	Salmonella	Absent in 1g
	S. aureus	10^4
	E. coli	10^5
Soft cheese made from heat treated milk	*L. monocytogenes*	Absent in 25g
	Salmonella	Absent in 1g
	S. aureus	10^3
	E. coli	10^3
	Coliforms	10^5
Fresh cheese	*L. monocytogenes*	Absent in 25g
	Salmonella	Absent in 1g
	S. aureus	100
Butter	*L. monocytogenes*	Absent in 25g
	Salmonella	Absent in 1g
	Coliforms	10
Powdered milk and milk based products	*L. monocytogenes*	Absent in 1g
	Salmonella	Absent in 1g
	S. aureus	100
	Coliforms	10
Frozen milk based products	*L. monocytogenes*	Absent in 1g
	Salmonella	Absent in 1g
	S. aureus	100
	Coliforms	100
	Total bacteria	10^5
Liquid milk based products	*L. monocytogenes*	Absent in 1g
	Salmonella	Absent in 1g
	Coliforms	5

Source: Council Directives 92/46 EEC (1992)

Table 7. Microbiological safety limits for selected milk products in community legislation in force by the European Commission

consumed raw, a more stringent standard is generally required because consumers of raw milk are at a greater risk for contracting a milk-borne illness such as salmonellosis. In some countries, standards adopted may depend on whether milk is refrigerated or merely water-cooled. For example, in North America, SPC values of $<10^6$ ml^{-1} or equivalent are acceptable for manufacturing grade 'A' milk. In contrast, in the UK no distinction is made between raw milk marketed for further processing and that marketed for fluid consumption (Chambers, 2002). Although on-farm testing and independent laboratory testing do not guarantee food safety, they are generally accepted means to monitor milk quality. In dairy developed countries, buying raw milk from a Grade 'A' herd assures that the milk is tested for pathogens on a regular basis therefore is fit for further processing and consumption (Walstra *et al.*, 2006). Quality related safety limits practiced in selected countries are presented in Table 6, while Table 7 depicts microbiological safety limits for selected milk products in community legislation in force by the European Commission.

7. Conclusion

The microbiological properties of marketed milk and milk products in different parts of Ethiopia are generally below standards. This is mainly due to unhygienic conditions at one or more of the stages in the dairy value chain from farm to table, which in turn might be attributed to inadequate dairy infrastructure coupled with limited knowledge on the hygienic production and handling of milk and milk products. Based on experiences from a number of countries, it is likely that problems with effective translation of knowledge to practice, rather than incomplete knowledge per se, are the more important constraints to national progress towards improved milk quality.

Currently, the Ethiopian dairy sector is developing and the involvement of the private sector is at the increase. Moreover, consumers are increasingly concerned about the quality of products and the production conditions. A concerted effort towards improving the qualities of milk and milk products and contributing to the betterment of the Ethiopian formal milk business is essential. This benefits both the producer through allowing entering into the competitive market and bringing increased income from the sale of quality products, and the consumer through creating access to products of acceptable quality.

From experiences of a number of countries, putting functional quality standards, quality control system and payment system based on quality in place resulted not only in improved quality of marketed milk but also the volume of milk delivered to collection centers and dairies. It is important that quality standards for milk and major milk products for Ethiopia, should take into consideration factors such as the prevailing conditions of facilities and infrastructures required for dairy development; the existing quality standards currently in use in different countries; and the actual qualities of milk and milk products being marketed in different parts of Ethiopia. Such an approach will improve the Ethiopian formal milk business.

8. References

Asfaw, M. M. (2008). Assessment of processing techniques and quality attributes of butter produced in Delebo water shade of Wolayita zone, Southern Ethiopia. Hawassa University. M.Sc. thesis.

Ashenafi M. (2002). The microbiology of Ethiopian foods and beverages: A review. SENET: Ethiopian Journal of Science. 25 (1):97-140.

Ashenafi, M. (1990). Microbiological quality of Ayib, a traditional Ethiopian cottage cheese. International Journal of Food Microbiology, 10:261-268.

Ashenafi, M. (2006). A review on the microbiology of indigenous fermented food and beverages of Ethiopia. Ethiopian Journal of Biological Sciences 5(2), 189-245.

Ashenafi, M. (1994). Fate of Listeria monocytogenes during the fermentation of Ergo, a traditional Ethiopian sour milk. Journal of Dairy Science 77, 696-702.

Assefa, E., Beyene, F. and Santhanam, A. (2008). Isolation and characterization of inhibitory substance producing lactic acid bacteria from Ergo, Ethiopian traditional fermented milk.

Beyene F. (1994). Present situation and future aspects of milk production, milk handling and processing of dairy products in Southern Ethiopia. Ph.D. Thesis. Department of Food Science, Agricultural University of Norway. Ås, Norway.

Bintsis, T., Angelidis A. S. and Psoni, L. (2008). Modern Laboratory Practices: Analysis of Dairy Products. In: Advanced dairy science and technology. Britz, T. J. and Robinson R. K. (Eds.). Blackwell Publishing Ltd, UK.

CDFA. (2008). New Coliform Standard for Milk Sold Raw to Consumers. California Department of Food and Agriculture (CDFA), Press Release on Raw Milk.

Chambers, J.V. (2002). The Microbiology of Raw Milk. Dairy Microbiology Handbook. Third Edition. Edited by Richard K. Robinson. John Wiley and Sons, Inc., New York.

Cody, S.H., Abbott, S.L., Marfin, A.A., Schulz, B., Wagner, P., Robbins, K., Mohle-Boetani, J.C., and Vugia, D.J. 1999. Two outbreaks of multidrug-resistant *Salmonella* serotype Typhimurium DT104 infections linked to raw-milk cheese in Northern California. JAMA. 281(19):1805-10. (Abs. PubMed).

Council Directives 92/46 EEC. (1992). Laying down the health rules for the production and placing on the market of raw milk, heat-treated milk and milk-based products. Official Journal of the European Communities, No L 268/1.

CSA. (2010). Agricultural Sample Survey. Livestock, Poultry and Beehives population (private peasant holdings). Federal Democratic Republic of Ethiopia Central Statistical Authority (CSA), Addis Ababa, Ethiopia.

Desenclos, J.C., Bouvet, F., Benz-Leloine, E., Grimont, F., Desqueyroux, H., Rebiere, I., and Grimont, P.A. (1996). Large outbreak of *Salmonella enterica* serotype Paratyphi B infection caused by a goats' milk cheese, France, 1993: a case finding and epidemiological study. *BM*, 312:91-94.

Duffy, G., Garvey, P. and Sheridan, J.J. (2002F). A European Study on Animal Food & Biomedical Aspects of *E. coli* 0157:H7. The National Food Centre, Dunsinea, Castleknock, Dublin, Irland.

ENA. (2004). Milk, Dairy Products Loss Of Five African, Middle East Countries Stands At 90 Mln. USD, Ethiopian News Agency (ENA), Addis Ababa, 10/22/2004.

FAO. (1990). The technology of traditional milk products in developing countries. FAO Animal Production and Health Paper 85. Food and Agriculture Organization of the United Nations, Rome, Italy. 333 pp.

FAO. (2010). Status and prospects for smallholder milk production – A global perspective, by T. Hemme and J. Otte. Rome.

Felleke G. (2003). Milk and Dairy Products, Post-harvest Losses and Food Safety in Sub-Saharan Africa and the Near East. A Review of the Small Scale Dairy Sector - Ethiopia. FAO Prevention of Food Losses Programme. FAO, Rome, Italy.

Francesconi G.N. (2006). Promoting milk quality of cooperative smallholders: Evidence from Ethiopia and implications for policy. In proc. of the 14th Annual conference of the Ethiopian Society of Animal Production (ESAP), Part II: Technical papers, held on September 5 – 7, 2006, Addis Ababa, Ethiopia. pp 31-41.

Gadaga, T.H., Mutukumira, A.N. and Narvhus, J.A. (2000). Enumeration and identification of yeasts isolated from Zimbabwean traditional fermented milk. International Dairy Journal 10; 459-466.

Giangiacomo, R. (2000). Milk testing, quality control, hygiene and safely. FAO e-mail conference on "Small-scale milk collection and processing in developing countries". June 6 - August 3, 2000. 108 p.

Godefay, B. and B. Molla. (2000). Bacteriological quality of raw cow's milk from four dairy farms and a milk collection center in and around Addis Ababa. Berl. Munch. Tierarztl. Wochenschr. 113:276-278.

Gonfa, A., Foster, H.A., Holzapfel, W.H. (2001). Field survey and literature review on traditional fermented milk products of Ethiopia. Int. J. Food Microbiol. 68, 173–186.

Ibrahim, H. and Olaluku, E. (2000). Improving cattle for milk, meat and traction. ILRI Manual 4. International Livestock Research Institute (ILRI), Nairobi, Kenya, pp. 135.

IDF. (1994). Recommendations for the hygienic manufacture of milk and milk based products. Bulletin of the International Dairy Federation (IDF). No. 292, 32 p.

IFCN. (2006). Dairy Report 2006. For a better understanding of milk production world-wide. International Farm Comparison Network (IFCN) Dairy Research Center, Kiel, Germany.

ILCA. (1992). Alternative milk processing and preservation techniques and the quality of market butter and cheese. Annual program report 1991. International Livestock Centre for Africa. Addis Ababa, Ethiopia. pp. 39-40.

Jones G.M. and Sumner S. (1999). Testing bulk milk samples. Dairy. Publication 404-405. Virginia Cooperative Extension. Virginia State University.

Kassa, B. E. (2008). Cottage cheese production in Shashemane and the role of Rue (Ruta chalepensis) and garlic (Allium sativum) on its quality and shelf life. Hawassa University. M.Sc. Thesis.

Kleinschmit, M., and Gompert, T. (2007). Raw Milk Use and Safety Fact Sheet. Center for Rural Affairs, Northeast Nebraska RC&D, Plainview, Nebraska.

Le Marc, Y., Valík, L. and Medveďová, A. (2009). Modelling the effect of the starter culture on the growth of Staphylococcus aureus in milk. International Journal of Food Microbiology 129: 306–311.

Mahari, T. and B.A. Gashe. (1990). A survey of the microflora of raw and pasteurized milk and the sources of contamination in a milk processin plant in Addis Ababa, J Dairy Res, 57(2):233-8.

Mamo, W. K. (2007). Composition, microbial quality and acceptability of butter produced from the milk of dairy cows in Hawassa, Southern Ethiopia. Hawassa university. M.Sc. thesis. Pp 89.

Mostert, J.F. and Jooste, P.J. (2002). Quality Control in The Dairy Industry. Dairy Microbiology Handbook. Third Edition. Edited by Richard K. Robinson. John Wiley and Sons, Inc., New York. P 655- 736.

Nebiyu, R.G. (2008). Traditional and improved milk and milk products handling practices and compositional and microbial quality of raw milk and buttermilk in Delebo water shade of Wolayita zone, Ethiopia. Hawassa University. M.Sc. thesis.

NRC. (1985). An evaluation on microbiological criteria for foods and food ingredients. Subcommittee on microbiological criteria, Committee on Food Protection, National Research Council (NRC).

O'Connor, C.B. (1993). Traditional cheese making manual. ILCA (International Livestock centre for Africa), Addis Ababa, Ethiopia. 43 pp.

O'Connor, C.B. (1994). Rural dairy technology. ILRI training manual 1. ILRI (International Livestock Research Institute), Addis Ababa, Ethiopia. pp. 133.

O'Connor, C.B. (1992). Rural smallholder milk production and utilization and the future for dairy development in Ethiopia. Dairy marketing in Sub-Saharan Africa. Proceeding of a symposium held at ILCA, Addis Ababa, Ethiopia. 26-30 November 1990. International Livestock Center for Africa, Addis Ababa, Ethiopia. pp. 123-130.

O'Mahony, F. and Peters, J. (1987). Sub-Saharan Africa. Options for smallholder milk processing. Food and Agriculture Organisation of the United Nations. World Animal Review. No. 62. pp.16-30.

Reda, T. (1998). Milk processing and marketing options for rural small-scale producers. In: National Conference of the Ethiopian Society of Animal Production (ESAP), pp. 61-67.

Ruegg P.L. (2003). Practical food safety interventions for Dairy Production. J. Dairy Sci. 86: (E. Suppl.):E1-E9.

Spreer, E. (1998). Milk and dairy product technology. Mixa, A (translator). Marcel Dekker, INC. ISBN: 0-8247-0094-5. New York, pp. 39-58.

Tola A. (2002). Traditional milk and milk products handling practices and raw milk quality in Eeastern Wollega. MSc thesis. Alemaya University, Alemaya, Ethiopia. 108 pp.

Walstra, P., Wouters. Jan T.M. and Geurts, T.J. (2006). Dairy Science and Technology Second Edition. CRC Press Taylor & Francis Group. P 763.

Yilma, Z. (1999). Smallholder Milk Production Systems and Processing Techniques in the central high lands of Ethiopia. MSc Thesis, Swedish University of Agricultural Sciences Uppsala, Sweden 132p.

Yilma, Z. (2003). Sanitary conditions and microbial qualities of dairy products in urban and peri-urban dairy shed of the central Ethiopia. DEA. Lyon, France.

Yilma, Z., Faye, B and Loiseau, G. (2005). Microbial properties of butter and Ethiopian cottage cheese (Ayib). Ethiop. Vet. J., 2005, 9 (1), 43-57.

Yilma, Z., Faye, B and Loiseau, G. (2007). Occurrence and distribution of species of *Enterobacteriaceae* in selected Ethiopian traditional dairy products: A contribution to epidemiology. Food Control 18 (2007) 1397–1404.

Yilma. Z. and Faye, B. (2006). Handling and Microbial Load of Cow's Milk and Irgo - Fermented Milk Collected from Different Shops and Producers in Central Highlands of Ethiopia. Eth. J. Anim. Prod. 6(2): 67-82.

Section 7

Epidemiology of Lymphoid Malignancy

16

Epidemiology of Lymphoid Malignancy in Asia

Zahra Mozaheb
Mashhad University of Medical Science
Iran

1. Introduction

Lymphoid malignancy is a remarkable disease because of its difference in epidemiology and etiology in different areas around the world. Several features of the epidemiology of lymphoid malignancy particularly stand out. The overall lymphoid malignancy incidence in Asian countries is relatively low. Histopathologic subtypes of lymphoma are different in eastern and western countries and generally similar among Asian countries. Differences in geographic distribution are striking for follicular lymphoma, which is less common in eastern countries than elsewhere. Asians have higher rates of aggressive NHL (Non-Hodgkin Lymphoma), T-cell lymphomas, and extra-nodal disease. Hodgkin's Lymphoma (HL) is relatively rare in Asian countries, and its subtypes are various in comparison with other areas.

While for most cancers incidence and mortality are decreasing, the incidence rates of all subtypes of NHL have increased during the second half of the twentieth century, but the reason is poorly understood. This rise has been noted worldwide, in both genders, particularly in the elderly, and increase in high-grade NHL is predominant. Increase in NHL may be attributed to immunodeficiency, radiation, various infections, blood transfusion, familial aggregation, genetic susceptibility to NHL, chemical exposures to pesticides and solvents, and diet. Some studies also suggest that association between risk factors and specific NHL subtypes may be stronger than association between the same risk factors and NHL in aggregate. In addition the mentioned risk factors are different in various areas; therefore it may cause different distribution of lymphoid malignancy around the world. Geographic variation in lymphoma rate suggests the importance of environmental and gens effects. Risks for developing NHL include immunosuppression a causal link between infectious agents and lymphomagenesis, which have also been determined, particularly for *human T-cell leukemia/lymphoma virus type1 (HTLV-1), Epstein– Barr virus (EBV), Helicobacter pylori* infections and *Hepatitis C Viruses (HCV)*infection, which are relatively frequent in our area. In addition to the incidence of non-Hodgkin's lymphoma and its histological subtypes in Asian migrants to the United States which is lower in first-generation migrants, confirmed this suggestion. Other exogenous factors which have been implicated in lymphomagenesis, mentioned earlier, are used more without any protection in developing countries. They may play an important role in these differences.

In this chapter we compare our findings with the data from other relevant studies available in literature from various parts of Asia, as well as with those of Western countries in an attempt to gain more insights into the differences between the Oriental and Western countries. In addition, because most different are related to etiologic factors, we also describe some of them.

2. Non-Hodgkin Lymphoma

Non-Hodgkin lymphoma is a heterogeneous group of B-cell and T-cell neoplasm that arise primarily in the lymph nodes with varied clinical and biologic feature. Current classification system include the Revised European-American Lymphoma (REAL) classification and the World Health Organization (WHO) classification of hematopoietic and lymphoid neoplasms (Alexander, et al., 2007). The distribution of NHL types varies internationally (Anderson, Armitage, & Weisenburger, 1998). Epidemiological investigation of the NHL and its etiology may result in a better understanding and hence prevention.

2.1 Descriptive epidemiology

Based on World Health Organization (WHO) classification,36 subtype of NHL (21 of B-cell and 15 of T-cell type) are recognized (Ekström-Smedby, 2006). NHL is the most common in the developed world, with the highest incidence in USA, Australia and New Zealand, and Europe, and the lowest in eastern and South central Asia (Ekström-Smedby, 2006). The age standardized incidence of NHL, around the year 2000, was estimated at approximately 10-14 per 100000 person-year in western countries, and 3 per 100000 in South central Asia (Parkin, Bray, Ferlay, & Pisani, 2005).

In recent decades, there has been a dramatic increase in NHL incidence worldwide, of about 2-4% annually (Baris & Zahm, 2000). This increase has been occurred in both males and females in all age groups except the very young and in black and whites (Weisenburger, 1994). Racial differences have not been observed in age-specific incidence curves until the age of 45 for males and 35 for females, however over these ages, NHL develops more frequently in whites than blacks (Müller, Ihorst, Mertelsmann, & Engelhardt, 2005). The highest increase was observed in western countries, but this increase is no limited to these countries, and it has been observed in eastern countries such as India, Japan, Singapore (Devesa & Fears, 1992). Several reasons including: recategorisation of borderline type of lymphoma; less histopathological misdiagnosis of NHL as Hodgkin's disease; greater use of immunohistological techniques to examine cancer of uncertain cell type and coding effects, may account for part of the increase (A. J. Swerdlow, 2003). The general trends in western countries has been a dramatic increase in incidence in young men in areas where AIDS has become common (Morton, et al., 2006).

The median age of NHL in Asian countries is significantly lower, compared to the population-based registration in western countries. The Hematological Malignancy Research Network reported that the median age of their patients was 68 years old (Smith, et al., 2010). However the median age in Asian countries is about 54 years old, in Iranian patients was 55 years old (Mozaheb, Aledavood, & Farzad, 2011), in the Korean patients 52 years (Y.-H. Ko, et al., 1998), in Taiwan 54 years (Lee, Tan, Feng, & Liu, 2005), and in a previous study in Japan 54.5 years (Aozasa, et al., 1985), but in a recent study in Japan it was 66 years (Aoki, et al., 2008). It is notable that the median age of Asian patients at the time of presentation was younger than in the western countries and it might be attributable to the lower frequency of lymph node type lymphoma, and higher frequency of T-cell lymphoma, which comes as follows.

Geographically related variation in the incidence of histopathologic distribution and clinical feature of NHL are well recognized (Shih & Liang, 1991). T-cell leukemia lymphoma occurs more frequently in southwest Japan, and the Caribbean basin (Takatsuki, 1990), northeast of Iran (Mashhad) (Abbaszadegan, et al., 2003); follicular lymphoma (FL) occurs less frequently in eastern countries (Intragumtornchai, et al., 1996; Mozaheb, et al., 2011; Ohshima, Suzumiya, & Kikuchi, 2002), and Immunoproliferative Small Intestinal Disease (IPSID) is the most prevalent in the Middle east and Africa (Khojasteh & Haghighi, 1990).

2.1.1 Immunologic characterization of non-Hodgkin's lymphoma

Although B-cell lymphomas are constantly more common around the world, T-cell lymphomas are proportionally more common in Asia than in western countries (Müller, et al., 2005). Despite a higher percentage of T-cell lymphomas in Asians compared with westerns, the absolute incidences of T-NHL in HTLV1 non endemic areas, and western countries are quite similar when calculated by age-adjusted incidence (Aoki, et al., 2008; Au, et al., 2005; Wang, Young, Win, & Taylor, 2005). In a Chinese (non endemic area for HTLV1) study T-cell lymphoma proportion was 28.1% (Wang, et al., 2005), and also in Taiwan which is not endemic for HTLV1, T/NK lymphoma incidence was 12.4% (Lee, Tsou, Tan, & Lu, 2005). In an Indian study T-cell lymphomas formed 16.2% of the total NHL (Naresh, Srinivas, & Soman, 2000). Previous Japanese studies have reported a higher proportion of T-cell lymphoma, accounting for approximately 32-38% of non-Hodgkin lymphoma (Kadin, Berard, Nanba, & Wakasa, 1983; Pathologists, 2000), but the recent findings in Japan show the decreased frequency of T/NK cell lineage (25%) (Aoki, et al., 2008). In endemic area for HTLV1 in Japan, T/NK-cell neoplasm accounted for a higher percentage of lymphoid neoplasm, in Kyushu (30%) and Okinawa (38%), compared with other areas of Japan (18–20%) (Aoki, et al., 2008). In one study in 1997 in Korea, in comparison with data reported in 1992, the proportion of T-lineage lymphoma was markedly decreased (25%). At that time, the T-lineage of lymphoma accounted for 35.2% of malignant lymphomas (Y. H. Ko, et al., 1998). It may be due to an increase in the frequency of B-cell lymphoma and an actual decrease in T/NK-cell, but the real reason remains unclear (Y. H. Ko, et al., 1998).

2.1.2 Histological subtype of non-Hodgkin's lymphoma

Diffuse Large B Cell Lymphoma. Among B-cell lymphomas, diffuse large B cell lymphoma (DLBCL) is the most common non-Hodgkin's Lymphoma representing approximately one third of all Non-Hodgkin's Lymphomas worldwide. This is one type of Non Hodgkin's Lymphoma in which the relative incidence does not seem to vary geographically (Mozaheb, et al., 2011). In almost all parts of the world this is the most frequent occurring non-Hodgkin's lymphoma (K. E. Hunt & Reichard, 2008). In some studies like a recent study in Mashhad, Iran (Mozaheb, et al., 2011) there was a higher rate of aggressive NHL specially, diffuse large B cell lymphoma which occurs more frequent than others. It may be related to the etiology of diffuse large B cell lymphoma such as immune deficient conditions and their treatments which in most instances caused aggressive non-Hodgkin's lymphoma, and we should consider that a comparative excess of DLBCL resulting in a deficit of follicular lymphoma. In addition genetic factors may have an important role in this difference.

Moreover it can represent the progression/transformation (referred to as secondary) of a less aggressive lymphoma, such as follicular lymphoma, marginal zone B-cell lymphoma, or nodular lymphocyte–predominant Hodgkin's lymphoma (K. E. Hunt & Reichard, 2008). All lymphoid cancers are more frequent in males than females among all age groups and in our study Diffuse large B cell lymphoma occurs about twice among men (Mozaheb, et al., 2011). This pattern suggests that the underlying environmental or behavioral factors are also important and must be more common in men. The most common subtypes of NHL in Various Geographic Locations are showed in table 1.

Follicular Lymphoma. Incidence rates of follicular lymphoma (FL) inexplicably vary markedly between Asian and Western countries (Biagi & Seymour, 2002). Follicular lymphoma was found more frequently in North America and Europe compared to other geographic sites (Kim, et al., 1992). The lowest rates of follicular lymphoma have been reported among Asian population (Anderson, et al., 1998; Mozaheb, et al., 2011). In addition, the risk was lower for the first generation of migrants from China and Japan into the US in comparison with the subsequent migrant generations, and in Japanese-Americans in Hawaii it was reported to be relatively high compared with that for native Japanese and close to the rate of North American Caucasians (Yanagihara, Blaisdell, Hayashi, & Lukes, 1989). The percentage of follicular lymphoma in our study in Mashhad, IRAN, was the lowest observed in any site (1.4%) (Mozaheb, et al., 2011), it was near the incidence rate of NHL in a previous study in Korea (1.6) (Y. H. Ko, et al., 1998). Although the exact reason for this difference is unknown, the results of several studies suggest differences in genes and environmental factors such as diet habits, infections and smoking, which plays an important role in follicular lymphoma, are responsible. Some cytogenetic changes such as a higher incidence of bcl-2 translocations are seen within follicular lymphoma among individuals in the US than for Asian populations (Shih & Liang, 1991). It conclude that a significant gradient exists in the *bcl-2* frequency between these FL populations, and therefore suggest that the relatively low incidence of FL in Asian populations is caused not by a lower frequency of *bcl-2* rearrangements in healthy populations but by distinct molecular pathways developing in different geographic regions that nonetheless culminate in FL, which is morphologically similar but molecularly distinct (Biagi & Seymour, 2002).

In a previous study in Japan the incidence rate of FL was 6.7% (Pathologists, 2000), but in a recent study in Japan they found a relatively high rate of FL (19%) similar to that of western countries (11-30%) (Aoki, et al., 2008). They suggest the following reasons for the relatively high rate of occurrence of follicular lymphomas. First, there have been improvements in the recognition and diagnostic accuracy for this subtype due to the development of comprehensive diagnostic methods including flow cytometry, immunohistochemistry, chromosome testing, gene testing and FISH. Second, the patients in their recent study comprised only initial visit cases and did not include consultation cases, because typical follicular lymphoma tends to be diagnosed at the initial visit and not during consultation, previous studies of patients in large hospitals may not have included initial visit cases and thus underestimated the frequency of follicular lymphoma. The third reason is the westernization of the Japanese lifestyle that may have contributed to an increase in follicular lymphoma (Aoki, et al., 2008). The rate of follicular lymphoma for Japanese- Americans in Hawaii was reported to be relatively high compared to that of native Japanese and close to the rate of North American Caucasians. A similar trend in completely follicular lymphoma has been reported for Korea. In one study in 1997 compared with the data reported in 1991, the increase in the relative frequency of Fl (1.6% vs 6.4%) over time suggests that the patterns of malignant lymphoma occurrence in the Republic of Korea might be gradually changing, probably due to westernization and other reasons which were mentioned previously (Y. H. Ko, et al., 1998).

Country/ year	IRAN	KOREA	TIWAN	INDIA	CHINA	THILAND	JAPAN	Asia	UK	USA
Lymphoma	2010	1991/1997	2000/2006	2000	2005	2004	2000/2008	1991	2001	2006
Total (No)	391	1165/1548	----/598		447	1983	3025/2260	9567	10580	
NHL %	92	94.7/94.7	----/93	2831	82.6%	92.1%	94/7/92.7		84.4	
B/T cell %		75/25	81.7/18.3 80.6/19.4	79/15.2	68.6/30.6	75/25	68/24, 65.2/25.4	76/24	93/7	90/10
DLBCL %	37.8	-/43.2	47.2/39	34	35.1	50.5	33/33	41.2	41.3	28
FL %	1.4	1.6/6.2	8.6/16.4	12.6	8.6	8.4	6.7/18.2	9.2	17	13
MCL %	2.2	-/1.5	----/4	3.4	2.6	1.5	2.7/2.7		3.7	2
MALT lymphoma%	2.2	-/0.6	6.1/5.6	8.2	11.7	5.5	8.4/4.2	8.7	3.6	3.7
SLL/CLL %	23.9	-/2.3		5.6	3.6	3.4	1.4/1.4			20
NK/T cell lymphoma %			----/12.4	0.9	30.6		1.5			5
Peripheral T cell lymphoma %	1.9	-/9.4	19.3/3.8	1.9	12	13.1	6.6/4.5	9.7	5.9	6
ATLL %	1.4	-/0.1		rare	rare		7.4/10		rare	rare
HL %	8	5.3/5.3	----/7		13.9	7.9	4.4/7.3		15.6	8

Table 1. The Most Common subtypes of NHL in Various Geographic Locations

In the analysis of 1983 cases of malignant lymphoma in Thailand shows that Bangkok has a significantly high frequency of FL, much higher than that the Central region. They suggest that the underlying reason for this observation is not known. Obviously, Metropolitan Bangkok has a more diverse population, migrated from various geographical locations, than people in the Central region (Sukpanichnant, 2004). A clinicopathological analysis of 598 Malignant Lymphomas in Taiwan during the period of 1995–2002 was retrieved, and their data showed a similar incidence of FL (16.4%) to that in Western countries (Lee, Tan, et al., 2005).

Mantle cell Lymphoma (MCL) in a case series has been between 2 and 10% of all NHL. The incidence rate is approximately similar around the world (table 1) and it is about 0.5 cases per 100000 person-year, with male to female ratio 2.3-2.5:1, and a median age at diagnosis is about 70 years. Relative association of MCL risk with *Borrelia burgdorferi* infection, family history of hematopoietic malignancies, and genetic variation in the interleukin 10 and tumor necrosis factor genes have been reported, but finding remain unconfirmed (Smedby & Hjalgrim., 2011).

T cell lymphomas are very complicated, based on WHO classification, there are various subtypes, and different types of them are different in various area of the world and some are extremely rare, occurring in a few patients per year throughout the world. Major T cell NHL types were reported in the international study in about 1300 patients 22 sites in different countries. Based on this study the most common subtype of T cell lymphoma in North American (NA) was PTCL (unspecified), in Europe was Angioimmunoblastic T cell lymphoma (AITL), and in Asia was Natural Killer T cell lymphoma (NKTCL) and ATLL (Foss, et al., 2011). This variation may reflect exposure or genetic susceptibility to pathogenic agents such as EBV and HTLV1 in Asian countries. Table 2 showed the major T cell subtype of NHL in different area (Vose, et al., 2008).

%	PTCL	AITL	Anaplastic	NKT CL	ATLL
NA	**34.4**	16	23.8	5.1	2
Europe	34.3	**28.7**	15.8	4.3	1
Asia	22.4	17.9	5.8	22.4	**25**

Table 2. Major subtype of T cell lymphoma by region

Generally speaking an increasing incidence in lymphoma reported from western countries is also seen in Asia, albeit at a lower rate (Shih & Liang, 1991).Essential differences in the incidence and distribution of major NHL subtypes among different geographic areas were seen which seems to be related to host, racial and environmental differences (Atichartakarn, et al., 1982), but these differences gradually changes in recent reports, this shows that the environmental factors probably are more important than the genes.

2.1.3 Extra-nodal non-Hodgkin Lymphoma

Non-Hodgkin lymphoma arises in lymphatic cell in other organs except lymphatic tissues, called extra-nodal lymphoma. Some authors believe that, specific local factors may play an etiologic role in the development of lymphomas at certain extra-nodal sites e.g., Helicobacter pylori infection is associated with primary gastric lymphoma, but not with lymphoma at other sites (Parsonnet, et al., 1994b; Wotherspoon, et al., 1993). There are geographical and ethnic differences in the incidence of extra-nodal lymphomas (Newton, Ferlay, Beral, & Devesa, 1997).

The frequency of primary extra-nodal NHL in Asia Varied from 28.5 to 45% (Shih & Liang, 1991), it is similar to Europe, but slightly more common than united states: Denmark 37% (d'Amore, et al., 1991), India 22% (Advani, et al., 1990), Hawaii-Japanese 34% (Yanagihara, et al., 1989), Lebanon 44% (P. Salem, et al., 1986), Chinese Hong Kong 28% (Ho, Todd, Loke, Ng, & Khoo, 1984), USA 25% (Freeman, Berg, & Cutler, 1972), Italy 48%, East Germany 47% (Newton, et al., 1997).

The incidence of extra-nodal NHL in Western countries has increased substantially in the last 40 years. This may be due to improved diagnostic procedures (particularly in gastrointestinal and brain lymphomas) and changes in classification systems, but the change is real and the AIDS epidemic in the 1980s does not completely explain this rise (Groves, Linet, Travis, & Devesa, 2000). The etiology of extra-nodal lymphomas appears to be multifactorial and includes immune suppression, infections both viral and bacterial, and exposure to pesticides and other environmental agents (Zucca, 2008). True geographic differences are, however, present for example, the incidence of Epstein–Barr virus and human T-cell lymphotropic virus 1-associated with T-cell lymphomas is higher in Asia than in Europe and North America (Zucca, 2008).

One study, which was done in 39 centers in 14 countries (USA, Europe, Asian) reported the most frequent extra-nodal sites of lymphoma are stomach and skin, followed by small intestine and tonsil (Newton, et al., 1997). In recent study extra-nodal lymphoma in Japan, was seen in 27% of cases, but in previous Japanese series it was 60% (Izumo, 1996). DLBCL was the most common type of extra-nodal lymphoma lesion primarily biopsied/resected (60%). The ear–nose–throat region (7.2%), gastrointestinal tract (6.0%), soft tissue (2.8%) and skin (2.6%) was reported in Japanese study (Aoki, et al., 2008). A clinical analysis in Republic Korea revealed that the rate of extra-nodal lymphoma exceeded that of lymph node lymphoma (63.3% vs. 36.7%) (Y.-H. Ko, et al., 1998). As in other Far East countries, Korea has a relatively high rate of angiocentric lymphomas, which more than 70% of them arise in the nose and paranasal sinus. EBV was positive in 80% of nasal and paranasal angiocentric lymphomas. (Ko & Lee, 1994, 1996). In a study in Thailand, extra-nodal involvement was found in 1072 of 1826 cases (58.7%) of NHL. The frequency of B-cell NHL in cases of NHL involving extra-nodal sites was 72.9%, whereas the frequency of nodal B-cell NHL was 78.0%. Thus, a higher frequency of T-cell NHL involving extra-nodal sites and a higher frequency of B-cell NHL involving lymph nodes were significant when compared to the overall NHL ($P < 0.05$). In the Thailand study, among the extra-nodal sites involved in NHL, the upper aerodigestive tract (including the tonsils, sinonasal region, oral cavity, and nasopharynx) was the most common site. The second most common site was the gastrointestinal tract, including the stomach and intestine (Sukpanichnant, 2004). These studies shows that extra-nodal NK/T cell lymphoma is more prevalent in far east and is closely related to EBV infection (Jaffe, 1999; Jaffe, et al., 1996).

Immunoproliferative small intestinal disease (IPSID) or α heavy chain disease is mostly found in young adults of low socioeconomic class in developing countries or in indigent immigrant population within western countries. Relatively high incidence rates of small intestinal lymphoma have been reported before in the Middle east, Mediterranean region, South and central Africa, Mexico, and South America, but is rare in Southeast Asia (Pramoolsinsap, Kurathong, Atichartakarn, & Nitiyanand, 1993).

IPSID was one of the most common small intestinal malignancy in the Middle East (Azar, 1962). Early infectious stress in infancy and chronic antigenic stimulation along with genetic factors are probably important in the pathogenesis of IPSID (Khojasteh, Haghshenass, & Haghighi, 1983). It showed that Campylobacter jejune were present in 5/7 cases of IPSID in one study and 12/27 (47%) cases in other and 14/87 (16%) cases of other intestinal lymphoma. Eradication of the organism with antibiotics lead to complete remission of IPSID (Du, 2007).

In one series of 161 patients with IPSID in Shiraz (Iran), they observed a dramatic decrease in the incidence of the disease over the past decade. After the Islamic revolution in Iran, improving sanitation in villages was one of the priorities of the many health strategies in Iran. Access to sanitary drinking water in rural areas increased from 35% before 1988 to 80% a decade later. Vaccination programs increased dramatically after the Islamic revolution, reaching more than 90% of children. Local health facilities increased significantly during the first two decades after the revolution. They suggest that improvement of health in general and decreasing childhood gastroenteritides in particular has resulted in a decrease in the incidence of IPSID. This report highlights the almost complete disappearance of a malignant disease from a region where it was once very common. This changes probably related to changes in environmental factors, decreasing exposure to infectious agents (Lankarani, et al., 2005). Other preliminary recent epidemiological data has also shown a decrease in the incidence of this disease in endemic areas; therefore, environmental factors are suspected to play an important role in its pathogenesis (P. A. Salem & Estephan, 2005).

2.2 Epidemiologic etiology

2.2.1 Immunodeficiency and autoimmune disease

Immunodeficiency, including acquired conditions and congenital disease, is the strongest factor known to increase NHL risk (Chiu & Weisenburger, 2003). About 25% of patients with congenital immunodeficiency syndromes such as Wiskott-Aldrich syndrome, ataxia telangiectasia and severe combined immunodeficiency, will develop tumors during their lifetime, which NHL accounting for 50% of them. It seems that these patients unable to promptly eliminate respiratory and gastrointestinal pathogens due to defects in formation of specific protective antibodies and are susceptible to chronic antigenic stimulation (Filipovich, Mathur, Kamat, & Shapiro, 1992).

High rate of NHL also have been observed among individual with iatrogenic immunosuppression (i.e. organ or blood stem cell transplantation recipients, long term survivors of Hodgkin's lymphoma), variety of autoimmune disease, and Acquired immunodeficiency syndrome (AIDS). Although immunosuppressive drug use in the treatment of these conditions may cause an increase in NHL incidence, evidence suggests that the persistent inflammatory activity of the autoimmune process may have a direct relation with increase risk of lymphomagenesis. One study showed that these conditions may be accompanied by impaired T-cell function, which interferes with an immune response to virus and emerging malignant cells. NHL due to secondary immunodeficiency is associated with the presence of EBV infection, and tumors are characterized by high grad, and proclivity for extra-nodal sites (Fisher & Fisher, 2004). Based on these data immunodeficiency may be more common in some area which aggressive lymphoma is more common such as Asian countries.

Autoimmune disorders that are strongly associated with NHL are Sjogren's syndrome, systemic lupus erythematosus (SLE), rheumatoid arthritis, and celiac disease (CD). There is no evidence to support excess risk of NHL in other autoimmune disorders. One study demonstrated a 25-fold increase in the risk of NHL among persons with highly inflammatory RA as compared to a similar group having low inflammatory disease; this risk was independent of treatment (Fisher & Fisher, 2004). Finding in the other study suggests that the excess risk of NHL in RA patients may be a result of the disease or its treatment, rather than shared genetic susceptibility (Ekström, et al., 2003; Kinlen, 1992).

Celiac disease is an autoimmune digestive disease which is caused by an immune response to the protein gluten. Untreated CD is associated with increased risk of lymphoma, mostly with origins from gastrointestinal mucosa. The pathogenesis behind this association is not fully understood, but greater permeability to environmental carcinogenesis, release of proinflammatory cytokines , and chronic antigenic stimulation are among the suggested

mechanisms. Also a correlation between the duration of gluten exposure and the incidence of lymphoma has been found. The relative risk of lymphoma is reduced by a gluten free diet (Jafroodi, Zargari, & Hoda, 2009). In a US cohort study, an increased risk of NHL was reported in patients with celiac disease (SMR = 9.1, 95% CI: 4.7-13.0). Similarly, a relative risk of 5.8 (95% CI: 1.58-14.86) was observed in a UK cohort (Alexander, et al., 2007).
The incidence of CD is increasing among certain populations in Africa (Saharawui population), Asia (India), and the Middle East (Cummins & Roberts Thomson, 2009). In Asian populations, including the Japanese, CD and the associated NHL have been supposed to be quite rare, and studies concerning the frequency of CD or its relationship with NHL are scarce. A Japanese case report describes a Japanese middle-aged man with intestinal diffuse large B-cell lymphoma associated with CD. Following multi-combined chemotherapy, the patient's lymphoma has received complete response, and his GI symptoms have improved with a gluten free diet (Makishima, et al., 2006). Also an Iranian case report describes a child with Hodgkin's disease and sever atopic dermatitis associated with CD (Arellano, et al., 2009). These cases suggest that the possibility of CD and its association with lymphoid malignancy should be kept in mind, even in Asian populations.

2.2.2 Infectious agents

Epidemiological studies pointed towards a viral and bacterial etiology on NHL. In this part we discuss about some of them which are more important.

Epstein-Barr virus (EBV). The *Epstein-Barr virus* has a worldwide distribution, which greater than 80% of people over the age of 30 are infected. Once *EBV* infection has occurred, it remains for the lifetime of the individual (Serraino, et al., 2005). Infection with this virus usually occurs in children, but can also occur in adolescence or adulthood. *EBV* asymptomatically establishes persistent infections however, due to effective immune control, only a minority of infected carriers develop spontaneous *EBV*-associated lymphoma (Heller, Steinherz, Portlock, & Munz, 2007). Infection by *EBV* is more common in developing countries where sanitation, hygiene, and cooking are not as sterile as nations such as the USA (Evans & Kaslow, 1997).

EBV has a unique set of genes that causes a growth activation of the B-cells that are infected. Sometime the growth activating genes may cause the infected B-cell to transform into cancer in certain people. The most common type of lymphoma caused by EBV are T-cell lymphoma, Post-transplant lymphoma, AIDS associated lymphoma, Burkitt's lymphoma (BL), and Hodgkin's lymphoma. These *EBV*-associated neoplasms are characterized by peculiar geographic distributions and distinctive epidemiologic features (Serraino, et al., 2005) .

In the endemic areas of Africa, BL is the leading childhood cancer, occurring as many as 4-5 cases per 100000. In areas where *EBV* infection occurs at a very early age and malaria is holoendemic, the incidence of association with BL is highest. In African countries in the lymphoma belt there is a very high association between BL and *EBV* (90%). However, in France and the US, the rare cases of BL are only associated with *EBV* in 10-15% of all reported cases (Frimpong-Boateng).

Induced immunosuppretion, necessary for the transplant to be accepted, leads to a loss of control over *EBV* infection. The lymphoma that is developed contains parts of the latent *EBV* genome. About half of NHL tumors accompanying *HIV1* infections are *EBV* positive.

These lymphoma are grouped into several categories: small non-cleaved-cell lymphoma, diffuse large cell lymphoma, anaplastic large cell lymphoma, and body-cavity based lymphoma (Gaidano, et al., 1996).

Several studies showed the association of Asian T cell lymphoma and evidence of *EBV* infections. Asian T-cell lymphomas are different from Western T-cell lymphoma, and are also associated with increased levels of cytokine production, including tumor necrosis factor (Dutcher, 2003). Aggressive NK-cell LGL leukemia is usually a rapidly progressive disorder associated with EBV, with a higher prevalence in Asia and South America (Sokol & Loughran, 2006).

Human T-Cell Lymphotrophic virus-1 (HTLV1). HTLV1, the first human retrovirus to be discovered, is estimated to infect 10-20 million people worldwide (De Thé & Bomford, 1993). Infection with *HTLV1* is strongly related to adult T-cell leukemia/ Lymphoma (Hinuma, et al., 1981) and *HTLV1* associated myelopathy (Morgan, Mora, Rodgers-Johnson, & Char, 1989). *HTLV1* is primarily transmitted by breast feeding, blood transfusion, Sharing of needles and sexual transmission. The predominance of vertical transmission results in clustering cases in familial or geographically discrete groups. It is endemic in southern Japan, the Caribbean, the Melanesian island, Papua New Guinea, the Middle East, central and southern Africa, and South America. In these endemic areas, seroprevalences range are different from about one percent in Mashhad in southeast Iran (1-3%) (Abbaszadegan, et al., 2003; Tarhini, et al., 2009) to 30 percent in rural Miyazaki in southern Japan. In table 3 we can see the prevalence rate of *HTLV1* in different countries.

Population *HTLV-I* seroprevalence increases with age and is twice as high in females. In Jamaica 17·4% of women over 70 and 9·1% of men over 70 were seropositive. In Japan, *HTLV-I* seroprevalence in persons over 80 was 50% in females and 30% in males. This gender difference usually emerges after 30 years of age and may be related to more efficient transmission of the virus from males to females in the sexually active years (Yamaguchi, 1994). Seroprevalence tends to increase with age and women are nearly twice as likely to be infected as men (Mueller, Okayama, Stuver, & Tachibana, 1996).

HTLV1 shows little genomic variability during the course of infection and between patients in the same geographic area. Mother/child and spouse pairs from Okinawa (Japan) have been shown to be infected with highly conserved viruses upon direct sequencing of viral genome (Kakuda, Ikematsu, Chong, Hayashi, & Kashiwagi, 2002). Studies in France (Gessain, Gallo, & Franchini, 1992) the Solomon Islands (Nerurkar, Song, Saitou, Melland, & Yanagihara, 1993) and Zaire (LIU, et al., 1994) have shown similarly low genomic variability based upon the less accurate sequencing of PCR products. Therefore, small strain variation is recognized between geographic areas. Risk of infection is higher (fourfold increase) in breast fed infants than in those who are bottle fed (HIRATA, et al., 1992). A longer duration of breast feeding increase transmission risk (Li, et al., 2004). Another important risk factor is provirus load in breast milk.

The infection is usually asymptomatic in the beginning and the disease typically manifests later in life; therefore silent transmission occurs. Since there are no prospects of vaccines and screening of blood banks and prenatal care settings are not universal, transmission is active in many areas such as parts of Africa, South and Central America, the Caribbean region, Asia, and Melanesia (Goncalves, et al., 2010).

country	Sample size	Prevalence of HTLV1	Group
rural Miyazaki, southern Japan		Up to 30%	General population
Iran (Mashhad)	1653	2.1	General population
Lebanon	3529	0.06	Blood donors
Taiwan	3700000	0.06	Blood donors
Korea	9281	0.13	Blood donors
Jamaica		3-6%	General population
Caribbean		6%	General population
Curacao	2524	1.92%	General population
Papua New Guinea	1221	0-14.6%	General population
Argentina	2082	1.9%	General population
U.S	1700000	0.01	Blood donors
Italy	14598	0.03	Blood donors
Germany	100852	0	Blood donors
U.K	570609	0.001	Blood donors

Table 3. Prevalence of *HTLV1* in different countries

Adult T-cell lymphoma leukemia (ATL) is an aggressive lymphoproliferative malignancy, with short survival in its acute form and an incidence of less than 5% in *HTLV-1*-infected people (Shimoyama, 1991). The cumulative incidence of ATL among Japanese HTLV1 carrier is about 2.5% (3-5% in male and 1-2% in female). Although women are more infected with HTLV1, but ATL is more common in men, it shows that other factors also should be responsible. At first ATL was described in Japan and later in the Caribbean region and South America (Uchiyama, Yodoi, Sagawa, Takatsuki, & Uchino, 1977). In the United States and Europe, ATL was diagnosed in immigrants from regions of endemicity. ATL occurs at least 20 to 30 years after the onset of *HTLV-1* infection and is more common in adult males. Individuals infected in childhood may be at a higher risk of developing ATL (Pawson, et al., 1998). The occurrence of ATL in the fourth decade predominates in Brazil and in Jamaica (Proietti, Carneiro-Proietti, Catalan-Soares, & Murphy, 2005), but in Japan, the fifth decade of life is predominant for the occurrence of ATL (Shimoyama, 1991). Possibly, local factors play a role in disease pathogenesis.

Helicobacter pylori (*H. pylori*). *Helicobacter pylori* colonizes gastric mucosa, leading to chronic Gastric infection, and induce peptic ulcer disease and gastric carcinoma, also may cause B-cell lymphomas, particularly mucosa-associated lymphoid tissue (MALT) tumors in the stomach, with the association being strongest in early lesion (Chiu & Weisenburger, 2003; Zucca, et al., 2000). In developing countries, where over 90% of the population may be infected, *H. pylori* infection usually occurs during childhood with chronic infection continuing throughout adulthood (Pounder & Ng, 1995). In contrast, although in developed countries the overall prevalence generally remains lower than in developing countries, the prevalence is low among children and rises with age in adults. *H. pylori* has been detected in more than 90% of patients with low-grade gastric MALT lymphoma, and in 40-75% of high-grade gastric lymphomas (Boot & Jong, 2002).

Direct fecal oral transmission is predominant in industrialized countries whereas other transmission routes such as contamination of water may be more important in developing countries. The bacteria is transmitted within families in early childhood (Farinha & Gascoyne, 2005). Parsonnet *et al.* (Parsonnet, et al., 1994a) and Vineis *et al.* (Vineis, et al., 1999) reported a significant positive association between *H. pylori* infection and risk of gastric NHL but not non-gastric NHL. Greater than 60% of MALT lymphomas regress with *H. pylori* eradication following treatment with antibiotics (R. Hunt, Sumanac, & Huang, 2001). Because the US prevalence of *H. pylori* infection is low and declining, *H. pylori* most likely did not play a significant role in the overall rising trend of NHL incidence in the US (Alexander, et al., 2007). H. pylori infection is more common in Asian countries, therefore as we can see in table 1, MALT lymphoma in most Asian countries are more common than western countries.

Hepatitis C Virus (HCV). Hepatitis C virus infection has been reported to be a prevalent disease since the second half of the 20th century (Strickland, 2006). Infection in different parts of Asia is similar, with an average seroprevalence of hepatitis C antibody less than 2.5% in the general population. The major routes of *HCV* transmission in Asia have been through blood transfusions and intravenous drug use, similar to the other countries. Other possible routes of transmission are medical intervention, tattooing, acupuncture, vertical and sexual transmission, accidental needle-stick and household contact. It is believed that *HCV* is still spreading in some areas of Asia because of the lack of routine screening of donated blood (Kao & Chen, 2000). *HCV* has been linked to lymphomagenesis in people with and without type II mixed cryoglobulinemia (Saadoun, Landau, Calabrese, & Cacoub, 2007). Increasing evidence indicates that the association between *HCV* infection and lymphoma may be due to viral infection related chronic antigenic stimulation. The chronic inflammation pathway would be consistent with the association between *HCV* and several types of lymphomas and with the regression of some lymphoma after eradicating the *HCV* infection (Hermine, et al., 2002; Vallisa, et al., 2005). One study showed that the association between *HCV* infection and risk of NHL subtypes included mostly countries with low background *HCV* prevalence. This study showed increased risks of DLBCL, marginal zone lymphoma and lymphoplasmacytic lymphoma associated with *HCV* infection (De Sanjose, et al., 2008). Another study revealed that there is no association between NHL and *HCV* infection (King, Wilkes, & DIAZ ARIAS, 1998). Prevalence of *HCV* in series of patients with NHL in studies from different countries was various, it was more common in Italy and Japan (Armstrong, et al., 2006). Based on these studies there are marked regional differences in the prevalence of *hepatitis C* infection in non-Hodgkin lymphoma. It seems that other factors including genetics, race, hormonal, and immunologic factors are required for malignant transformation. Several studies showed the frequency was higher in older women. Lymphoma associated with *HCV* infection more frequently present as primary extra-nodal lymphoma, especially in the liver, spleen and salivary glands (Armstrong, et al., 2006).

Human Immunodeficiency Virus (HIV). The relationship between human immunodeficiency *virus*/acquired immunodeficiency syndrome (HIV/AIDS) and the risk of developing NHL has been observed with strong positive associations in numerous studies. (Hooper, Holman, Clarke, & Chorba, 2001; Ragni, et al., 1993). The relative risk of NHL among persons infected with *HIV* has been reported to be over 100, (Coté, et al., 1997; Goedert, et al., 1998) with the greatest risk for B-cell lymphomas and high-grade histology (Coté, et al., 1997; A. Swerdlow, 2003). Chronic antigenic stimulation and immune deficiency may be responsible for the increased risk of *NHL* among *HIV*-infected persons. *HIV* may act by inducing immunodysregulation, affecting genes responsible for cell regulation and failing to control other viruses, which may result in opportunistic infection and replication of oncogenic viruses (Coté, et al., 1997). In AIDS patients NHL has been reported in approximately 2-3% of patients with AIDS, but AIDS accounts only for a small fraction of all NHL (Biggar & Rabkin, 1992; Rabkin & Yellin, 1994). In an international collaboration on *HIV* and cancer, incidence data from 23 prospective studies were used to compare incidence rates of NHL in *HIV*-infected persons in 1997–1999 with those in 1992–1996 (Coutinho, 2000). The incidence rates for NHL declined from 6.2 per 1,000 person-years to 3.6 per 1,000 person-years. Grulich *et al.* (Grulich, et al., 2001) reported a significantly lower relative risk of NHL in persons with *HIV* in the period of highly active antiretroviral therapy (HAART) availability than in the period immediately prior (RR = 0.58, 95% CI: 0.36–0.92) *(Alexander, et al., 2007).*

In one study in Japan the incidence of AIDS-related lymphoma detected at autopsy was higher in Japan (27%) than in the US (12%). However, histological subtypes of AIDS-related lymphoma in Japan seem to be similar to those in western countries and DLBCL is also the most common subtype of AIDS-related lymphoma in Japan. A large number of AIDS-related lymphoma cases were categorized into EBV-associated opportunistic lymphoma in Japan. The incidences detected by autopsy did not differ statistically between the pre-HAART era and the HAART era ($P = 0.31$), and the histological subtype of DLBCL was stable in both the pre-HAART era (78%) and the HAART era (77%) . In contrast, they found an increase in patients with BL from 2% in the pre-HAART era to13% in the HAART era. (Hishima, et al., 2006). Despite the high rate of human immunodeficiency virus infection in Thailand, only 5 cases of documented AIDS-associated lymphoma were noted in one study (5 of 389 NHL; 1.3%). Similarly, Kaposi's sarcoma is not common in AIDS patients in Thailand. The underlying reason for this unique feature of AIDS-related lymphoma in Thailand is not known and further investigation is needed (Sukpanichnant, et al., 1998). In one study in India the proportional incidence ratio (PIR) for NHL was significantly increased in *HIV* era (PIR in males = 17.1, 95%CI 13.33-21.84, females = 10.3, 95%CI 6.10-17.41), and their finding was similar to that reported by other studies (Dhir, et al., 2008). In one study in Singapore when comparing the age-standardized rates for males and female in 1998 - 2002 which are 8.2 and 5.0 per 100,000 respectively compared with 7.5 and 4.4 per 100,000 in 1993-1997 and 3.1 and 1.9 per 100,000 in 1968-1972, this may be partly due to *HIV*/AIDS, changes in pathological classification and improved diagnostic capabilities (Seow & Registry, 2004). Except for one study in Thailand, *HIV*/AIDS lead to increase incidence rate of lymphoma in both eastern and western countries.

Human herpesvirus-8 (HHV-8). Human herpesvirus-8, is endemic in regions of the Mediterranean and Africa (Kamiyama, et al., 2004), but the seroprevalence of *HHV-8* which has been studied in Malaysia, India, Sri Lanka, Thailand, Trinidad, Jamaica and the USA, in both healthy individuals and those infected with *HIV*, was found to be low in these countries in both the healthy and the *HIV*-infected populations (Ablashi, et al., 1999). *HHV-8* is generally accepted to be associated with development of primary effusion lymphoma (PEL), a rare B-cell lymphoma that almost exclusively affects *HIV*-positive patients (Ascoli, et al., 2002). However this lymphoma is often associated with both *HHV-8* and *EBV*, limiting the understanding of the pathogenic role of *HHV-8* (Ascoli, et al., 2002). Within B-cell lymphomas, however, *HHV-8* infection was associated significantly and positively with risk of lymphoplasmacytic lymphoma (OR = 4.47, 95% CI: 1.34–14.85) or low-grade B-cell lymphoma and lymphoma not otherwise specified (OR = 5.82, 95% CI: 1.07-31.73) (Feuillard, et al., 1997).

Simian Virus 40 (SV40). Simian Virus 40 is the most well characterized member of the Polyomaviridae family, and is closely related to two human polyomaviruses (Poulin & DeCaprio, 2006).It induces an inapparent infections in immunocompetent hosts, but can produces pathologic effects in immunocompromised individuals through the destruction of infected cells (Imperiale, 2000).*Simian virus 40*, an agent that infects *Asian* ma- caques, contaminated the early poliovirus vaccines used in the United States, Europe, and other region during the mass immunization program for poliovirus in the late 1950 and early 1960 (Strickler, et al., 2003). The Norwegian study shows that between 1953 and 1997, the incidence rate of lymphoproliferative diseases increased about 3-fold in both males and females (Thu, et al., 2006), and the other study report that *polyomavirus SV40* is significantly associated with non-Hodgkin lymphoma in *HIV-1*-infected and *HIV-1*-uninfected patients and might have a role in the development of these hematological malignancies (Vilchez, et al., 2002). These observations suggest that *polyomavirus SV40* might be causing infections in human beings long after the use of the contaminated vaccines. There is no documented study around it in Asian countries.

2.2.3 Genetic factors and family history

Family history and genetic factors increase risk of NHL in people whose relatives previously were diagnosed with NHL, but hereditary factors are hypothesized to account only for a small percentage of NHL and are unlikely to explain the increase in NHL incidence. Tumor suppressor genes, oncogenes and DNA repair genes may play a role in NHL carcinogenesis, and some genes may interact with environmental exposures that affect NHL risk (Fisher & Fisher, 2004). In a US multicenter case-control study, Chatterjee *et. al* showed *(Chatterjee, et al., 2004)* the strongest associations were found among siblings (HR = 7.6, 95% CI: 0.98–58.8) and male relatives (HR = 6.2, 95% CI: 0.77–50.0) of NHL cases. For a parental history of histopathologically concordant lymphoma, the strongest associations with lymphoma risk among offspring were found for B-cell lymphoma (SIR = 11.8, 95% CI: 2.2–34.8) and follicular lymphoma (SIR = 6.1, 95% CI: 1.1–18.0) *(Altieri, Bermejo, & Hemminki, 2005).*

Several genetic polymorphisms associated with the risk of NHL suggest that single nucleotide polymorphisms (SNPs) in tumor necrosis factor (TNF) and interleukin-10 (IL10) are associated with risk of NHL, especially diffuse large B –cell lymphoma. Relatively few studies have examined the potential interaction between germline susceptibility and environmental or lifestyle factors in the etiology of NHL (Alexander, et al., 2007). The mechanism (s) by which genetic predisposition or gene-environment interactions may enhance or reduce the risk of developing NHL remains a largely unexplored area of research (Alexander, et al., 2007).

2.2.4 Lifestyle and personal and environmental factors

Results from studies that evaluated lifestyle and personal factors are generally inconsistent, with few exceptions. Alcohol consumption appears to be inversely associated with NHL, based primarily on results from case–control studies (Chiu, et al., 1999; Chiu, et al., 2002). Further evidences from cohort studies are needed. Smoking does not appear to play an important role in the etiology of NHL overall; however, it has relation with follicular lymphoma (Bracci & Holly, 2005). Fish intake has been associated consistently with a nonsignificantly decreased risk of NHL in several studies (Zhang, et al., 1999), but intake of omega-3 fatty acids from fish was not associated with reduced risk of NHL in one cohort study (Purdue, Bassani, Klar, Sloan, & Kreiger, 2004). Several but not all studies have reported positive association with red meat intake. Data are limited, and results have not been consistent, for estimates of associations with specific types of red meat or with preparation or cooking methods (Chang, et al., 2006; Ward, et al., 1994). Saturated fat intake was associated positively (Chang, et al., 2006), however vegetable consumption was associated inversely, with NHL risk in most studies (Chang, et al., 2005; Mozaheb & Aledawood, 2011). Biological mechanisms for these dietary factors have not been established. Neither obesity nor physical activity has been associated consistently with NHL (Alexander, et al., 2007).

Certain workers have a slightly increased risk of developing NHL, including farmers; pesticide applicator; miller; meat worker; wood and forestry worker; chemists; painters; mechanics; printers; and worker in the petroleum, rubber, plastics, and synthetics industries (Alexander, et al., 2007). Some of these occupations are more common in Asian countries such as farmers, pesticide applicator, wood worker, worker in petroleum; on the other hand exposure is more because of low educational program in these places. Also There is significant relationship between hair dye use and NHL risk (Altekruse, Jane Henley, & Thun, 1999).

3. Hodgkin's Lymphoma

Hodgkin lymphoma is a neoplastic disease of the lymphoid tissue characterized by the present of multinucleated giant cell of B-cell origin, known as Red-Stenberg cell, in background of numerous reactive lymphocyte (Classical, 2009). HL is less common in Asians, especially at the young adult ages. There is incidence variation by age, social class, geographic location in HL. Thus, the comparison of HL rates in Asian and western countries could inform the relative importance of environmental factors and genetic to disease etiology.

3.1 Descriptive epidemiology

The epidemiology of Hodgkin's lymphoma is complex. Hodgkin Lymphoma demonstrates different histologic findings, clinical presentation, and outcome. Hodgkin's lymphoma is relatively uncommon, but at young adult ages it is one of the most common malignancies. Increasingly there is a great difference in incidence between developing and western developed countries. In developing countries, the disorder appear predominantly during childhood and its incidence decreases with age (Thomas, Re, Zander, Wolf, & Diehl, 2002). The annual age adjusted incidence rates of 2.8 and 2.4 per 100,000 in the USA and UK respectively (RiesLAG, HankeyBF, & HarrasA, 1994).

Hodgkin's lymphoma has been reported to be rare in Asians. One study in the US from 2000 to 2007, 16,710 cases of HL reported that black and Asians had low incidence (black/white incidence rate ratio (IRR) 0.86, $P<0.01$; Asian/White IRR 0.43, $P<0.01$). The bimodal pattern of incidence was less prominent for black males. Asian and black presented at a mean age of 38 years compared to 42 years for Whites ($P<.001$) (Pareen, Alison, Neha, & Christopher, 2010).There are few studies in exploring the relative contributions of environmental and hereditary etiology of Hodgkin's lymphoma, and individual risk factors in an Asian population. The other study which compared HL incidence rate in Japanese, Chinese,

Filipino, and Asian Indian in the US and in Asia reports HL incidence rates were quite low in all Asian subgroups but approximately double in US Asian. The consistently low rates of HL in Asians suggest genetic resistance to the disease development, possibly associated with HLA type. In addition environmental and lifestyle differences between the USA and Asia are important. In some study from Eastern Asia and among Chinese immigrants in North America indicate increasing incidence trends for HL being associated with westernization (Caporaso, Goldin, Anderson, & Landgren, 2009). International and inter-ethnic differences and risk factor patterns in case-control data, implicate environmental influences in the etiology of HL (Glaser & Hsu, 2002).

Incidence rate of HL are usually grater in male than in female (Correa & O'Conor, 1971). In western countries the young adult peak largely consist of nodular sclerosis tumors, whereas the rise at older ages are largely mixed cellularity and lymphocytic-depleted histology (Spitz, et al., 1986). Hodgkin's lymphoma tends to be more common in young adult with higher socio-economic classes (Correa & O'Conor, 1971). Pattern of low social class determinants in children and older adult with HL, the age groups at risk for mixed cellularity (MC), support involvement of underling infectious agent given intense exposure, and EBV is a likely candidate based on its high prevalence in these groups (Glaser & Jarrett, 1996). Based on different studies the most common subtype of HL in the most Asian countries such as Iran, Korea, Thailand, Japan is mixed cellularity and relative paucity of NS subtype, particularly in males (Glaser & Hsu, 2002), which seems to be related to the etiologic factors (environment and/or inheritance) of disease. Subtypes of HL in different countries are showed in table 4.

HL	Iran No (%)	Korea No (%)	Thailand No (%)	Taiwan	Japans No (%)	US %	UK %
NS	10 (31.2)	26 (31.7)	58 (36.9)	29 (69)	70 (42.4)	Up to 08	60
MC	16 (50)	38 (46.3)	64 (40.8)	2 (4.7)	51 (31)	<10	15
LD	3 (9.3)	6 (7.3)	14 (8.9)	0	8 (5)	1	rare
LP	1 (3.1)	4 (2.6)	18 (11.5)	2 (4.7)	18 (11)	6	10
NLPHD	2 (6.3)	8 (9.8)	3 (1.9)	3 (7.1)	8 (5)	5	5

Table 4. Subtypes of Hodgkin's disease in various countries

A shift from MC-dominant histologic subtype of HL was observed over 20-year period within Japan, particularly in young adults (Aozasa, Ueda, Tamai, & Tsujimura, 1986). As NS and MC have been shown to have different environmental cofactors, including socioeconomic status and degree of *EBV* tumor-cell presence, geographic variation in HL is likely to reflect change in socioeconomically determined exposures whenever possible.

3.2 Etiologic epidemiology

The differences in descriptive epidemiology of Hodgkin's lymphoma between children, young adults and older adults may reflect differences in etiology between these age groups.

3.2.1 Environment

Infections. Systemic analysis of epidemiological data pointed towards an infectious agent as a potential cause for Hodgkin's lymphoma. Recognition of an association of infectious mononucleosis with Hodgkin's disease predate the discovery of **EBV** (Richard F. Ambinder, 2007). Investigators have reported that EBV infectious mononucleosis is associated with a lifelong "immunologic scar" (Sauce, et al., 2007). The statistical analysis suggested that HL tended to occur 2.9 years after infectious mononucleosis (R.F. Ambinder, 2007). Remarkably, the change in lymphocyte cell population is sustained over years or longer (Richard F. Ambinder, 2007). There are new insights into infectious mononucleosis and disturbances in cellular immunity, new insight relating to the role that viruses may play in molecular pathogenesis of HL, an emerging appreciation of the increased incidence of HL in *HIV* and its relationship to immune suppression (Richard F. Ambinder, 2007). A role for suppression T cell suggested in the 1970s, and increasing evidence shows a role for this cells in suppressing antitumor immune responses (Hjalgrim, et al., 2007).

In western countries, about 50% of all cases of classical HL are *EBV* positive, means the virus is carried within the tumor cells. Detection of *EBV* in tumors in these region are least common in young adult disease. In some parts of Latin America, Africa, and Asia, the percentage is much higher with the percentage in children approaching 90- 100% (Glaser, et al., 1997; Zarate Osorno, Roman, Kingma, Meneses Garcia, & Jaffe, 1995). The MC subtype harboring *EBV* DNA in up to 70% of cases and the NS subtype being positive in 15-30% of cases (Brousset, et al., 1991). Also detection of *EBV* in HL in most Asian countries are less in young adults and are more detectable in children and older ages. Because of these differences infectious cofactors other than *EBV* have been suggested, but no consensus in support of any other particular association have emerge (Wilson, et al., 2007).

As we mentioned *EBV* induce immune suppression, and in an *EBV* positive person, MC subtype is more common (like *HIV* positive), therefore in MC subtype of HL, which is more common in Asian countries, immunodeficiency has more important role in comparison with other subtypes.

HIV. Hodgkin's lymphoma in the setting of *HIV* has distinctive features and is usually associated with EBV infection (Glaser, et al., 2003). HL in patients with *HIV* tends to present at an advanced stage with associated B symptoms and extra-nodal involvement and is most often a mixed cellularity subtype. Model fitting suggested that for persons with AIDS with moderate immunosuppretion at the onset of AIDS, HL risk was 15-fold higher than in the general population. Lower CD4 counts were associated with less risk, the risk fall as CD4 count fall (R.F. Ambinder, 2007).

3.2.2 Inheritance

The risk of developing HL among family member of patients affected by HL increase from three-to nine-fold (Haim, Cohen, & Robinson, 1982). One study showed a significant association between HL and parental consanguinity and pointed to the possible etiologic role of recessive inheritance (Abramson, Pridan, Sacks, Avitzour, & Peritz, 1978).

The relative risk for HL among first degree relatives of cases compared with controls was 3.1. Relative risks were higher in males compared with females, and in siblings of cases compared with parents and offspring. Identifying inherited susceptibility genes is an important step towards defining the pathway leading to development of HL and understanding its etiology. There are many studies of somatic mutations in HL tumor cells, but although there are associations with HLA types, specific germline genes causing susceptibility have not yet been identified. On the other hand it is not known whether or how extrinsic risk factors interact with genetic susceptibility (Goldin, et al., 2005).

Oza et al. in the single study of HL-HLA relationship found that HLA-DPB1*0301 inreased risk of HL in all ethnic groups, while HLA-DPB1*0401 was associated with a lowered risk of HL in Japanese and Chinese and an elevated risk for US whites and Israelis (Oza, et al., 1994). Therefore; HLA-DPB1*1401, or factors related to it, could explain some of the lower incidence of HL in certain Asian ethnic groups, although environmental factors involves as well and indicate that HL etiology is complex.

4. Conclusion

There is evidence of etiologic heterogeneity among types of NHL, with different incidence patterns according to age, sex, race and specially geography. The extent to which these differences reflect differences in etiology needs further study.

Epidemiologic studies indicate that environmental factors may play an important role in the etiology of non-Hodgkin's lymphoma. Given the recognition that transmissible agents, especially in the developing world, are a significant cause of some kind of lymphoma, focusing on effective strategies to prevent infection altogether will go a long way to diminish the lymphoma. Additionally, effective strategies for toxic and occupational exposure and changing global lifestyles will yield huge dividends. Future epidemiologic research on NHL will be enhanced by analyses of subtypes of NHL, improved reliability and validity of exposure assessment tools to evaluate occupational, environmental and personal exposures, and evaluation of susceptible subgroups of individuals whose risk of NHL may differ from that of the general population. Finding the relation between environmental factors and genes in lymphomagenesis also important and it needs more investigation.

Lower rate of HL in Asians suggestive of genetic resistance, in addition international and inter-ethnic differences implicate environmental influence. Additional insight into the balance of genetic and environment factors on HL risk should be forthcoming. Differences in HL risk reported in several studies indicate that such studies of HL risk factors should be conducted for specific Asian population.

Overall in developing countries the most common subtype of lymphoid malignancies both HL and NHL are those subtype which immunodeficiency have an important role in their pathogenesis.

5. References

Abbaszadegan, M. R., Gholamin, M., Tabatabaee, A., Farid, R., Houshmand, M., & Abbaszadegan, M. (2003). Prevalence of human T-lymphotropic virus type 1 among blood donors from Mashhad, Iran. *Journal of clinical microbiology, 41* (6), 2593, ISSN 0095-1137.

Ablashi, D., Chatlynne, L., Cooper, H., Thomas, D., Yadav, M., Norhanom, A., et al. (1999). Seroprevalence of human herpesvirus-8 (HHV-8) in countries of Southeast Asia compared to the USA, the Caribbean and Africa. *British journal of cancer, 81* (5), 893, ISSN 0007-0920.

Abramson, J., Pridan, H., Sacks, M., Avitzour, M., & Peritz, E. (1978). A case-control study of Hodgkin's disease in Israel. *Journal of the National Cancer Institute, 61* (2), 307, ISSN 0027-8874.

Advani, S. H., Banavali, S. D., Agarwala, S., Gopal, R., Dinshaw, K. A., Borges, A., et al. (1990). The pattern of malignant lymphoma in India: a study of 1371 cases. *Leukemia and Lymphoma, 2* (5), 307-316, ISSN 1042-8194.

Alexander, D. D., Mink, P. J., Adami, H. O., Chang, E. T., Cole, P., Mandel, J. S., et al. (2007). The non Hodgkin lymphomas: A review of the epidemiologic literature. *International journal of cancer, 120* (S12), 1-390, ISSN 020-7136.

Altekruse, S. F., Jane Henley, S., & Thun, M. J. (1999). Deaths from hematopoietic and other cancers in relation to permanent hair dye use in a large prospective study (United States). *Cancer Causes and Control, 10* (6), 617-625, ISSN 0957-5243.

Altieri, A., Bermejo, J. L., & Hemminki, K. (2005). Familial risk for non-Hodgkin lymphoma and other lymphoproliferative malignancies by histopathologic subtype: the Swedish Family-Cancer Database. *Blood, 106* (2), 668, ISSN 0006-4971.

Ambinder, R. F. (2007). Epstein-Barr Virus and Hodgkin Lymphoma. *Hematology, 2007* (1), 204-209, ISSN 1024-5332 .

Anderson, J. R., Armitage, J. O., & Weisenburger, D. D. (1998). Epidemiology of the non-Hodgkin's lymphomas: Distributions of the major subtypes differ by geographic locations. *Annals of Oncology, 9* (7), 717, ISSN 0923-7534.

Aoki, R., Karube, K., Sugita, Y., Nomura, Y., Shimizu, K., Kimura, Y., et al. (2008). Distribution of malignant lymphoma in Japan: analysis of 2260 cases, 2001-2006. *Pathology International, 58* (3), 174-182, ISSN 1320-5463.

Aozasa, K., Tsujimoto, M., Sakurai, M., Honda, M., Yamashita, K., Hanada, M., et al. (1985). Non-Hodgkin's lymphomas in Osaka, Japan. *European Journal of Cancer and Clinical Oncology, 21* (4), 487-492, ISSN 0959-8049.

Aozasa, K., Ueda, T., Tamai, M., & Tsujimura, T. (1986). Hodgkin's disease in Osaka, Japan (1964-1985). *European Journal of Cancer and Clinical Oncology, 22* (9), 1117-1119, ISSN 0959-8049.

Arellano, F. M., Arana, A., Wentworth, C. E., Fernández-Vidaurre, C., Schlienger, R. G., & Conde, E. (2009). Lymphoma among patients with atopic dermatitis and/or treated with topical immunosuppressants in the United Kingdom. *Journal of Allergy and Clinical Immunology, 123* (5), 1111-1116. e1113, ISSN 0091-6749.

Armstrong, G. L., Wasley, A., Simard, E. P., McQuillan, G. M., Kuhnert, W. L., & Alter, M. J. (2006). The prevalence of hepatitis C virus infection in the United States, 1999 through 2002. *Annals of Internal Medicine, 144* (10), 705, ISSN 0003-4819.

Ascoli, V., Lo Coco, F., Torelli, G., Vallisa, D., Cavanna, L., Bergonzi, C., et al. (2002). Human herpesvirus 8-associated primary effusion lymphoma in HIV--patients: a clinicopidemiologic variant resembling classic Kaposi's sarcoma. *haematologica, 87* (4), 339, 0390-6078.

Atichartakarn, V., Kurathong, S., Nitiyanand, P., Kiatikajornthada, N., Petchclai, B., Ou, D., et al. (1982). Alpha chain disease in the Thai man. *The Southeast Asian journal of tropical medicine and public health, 13* (1), 120.

Au, W. Y., Ma, S. Y., Chim, C. S., Choy, C., Loong, F., Lie, A., et al. (2005). Clinicopathologic features and treatment outcome of mature T-cell and natural killer-cell lymphomas diagnosed according to the World Health Organization classification scheme: a single center experience of 10 years. *Annals of Oncology, 16* (2), 206, ISSN 0923-7534.

Azar, H. A. (1962). Cancer in Lebanon and the near east. *Cancer, 15* (1), 66-78, ISSN 1097-0142.

Baris, D., & Zahm, S. H. (2000). Epidemiology of lymphomas. *Current Opinion in Oncology, 12* (5), 383-394, ISSN 1040-8746.

Biagi, J. J., & Seymour, J. F. (2002). Insights into the molecular pathogenesis of follicular lymphoma arising from analysis of geographic variation. *Blood, 99* (12), 4265, ISSN 0006-4971.

Biggar, R. J., & Rabkin, C. S. (1992). The epidemiology of acquired immunodeficiency syndrome-related lymphomas. *Current Opinion in Oncology, 4* (5), 883, ISSN 1040-8746.

Boot, H., & Jong, D. (2002). Gastric lymphoma: the revolution of the past decade. *Scandinavian Journal of Gastroenterology, 37* (230), 27-36, ISSN 0036-5521.

Bracci, P. M., & Holly, E. A. (2005). Tobacco use and non-Hodgkin lymphoma: results from a population-based case-control study in the San Francisco Bay Area, California. *Cancer Causes and Control, 16* (4), 333-346, ISSN 0957-5243.

Brousset, P., Chittal, S., Schlaifer, D., Icart, J., Payen, C., Rigal-Huguet, F., et al. (1991). Detection of Epstein-Barr virus messenger RNA in Reed-Sternberg cells of Hodgkin's disease by in situ hybridization with biotinylated probes on specially processed modified acetone methyl benzoate xylene (ModAMeX) sections [see comments]. *Blood, 77* (8), 1781, ISSN 0006-4971.

Caporaso, N. E., Goldin, L. R., Anderson, W. F., & Landgren, O. (2009). Current insight on trends, causes, and mechanisms of Hodgkin's lymphoma. *The Cancer Journal, 15* (2), 117, ISSN 0340-7004.

Chang, E. T., Bälter, K. M., Torrång, A., Smedby, K. E., Melbye, M., Sundström, C., et al. (2006). Nutrient intake and risk of non-Hodgkin's lymphoma. *American journal of epidemiology, 164* (12), 1222, ISSN 0002-9173.

Chang, E. T., Ekström Smedby, K., Zhang, S. M., Hjalgrim, H., Melbye, M., Öst, Å., et al. (2005). Dietary factors and risk of non-Hodgkin lymphoma in men and women. *Cancer Epidemiology Biomarkers & Prevention, 14* (2), 512, ISSN 1055-9965.

Chatterjee, N., Hartge, P., Cerhan, J. R., Cozen, W., Davis, S., Ishibe, N., et al. (2004). Risk of non-Hodgkin's lymphoma and family history of lymphatic, hematologic, and other cancers. *Cancer Epidemiology Biomarkers & Prevention, 13* (9), 1415, ISSN 1055-9965.

Chiu, B. C. H., Cerhan, J., Gapstur, S., Sellers, T., Zheng, W., Lutz, C., et al. (1999). Alcohol consumption and non-Hodgkin lymphoma in a cohort of older women. *British journal of cancer, 80* (9), 1476, ISSN 0007-0963.

Chiu, B. C. H., & Weisenburger, D. D. (2003). An update of the epidemiology of non-Hodgkin's lymphoma. *Clinical Lymphoma, Myeloma & Leukemia, 4* (3), 161-168.

Chiu, B. C. H., Weisenburger, D. D., Cantor, K. P., Zahm, S. H., Holmes, F., Burmeister, L. F., et al. (2002). Alcohol consumption, family history of hematolymphoproliferative cancer, and the risk of non-Hodgkin's lymphoma in men. *Annals of epidemiology, 12* (5), 309-315, ISSN 0007-0963.

Classical, H. (2009). Michael Craig, Jame Abraham, Wyndham H. Wilson, and Elaine S. Jaffe. *Bethesda Handbook of Clinical Hematology*, 184.

Correa, P., & O'Conor, G. T. (1971). Epidemiologic patterns of Hodgkin's disease. *International journal of cancer, 8* (2), 192-201, ISSN 0020-7128.

Coté, T. R., Biggar, R. J., Rosenberg, P. S., Devesa, S. S., Percy, C., Yellin, F. J., et al. (1997). Non Hodgkin's lymphoma among people with AIDS: Incidence, presentation and public health burden. *International journal of cancer, 73* (5), 645-650, ISSN 0020-7128.

Coutinho, R. (2000). Highly active antiretroviral therapy and incidence of cancer in human immunodeficiency virus-infected adults. *J NATL CANCER I, 92* (15), 1823-1830, ISSN 0027-8874.

Cummins, A. G., & Roberts Thomson, I. C. (2009). Prevalence of celiac disease in the Asia–Pacific region. *Journal of Gastroenterology and Hepatology, 24* (8), 1347-1351, ISSN 0815-9319.

d'Amore, F., Christensen, B. E., Brincker, H., Pedersen, N. T., Thorling, K., Hastrup, J., et al. (1991). Clinicopathological features and prognostic factors in extranodal non-Hodgkin lymphomas. *European Journal of Cancer and Clinical Oncology, 27* (10), 1201-1208, ISSN, 0959-8049.

De Sanjose, S., Benavente, Y., Vajdic, C. M., Engels, E. A., Morton, L. M., Bracci, P. M., et al. (2008). Hepatitis C and non-Hodgkin lymphoma among 4784 cases and 6269 controls from the International Lymphoma Epidemiology Consortium. *Clinical Gastroenterology and Hepatology, 6* (4), 451-458, ISSN 1542-3565.

De Thé, G., & Bomford, R. (1993). An HTLV-I vaccine: why, how, for whom? *AIDS research and human retroviruses, 9* (5), 381-386, ISSN 0889-2229.

Devesa, S. S., & Fears, T. (1992). Non-Hodgkin's Lymphoma Time Trends: United States and International Data. *Cancer Research, 52* (19 Supplement), 5432s-5440s, ISSN 0008-5472.

Dhir, A. A., Sawant, S., Dikshit, R. P., Parikh, P., Srivastava, S., Badwe, R., et al. (2008). Spectrum of HIV/AIDS related cancers in India. *Cancer Causes and Control, 19* (2), 147-153, ISSN 0957-5243.

Du, M. Q. (2007). MALT lymphoma: recent advances in aetiology and molecular genetics. *Journal of Clinical and Experimental Hematopathology, 47* (2), 31-42, ISSN .

Dutcher, J. P. (2003). The role of Epstein-Barr virus and elevated levels of tumor necrosis factor in determining prognosis in Asian peripheral T-cell lymphomas. *Leukemia Research, 27* (6), 467-469, ISSN 0145-2126.

Ekström-Smedby, K. (2006). Epidemiology and etiology of non-Hodgkin lymphoma - a review. *Acta Oncologica, 45* (3), 258-271, ISSN 0284-186X .

Ekström, K., Hjalgrim, H., Brandt, L., Baecklund, E., Klareskog, L., Ekbom, A., et al. (2003). Risk of malignant lymphomas in patients with rheumatoid arthritis and in their first degree relatives. *Arthritis & Rheumatism, 48* (4), 963-970.

Evans, A. S., & Kaslow, R. A. (1997). *Viral infections of humans: epidemiology and control*: Springer Us, ISBN-13:978-0306448560.

Farinha, P., & Gascoyne, R. D. (2005). Helicobacter pylori and MALT lymphoma. *Editorial board A4, 128*, 1579-1605.

Feuillard, J., Aubin, J. T., Poirel, L., Davi, F., Kujas, M., Rousselet, M. C., et al. (1997). Detection rate and intratumoral virus load of human herpesvirus 8 in immunodeficiency related B cell lymphoid malignancies. *Journal of medical virology, 53* (3), 277-281, ISSN 0146-6615.

Filipovich, A., Mathur, A., Kamat, D., & Shapiro, R. (1992). Primary immunodeficiencies: genetic risk factors for lymphoma. *Cancer Research, 52* (19 Supplement), 5465s, ISSN 0939-5213.

Fisher, S. G., & Fisher, R. I. (2004). The epidemiology of non-Hodgkin's lymphoma. *Oncogene, 23* (38), 6524-6534, ISSN 6524-6534.

Foss, F. M., Zinzani, P. L., Vose, J. M., Gascoyne, R. D., Rosen, S. T., & Tobinai, K. (2011). Peripheral T-cell lymphoma. *Blood, 117* (25), 6756, ISSN 0006-4971.

Freeman, C., Berg, J. W., & Cutler, S. J. (1972). Occurrence and prognosis of extranodal lymphomas. *Cancer, 29* (1), 252-260, ISSN 1097-0142.

Frimpong-Boateng, K. Infectious Disease and Cancer in Africa–A medical and Demographical Reality.

Gaidano, G., Pastore, C., Gloghini, A., Volpe, G., Ghia, P., Saglio, G., et al. (1996). AIDS-related non-Hodgkin's lymphomas: molecular genetics, viral infection and cytokine deregulation. *Acta haematologica, 95* (3-4), 193-198, ISSN 0001-5792.

Gessain, A., Gallo, R. C., & Franchini, G. (1992). Low degree of human T-cell leukemia/lymphoma virus type I genetic drift in vivo as a means of monitoring viral transmission and movement of ancient human populations. *Journal of virology, 66* (4), 2288, ISSN 0022-838X.

Glaser, S. L., Clarke, C. A., Gulley, M. L., Craig, F. E., DiGiuseppe, J. A., Dorfman, R. F., et al. (2003). Population based patterns of human immunodeficiency virus related Hodgkin lymphoma in the Greater San Francisco Bay Area, 1988–1998. *Cancer, 98* (2), 300-309, ISSN 1097-0142.

Glaser, S. L., & Hsu, J. L. (2002). Hodgkin's disease in Asians: incidence patterns and risk factors in population-based data. *Leukemia Research, 26* (3), 261-269, ISSN 0135-2126.

Glaser, S. L., & Jarrett, R. F. (1996). 1 The epidemiology of Hodgkin's disease. *Baillière's clinical haematology, 9* (3), 401-416, ISSN 1521-6926.

Glaser, S. L., Lin, R. J., Stewart, S. L., Ambinder, R. F., Jarrett, R. F., Brousset, P., et al. (1997). Epstein Barr virus associated Hodgkin's disease: epidemiologic characteristics in international data. *International journal of cancer, 70* (4), 375-382, ISSN 0020-7136.

Goedert, J. J., Coté, T. R., Virgo, P., Scoppa, S. M., Kingma, D. W., Gail, M. H., et al. (1998). Spectrum of AIDS-associated malignant disorders. *The Lancet, 351* (9119), 1833-1839, ISSN 0140-6736.

Goldin, L., McMaster, M., Ter-Minassian, M., Saddlemire, S., Harmsen, B., Lalonde, G., et al. (2005). A genome screen of families at high risk for Hodgkin lymphoma: evidence for a susceptibility gene on chromosome 4. *Journal of medical genetics, 42* (7), 595, ISSN 0022-2593.

Goncalves, D. U., Proietti, F. A., Ribas, J. G. R., Araujo, M. G., Pinheiro, S. R., Guedes, A. C., et al. (2010). Epidemiology, treatment, and prevention of human T-cell leukemia virus type 1-associated diseases. *Clinical Microbiology Reviews, 23* (3), 577, ISSN 0893-8512.

Groves, F. D., Linet, M. S., Travis, L. B., & Devesa, S. S. (2000). Cancer surveillance series: non-Hodgkin's lymphoma incidence by histologic subtype in the United States from 1978 through 1995. *Journal of the National Cancer Institute, 92* (15), 1240, ISSN 0027-8874.

Grulich, A. E., Li, Y., McDonald, A. M., Correll, P. K., Law, M. G., & Kaldor, J. M. (2001). Decreasing rates of Kaposi's sarcoma and non-Hodgkin's lymphoma in the era of potent combination anti-retroviral therapy. *Aids, 15* (5), 629, ISSN 0269-9370.

Haim, N., Cohen, Y., & Robinson, E. (1982). Malignant Lymphoma in First Degree Blood Relatives. *Cancer, 49* (10), 2197-2200, ISSN 1097-0142.

Heller, K., Steinherz, P., Portlock, C., & Munz, C. (2007). EBV-positive lymphoma patients have a selective deficiency in EBV immunity. *Journal of Clinical Oncology, 25* (18_suppl), 21032, ISSN 0732-183X.

Hermine, O., Lefrère, F., Bronowicki, J. P., Mariette, X., Jondeau, K., Eclache-Saudreau, V., et al. (2002). Regression of splenic lymphoma with villous lymphocytes after treatment of hepatitis C virus infection. *New England Journal of Medicine, 347* (2), 89-94.

Hinuma, Y., Nagata, K., Hanaoka, M., Nakai, M., Matsumoto, T., Kinoshita, K. I., et al. (1981). Adult T-cell leukemia: antigen in an ATL cell line and detection of antibodies to the antigen in human sera. *Proceedings of the National Academy of Sciences, 78* (10), 6476.

Hirata, M., Hayashi, J., Noguchi, A., Nakashima, K., Kajiyama, W., Kashiwagi, S., et al. (1992). The effects of breastfeeding and presence of antibody to p40tax protein of human T cell lymphotropic virus type-I on mother to child transmission. *International journal of epidemiology, 21* (5), 989, ISSN 0300-5771.

Hishima, T., Oyaizu, N., Fujii, T., Tachikawa, N., Ajisawa, A., Negishi, M., et al. (2006). Decrease in Epstein-Barr virus-positive AIDS-related lymphoma in the era of highly active antiretroviral therapy. *Microbes and infection, 8* (5), 1301-1307, ISSN 1286-4576.

Hjalgrim, H., Ekström Smedby, K., Rostgaard, K., Molin, D., Hamilton-Dutoit, S., Chang, E. T., et al. (2007). Infectious mononucleosis, childhood social environment, and risk of Hodgkin lymphoma. *Cancer Research, 67* (5), 2382, ISSN 0008-543X.

Ho, F., Todd, D., Loke, S., Ng, R., & Khoo, R. (1984). Clinico pathological features of malignant lymphomas in 294 Hong Kong Chinese patients, retrospective study covering an eight year period. *International journal of cancer, 34* (2), 143-148, ISSN 0020-7136.

Hooper, W. C., Holman, R. C., Clarke, M., & Chorba, T. L. (2001). Trends in non hodgkin lymphoma (NHL) and HIV associated NHL deaths in the United States. *American journal of hematology, 66* (3), 159-166, ISSN 0361-8609.

Hunt, K. E., & Reichard, K. K. (2008). Diffuse large B-cell lymphoma. *Archives of pathology & laboratory medicine, 132* (1), 118-124, ISSN 0003-9969.

Hunt, R., Sumanac, K., & Huang, J. Q. (2001). Review article: should we kill or should we save Helicobacter pylori? *Alimentary pharmacology & therapeutics, 15*, 51-59, ISSN 0269-2813.

Imperiale, M. J. (2000). The human polyomaviruses, BKV and JCV: molecular pathogenesis of acute disease and potential role in cancer. *Virology (New York), 267* (1), 1-7, ISSN 0042-6822.

Intragumtornchai, T., Wannakrairoj, P., Chaimongkol, B., Bhoopat, L., Lekhakula, A., Thamprasit, T., et al. (1996). Non Hodgkin's lymphomas in Thailand: A retrospective pathologic and clinical analysis of 1391 cases. *Cancer, 78* (8), 1813-1819, ISSN 1097-0142.

Izumo, T. (1996). Malignant lymphoma in Japanese HTLV1-non endemic area based on the REAL classification. *Ann. Oncol., 7* (3), 342, ISSN 0923-7534.

Jaffe, E. S. (1999). Hematopathology: integration of morphologic features and biologic markers for diagnosis. *Modern pathology: an official journal of the United States and Canadian Academy of Pathology, Inc, 12* (2), 109, ISSN 0893-3952.

Jaffe, E. S., Chan, J. K. C., Su, I. J., Frizzera, G., Mori, S., Feller, A., et al. (1996). Report of the workshop on nasal and related extranodal angiocentric T/natural killer cell lymphomas: definitions, differential diagnosis, and epidemiology. *The American journal of surgical pathology, 20* (1), 103, ISSN 0147-5185.

Jafroodi, M., Zargari, O., & Hoda, S. (2009). Concomitant Hodgkin's Lymphoma and Atopic Dermatitis in a Child with Celiac Disease. *Archives of Iranian Medicine, 12* (3), 317-319, ISSN 1029-2977.

Kadin, M. E., Berard, C. W., Nanba, K., & Wakasa, H. (1983). Lymphoproliferative diseases in Japan and Western countries: proceedings of the United States-Japan seminar, september 6 and 7, 1982, in Seattle, Washington= Les affections lymphoprolifératives au Japon et dans les régions occidentales. Comptes-rendus du séminaire Etats-Unis-Japon du 6 au 7 septembre 1982 Seattle, Washington. *Human pathology, 14* (9), 745-772, ISSN 0046-8177.

Kakuda, K., Ikematsu, H., Chong, W. L. Y., Hayashi, J., & Kashiwagi, S. (2002). Molecular epidemiology of human T lymphotropic virus type 1 transmission in Okinawa, Japan. *The American journal of tropical medicine and hygiene, 66* (4), 404, ISSN 0002-9637.

Kamiyama, K., Kinjo, T., Chinen, K., Iwamasa, T., Uezato, H., Miyagi, J., et al. (2004). Human herpesvirus 8 (HHV8) sequence variations in HHV8 related tumours in Okinawa, a subtropical island in southern Japan. *Journal of clinical pathology, 57* (5), 529, ISSN 0021-9746.

Kao, J. H., & Chen, D. S. (2000). Transmission of hepatitis C virus in Asia: past and present perspectives. *Journal of Gastroenterology and Hepatology, 15*, E91-E96, ISSN 0815-9319.

Khojasteh, A., & Haghighi, P. (1990). Immunoproliferative small intestinal disease: portrait of a potentially preventable cancer from the Third World. *The American journal of medicine, 89* (4), 483-490, ISSN 0002-9343.

Khojasteh, A., Haghshenass, M., & Haghighi, P. (1983). Immunoproliferative small intestinal disease. *New England Journal of Medicine, 308* (23), 1401-1405, ISSN 0028-3635.

Kim, C. W., Kim, I., Ko, Y. H., Cho, H., Yang, W. I., Kwon, G. Y., et al. (1992). Clinicopathologic and immunophenotypic study of non-Hodgkin's lymphoma in Korea. Lymphoreticular Study Group of the Korean Society of Pathologists. *Journal of Korean medical science, 7* (3), 193, ISSN 1011-8934.

King, P., Wilkes, J., & DIAZ ARIAS, A. (1998). Hepatitis C virus infection in non Hodgkin's lymphoma. *Clinical & Laboratory Haematology, 20* (2), 107-110, ISSN 1751-5521.

Kinlen, L. (1992). Immunosuppressive therapy and acquired immunological disorders. *Cancer Research, 52* (19 Supplement), 5474s, ISSN 0008-5472.

Ko, Y. H., Kim, C. W., Park, C. S., Jang, H. K., Lee, S. S., Kim, S. H., et al. (1998). REAL classification of malignant lymphomas in the Republic of Korea. *Cancer, 83* (4), 806-812, ISSN 1097-0142.

Ko, Y. H., & Lee, J. D. (1994). EBV in situ hybridization study for non-Hodgkin's lymphomas. *Journal of Korean medical science, 9* (3), 224.

Ko, Y. H., & Lee, J. D. (1996). Epstein-Barr virus in Korean malignant lymphomas. *The Korean Journal of Pathology, 30* (11), 1011-1017.

Lankarani, K., Masoompour, S., Masoompour, M., Malekzadeh, R., Tabei, S., & Haghshenas, M. (2005). Changing epidemiology of IPSID in Southern Iran. *Gut, 54* (2), 311, ISSN 0017-5749.

Lee, M. Y., Tan, T. D., Feng, A. C., & Liu, M. C. (2005). Clinicopathological analysis of malignant lymphoma in Taiwan, defined according to the World Health Organization classification. *haematologica, 90* (12), 1703, ISSN 0390-6078.

Lee, M. Y., Tsou, M. H., Tan, T. D., & Lu, M. C. (2005). Clinicopathological analysis of T cell lymphoma in Taiwan according to WHO classification: high incidence of enteropathy type intestinal T cell lymphoma. *European journal of haematology, 75* (3), 221-226, ISSN 0902-4441.

Li, H. C., Biggar, R. J., Miley, W. J., Maloney, E. M., Cranston, B., Hanchard, B., et al. (2004). Provirus load in breast milk and risk of mother-to-child transmission of human T lymphotropic virus type I. *Journal of Infectious Diseases, 190* (7), 1275, ISSN 0022-1899.

LIU, H. F. U., Vandamme, A. M., KAZADI, K., Carton, H., Desmyter, J., & GOUBAU, P. (1994). Familial transmission and minimal sequence variability of human T-lymphotropic virus type I (HTLV-I) in Zaire. *AIDS research and human retroviruses, 10* (9), 1135-1142, ISSN 0889-2229.

Makishima, H., Ito, T., Kodama, R., Asano, N., Nakazawa, H., Akamatsu, T., et al. (2006). Intestinal diffuse large B-cell lymphoma associated with celiac disease: a Japanese case. *International journal of hematology, 83* (1), 63-65, ISSN 0925-5710.

Morgan, O. S., Mora, C., Rodgers-Johnson, P., & Char, G. (1989). HTLV-1 and polymyositis in Jamaica. *The Lancet, 334* (8673), 1184-1187, ISSN 0140-2381.

Morton, L. M., Wang, S. S., Devesa, S. S., Hartge, P., Weisenburger, D. D., & Linet, M. S. (2006). Lymphoma incidence patterns by WHO subtype in the United States, 1992-2001. *Blood, 107* (1), 265, ISSN 0006-4971.

Mozaheb, Z., Aledavood, A., & Farzad, F. (2011). Distributions of major sub-types of lymphoid malignancies among adults in Mashhad, Iran. *Cancer epidemiology, 35* (1), 26-29, ISSN 1877-7821.

Mozaheb, Z., Aledavood, A. (2011). Diet and non-Hodgkin Lymphoma risk, *Proceeding of EHA, 16th Congress of the Europian Hematologic Association,* pp s615, ISSN 0390-6078, LONDON,UK, June 9-12, 2011

Mueller, N., Okayama, A., Stuver, S., & Tachibana, N. (1996). Findings from the Miyazaki cohort study. *JAIDS Journal of Acquired Immune Deficiency Syndromes, 13,* S2, ISSN 1525-4135.

Müller, A. M. S., Ihorst, G., Mertelsmann, R., & Engelhardt, M. (2005). Epidemiology of non-Hodgkin's lymphoma (NHL): trends, geographic distribution, and etiology. *Annals of Hematology, 84* (1), 1-12.

Naresh, K., Srinivas, V., & Soman, C. (2000). Distribution of various subtypes of non-Hodgkin's lymphoma in India: a study of 2773 lymphomas using REAL and WHO Classifications. *Annals of Oncology, 11* (suppl 1), S63, ISSN 0923-7534.

Nerurkar, V. R., Song, K. J., Saitou, N., Melland, R. R., & Yanagihara, R. (1993). Interfamilial and intrafamilial genomic diversity and molecular phylogeny of human T-cell lymphotropic virus type I from Papua New Guinea and the Solomon Islands. *Virology, 196* (2), 506-513, ISSN 0042-6822.

Newton, R., Ferlay, J., Beral, V., & Devesa, S. S. (1997). The epidemiology of non Hodgkin's lymphoma: Comparison of nodal and extra nodal sites. *International journal of cancer, 72* (6), 923-930, ISSN 0020-7128.

Ohshima, K., Suzumiya, J., & Kikuchi, M. (2002). The World Health Organization classification of malignant lymphoma: Incidence and clinical prognosis in HTLV 1 endemic area of Fukuoka. *Pathology International, 52* (1), 1-12, ISSN 1320-5463.

Oza, A. M., Tonks, S., Lim, J., Fleetwood, M. A., Lister, T. A., Bodmer, J. G., et al. (1994). A clinical and epidemiological study of human leukocyte antigen-DPB alleles in Hodgkin's disease. *Cancer Research, 54* (19), 5101, ISSN 0008-5472.

Pareen, S., Alison, M., Neha, M., & Christopher, R. (2010). Incidence Patterns and Outcomes for Hodgkin Lymphoma Patients in the United States. *Advances in Hematology, 2011.*

Parkin, D. M., Bray, F., Ferlay, J., & Pisani, P. (2005). Global Cancer Statistics, 2002. *CA: A Cancer Journal for Clinicians, 55* (2), 74-108.

Parsonnet, J., Hansen, S., Rodriguez, L., Gelb, A. B., Warnke, R. A., Jellum, E., et al. (1994a). Helicobacter pylori infection and gastric lymphoma. *New England Journal of Medicine, 330* (18), 1267-1271, ISSN 0028-7493.

Pathologists, L. S. G. o. J. (2000). The World Health Organization classification of malignant lymphomas in Japan: incidence of recently recognized entities. *Pathol Int, 50,* 696-702, ISSN 1320-5463.

Pawson, R., Richardson, D. S., Pagliuca, A., Kelsey, S. M., Hoque, S., Breuer, J., et al. (1998). Adult T-cell leukemia/lymphoma in London: clinical experience of 21 cases. *Leukemia & lymphoma, 31* (1-2), 177-185, ISSN 1042-8194.

Poulin, D. L., & DeCaprio, J. A. (2006). Is there a role for SV40 in human cancer? *Journal of Clinical Oncology, 24* (26), 4356, ISSN 0732-183X.

Pounder, R., & Ng, D. (1995). The prevalence of Helicobacter pylori infection in different countries. *Alimentary pharmacology and therapeutics, 9* (2), 33-40, ISSN 0269-2813.

Pramoolsinsap, C., Kurathong, S., Atichartakarn, V., & Nitiyanand, P. (1993). Immunoproliferative small intestinal disease (IPSID) in Thailand. *The Southeast Asian journal of tropical medicine and public health, 24* (1), 11.

Proietti, F. A., Carneiro-Proietti, A. B. F., Catalan-Soares, B. C., & Murphy, E. L. (2005). Global epidemiology of HTLV-I infection and associated diseases. *Oncogene, 24* (39), 6058-6068, ISSN 0950-9232.

Purdue, M. P., Bassani, D. G., Klar, N. S., Sloan, M., & Kreiger, N. (2004). Dietary factors and risk of non-Hodgkin lymphoma by histologic subtype: a case-control analysis. *Cancer Epidemiology Biomarkers & Prevention, 13* (10), 1665, ISSN 1055-9965.

Rabkin, C. S., & Yellin, F. (1994). Cancer incidence in a population with a high prevalence of infection with human immunodeficiency virus type 1. *Journal of the National Cancer Institute, 86* (22), 1711, ISSN 0027-3864.

Ragni, M. V., Belle, S. H., Jaffe, R. A., Duerstein, S. L., Bass, D. C., McMillan, C. W., et al. (1993). Acquired immunodeficiency syndrome-associated non-Hodgkin's lymphomas and other malignancies in patients with hemophilia. *Blood, 81* (7), 1889, ISSN 0006-4971.

RiesLAG, M. B. A., HankeyBF, K. C. L., & HarrasA, E. B. K. (1994). SEER cancer statistics review, 1973–1991: tables and graphs. *Bethesda (MD): National Institutes of Health, National Cancer Institute.*

Saadoun, D., Landau, D., Calabrese, L., & Cacoub, P. (2007). Hepatitis C-associated mixed cryoglobulinaemia: a crossroad between autoimmunity and lymphoproliferation. *Rheumatology, 46* (8), 1234, ISSN 1462-0324.

Salem, P., Anaissie, E., Allam, C., Geha, S., Hashimi, L., Ibrahim, N., et al. (1986). Non Hodgkin's lymphomas in the Middle East. A study of 417 patients with emphasis on special features. *Cancer, 58* (5), 1162-1166, ISSN 1097-0142.

Salem, P. A., & Estephan, F. F. (2005). Immunoproliferative small intestinal disease: Current concepts. *The Cancer Journal, 11* (5), 374, ISSN 1097-0142.

Sauce, D., Larsen, M., Leese, A., Millar, D., Khan, N., Hislop, A., et al. (2007). IL 7R versus CCR7 and CD45 as Markers of Virus Specific CD8+ T Cell Differentiation: Contrasting Pictures in Blood and Tonsillar Lymphoid Tissue. *Journal of Infectious Diseases, 195* (2), 268, ISSN 0022-1899.

Seow, A., & Registry, S. C. (2004). *Trends in cancer incidence in Singapore, 1968-2002*: Singapore Cancer Registry.

Serraino, D., Piselli, P., Angeletti, C., Scuderi, M., Ippolito, G., & Capobianchi, M. (2005). Infection with Epstein-Barr virus and cancer: an epidemiological review. *Journal of biological regulators and homeostatic agents, 19* (1-2), 63-70, ISSN 0393-974X.

Shih, L., & Liang, D. (1991). Non-Hodgkin's lymphomas in Asia. *Hematology/oncology clinics of North America, 5* (5), 983, ISSN 0889-8588.

Shimoyama, M. (1991). Diagnostic criteria and classification of clinical subtypes of adult T cell leukaemia lymphoma. *British Journal of Haematology, 79* (3), 428-437, ISSN 0007-1048.

Smedby KE, Hjalgrim H. (2011). Epidemiology and etiology of mantle cell lymphoma and other non-Hodgkin lymphoma subtype. *Semin Cancer Biol,*21 (5),293-298, ISSN 1044-579X.

Smith, A., Roman, E., Howell, D., Jones, R., Patmore, R., Jack, A., et al. (2010). The Haematological Malignancy Research Network (HMRN): a new information strategy for population based epidemiology and health service research. *British Journal of Haematology, 148* (5), 739-753, ISSN 0007-1048.

Sokol, L., & Loughran, T. P. (2006). Large granular lymphocyte leukemia. *The oncologist, 11* (3), 263, ISSN 1083-7159.

Spitz, M., Sider, J., Johnson, C., Butler, J., Pollack, E., & Newell, G. (1986). Ethnic patterns of Hodgkin's disease incidence among children and adolescents in the United States, 1973-82. *Journal of the National Cancer Institute, 76* (2), 235, ISSN 0287-8874.

Strickland, G. T. (2006). Liver disease in Egypt: hepatitis C superseded schistosomiasis as a result of iatrogenic and biological factors. *Hepatology, 43* (5), 915-922, ISSN 1024-5332.

Strickler, H. D., Goedert, J. J., Devesa, S. S., Lahey, J., Fraumeni, J. F., & Rosenberg, P. S. (2003). Trends in US pleural mesothelioma incidence rates following simian virus 40 contamination of early poliovirus vaccines. *Journal of the National Cancer Institute, 95* (1), 38, ISSN 0287-8874.

Sukpanichnant, S. (2004). Analysis of 1983 cases of malignant lymphoma in Thailand according to the World Health Organization classification. *Human pathology, 35* (2), 224-230, ISSN 0046-8177.

Sukpanichnant, S., Sonakul, D., Piankijagum, A., Wanachiwanawin, W., Veerakul, G., Mahasandana, C., et al. (1998). Malignant lymphoma in Thailand. *Cancer, 83* (6), 1197-1204, ISSN 1097-0142.

Swerdlow, A. J. (2003). Epidemiology of Hodgkin's disease and non-Hodgkin's lymphoma. *European Journal of Nuclear Medicine and Molecular Imaging, 30* (0), S3-S12, ISSN 1619-7070.

Takatsuki, K. (1990). Adult T-cell leukemia/lymphoma. *Adult T-Cell Leukaemia in Japan: A Special Issue of the Journal Hematology Reviews and Communications*, 201, ISBN-13:978-3718649334.

Tarhini, M., Kchour, G., Zanjani, D. S., Rafatpanah, H., Otrock, Z. K., Bazarbachi, A., et al. (2009). Declining tendency of human T cell leukaemia virus type I carrier rates among blood donors in Mashhad, Iran. *Pathology, 41* (5), 498, ISSN 0031-3025.

Thomas, R., Re, D., Zander, T., Wolf, J., & Diehl, V. (2002). Epidemiology and etiology of Hodgkin's lymphoma. *Annals of Oncology, 13* (suppl 4), 147, ISSN 0923-7534.

Thu, G. O., Hem, L. Y., Hansen, S., Møller, B., Norstein, J., Nøkleby, H., et al. (2006). Is there an association between SV40 contaminated polio vaccine and lymphoproliferative disorders? An age-period-cohort analysis on Norwegian data from 1953 to 1997. *International journal of cancer, 118* (8), 2035-2039, ISSN 0020-7136.

Uchiyama, T., Yodoi, J., Sagawa, K., Takatsuki, K., & Uchino, H. (1977). Adult T-cell leukemia: clinical and hematologic features of 16 cases. *Blood, 50* (3), 481, ISSN 0006-4971.

Vallisa, D., Bernuzzi, P., Arcaini, L., Sacchi, S., Callea, V., Marasca, R., et al. (2005). Role of anti-hepatitis C virus (HCV) treatment in HCV-related, low-grade, B-cell, non-Hodgkin's lymphoma: a multicenter Italian experience. *Journal of Clinical Oncology, 23* (3), 468, ISSN 0732-183X.

Vilchez, R. A., Madden, C. R., Kozinetz, C. A., Halvorson, S. J., White, Z. S., Jorgensen, J. L., et al. (2002). Association between simian virus 40 and non-Hodgkin lymphoma. *The Lancet, 359* (9309), 817-823, ISSN 0140-6736.

Vineis, P., Crosignani, P., Sacerdote, C., Fontana, A., Masala, G., Miligi, L., et al. (1999). Hematopoietic cancer and peptic ulcer: a multicenter case-control study. *Carcinogenesis, 20* (8), 1459, ISSN 0143-3334.

Vose J, Armitage J, Weisenburger D. (2008) International peripheral T cell and natural killer T cell lymphoma study: pathology findings and clinical outcomes. *Journal clinical oncology,* 26 (25),4124-4130, ISSN 0732-183X.

Wang, J., Young, L., Win, W., & Taylor, C. R. (2005). Distribution and ZAP-70 expression of WHO lymphoma categories in Shanxi, China: a review of 447 cases using a tissue microarray technique. *Applied Immunohistochemistry & Molecular Morphology, 13* (4), 323, ISSN 1062-3345.

Ward, M. H., Hoar Zahm, S., Weisenburger, D. D., Gridley, G., Cantor, K. P., Saal, R. C., et al. (1994). Dietary factors and non-Hodgkin's lymphoma in Nebraska (United States). *Cancer Causes and Control, 5* (5), 422-432, ISSN 0957-5243.

Weisenburger, D. D. (1994). Epidemiology of non-Hodgkin's lymphoma: Recent findings regarding an emerging epidemic. *Annals of Oncology, 5* (suppl 1), S19-S24, ISSN 0923-7534.

Wilson, K., Freeland, J., Gallagher, A., Cosby, S., Earle, J., Alexander, F., et al. (2007). Measles virus and classical Hodgkin lymphoma: no evidence for a direct association. *International journal of cancer, 121* (2), 442-447, ISSN 0020-7136.

Wotherspoon, A., Diss, T., Pan, L., Isaacson, P., Doglioni, C., Moschini, A., et al. (1993). Regression of primary low-grade B-cell gastric lymphoma of mucosa-associated lymphoid tissue type after eradication of Helicobacter pylori. *The Lancet, 342* (8871), 575-577, ISSN 0140-6736.

Yamaguchi, K. (1994). Human T-lymphotropic virus type I in Japan. *The Lancet, 343* (8891), 213-216, ISSN 0140-6736.

Yanagihara, E. T., Blaisdell, R. K., Hayashi, T., & Lukes, R. J. (1989). Malignant lymphoma in Hawaii Japanese: A retrospective morphologic survey. *Hematological oncology, 7* (3), 219-232, ISSN 0278-0232.

Zarate Osorno, A., Roman, L. N., Kingma, D. W., Meneses Garcia, A., & Jaffe, E. S. (1995). Hodgkin's disease in Mexico. Prevalence of Epstein Barr virus sequences and correlations with histologic subtype. *Cancer, 75* (6), 1360-1366, ISSN 1097-0142.

Zhang, S., Hunter, D. J., Rosner, B. A., Colditz, G. A., Fuchs, C. S., Speizer, F. E., et al. (1999). Dietary fat and protein in relation to risk of non-Hodgkin's lymphoma among women. *Journal of the National Cancer Institute, 91* (20), 1751, ISSN 0027-8874.

Zucca, E. (2008). Extranodal lymphoma: a reappraisal. *Annals of Oncology, 19* (suppl 4), iv77, ISSN 0923-7534.

Zucca, E., Roggero, E., Maggi-Solcà, N., Conconi, A., Bertoni, F., Reilly, I., et al. (2000). Prevalence of Helicobacter pylori and hepatitis C virus infections among non-Hodgkin's lymphoma patients in Southern Switzerland. *haematologica, 85* (2), 147, ISSN 0390-6078.

Section 8

Epidemiology of Primary Immunodeficiency Diseases

17

Primary Immunodeficiency Diseases in Latin America: Epidemiology and Perspectives

Paolo Ruggero Errante and Antonio Condino-Neto*
Department of Immunology, Institute of Biomedical Sciences
University of São Paulo, São Paulo
Brazil

1. Introduction

Primary immunodeficiencies (PID) are genetic disorders of immunity whose incidence varies from 1:250 to 1:1,000,000 depending of disease and study population. Because of incomplete records of immunodeficiency in the world, is estimated that the prevalence of 1:5,000 to 1:100,000 (Geha *et al.*, 2007; Boyle & Buckley, 2007; Notarangelo,*et al.*, 2010). Thus, the PID is a important group to public health as other genetic diseases that rely government support in a neonatal screening program such phenylketonuria (PKU) with incidence of 1/15.000 (de Carvalho *et al.*, 2007) and congenital hypothyroidism, with incidence of 1/4.000 (American Academy of Pediatrics, 1993; Olivieri, 2009). The PID are classified in defective immune deficiency prevalent in predominantly antibody; combined immunodeficiencies, cellular immunodeficiencies, phagocyte defects, immune deficiencies associated with lymphoproliferative diseases, and deficiencies of complement system or secondary immunodeficiencies associated with other diseases. This classification is updated periodically by the International Union of Immunological Societies (IUIS), associated with the World Health Organization (WHO) (Geha *et al.*, 2007; Notarangelo,*et al.*, 2010).

This classification is progressively adjusting to the rapid evolution of the field. Many new phenotypes (e.g. hemophagocytosis, thrombotic purpura, herpes encephalitis, Mendelian susceptibility to mycobacterial infection, epidermodysplasia verruciformis, chronic mucocutaneous candidiasis, autoinflammatory disorders, and anhidrotic ectodermal dysplasia with immunodeficiency) have emerged as reflecting new PID.

Knowledge of PID is still deficient in many countries and within many countries, since doctors and health authorities are often poorly informed about their clinical presentations, diagnosis, importance and health impact of these diseases, and geographic factors that influence the release of same around the world (Sewell, 2006). Recent estimates of PID made by the European Parliament showed that approximately 1 in 800 to 10,000 people have PID that significantly affects your health, PID affect at least 10 million people worldwide, the true prevalence of PID in some forms of general population is estimated between 1 in 250 and 1 in 500, data comparable with type I diabetes (1 in 700) and multiple sclerosis (1 in

* Corresponding Author

1000), although more than 200 PID have been discovered, some are more common than leukemia and lymphoma in children (Banks, 2010).

Initial efforts in classification of PID left WHO in 1970, where this first meeting was identified and classified 14 different entities, and in 2006, more than 100 types (Bonilla & Geha, 2006). Currently, they comprise more than 200 different types of genetic diseases that predispose the human host to recurrent infections, which may be associated with other disorders (Notarangelo *et al.,* 2010), but also to chronic and systemic inflammation, hypersensitivity reactions, autoimmunity, and cancer. Advances in biological sciences and biotechnology are now making possible for the first time, to systematically assess the actual impact of PID in human health, and this promises to revolutionize the way we look at these diseases.

Patients with PID have higher susceptibility to infection often accompanied by inflammatory disorders, hypersensitivity reactions, autoimmunity and cancer (Morimoto & Routes, 2008; Notarangelo 2010). The clinical presentation of patients is extremely broad, with asymptomatic individuals who have fulminating infection, which if not diagnosed and treated properly evolution to death (Chapel 2005; Bustamante *et al.,* 2008a). Patients with PID have consequence of delay diagnosis and treatment permanent damage of body. This involves disabling from attending school and/or work, reducing the number of people with productive capacity, increasing the number of people hospitalized with high cost to government, increased mortality rate in children and adults of working age (Yarmohammadi *et al.,* 2004; Bonilla *et al.,* 2005). The delay in diagnosis leads to pulmonary complications such bronchiectasis and irreversible change in the quality of life of patients and their families (Kainulainen *et al.,* 2001; Champi, 2002).

Although this delay in diagnosis of PID is evident in countries or disadvantaged regions, also occurs in developed countries after multiple hospitalizations of patients. Thus, is recommended research and education in PID, since the prognosis of many patients can be improved by early diagnosis and appropriate access to care and treatment (Bonilla *et al.,* 2005; Turvey & Bonilla, 2009). In medical terms, there are three important reasons for understanding the PID, first, a high index of suspicion and early diagnosis may lead to treatments that save lives or bring significant improvement in quality of life, secondly the discovery of genetic defects in immunity makes possible family counseling and prenatal diagnosis, and thirdly, the study of the pathophysiology of genetic and immunological defects provides important tools to understanding the regulation of the human immune system (Bustamante *et al.,* 2008b; Casanova *et al.,* 2008; Lee & Lau, 2009; Fried & Bonilla, 2009). In recent decades, no other field of immunology had so much progress in understanding how pathophysiology of primary immunodeficiencies. These developments have resulted not only in understanding of immunodeficiencies, but understanding of immune system in humans (Boufisha *et al.,* 2010). Patients with PID are considered not successful experiments of nature that brought many benefits to medicine in the installation of diagnostic protocols and rational treatment, location of targets for gene therapy and assessment of need for bone marrow transplantation and its benefits (Griffith *et al.,* 2009; Neven *et al.,* 2009; Pessach *et al.,* 2009; Kohn 2010). This knowledge was translated into association of specific defects of immunity with signs and symptoms that can establish correct diagnosis of disease, beyond the description of new immunodeficiency (Cassimos *et al.,* 2010). Since the PID diseases are congenital and hereditary character, children are overweight patients, however, a greater number of adults have been diagnosed as children grow and become adults (Bustamante *et al.*, 2008a). How healthy children have on average 6-8 mild respiratory infections, especially upper airway in first year of life and more than six episodes of otitis and gastroenteritis per year in the first three years of life, young children with high environmental exposure or with siblings who attend schools may exceed these averages by one to two years, the diagnosis of PID is often underestimated (Puck, 1997). But they may be observed in children with normal development, which may harbor latent PID or low impact on the immune system. Pediatrics specialize in PID ensure that half children are taken by parents to the doctor with a history of recurrent infections are normal, and other 50%, 30% have allergies, 10% other diseases and 10% PID (Grumach *et al.*, 1997). To aid diagnosis and reporting of PID, the American Red Cross and Jeffrey Model Foundation developed the 10 warning signs suspected for PID. For experts (Modell, 2007a; Modell, 2007b), these signs are considered extremely important, since the prognosis and therapeutic success depends upon prompt diagnosis, and most are performed in referral centers. However, some authors consider the 10 warning signs not sensitive or specific, since a third of patients do not present single warning sign (Aloi *et al.*, 2007). Once diagnosed with PID, the patient is referred to clinical immunologist who directs specific treatment, immunizations, and definitive and specific diagnosis. Thus, there is a gain in quality life of patients and their families, avoiding sequels, unnecessary suffering and high social cost. The therapeutic treatment these patients involve three basic tenets: reduce the exposure to the infectious agent, effective or prophylactic antimicrobial therapy, replacement of deficient immune functions (Garcia *et al.*, 2007). During the evaluation of PID is essential documentation of the patient's clinical history, frequency, duration and complications of infections, outbreaks of infection, microorganisms involved and response to treatment, and anatomical defects, allergic processes and metabolic disorders (Bonilla *et al.*, 2005). A detailed family history should be taken into consideration, since many PID are linked with X chromosome and the presence of children in maternal family with recurrent infections, or death in childhood due to severe infection indicates the possibility of PID. Initially, screening tests are indicated or initial and advanced testing as suspected PID (Sewell *et al.*, 2006). In general, immune assessment requires specialized laboratory and high financial cost, and it comes to pediatric patients, should be chosen methods that can be executed with low amount of blood (Oliveira & Fleisher, 2010). The diagnosis of some PID may be removed if they are used and selected screening tests such blood test for congenital neutropenia, leukocyte adhesion deficiency (LAD), severe combined immunodeficiency (SCID) and Wiskott-Aldrich Syndrome (WAS), or immunoglobulin's quantification in suspected predominantly antibody defects (Gill, 2002). The diagnostic criteria are divided into three categories, definite, probable and possible. In ensuring inclusion of patients with polymorphic variants in genes associated with PID and specific clinical and laboratory changes, the patient must meet all criteria characteristic of the disease (Conley *et al.*, 1999). The delay in diagnosis is often associated with limited access to specialized resources (Lindegren, 2004), is not unique to developing countries (Liang *et al.*, 2008), leading to large variation between numbers of cases (Stihem, 2004). In Finland, the common variable immunodeficiency (CVID) showed delay time diagnosis of 5 years in 2/3 of patients and 10 years in 1/3 these (Kainulainen *et al.*, 2001), in United Kingdom this delay was 6.2 years during 1989 to 1995, and decreased 3.5 years after implantation of government program to guide distribution of national guidance on recognition and diagnosis of PID, after a study conducted between 1996 to 2002 (Seymour *et al.,* 2005). To be assured diagnostic quality indicators should be generated which include patient registration data, which together form the field and field set and its variables called record. These cases are based registry designed to improve patient care, but are useful for studying diseases. An example is early records of 368 patients with chronic granulomatous disease (GCD) by American Foundation for Immunodeficiencies started in 1993, allowing a calculation of incidence of the disease for USA born in 1/200.000 (Winkelstein *et al.,* 2000). In 1997, this study has been expanded to Common Variable Immunodeficiency (CVID), Wiskott-Aldrich Syndrome (WAS), Severe Combined Immunodeficiency (SCID), Leukocyte Adhesion Deficiency (LAD), DiGeorge Syndrome, Hyper-IgM Syndrome (HIGM) (Winkelstein *et al.,* 2003) and X-Linked Agammaglobulinemia (XLA) (Winkelstein *et al.,* 2006), showing concern in development systems of records, population data for estimating incidence, prevalence and characteristics of disease. These data are important to maintain epidemiological studies and research and design of new clinical trials, reducing mortality, increasing survival and improved quality of life. In Europe, this service is performed by European Society for Immunodeficiency-ESID non-governmental organization that aims, to facilitate exchange of information between doctors, nurses, researchers, patients and their families, promote research into causes, mechanisms and treatment of PID (Sewel *et al.,* 2006; de Vries, 2006; Guzman *et al.,* 2007; Gathmann *et al.,* 2009). This group was established in 1993, Society in 1994, and receives data from 66 specialized centers in 26 European countries. In 2005 record showed amount of 10,000 patients from 26 countries with prevalence of 4-47/1.000.000, and the European internet-based patient and research database for primary immunodeficiencies results in 7,047 patients with PID in 30 countries (Knerr *et al.,*2008) and 7430 patients from 39 countries have been documented in the ESID database (Gathmann *et al.,* 2009).

In Latin America in 1993, was created the Latin American Group for Immunodeficiencies (LAGID) to study the prevalence of PID in different regions of Latin America and promote awareness of these diseases. There are also databases online with identification of mutations locus in specific cases of PID that are established by ESID and extended by others researchers. This was initiated in 1995 to collect data in Bruton's tyrosine kinase mutations (BTK) in XLA (Lindegren *et al.,* 2004). This occurred in Brazil, through the creation of Brazilian Group of Primary Immunodeficiencies (BRAGID), which through information campaigns, increased the number of 314 cases in 2000 to 536 cases in 2004 with Southeast region responsible for 70% total cases. Another relevant factor in understanding the epidemiology of PID is introduction of specialized care networks. In England there is the National Specialist Advisory Group Comissionary (NSCAG) of National Health System (NHS), which tracks PID complex cases, such the Great Ormond Street Hospital (Jones & Gaspar, 2000) and Newcastle General Hospital (Slatter & Gennery, 2010).

Several international initiatives are currently underway to promote awareness PID and increase number of diagnosis and registration of PID (http://www.primaryimmune.org/resources/resources.htm) (Modell, 2007a; Modell, 2007b; Pickett *et al.,* 2008). Considering the increasingly frequent recognition of these diseases and their valuable contribution to understanding human immune system and mechanisms of defense against infections (more frequent medical care in worldwide) (Alcais *et al.,* 2009), it is essential establish the frequency and type in population (Casanova & Abel, 2007; Ballow *et al.,* 2009). The lack of proper diagnosis and treatment are the main problems in patients with PID in Latin America. These are related to lack of proper training of pediatrics, leading to misdiagnosis or late diagnosis, lack of proper screening, lack of government resources to implementation of diagnostic centers and disinterest of private institutions in diagnosis of PID, regional variability access to educational program and establishment of diagnostic and treatment center (Pickett *et al.*, 2008; Condino-Neto *et al.*, 2011; Leiva *et al.*, 2011).

2. Difficulties in diagnosis, treatment and education of PID in Latin America

2.1 Argentina

The main diagnostic centers in Argentina are located in Buenos Aires, and other centers are located in La Plata, Rosario, Cordoba and Mendoza. These centers are accessible and without cost to the community, provided that patients are referred by doctor. Private hospitals in Argentina offer only partial diagnosis, because no they have laboratories and professionals specialized in PID. Patients in Paraguay, Bolivia and Uruguay are also diagnosed and treated in Buenos Aires since these countries do not have adequate support. As their countries do not encourage their costs, or they do not have health insurance, this burden financially immunology centers in Argentina (Maceira *et al.*, 2010). Patients with PID who need IVIG are usually met in Buenos Aires, and treatment is not automatically continued in the pediatric patient who came into adults, it should be transferred from pediatric hospital to hospital for adults, interrupting treatment (Krasovec *et al.*, 2007). In Argentina, immunologists are not recognized experts by the Ministry of Health, and only two hospitals in Buenos Aires offer scholarships programs and post-graduate training in immunology funded by government agencies (Galicchio *et al.*, 2010; Condino-Neto *et al.*, 2011).

2.2 Brasil

It is estimated that Brazil has 2,000 patients on treatment and approximately 20,000 patients with PID (Leiva *et al.*, 2007). Immunological diagnosis is supported by numerous centers located in São Paulo, Minas Gerais, Paraná, Rio Grande do Sul, Bahia and Rio de Janeiro (Grumach *et al.*, 1997; Leiva *et al.*, 2007). Centers located in southeast of country have specialized researchers, structure and molecular diagnostics. In Brazil, the federal government assists the movement of patients from regions without infrastructure to specialized centers, and coverage for certain screening tests of PID (Ocké-Reis & Marmor, 2010; Paim *et al.*, 2011). High costs and access to specialized laboratories are considered major problems by doctors for the diagnosis of PID (results available http://www.bragid.org.br/download/graphicos.pps), with strong educational, whose website presents PID centers throughout Brazil, journals, reviews and articles, case discussions, and announcements of meetings. This is supported by St. Jude's Hospital children and government agencies FAPESP and CNPq. Activities of this group include completion of first and second Summer School of PID by LAGID, implementation of Electronic Registration of Latin America Immunodeficiencies (http://imuno.unicamp.br:8080/) with installation of hardware in UNICAMP center computing support of ESID. The Federal University of São Paulo-UNIFESP, in partnership with Jeffrey Modell Foundation and Baxter International, created the first Jeffrey Modell Diagnostic Center for PID in Latin America; with goal of enabling physicians perform diagnostic, treatment and education of patients and PID cases reported in Brazil and Latin America. Patients with PID who need IVIG in Brazil receive government financial support, and not institutions or private health insurance, where patients should be initially admitted for diagnostic and treatment center. In Brazil, there are numerous funding agencies to residency programs in allergy and immunology, although only few centers are able to train professionals and PID treatment, located in São Paulo (Costa-Carvalho *et al.*, 2011; Condino-Neto *et al.*, 2011).

2.3 Chile

The best laboratories for diagnosis of PID in Chile are located in Santiago, Temuco, Valparaiso and Concepcion. Initial screening tests for PID can be performed in large hospitals, although it does not receive government financial support (Goic & Armas, 2010). As in most underdeveloped countries in Latin America, the diagnosis of PID is often performed after numerous episodes of infection and treatment, and patient referral to specialist in infectious diseases, and finally to immunology center. Patients with PID, who need IVIG, are not reimbursed by the public health system for PID, burdening the costs to patients, which makes the treatment is not performed or interrupted. Chile has a three-year residency in immunology at the University of Santiago of Chile, providing training care of adult and pediatric patients (Condino-Neto *et al.*, 2011).

2.4 Colombia

Colombia has a national PID referral center located in University of Antioquia in Medellin, which has laboratory equipped to perform molecular and immunological diagnosis of PID, and other centers and programs are being developed in Bogota, Cali, Cartagena and Barranquila. Currently, 80% of cases of PID in Colombia come from Antioquia (Montoya *et al.*, 2002; Obando *et al.*, 2005) and neighboring states, which represents less than 20% of Colombia population. Most clinical laboratories in Colombia are able to perform initial PID screening, but specific tests are only available in Medellin and Bogota (Montoya *et al.*, 2002; Diaz *et al.*, 2008). In Colombia, the government Compulsory Health Plan (POS) provides basic coverage for PID and additional coverage can be obtained from private insurance companies (Gonzáles *et al.*, 1999; Cardona & Segura, 2011). Patients with PID, who need IVIG, are not refunded by POS, but IVIG treatments are covered by private insurance companies, who refunded through government's national fund FOSYGA. In this country there is Foundation for Diana Garcia de Olarte PID, which supports and develops educational programs, provides infrastructure for IVIG treatment centers and offers legal advice for patients who need IVIG (Montoya & Sorensen, 2001). The University of Antioquia in Medellin has immunology program for medical residents, and like Latin American countries, this prefer specialize in other areas, since the financial return is greater (Condino-Neto *et al.*, 2011).

2.5 Honduras

Honduras has two PID diagnostic centers, located in Tegucigalpa and San Pedro Sula, accessible to entire community, first laboratory support specific PID, and country have serious problems in laboratory diagnosis and access costs (Leon, 2003), availability of IVIG and cost. Only two hospitals in Tecigalpa, including National Institute of Social Security, provide treatment with IVIG. The country has no specific PID program residency, and receives training only three months on basic immunology, autoimmunity, allergy and immunodeficiency (Condino-Neto *et al.*, 2011).

2.6 Mexico

Mexico has specialized centers diagnosis of PID in Mexico City, Monterrey and Guadalajara, and molecular diagnosis of some PID can be performed only in Mexico City. Mexico has serious access problems to laboratory tests, cost and medical education in PID (Romero-Márquez & Romero-Zepeda, 2010; Yavich *et al.*, 2010). The Access to IVIG is extended to public health system and is administered in public hospitals and clinics, but doctors do not follow specific guidelines for the administration of IVIG. The use of IVIG represents 20% of coast in obtaining drugs by National Institute of Pediatrics in Mexico City. In Mexico, there are plenty residency programs in allergy and immunology, with emphasis on allergies. Only the National Institute of Pediatrics in Mexico City has residency program with emphasis on pediatric allergy and immunology (Condino-Neto *et al.*, 2011).

3. Latin American group of immunodeficiency

One of major problems of records diseases in underdeveloped countries has been limitation of diagnostic and treatment, and send reports of cases by physicians, resulting in overestimation in certain clinical centers in collection of samples, since most of these centers is reference to some types of PID, and lack of standardized definitions of cases makes it impossible to calculate rates of healthy population from this source, by only reporting positive cases without reference population data (Condino-Neto *et al.*, 2011).

The PID diagnosis is performed in immunology centers, usually located in major cities of Latin American countries, and the vast majority of pediatricians and general practitioners are not prepared to establish PID diagnosis. The medical community educator has a role in awareness of population and health professionals in PID. In 1997, the University of São Paulo, Brazil, 166 cases of PID were registered with frequency of predominantly humoral defects (60.8%), T cell defects (4.9%), combined T-and B-cell deficiencies (9, 6%), phagocyte disorders (18.7%) and complement deficiency (6%). During observed period, 13.8% of children died, primarily of recurrent infections. In comparison with other reports, was higher relative frequency of phagocyte and complement deficiency. This is the first report on PID over 15 year's observation (1981-1996) (Grumach *et al.*, 1997). In 1998, a Colombia study with 83 PID patients demonstrated most common disturbance was antibody deficiency (74,6%), followed abnormalities of unspecific mechanisms (13,3%), deficiencies of cell mediated immunity (9,6%), and mortality ratio was 6% especially in patients with cellular deficiency (Núñes, 1988).

In Antioquia, Colombia, between August of 1994 and July of 2002, 98 patients was registered with diagnosis of PID, with most frequent report antibodies deficiency (40,8%), followed by combined deficiencies (21,4%)(Montoya *et al.*, 2002). In Latin America, in 1993, immunologists from four Latin American countries (Argentina, Brazil, Chile, Colombia), created the Latin American Group for Immunodeficiencies (LAGID) to study the frequency of PID and promote knowledge by general practitioners and specialists in allergy and immunology, including Latin American countries, creating a record in each participating country. Currently, 14 countries belong to this group, which had record 3321 patients in 2004.

LAGID was implemented in 1993 with the mission to include several Latin American countries, spread the educational and awareness programs, establish PIDD registries, and promote annual scientific meetings with the participation of well-recognized international authorities in the PID field, This environment made possible the intensive interaction among Latin American doctors which in turn interacted with North American and European investigators resulting in a network, significant scientific development in Latin America, and the several resultant publications, starting with the clinical studies based on the LAGID registries

In order to encourage the registration of cases by LAGID, this sets out on its website (http://www.lagid.lsuhsc.edu) the objectives:

1. Knowing the frequency of different PID
2. Compare the frequency of different PID by region and country
3. Knowing the time that elapses between the onset of symptoms and diagnosis and measure whether this time can be shortened through the dissemination of knowledge about PID
4. Create awareness in importance of PID in primary care physicians, educators from basic and clinical science and health authorities to decide how to allocate resources for diagnosis and treatment of diseases in diverse groups
5. Promote research in various aspects of specific PID that would not be possible to settle in very small groups of patients
6. Disseminate the findings in field of Latin American PID to medical and international immune community
7. Facilitate the formation of support groups for parents and sponsors

The first LAGID published a series of studies in 1998, recording instances of medical services totaling 1428 patients of eight countries (Argentina, Brazil, Chile, Colombia, Costa Rica, Mexico, Paraguay, Uruguay), concluding that predominantly antibody deficiencies were reported in 58% patients, followed by cellular and antibody immunodeficiencies associated with others abnormalities in 18%, immunodeficiency syndromes associated with granulocyte dysfunction in 8%, phagocytic disorders in 9%, combined cellular and antibody immunodeficiencies in 5%, and complement deficiencies in 2% of patients (Zelazko *et al.*, 1998).

In a second step, this same group published a second series of studies in 2007, documenting 3.321 cases of 12 Latin American countries (Argentina, Bolivia, Brazil, Chile, Colombia, Costa Rica, Ecuador, Mexico, Peru, Paraguay, Uruguay and Venezuela). The most common form of PID was predominantly antibody deficiency (53,2%), other well-defined PID syndromes such ataxia telangiectasia, Hyper IgE and Di George (22,6%), Combined T- and B-cell Immunodeficiency (9,5%), phagocytic disorders (8,6%), diseases of immune dysregulation (3,3%) and complement deficiencies (2,8%). All countries that participated in the first publication in 1998 reported increase in PID register cases, ranging between 10 and 80% (Leiva *et al.*, 2007).

In second LAGID record, Argentina recorded 852 cases of predominantly antibody deficiency, and Brazil 404 with predominates isothype deficiencies of light chain with normal numbers of B cells. Brazil reported 75 cases of Combined T-and B-cell Immunodeficiency and Argentina 69 cases. Like other well-defined syndromes, Argentina reported 60 cases of Di George Syndrome, 42 of Hyper IgE Syndrome and 40 of Wiskott-Aldrech Syndrome, Costa Rica 82 cases of DNA repair defects and Brazil 37 cases of Chronic

Mucocutaneous Candidiasis. Representing diseases of immune dysregulation, Argentina reported 22 cases of Immunodeficiency with Hypopigmentation, followed by 14 cases of Brazil. Congenital defects of phagocytic number, function or both, Brazil reported 50 cases of cyclic neutropenia and 42 cases of Chronic Granulomatous Disease (CGD), and Argentina 46 cases. Brazil reported 50 cases of deficiency complement, followed by 13 reports of Argentina (Leiva *et al.,* 2007). Like others studies, predominantly antibody deficiency was the principal PID observed in Latin America, Australia (Baumgart *et al.,* 1997; Kirkpatrick et al., 2007), China (Zhao *et al.,* 2006; Wang *et al.,* 2011), Egypt (Reda *et al.,* 2009), French (CEREDIH, 2010), Hong Kong (Lam *et al.,* 2005), Iran (Aghamohammadi *et al.,* 2002; Farhoudi *et al.,* 2005; Rezaei *et al.,* 2006), Italy (Luzi *et al.,* 1983), Kuwait (Al-Herz, 2008), Netherland (Zegers *et al.,* 1994), Norway (Stray-Pedersen *et al.,* 2000), Poland (Bernatowska *et al.,* 1998), Republic of Ireland (Abuzakouk *et al.,* 2005), Spain (Matamoros *et al.,* 1997; Milá *et al.,* 2001), Swiss (Ryser *et al.,* 1998), Taiwan (Lee *et al.,* 2011), Thailand (Benjasupattananan *et al.,* 2009), Tunisia (Bejaoui *et al.,* 1997) and USA (Javier *et al.,* 2000; Stiehm, 2007), Studies in other countries reveled major number of granulocyte dysfunction in India (Verma *et al.,* 2008), and Combined T-and B-cell Immunodeficiency in Turk (Shabestari *et al.,* 2007).

On October 14, 2009, a group of experts from six Latin American countries (Argentina, Brazil, Chile, Colombia, Honduras and Mexico) and representatives of LASID meet in Cartagena de Indias in Colombia to discuss particular needs of each country about PID. Also this year, was created on-line Program Registration in Latin America (Registration of Society for Immunodeficiencies Latin American-LASID) in site http://deficiencia.unicamp.br:8080/, to provide information of PID epidemiology in Latin America. This meeting was held on 28 and 29 April in São Paulo, with the participation of 90 participants from Argentina, Brazil, Chile, Colombia, Honduras and Mexico, three faculty members from the USA and a faculty member of ESID. The online registration for Latin America was adapted from the record set ESID in Europe; Latin America is supported by Jeffrey Modell Foundation and National Council for Scientific and Technological Development (CNPq) of Brazil. From this date, 24 centers were enrolled in diagnosis, treatment and research, with more than 600 registered patients. In others countries, the online database network make good results in records of PID (Eades-Perner *et al.,* 2007; Guzman *et al.,*; 2007; Gathmann *et al.,* 2009),

The LAGID has published four reports and proceedings; the first two papers focused on the prevalence and characteristics of PID patients in Latin America (Zelazco *et al.,* 1998; Leiva *et al.,* 2007); the third and fourth summarized deficiencies in PID diagnosis and treatment in Latin America and described features of educational outreach program, immunology fellowship program, and laboratory network aimed at correcting these deficiencies (Condino-Neto *et al.,* 2011; Leiva *et al.,* 2011). From July 2009 to September 2010, the LAGID recorded 838 cases of PID.

In April 2011, the registry of Immunodeficiencies completed two years, with more than 1000 cases reported from 35 centers representing various Latin America countries. Recently, the Committee decided to hold LASID collaborative studies with the recorded data to better understand profile of prevalent PID, such XLA, HIgM, and CGD, filling out form and sending data to protocololasidxla@bragid.org.br or protocololasidhim@bragid.org.br or protocololasiddgc@bragid.org.br depending on PID. The group also offers financial education programs in PID, with projects submitted to e-mail info@imunopediatria.org.br.

Those studies contributed with new insights on clinical presentation and impacted positively on the molecular diagnosis of PID. All together the Latin American experience shows that BCG complications is prevalent among SCID, T-cell deficiencies, and CGD patients; that fungal infections is highly prevalent among X-linked HIGM patients, and that ataxia-teleangiectasia is especially frequent in Mexico and Costa Rica. Currently Chile is building a new diagnostic center at University La Frontera that will interact with research centers in Argentina, Brazil, and Colombia. This strategy will strength even more the interaction among the several Latin American research centers.

Studies by LAGID showed numerous factors responsible for delay in diagnosis and treatment of patients with PID. Most pediatricians and family physicians in Latin America are not sufficiently trained to carry out the diagnosis of PID, there is a low amount of specialized installations for specific immunological tests, there is limited coverage for screening tests given by the government or private institutions, regional variability access to health and failure to comply with guidelines in certain countries and regions. To improve some of these aspects, diagnosis and treatment of patients with PID, experts from Latin America and the USA meet to discuss three specific programs, educational program (The L-Project), scholarships program and establishing of laboratory network to expand access to data (The Latin América Advisory Board on Primary Immunodeficiencies) (Leiva *et al.*, 2011; Condino-Neto *et al.*, 2011).

3.1 Educational program

The educational program (L-Project) was established to create increased awareness of general public, continuing education network on PID, promote basic and clinical research of PID and inform government officials in impact of PID on health published in Latin America. This program covers students, residents, pediatricians, nurses and officials involved in health system. It also emphasizes encouragement medical students seeking academic placement of teaching, research and clinical PID. These programs include summer school, containing cases and report on short-term programs associated with PID infection, dissemination of information by radio, television, websites, newspapers, magazines and educational material for community (Marodi & Casanova, 2009; Leiva *et al.*, 2011). This proposal directly contributes to knowledge generation and increase technological capacity of Latin America in this field. It is virtuous chain where all the researchers and the community involved propagate their knowledge acquired in other centers of reference, allowed expansion of existing lines of research in Brazil.

3.2 Summer school

Creating of Summer school is considered a viable solution to promote scientific interaction, and standardization of PID knowledge in different member countries because educational systems and medical residents differ in each country member (Condino-Neto *et al.*, 2011; Leiva *et al.*, 2011). In Brazil, São Paulo in 2006 was held the first Summer School, based on model proposed by ESID and CIS. This meeting was attended by 12 teachers of LAGID, ESID and CIS experts PID and 12 students, where they were focused biochemical and molecular diagnosis PID, major PID in Latin America; IVIG therapy guidelines, hematopoietic bone marrow transplantation; communication network LAGID. New meeting was held in 2008 in Temuco, Chile, and recently in 2010, Bahia, Brazil, with inclusion of 90 students from different Latin America countries.

3.3 Scholarship program offer

One of great difficulties encountered in developing countries for training professionals in PID is to awaken academic and professional interests, without compromising quality of life and survival of students and health professionals. Thus, different Latin American countries offer scholarships funded by educational institutions and other entities, governmental or private, with development of people involved and trained in specific areas of health. One of major problems seen in developing countries is the absence of jobs, which means that many students, just looking for graduate services that offer post-graduate scholarships, forgetting commitment they have with the community. Another problem in Latin America is formation of highly trained and qualified for certain areas of education and research, which are not absorbed by countries, end migrating to other parts of world. To resolve these problems, the Advisory Council LAGID determined availability of scholarships for doctors interested in area of clinical PID, as well doctors and teachers interested in immunology. The participating institutions were willing to participate in record LAGID, and grant applicants to submit personal statement, career development plan, and mentor involved with project statement of no conflict of financial interest and letters of recommendation. In this agreement, it was established that no country could be assigned more than two grants during period of two years, and beneficiaries of scholarship must publish report on its activities or clinical results or research (Leiva *et al.,* 2011).

3.4 Creation of centers of education, diagnosis and treatment

One of the major problems encountered in developing countries is lack of proper training of physicians and pediatric regional variability in access to educational program and establishment of diagnostic and treatment center. Thus, education and training are needed for specialists, pediatricians, general practitioners from different countries and regions of Latin America, ensuring that they are able to recognize warning PID signs. This includes creation of Summer School, symposia and conferences of PID. These educational efforts should also be understood to medical students, nurses and general public. For that, programs are needed government and private funding, and network (Leiva *et al.,* 2011). In Brazil, the Jeffrey Modell Foundation, and Baxter pharmaceutical industry, created on April 29, 2009 at Federal University of São Paulo-UNIFESP, the first Jeffrey Modell Diagnostic Center for PID in Latin America, based in field of Immunology pediatric UNIFESP, with working points in different parts of the country. The Jeffrey Modell Diagnostic Center operates in front of medical education, diagnosis and records of PID and patient education (Modell, 2007a; Modell, 2007b). Other diagnostic centers sponsored by the Jeffrey Modell will be opened in Mexico, Argentina, Colombia and Chile. Advancing educational model for educational outreach in Latin America is observed in the Brazilian Group of Human Immunodeficiency (BRAGID) (http://www.bragid.org.br), whose number of registered doctors increased from 190 in 2002 to 2.500 in 2009, after creation of local seminars on dating PID. The BRAGID provides information on warning PID, different clinical presentation PID of and diagnostic laboratories. Offer clinical cases that can be discussed in Internet. This model is followed in Colombia, which has specialized site that shows warning PID signs, types of PID and use of IVIG. In other Latin American countries, government agencies related to areas of health are more concerned with control of infectious diseases, and most professionals in the field of immunology work independently.

4. Conclusion

The PID are congenital and inherited diseases that affect the immune system, which occurrence in population varies by type of study and study group. Recent studies indicate that these values in the general population are underestimated and are one of the biggest problems and lack of knowledge, both worldwide and Latin America. Many factors compromise its knowledge, such as lack of education centers, professional structure, and laboratory records. The incidence of PID in Latin America is similar to that observed in different parts of the world, with predominantly antibody defects. In Latin America, adds to these, the lack of government support and private initiative. To redress this problem was created LAGID, which hosts Latin American countries concerned with knowledge of incidence, diagnosis, treatment and discovery of new PID. For this, congresses are held, online records and establishing laboratory training, diagnosis and treatment of PID, based on the model established in Europe.

5. References

Aghamohammadi, A., Moein, M., Farhoudi, A., Pourpak, Z., Rezaei, N., Abolmaali, K., Movahedi, M., Gharagozlou, M., Ghazi, B.M., Mahmoudi, M., Mansouri, D., Arshi, S., Trash, N.J., Akbari, H., Sherkat, R., Hosayni, R.F., Hashemzadeh, A., Mohammadzadeh, I., Amin, R., Kashef, S., Alborzi, A., Karimi, A., Khazaei, H. (2002). Primary immunodeficiency in Iran: first report of the National Registry of PID in Children and Adults. *Journal of Clinical Immunology,* Vol. 22 (November 2002), No. 6, pp. 375-80, ISSN 1573-2592.

Abuzakouk, M., Feighery, C. (2005). Primary immunodeficiency disorders in the Republic of Ireland: first report of the national registry in children and adults. *Journal of Clinical Immunology,* Vol. 25 (January 2005), No. 1, pp. 73-7, ISSN 1573-2592.

Alcaïs, A., Abel, L., Casanova, J.L. (2009). Human genetics of infectious diseases: between proof of principle and paradigm. *Journal of Clinical Investigation,* Vol. 119 (September 2009), No. 9, pp. 2506–14, ISSN 00219738.

Al-Herz, W. (2008). Primary immunodeficiency disorders in Kuwait: first report from Kuwait National Primary Immunodeficiency Registry (2004-2006). *Journal of Clinical Immunology,* Vol. 28 (March 2008), No. 2, pp.186-93, ISSN 1573-2592.

Aloei, F.P., Mishra, S.S., MacGinitie, A.J. (2007). Guidelines for "10 warning signs of primary immunodeficiency" neither sensitive nor specific. The *Journal of Allergy and Clinical Immunology,* Vol. 119 (January 2007), No. 1, Suppl. pp. S14-S14F, ISSN 0091-6749.

American Academy of Pediatrics. (1993). Newborn screening for congenital hypothyroidism: Recomended guidelines. *Pediatrics,* Vol.91 (June 1993), No. 6, pp.1203-1209, ISSN 0031-4005.

Ballow, M., Notarangelo, L., Grimbacher, B., Cunningham-Rundles, C., Stein, M., Helbert, M., Gathmann, B., Kindle, G., Knigth, A.K., Ochs, H.D., Sullivan, K., Franco, J.L. (2009). Immunodeficiencies. *Clinical and Experimental Immunology,* Vol. 158 (December 2009), Suppl. 1, pp. 14–22, ISSN 0009-9104.

Banks, M. (2010). Deficient diagnosis. *Parliament Magazine,* Vol. 3 (May 2010), pp. 24-25, ISSN 1372-7966.

Baumgart, K.W., Britton, W.J., Kemp, A., French, M., Roberton, D. (1997). The spectrum of primary immunodeficiency disorders in Australia. *Journal of Allergy and Clinical Immunology,* Vol. 100 (September 1997), No. 3, pp. 415-23, ISSN 0091-6749.

Bejaoui, M., Barbouche, M.R., Sassi, A., Larguche, B., Miladi, N., Bouguerra, A., Dellagi, K. (1997). Primary immunodeficiency in Tunisia: study of 152 cases. *Archives de Pédiatrie,* Vol. 4 (September 1997), No. 9, pp. 827-31, ISSN 0929-693X.

Benjasupattananan, P., Simasathein, T., Vichyanond, P., Leungwedchakarn, V., Visitsunthorn, N., Pacharn, P., Jirapongsananuruk, O. (2009). Clinical characteristics and outcomes of primary immunodeficiencies in Thai children: an 18-year experience from a tertiary care center. *Journal of Clinical Immunology,* Vol. 29 (May 2009), No. 3, pp. 357-64, ISSN 1573-2592.

Bernatowska, E., Madalinski, K., Michalkiewicz, J., Gregorek, H. (1988). Primary immunodeficiency diseases in children treated in the Children's Memorial Hospital, Poland. *Immunological Investigations,* Vol. 17 (April 1988), No. 2, pp. 107-20, ISSN 0882-0139.

Bonilla, F.A., Bernstein, I.L., Khan, D.A., Ballas, Z.K., Chinen, J., Frank, M.M., Kobrynski, L.J., Levinson, A.I., Mazer, B., Nelson, R.P.Jr, Orange, J.S., Routes, J.M., Shearer, W.T., Sorensen, R.U.; American College of Allergy, Asthma and Immunology; Joint Council of Allergy, Asthma and Immunology. (2005). Practice parameter for the diagnosis and management of primary immunodeficiency. *Annals of Allergy Asthma Immunology,* Vol. 94 (May 2005), No. 5, pp.S1-63, ISSN 1081-1206.

Bonilla, F.A., Geha, R.S. (2006). Update on primary immunodeficiency diseases. *Journal of Allergy and Clinical Immunology,* Vol. 117 (February 2006), No. 2 (Suppl Mini-Primer), pp. S435-41, ISSN 0091-6749.

Bousfiha, A., Picard, C., Boisson-Dupuis, S., Zhang, S.Y., Bustamante, J., Puel, A., Jouanguy, E., Ailal, F., El-Baghdadi, J., Abel, L., Casanova, J.L. (2010). Primary immunodeficiencies of protective immunity to primary infections. *Clinical Immunology,* Vol. 135 (May 2010), No.2, pp. 204-9, ISSN 1521-6616.

Boyle, J.M., Buckley, R.H. (2007). Population prevalence of diagnosed primary immunodeficiency diseases in the United States. *Journal of Clinical Immunology,* Vol. 27 (September 2007), No. 5, pp. 497-502, ISSN 1573-2592.

Bustamante, J., Boisson-Dupuis, S., Jouanguy, E., Picard, C., Puel, A., Abel, L., Casanova, J.L. (2008a). Novel primary immunodeficiencies revealed by the investigation of paediatric infectious diseases. *Current Opinion in Immunology,* Vol. 20 (February 2008), No. 1, pp. 39-48, ISSN 0952-7915.

Bustamante, J., Zhang, S., von Bernuth, H., Abel, L., Casanova, J.L. (2008b). From Infectious diseases to primary immunodeficiencies. *Immunology Allergy Clinical North America,* Vol. 28 (May 2008), No. 2, pp. 235–58. ISSN 0889-8561.

Cardona, A. D., Segura C.A.M. (2011). Public health policies as regards the elderly in Colombia. *Revista Espanola Geriatria y Gerontologia,* Vol. 46 (March-April 2011), No. 2, pp. 96-9, ISSN 0211-139X.

Casanova, J.L., Abel, L. (2007). Primary Immunodeficiencies: A Field in Its Infancy. *Science,* Vol 317 (August 2007), No. 5838, pp. 617-19, ISSN 0036-8075.

Casanova, J.L., Fieschi, C., Zhang, S., Abel, L. (2008). Revisiting human primary immunodeficiencies. *Journal of Internal Medicine,* Vol. 264 (August 2008), No. 2, pp. 115-27, ISSN 0954-6820.

Cassimos, D.C., Liatsis, M., Stogiannidou, A., Kanariou, M. (2010). Children with frequent infections: A proposal for a stepwise assessment and investigation of the immune system. The immune defense to foreign invaders Symphony. Which instrument is out of tune? *Pediatric Allergy and Immunology,* Vol. 21 (May 2010), No. 3, pp. 463–73, ISSN 0905-6157.

CEREDIH: The French PID study group. (2010). The French national registry of primary immunodeficiency diseases. *Clinical Immunology,* Vol. 135 (May 2010), No. 2, pp. 264-72, ISSN 1521-6616.

Champi, C. (2002). Primary immunodeficiency disorders in children: prompt diagnosis can lead to lifesaving treatment. *Journal of Pediatric Health Care,* Vol. 16 (January-February 2002), No. 1, pp. 16-21, ISSN 0891-5245.

Chapel, H.H. (2005). Primary immune deficiencies-improving our understanding of their role in immunological disease. *Clinical and Experimental Immunology,* Vol. 139 (January 2005), No. 1, pp. 11-12, ISSN 0009-9104.

Condino-Neto, A., Franco, J.L., Trujillo-Vargas, C., Espinosa-Rosales, F.J., Leiva, L.E., Rodriguez-Quiroz, F., King, A., Lagos, M., Oleastro, M., Bezrodnik, L., Grumach, A.S., Costa-Carvalho, B.T., Sorensen, R.U. (2011). Critical issues and needs in management of primary immunodeficiency diseases in Latin America. *Allergology Immunopathology* (Madr), Vol. 39 (January-February 2011), No. 1, pp. 45-51, ISSN 0301-0546.

Conley, M.E., Notarangelo, L.D., Etzioni, A. (1999). Diagnostic criteria for primary immunodeficiencies. *Clinical Immunology,* Vol. 93 (December 1999), No. 3, pp. 190-7, ISSN 1521-6616.

Costa-Carvalho, B.T., Waldalsen, G.F., Pulici, G., Aranda, C.S., Solé, D., C. (2011). Pulmonary complications in patients with antibody deficiency. *Allergology Immunopathology* (Madr), Vol. 39 (May-June 2011), No. 3, pp. 128-32, ISSN 0301-0546.

de Carvalho, T.M., dos Santos. H.P., dos Santos, I.C., Vargas, P.R., Pedrosa, J. (2007). Newborn screening: a national public health programme in Brazil. *Journal of Inherited of Metabolic Disease,* Vol. 30 (August 2007), No. 4, pp. 615, ISSN 0141-8955.

de Vries, E. (2006). For the Clinical Working Party of the European Society for Immunodeficiencies (ESID). Patient-centred screening for primary immunodeficiency: a multi-stage diagnostic protocol designed for non-immunologists. *Clinical and Experimental Immunology,* Vol. 145 (August 2006), No. 2, pp. 204-14, ISSN 0009-9104.

Díaz, M.A., Sarrazola, D.M., Orrego, J.C. Caracterización epidemiológica, clínica y de algunos parámetros inmunológicos del síndrome de infección recurrente en niños y adolescentes desplazados a la ciudad de Cúcuta. *Asociación Colombiana de Infectología,* Vol. 12 (February 2008), No. 1, pp. 254-63, ISSN 0123-9392.

Eades-Perner, A.M., Gathmann, B., Knerr, V., Guzman, D., Veit, D., Kindle, G., Grimbacher, B. (2007). ESID Registry Working Party. The European internet-based patient and research database for primary immunodeficiencies: results 2004-06. *Clinical and Experimental Immunology,* Vol. 147 (February 2007), No. 2, pp. 306-12, ISSN 0009-9104.

Farhoudi, A., Aghamohammadi, A., Moin, M., Rezaei, N., Pourpak, Z., Movahedi, M., Gharagozlou, M., Amir, T.S., Mir, S.G.B., Mahmoudi, M., Kouhi, A., Atarod, L.,

Ahmadi, A.A., Bazargan, N., Isaeian, A. (2005). Distribution of primary immunodeficiency disorders diagnosed in the Children's Medical Center in Iran. *Journal of Investigational Allergology and Clinical Immunology,* Vol. 15 (2005), No. 3, pp. 177-82, ISSN 1018-9068.

Fried, A.J., Bonilla, F.A. (2009). Pathogenesis, diagnosis, and management of primary antibody deficiencies and infections. *Clinical Microbiology Reviews,* Vol. 22 (July 2009), No. 3, pp. 396-414, ISSN 0893-8512.

Galicchio, M.F., Ornani, A., Bezrodnik, L., Di Giovanni, D., Gómez Raccio, A., Paz, R., Regairaz, L., Belardinelli, G., Basile, N., Oleastro, M., Ruprecht, B., Rosenzweig, S., Zelazko, M., Liberatore, D., Galicchio, M.F., Pérez, N., Cantisano, C., Díaz, H., Riganti, C.G., Gentile, Á., Bazán, V., Uboldi, A., Del Pont, J.M., Califano, G. (2010). Guías de manejo: Vacunas en pacientes con inmunodeficiencias primarias. *Archivos Argentinos de Pediatria,* Vol. 108 (May 2010), No. 5, pp. 454-64, ISSN 0325-0075.

García, J.M., Español, T., Gurbindo, M.D., Casas, C.C. (2007). Update on the treatment of primary immunodeficiencies. *Allergology Immunopathology,* Vol. 35 (September-October 2007), No. 5, pp.184-92, ISSN 0301-0546.

Gathmann, B., Grimbacher, B., Beauté, J., Dudoit, Y., Mahlaoui, N., Fischer, A., Knerr, V., Kindle, G. (2009). The European internet-based patient and research database for primary immunodeficiencies: results 2006–2008. *Clinical and Experimental Immunology,* Vol. 157 (September 2009), Suppl 1, pp. 3-11, ISSN 0009-9104.

Geha, R.S., Notarangelo, L.D., Casanova, J.L., Chapel, H., Conley, M.E., Fischer, A., Hammarstrom, M.D., Nonoyama, S., Ochs, H.D., Puck, J.W., Roifman, C., Seger, R., Wedgwood, J. (2007). Primary immunodeficiency diseases: an update from the International Union of Immunological Societies Primary Immunodeficiency Diseases Classification Committee. *Journal of Allergy and Clinical Immunology,* Vol. 120 (October 2007), No. 4, pp. 776-94, ISSN 0091-6749.

Gill, B. (2002). Specialised clinical immunology services. Definition No 16 & 17. *CPD Bulletin Immunology and Allergy,* Vol. 2 (2002), No. 2, pp. 33-68; Vol. 3 (2003), No. 3, pp. 69-100, ISSN 1367-8949.

Goic, A., Armas, R. (2010). The ALANAM statement on public health policy. *Revista Medica de Chile,* Vol. 138 (December 2010), No. 12, pp. 1558-60, ISSN 0034-9887.

Gonzáles, M. (1998). Análisis de la demanda de servicios y la morbidad en la atención en salud a la población desplazada por la violencia, prestada por la red de hospitales de Sant Fé de Bogotá D.C. en convenio con el Ministerio de Salud durante los primeiros 11 meses de 1998. Bogotá, D.C.: 1999.

Griffith, L.M., Cowan, M.J., Notarangelo, L.D., Puck, J,M,, Buckley, R,H,, Candotti, F., Conley, M.E., Fleisher, T.A., Gaspar, H.B., Kohn, D.B., Ochs, H.D., O'Reilly, R.J., Rizzo, J.D., Roifman, C.M., Small, T.N., Shearer, W.T. (2009). Workshop Participants. Improving cellular therapy for primary immune deficiency diseases: recognition, diagnosis, and management. *Journal of Allergy and Clinical Immunology,* Vol. 124 (December 2009), No. 6, pp. 1152-60, ISSN 0091-6749.

Grumach, A.S., Duarte, A.J., Bellinati-Pires, R., Pastorino, A.C., Jacob, C.M., Diogo, C.L., Condino-Neto, A., Kirschfink, M., Carneiro-Sampaio, M.M. (1997). Brazilian report on primary immunodeficiencies in children: 166 cases studied over a follow-up time of 15 years. *Journal of Clinical Immunology,* Vol. 17 (July 1997), No. 4, pp. 340-5, ISSN 1573-2592.

Guzman, D., Veit, D., Knerr, V., Kindle, G., Gathmann, B., Eades-Perner, A.M., Grimbacher, B. (2007). The ESID Online Database network. *Bioinformatics*, Vol. 23 (March 2007), No. 5, pp. 654-5, ISSN 1367-4803.

Javier, F.C. 3rd, Moore, C.M., Sorensen, R.U. (2000). Distribution of primary immunodeficiency diseases diagnosed in a pediatric tertiary hospital. *Annals of Allergy, Asthma and Immunology*, Vol. 84 (January 2000), No. 1, pp. 25-30, ISSN 1081-1206.

Jones, A.M., Gaspar, H.B. (2000). Immunogenetics: changing the face of immunodeficiency. *Journal of Clinical Pathology*, Vol. 53 (January 2000), No. 1, pp. 60-5, ISSN 0021-9746.

Kainulainen, L., Nikoskelain, J., Ruuskanen, O. (2001). Diagnostic finding in 95 Finish patients with common variable immunodeficiency. *Journal of Clinical Immunology*, Vol. 21 (March 2001), No. 2, pp. 145-9, ISSN 1573-2592.

Kirkpatrick, P., Riminton, S. (2007). Primary immunodeficiency diseases in Australia and New Zealand. *Journal of Clinical Immunology*, Vol. 27 (September 2007), No. 5, pp. 517-24, ISSN 1573-2592.

Knerr, V., Gathmann, B., Eades-Perner, A.M., Kindle, G., Grimbacher, B. (2008). The ESID Online Database for primary immunodeficiencies. First analyses with regard to Germany and Europe. *Medizinische Klinik* (Munich), Vol. 103 (September 2008), No. 9, pp. 620-7, ISSN 0723-5003.

Kohn, D.B. (2010). Update on gene therapy for immunodeficiencies. *Clinical Immunology*, Vol. 135, (May 20100), No. 2, pp. 247–54, ISSN 1521-6616.

Krasovec, S., Ornani, A., Oleastro, M. (2007). Efficacy and tolerability of an Argentine intravenous immunoglobulin in pediatric patients with primary immunodeficiency diseases. *Journal of Clinical Immunology*, Vol. 27 (March 2007), No. 2, pp. 227-32, ISSN 1573-2592.

Lam, D.S., Lee, T.L., Chan, K.W., Ho, H.K., Lau, Y.L. (2005). Primary immunodeficiency in Hong Kong and the use of genetic analysis for diagnosis. *Hong Kong Medical Journal*, Vol. 11 (April 2005), No. 2, pp. 90-6, ISSN 1024-2708.

Lee, P.P., Lau, Y.L. (2009). Primary immunodeficiencies: "new disease in an old century" *Cellular and Molecular Immunology*, Vol. 6 (December 2009), No. 6, pp. 397-406, ISSN 1672-7681.

Lee, W.I., Huang, J.L., Jaing, T.H., Shyur, S.D., Yang, K.D., Chien, Y.H., Chiang, B.L., Soong, W.J., Chiou, S.S., Shieh, C.C., Lin, S.J., Yeh, K.W., Chen, L.C., Ou, L.S., Yao, T.C., Lin, T.Y., Chiu, C.H., Huang, Y.C., Wu, K.H., Lin, C.Y., Yu, H.H., Yang, Y.H., Yu, H.R., Yen, H.J., Hsieh, M.Y., Kuo, M.L., Hwu, W.L., Tsai, Y.C., Kuo, H.C., Lin, Y.L., Shih, Y.F., Chang, K.W. (2001). Distribution, clinical features and treatment in Taiwanese patients with symptomatic primary immunodeficiency diseases (PIDs) in a nationwide population-based study during 1985-2010. *Immunobiology*, vol. 216 (December 2011), No. 12, pp. 1286-94, ISSN 0171-2985.

Leiva, L.E., Bezrodnik, L., Oleastro, M., Condino-Neto, A., Costa-Carvalho, B.T., Sevciovic Grumach, A., Espinosa-Rosales, F.J., Luis Franco, A., King, J., Inostroza., Quezada, A., Porras, O., Sorensen, R.U. (2011). Primary immunodeficiency diseases in Latin America: proceedings of the second Latin America Society for Immunodeficiencies (LASID) Advisory Board. *Allergology Immunopathology* (Madr), Vol. 39 (March-April 2011), No. 2, pp.106-10, ISSN 0301-0546.

Leiva, L.E., Zelazco, M., Oleastro, M., Carneiro-Sampaio, M., Condino-Neto, A., Costa-Carvalho, B.T., Grumach, A.S., Quezada, A., Patiño, P., Franco, J.L., Porras, O., Rodríguez, F.J., Espinosa-Rosales, F.J., Espinosa-Padilla, S.E., Almillategui, D., Martínez, C., Tafur, J.R., Valentín, M., Benarroch, L., Barroso, R., Sorensen, R.U. (2007). Primary immunodeficiency diseases in Latin America: the second report of the LAGID registry. *Journal of Clinical Immunology*, Vol. 27 (January 2007), No. 1, pp. 101-8, ISSN 1573-2592.

Leon, M. (2003). Perceptions of health care quality in Central America. *International Journal of Quality Health Care* Quality Assurance, Vol. 15 (February 2003), No. 1, pp. 67-71, ISSN 0952-6862.

Liang, F.C., Wei, Y.C., Jiang, T.H., Hsiehi, M.Y., Wen, Y.C., Chiou, Y.S., Wu, S.H., Chen, L.C., Huang, J.L., Lee, W.I. (2008). Current classification and status of primary immunodeficiency diseases in Taiwan. *Acta Paediatrica Taiwanica*, Vol. 49 (January-February 2008), No. 1, pp. 3-8, ISSN 1608-8115.

Lindegren, M.L., Kobrynski, L., Rasmussen, S.A., Moore, C.A., Grosse, S.D., Vanderford, M.L., Spira, T.J., McDougal, J.S., Vogt, R.F.Jr., Hannon. W.H., Kalman, L.V., Chen, B., Mattson, M., Baker. T.G., Khoury. M. (2004). Applying public health strategies to primary immunodeficiency diseases: a potential approach to genetic disorders. MMWR *Recommendations and Reports*, Vol. 16 (January 2004), No. 53, pp. 1-29, ISSN 1057-5987.

Luzi, G., Businco, L., Aiuti, F. (1983). Primary immunodeficiency syndromes in Italy: a report of the national register in children and adults. *Journal of Clinical Immunology*, Vol. 3 (October 1983), No. 4, pp. 316-20, ISSN 1573-2592.

Maceira, D., Paraje, G., Aramayo, F., Masi, S.D., Sánchez, D. (2010). Public financing of health research in five Latin American countries. *Revista Panamericana de la Salud Publica*, Vo. 27 (June 2010), No. 6, pp. 442-51, ISSN 1020-4989.

Maródi, L., Casanova, J.L. (2009). Primary immunodeficiency diseases: the J Project. *Lancet*, Vol. 373 (June 2009), No. 9682, pp. 2179-81, ISSN 0140-6736.

Matamoros, F.N., Mila, L.J., Español, B.T., Raga, B.S., Fontan, C.G. (1997). Primary immunodeficiency syndrome in Spain: first report of the National Registry in Children and Adults. *Journal of Clinical Immunology*, Vol. 17 (July 1997), No. 4, pp. 333-9, ISSN 1573-2592.

Milá, L.J., Etxagibel, G.A., Matamoros, F.N. (2001). The Spanish Registry of Primary Immunodeficiencies (REDIP). *Allergologia et Immunopathologia* (Madr), Vol. 29 (May-June 2001), No. 3, pp. 122-5, ISSN 0301-0546.

Modell, F. (2007a). Immunology today and new discoveries: building upon legacies of Dr. Robert A. Good. *Immunologic Research*, Vol. 38 (2007), No. 1-3, pp. 48-50, ISSN 0257-277X.

Modell, V. (2007b). The impact of physician education and public awareness on early diagnosis of primary immunodeficiencies: Robert A. Good Immunology Symposium. *Immunologic Research*, Vol. 38 (2007), No. 1-3, pp. 43-7, ISSN 0257-277X.

Montoya, C.J., Henao, J., Salgado, H., Olivares, M.M., López, J.A., Rugeles, C., Franco, J.L., Orego, J., Garcia, D.M., Patino, P.J. (2002). Phenotypic diagnosis of primary immunodefiencies in Antioqua, Colômbia 1994-2002. *Biomédica*, Vol. 22 (December 2002), No. 4, pp. 510-18, ISSN 0120-4157.

Montoya, C.J., Sorensen, R.U. Lecciones sobre el uso de gammaglobulina humana endovenosa. Boletin LAGID. 23 de fevereiro de 2001. Disponible [on-line]:http//www.lagid.lsuhsc.edu/Tratamientos/971-010.htm2001.

Morimoto, Y., Routes, J.M. (2008). Immunodeficiency Overview. *Primary Care*, Vol. 35 (March 2008), No. 1, pp. 159–73, ISSN 0095-4543.

Neven, B., Leroy, S., Decaluwe, H., Le Deist, F., Picard, C., Moshous, D., Mahlaoui, N., Debré, M., Casanova, J.L., Dal Cortivo, L., Madec, Y., Hacein-Bey-Abina, S., de Saint Basile, G., de Villartay, J.P., Blanche, S., Cavazzana-Calvo, M., Fischer, A. (2009). Long-term outcome after hematopoietic stem cell transplantation of a single-center cohort of 90 patients with severe combined immunodeficiency. *Blood*, Vol. 113 (April 2009), No. 17, pp. 4114-24, ISSN 0006-4971.

Notarangelo, L.D. (2010). PIDs and cancer: an evolving story. *Blood*, Vol. 116 (August 2010), No. 8, pp. 1189-90, ISSN 0006-4971.

Núñes, R.M. (1988). Primary immunodeficiency in Colombian children. *Allergologia et Imunopathologia (Madr)*, Vol. 16 (July-August 1988), No. 4, pp. 273-5, ISSN 0301-0546.

Notarangelo, L.D., Fischer, A., Geha, R.S., Casanova, J.L., Conley, M.E., Cunningham-Rundles, C., Etzioni, A., Hammartrom, L., Nonoyama, S., Ochs, HD., Puck, J., Roifmann, C., Seger, R., Wedgwood, J. (2010). Primary imunodeficiencis: 2009 update. International Union of Immunological Societies Expert Committee on Primary Immunodeficiencies. *Journal of Allergy and Clinical Immunology*, Vol. 124 (December 2009), No. 6, pp. 1161-78. Erratum in: *Journal of Allergy and Clinical Immunology*, Vol. 125 (March 2010), No. 3, pp. 771-3, ISSN 0091-6749.

Obando, L.E.E., Orrego, A.J.C.O., Restrepo, J.L.F., Olivares, M.C.J., Olivares, M.M., Salgado, H., Gomez, R.D., Grajales, P.J.P. (2005). Caracterización epidemiológica de pacientes con immunodeficiencias primarias en el Programa de Detección y Manejo del Síndrome de Infección Reccurrente del Grupo de Inmunodeficiencias Primarias-Universidad de Antioqua. *Revista Inmunoalergia*, Vol. 13 (2005), No. 5, pp. 142-3, ISSN 0123-6849.

Ocké-Reis, C.O., Marmor, T.R. (2010). The Brazilian national health system: an ununfulfilled promise? *International Journal of Health Planning and Management*, Vol. 25 (October-December 2010), No. 4, pp. 318-29, ISSN 0749-6753.

Oliveira, J.B., Fleisher, T.A. (2010). Laboratory evaluation of primary immunodeficiencies. *Journal of Allergy and Clinical Immunology*, Vol. 125 (February 2010), No. 2 (Suppl 2), pp. S297-305, ISSN 0091-6749.

Olivieri, A. (2009). The Study Group for Congenital Hypothyroidism. The Italian National Register of infants with congenital hypothyroidism: twenty years of surveillance and study of congenital hypothyroidism. *Rivista Italiana di Pediatria*, Vol. 35 (February 2009), No. 1, pp. 2, ISSN 0390-671X.

Paim, J., Travassos, C., Almeida, C., Bahia, L., Machinko, J. (2011). The Brazilian healt system: history, advances, and challenges. *Lancet*, Vol. 377 (May 2011), No. 9779, pp. 1778-97, ISSN 0140-6736.

Pessach, I., Walter, J., Notarangelo, L.D. (2009). Recent Advances in Primary Immunodeficiencies: Identification of Novel Genetic Defects and Unanticipated Phenotypes. *Pediatric Research*, Vol. 65 (May 2009), No. 5 Pt 2, pp. 3R–12R, ISSN 0031-3998.

Pickett, D., Modell, V., Leighton, I., Modell, F. (2008). Impact of a physician education and patient awareness campaign on the diagnosis and management of primary immunodeficiencies. *Immunologic Research,* Vol. 40 (2008), No. 1, pp. 93-4, ISSN 0257-277X.

Puck, J.M. (1997). Primary immunodeficiency disease. *The Journal of the American Medical Association,* Vol. 278 (December 1997), No. 22, pp. 1835-41, ISSN 0098-7484.

Reda, S.M., Afifi, H.M., Amine, M.M. (2009). Primary immunodeficiency diseases in Egyptian children: a single-center study. *Journal of Clinical Immunology,* Vol. 29 (May 2009), No. 3, pp. 343-51, ISSN 1573-2592.

Rezaei, N., Aghamohammadi, A., Moin, M., Pourpak, Z., Movahedi, M., Gharagozlou, M., Atarod, L., Ghazi, B.M,, Isaeian, A., Mahmoudi, M., Abolmaali, K., Mansouri, D., Arshi, S., Tarash, N.J.,Sherkat, R., Akbari, H., Amin, R., Alborzi, A., Kashef, S., Farid, R., Mohammadzadeh, I., Shabestari, M.S., Nabavi, M., Farhoudi, A. (2006). Frequency and clinical manifestations of patients with primary immunodeficiency disorders in Iran: update from the Iranian Primary Immunodeficiency Registry. *Journal of Clinical Immunology,* Vol. 26 (November 2006), No. 6, pp. 519-32, ISSN 1573-2592.

Romero-Márquez, R.S., Romero-Zepeda, H. (2010). Quality of life relation to public health and the health system reflections. Revista Médica del Instuto Mexicano de Seguro Social. Vol. 48, (January-February 2010), No. 1, pp. 91-102, ISSN 0443-5117.

Ryser, O., Morell, A., Hitzig, W.H. (1998). Primary immunodeficiencies in Switzerland: first report of the national registry in adults and children. *Journal of Clinical Immunology,* Vol. 8 (November 1988), No. 6, pp. 479-85, ISSN 1573-2592.

Seymour, B., Miles, J., Haeney, M. (2005). Primary antibody deficiency and diagnostic delay. *Journal of Clinical Pathology,* Vol. 58 (May 2005), No. 5, pp. 546-7, ISSN 0021-9746.

Sewell, W.A.C., Khan, S., Doré, P.C. (2006). Early indicators of immunodeficiency in adults and children: protocols for screening for primary immunological defects. *Clinical and Experimental Immunology,* Vol. 145 (August 2006), No. 2, pp. 201-3, ISSN 0009-9104.

Shabestari, M.S., Maljaei, S.H., Baradaran, R., Barzegar, M., Hashemi, F., Mesri, A., Rezaei, N. (2007). Distribution of primary immunodeficiency diseases in the Turk ethnic group, living in the northwestern Iran. *Journal of Clinical Immunology,* Vol. 27 (September 2007), No. 5, pp. 510-6, ISSN 1573-2592.

Slatter, M.A., Gennery, A.R. (2010). Primary immunodeficiency syndromes. *Advances in Experimental Medicine and Biology,* Vol. 685 (2010), pp. 146-65, ISSN 0065-2598.

Stiehm, R.E. (2007). The four most common pediatric immunodeficiencies. *Advances in Experimental Medicine and Biology,* Vol. 601 (April 2007), pp. 15-26, ISSN 0065-2598.

Stihem, E.R., Ochs, H.D., Winkelstein, J.A. (2004). Immunologycal disorders: General considerations. In: Immunodeficiency disorders in Infants & Children. ER Stihem, HD Ochs, JA Winkelstein, pp. 29-355. WB Sauders Company, ISBN 0-7216-4948-3, Philadelphia, Pennsylnania, USA.

Stray-Pedersen, A., Abrahamsen, T.G., Frøland, S.S. (2000). Primary immunodeficiency diseases in Norway. *Journal of Clinical Immunology,* Vol. 20 (November 2000), No. 6, pp. 477-85, ISSN 1573-2592.

Turvey, S.E., Bonilla, F.A., Junker, A.K. (2009). Primary immunodeficiency diseases: a practical guide for clinicians. *Postgraduated Medical Journal*, Vol. 85 (December 2009), No. 1010, pp. 660-6, ISSN 0032-5473.

Verma, S., Sharma, P.K., Sivanandan, S., Rana, N., Saini, S., Lodha, R., Kabra, S.K. (2008). Spectrum of primary immune deficiency at a tertiary care hospital. *Indian Journal of Pediatrics*, Vol. 75 (February 2008), No. 2, pp. 143-8, ISSN 0019-5456.

Yarmohammadi, H., Estrella, L., Cunningham-Rundles, C. (2004). Diagnosis of Primary Immunodeficiency; Can Review of Medical History Help? *Journal of Allergy and Clinical Immunology*, Vol. 113 (February 2004), No. 2, Suppl. pp. s47, ISSN 0091-6749.

Yavich, N., Báscolo, E.P., Hargerty, J. (2010). Bulding a PHC evaluation framework for Latin America. *Salud Publica Mexico*, Vol. 52 (January-February 2010), No. 1, pp. 39-45, ISSN 0036-3634.

Wang, L.L., Jin, Y.Y., Hao, Y.Q., Wang, J.J., Yao, C.M., Wang, X., Cao, R.M., Zhang. H., Chen. Y., Chen, T.X. (2011). Distribution and clinical features of primary immunodeficiency diseases in chinese children (2004-2009). *Journal of Clinical Immunology*, Vol. 31 (June 2011), No. 3, pp. 297-308, ISSN 1573-2592.

Winkelstein, J.A., Marino, M.C., Johnston, R.B. Jr., Boyle, J., Curnutte, J., Gallin, J.I., Malech, H.L., Holland, S.M., Ochs, H., Quie, P., Buckley, R.H., Foster, C.B., Chanock, S.J., Dickler, H. (2000). Chronic granulomatous disease. Report on a national registry of 368 patients. *Medicine* (Baltimore), Vol. 79 (May 2000), No. 3, pp.155-69, ISSN 0025-7974.

Winkelstein, J.A., Marino, M.C., Lederman, H.M., Jones, S.M., Sullivan, K., Burks, A.W., Conley, M.E., Cunningham-Rundles, C., Ochs, H.D. (2006). X-linked agammaglobulinemia: report on a United States registry of 201 patients. *Medicine* (Baltimore), Vol. 85 (July 2006), No. 4, pp. 193-202, ISSN 0025-7974.

Winkelstein, J.A., Marino, M.C., Ochs, H., Fuleihan, R., Scholl, P.R., Geha, R., Stiehm, E.R., Conley, M.E. (2003). The X-linked hyper-IgM syndrome: clinical and immunologic features of 79 patients. *Medicine* (Baltimore), Vol. 82 (November 2003), No. 6, pp. 373-84, ISSN 0025-7974.

Zegers, B.J., Weemaes, C.M., Weening, R.S., van der Meer, J.W., Vossen, J,M. (1994). Immunodeficiency in The Netherlands: clinical and immunological survey, 1970-1983. Interfacultaire werkgroep Immunodeficiëntie. *Nederlands Tijdschrift voor Geneeskunde*, Vol. 138 (February 1994), No. 7, pp. 354-9, ISSN 0028-2162.

Zelazko, M., Carneiro-Sampaio, M., C., Cornejo de Luigi, M., Garcia de Olarte, D., Porras Madrigal, O., Berrón Perz, R., Cabello, A., Rostan, M.V., Sorensen, R.U. (1998). Primary immunodeficiency diseases in Latin America: first report from eight countries partipating in the LAGID. Latin American Group for Primary Immunodeficiency Diseases. *Journal of Clinical Immunology*, Vol. 18 (March 1998) No. 2, pp. 161-6, ISSN 1573-2592.

Zhao, H.J., Chen, T.X., Hao, Y.Q., Zhou, Y.F., Ying, D.M. (2006). Overview of clinical occurrence of primary immunodeficiency disorders in children. Zhonghua Er Bi Yan Hou Ke Za Zhi. *Chinese Journal of Pediatrics*, Vol. 44 (June 2006), No. 6, pp. 403-6, ISSN 0412-3948.

Section 9

Genetic Epidemiology Family-Based

18

On Combining Family Data from Different Study Designs for Estimating Disease Risk Associated with Mutated Genes

Yun-Hee Choi
University of Western Ontario
Canada

1. Introduction

Genetic disorders caused primarily by abnormalities in genes or chromosomes are rare in the general population. The associated putative mutations that lead to a high risk of developing such diseases are even rarer. In order to study disease risks associated with mutated genes, families sampled under different study designs are commonly used in association studies. This is because family data recruited via affected individuals (probands) would be expected to contain more affected individuals and mutation carriers than families randomly sampled from a general population, thus leading to increased statistical efficiency in estimating the disease risk. The disease risk associated with a mutated gene can be measured on a relative or absolute scale. As the event we consider is disease with its age of onset, the relative risk can be measured as a ratio of two hazards of developing disease between mutation carriers and non-carriers, and the absolute risk as a function of age, i.e., the cumulative risk of developing disease by a given age, which is also termed penetrance.

Several family-based study designs have been used for estimating the disease risk associated with a gene mutation when onset varies with age. Gong & Whittemore (2003) discussed two basic types of family-based sampling schemes: population-based and clinic-based designs. For population-based designs, families are ascertained for study inclusion based on affected family members who are randomly sampled from the disease population. The proband is usually genotyped to determine if s/he carries the disease risk gene and additional genotype and phenotype data can then be collected from other family members. A kin-cohort design described by Wacholder et al. (1998) is an example of the population-based design as families are sampled through a volunteer (either affected or unaffected) who agrees to be genotyped and provides the disease history of her or his first-degree relatives through a questionnaire. Not restricted to including the first degree relatives and genotyping only probands, a kin-cohort design can be easily extended to case-family studies to include more extended family members and their genotype information. Case-control family studies have been widely used to analyse the ages of onset of disease in relation to genetic risk (Li et al., 1998; Shih & Chatterjee, 2000; Hsu & Gorfine, 2006), where case families are recruited via population-based cases and their matching control families are randomly sampled from the population.

For clinic-based designs, on the other hand, families are ascertained into the study based on having multiple affected family members in addition to the affected probands. Pedigrees with many cases are highly informative because they are more likely to carry the disease gene mutation, but typically have not been ascertained in any population-based manner. Such families are often identified from high-risk disease clinics and provide substantial information to estimate the disease risk (for example, Kopciuk et al., 2009). Multistage designs (Whittemore & Halpern, 1997; Siegmund et al., 1999) provide an alternative way to efficiently recruit high risk families, often using disease family registries, where families are sampled from more informative groups via several stages. Studies based on these high-risk families can be effective for characterizing the prevalence and penetrance of mutated genes, but it is well known that without proper ascertainment corrections statistical inference would lead to biased estimations of population attributes such as allele frequency, disease risks, and penetrance of the mutated genes.

To allow population-based inference for estimating disease risks associated with mutated genes, family data can be analyzed using various likelihood-based methods (Thomas, 2004). In particular, ascertainment-corrected likelihood approaches have been developed by several authors (for example, Choi et al., 2008; Carayol & Bonaïti-Pellié, 2004; Kraft & Thomas, 2000; Le Bihan et al., 1995). Based on the survival approach, Le Bihan et al. (1995) formulated a prospective likelihood for modeling phenotypes as the age of onset and disease status given genotypes, and corrected the likelihood by the probability of families being ascertained for study. This approach is natural as it models phenotypes as a function of genotype and covariates, but the ascertainment scheme has to be clearly known and simple enough to make proper correction. On the other hand, the retrospective likelihood models genotypes conditioning on the phenotypes of all family members (Carayol & Bonaïti-Pellié, 2004; Kraft & Thomas, 2000; Schaid et al., 2010). Although this approach provides the most robust way to obtain consistent estimates of relative risk even with the ascertainment schemes that are imprecisely defined or complex, it encounters the computational burden of summing over possible genotypes of all family members and a decreased efficiency resulting from conditioning. Choi et al. (2008) adapted the retrospective likelihood conditioning only on phenotypes of individuals who were involved in the ascertainment criteria; for families sampled from the population-based designs, only probands were used to correct for the ascertainment, whereas for families from the clinic-based designs, the probands and their parents and sibs were used for ascertainment correction. Moreover, Schaid et al. (2010) accommodated the composite likelihood approach to obtaining the retrospective likelihood based on all possible pairs of individuals in families to reduce the computational burden.

The main objectives of this article are first, to examine the effects of misspecification of study designs when more appropriate study designs have been ignored or incorrectly specified in the analysis; second, to provide simple and easy to apply adjustment schemes for estimating disease risks by combining family data from different study designs; and third, to develop an Expectation-Maximization algorithm to infer missing genotypes in the estimation of disease risks. We start with describing ascertainment-corrected likelihood methods to take the study design into account and propose a likelihood-based approach to estimating the disease risks for combined family data collected under different study designs. The performance of these ascertainment-corrected likelihood methods is evaluated in terms of bias and efficiency. The effect of design misspecification is examined for estimating the disease risks associated with mutated genes. The bias and efficiency involved in estimating two disease risks are compared when only probands for the families from the clinic-based study are adjusted for, and when the probands and other affected family members for the families from the population-based design are used for ascertainment correction. For the combined family data, the two design correction methods (population-based and clinic-based) are applied and compared respectively with our proposed combined likelihood method in terms of their accuracies and efficiencies for disease risk estimation.

This chapter includes the following sections. Section 2 introduces two family-based study designs—the population- and clinic-based study designs and their ascertainment-corrected likelihood methods for modeling ages at onset for family members in disease risk estimation. We propose a likelihood-based approach for the combined family data obtained from different study designs. In Section 3, an Expectation-Maximization (EM) algorithm is incorporated to account for the missing genotype information, where the missing genetic covariates are inferred from their conditional expectation given the observed genotypes and phenotypes of other family members. Moreover, a robust variance estimator is proposed to account for the dependence of individuals within families. Using simulation studies in Section 4, we examine the effects of study design misspecification for estimating the disease risks and investigate the properties of our proposed likelihood approach for combined families from different study designs. In Section 5, we illustrate our proposed approaches through an application to family data obtained from the combination of two studies of Lynch Syndrome—first, Newfoundland data from the clinic-based design and second, Ontario data based on the population-based design. Final remarks and possible extensions of this work will follow in Section 6.

2. Methods

2.1 Defining disease risks

For diseases caused by mutated genes, the phenotype of interest varies in age at onset, i.e., time to an event such as death or disease diagnosis. We denote the age at onset by T, the affection status at age of examination by δ. Then, the phenotype is given by $D = (T, \delta)$. Under the Cox's proportional hazards model, the hazard function for individual i conditional on mutation gene G and other risk factors X is assumed to take the form

$$h(t_i | g_i, \boldsymbol{x}_i) = h_o(t) \exp(\beta_g G + \beta_x X),$$

where $h_o(t)$ is a baseline hazard function and β_g and β_x are unknown regression parameters.

Based on this model, we consider two types of disease risk associated with a mutated gene—relative risk and absolute risk, the latter is also called penetrance.

(1) the relative risk in survival analysis is defined by the hazards ratio for an individual with a mutated gene compared to an individual free from the mutation, that is

$$Relative\, Risk = \exp(\beta_g).$$

(2) the penetrance function for the disease susceptibility gene is defined as the age-specific cumulative risk function conditional on the disease susceptibility gene G and other relevant covariates X,

$$Penetrance = P(T < t | G, X).$$

Design	Ascertainment Criteria
POP	Proband is affected
POP+	Proband is affected and mutation-carrier
CLI	Proband is affected and at least one parent and one sib are affected
CLI+	Proband is affected mutation-carrier and at least one parent and one sibling are affected

Table 1. Family-based study designs

The disease risks can be estimated by maximizing a likelihood function with proper ascertainment adjustment of the families. In a crude analysis of family data, their ascertainments are often corrected by simply excluding the probands from the analysis to prevent overestimating the risk. However, more prudent approaches such as likelihood methods would not simply drop out the probands because they include other important information about the disease risks. Rather they would adjust for the sampling process, allowing their contributions to the likelihood. To accommodate study designs and the ascertainment process properly, both the design and the ascertainment criteria should be known clearly. However, such designs or criteria in many cases are unclear or too complex to allow adjustment at the analysis stage. Moreover, family data could come from different sources where families were recruited using different designs or ascertainment criteria.

2.2 Family-based study designs

We consider the two most commonly used family-based study designs—population-based designs and clinic-based designs. The population-based study design uses the affected cases (probands) to sample their families while the clinic-based study design is based on the probands with a high family history of disease risk. Thus, the clinic-based families likely include more disease cases and mutation carriers compared to the families from population-based designs.

The ascertainment criteria for the population-based study are based on the affected probands who are randomly sampled from the diseased population; for example, cancer registries. To increase the power to study the effect of the mutated gene of interest, one can apply stringent criteria to recruit the probands to be not only affected but also be a mutation-carrier. Similarly, the clinic-based study designs can have two variants: one with random probands with multiple case family members and the other with carrier probands with multiple case family members. Such families can be recruited from cancer registries or cancer clinics.

Table 1 summarizes the four study designs and their sampling criteria used to ascertain families. Population-based designs correspond to ascertainment criteria POP and POP+. They are similar to a kin-cohort design but are more like case-family designs that include extended family members and their genotype information. Ascertainment criteria CLI and CLI+ correspond to clinic-based designs which have multiple disease occurrences among family members. Important to note is that ascertainment criteria for the POP+ and CLI+ designs include families who have at least one member (proband) who carries the mutated gene of interest.

2.3 Likelihood approaches for family-based study designs

This section describes the likelihood-based approaches for modeling ages at onset and genetic covariates using family data via population-based and clinic-based study designs. We propose a combined likelihood approach for family data arising from the two different study designs.

2.3.1 Ascertainment-corrected retrospective likelihood

The retrospective likelihood corrects for the ascertainment by conditioning on the phenotypes. Define $D = (d_1, \ldots, d_n)$ as a vector of phenotypes, $G = (g_1, \ldots, g_n)$ as a vector of genotypes, $X = (x_1, \ldots, x_n)$ a vector of covariates other than genotypes, and A the ascertainment event. The likelihood contribution L_f for a single family f can be written as

$$\begin{aligned} L_f &= P(G_f|D_f, X_f, A_f) \\ &= \frac{P(A_f|D_f, X_f, G_f)P(D_f|X_f, G_f)P(G_f)}{P(D_f, A_f|X_f)} \\ &\propto \frac{P(D_f|X_f, G_f)P(G_f)}{P(D_f, A_f|X_f)}, \end{aligned} \tag{1}$$

where we assume that $P(A_f|D_f, X_f, G_f)$ is equal to 1 if the vector D_f qualifies for ascertainment, and 0 otherwise, and so is independent of the parameter of interest.

We further assume that individuals' phenotypes are independent conditionally given their genotypes and covariates. Thus, we can express the numerator as

$$P(D_f|X_f, G_f) = \prod_{i=1}^{n_f} P(d_i|x_i, g_i),$$

and

$$P(G_f) = \prod_{i=1}^{n_f} \begin{cases} P(g_i), & \text{if individual } i \text{ is a founder,} \\ P(g_i|g_{m_i}, g_{f_i}), & \text{if individual } i \text{ is a nonfounder.} \end{cases}$$

Here $P(g_i)$ is based on Hardy-Weinberg Equilibrium (HWE) and depends on the population allele frequency, $P(g_i|g_{m_i}, g_{f_i})$ is the Mendelian transmission probability given parents' genotypes (g_{m_i}, g_{f_i}) of individual i.

The denominator is the correction term used to account for the study designs. In the population-based study, the ascertainment correction is based on the proband's phenotype in that it equals the probability of the proband, p, being affected before his/her age at examination, a_p, i.e.,

$$P(D_f, A_f|X_f) = \sum_g P(T_p < a_p|g)P(g),$$

where the sum is over all possible genotypes of the proband. For POP+ design, the sum takes place by assuming the proband is a mutation carrier.

In the clinic-based study, the denominator is based on the phenotypes of four individuals, two parents and two sibs, who involved in their family's ascertainment process. It can be expressed as

$$P(D_f, A_f|X_f) = \sum_{G_\omega} P(T_f < a_f|x_f, g_{\omega_f})^{\delta_f} P(T_f \geq a_f|x_f, g_{\omega_f})^{1-\delta_f} \times$$
$$P(T_m < a_m|x_m, g_{\omega_m})^{\delta_m} P(T_m \geq a_m|x_m, g_{\omega_m})^{1-\delta_m} P(g_{\omega_f}, g_{\omega_m}|g_{\omega_p}) \times$$
$$P(T_s < a_s|x_s, g_{\omega_s}) P(g_{\omega_s}|g_{\omega_p}) P(T_p < a_p|x_p, g_{\omega_p}) P(g_{\omega_p}),$$

where indices f, m, s, p represent father, mother, sib and proband, respectively, δ indicates the affection status, and $G_\omega = (g_{\omega_f}, g_{\omega_m}, g_{\omega_p}, g_{\omega_s})$ includes all possible genotypes of the four individuals in the ascertainment set. For CLI+ design, the sum in the denominator is taken over all possible genotypes, provided that the proband carries a mutated allele of the major gene. The conditional probabilities $P(g_{\omega_f}, g_{\omega_m}|g_{\omega_p} = 1)$ and $P(g_{\omega_s}|g_{\omega_p} = 1)$ are obtained based on the HWE and Mendelian transmission probabilities using Bayes theorem.

2.3.2 Combined population- and and clinic-based study designs

Consider a study where the families are sampled via different study designs, say n_p families from a population-based design and n_c families from a clinic-based design. When their study designs are known, we can construct the likelihoods based on their study designs. Let L_p and L_c be the likelihood functions based on the population-based design and clinic-based design, respectively. We propose the combined likelihood for the families from the two designs as

$$L_{comb}(\theta|D, G, X) = L_p(\theta|D^p, G^p, X^p) L_c(\theta|D^c, G^c, X^c),$$

where the superscripts p and c denote the population- and clinic-based study designs, respectively, and the likelihoods L_p and L_c are obtained using the retrospective likelihood approach in expression (1). Therefore, the combined likelihood using the retrospective likelihood approach can accommodate both population- and clinic-based designs.

Even when the sampling schemes are not clearly defined, we can still employ this combined likelihood approach by dividing the families into two groups—high risk and low risk families, according to the number of cases observed in the family. For example, a family would be classified as a high risk family if it includes at least three cases among family members, otherwise it would be classified as a low risk family.

3. Missing genotypes

In practice, family data often include some missing information, particularly, missing genotypes. In the presence of missing genotype information, we estimate the disease risks associated with a known gene mutation in the families. Suppose data include genetic covariates that consist of observed genotypes and missing genotypes and phenotypes as time-of-onset responses with no missing. To infer the unobserved genotypes in the family, we implement an expectation-maximazation (EM) algorithm (Dempster et al., 1977) and estimate the parameters in the likelihood. The EM algorithm is an iterative procedure that computes the maximum likelihood estimates (MLEs) in the presence of missing data.

3.1 Expectation-maximazation algorithm

Suppose a genetic covariate G_f in family f consists of observed genotypes G_{fo} and missing genotypes G_{fm} and the vector of unknown parameters θ includes both regression parameters and baseline hazard parameters. In our situation, the expectation of the complete data (D_f, X_f, G_f), $f = 1, \ldots, n$, is taken with respect to the conditional distribution of missing genotypes G_{fm} given observed data (D_f, X_f, G_{fo}) and current estimates of θ. Then the parameter estimates are updated by maximizing the likelihood function using the estimate of missing data in the expectation step. These two steps iterate until convergence to obtain the MLEs, where the algorithm is guaranteed to increase the likelihood at each iteration.

The conditional expectation of the log-likelihood function $\ell(\theta|D, G, X)$ of the complete data (D, G, X) given the observed phenotypes D_o and genotypes G_o, or Q function for the kth iteration is given by:

$$Q(\theta|\theta^{(k)}) = E_{\theta^{(k)}}\left[\ell(\theta|D, G, X)|D_o, G_o\right] . \tag{2}$$

For the ith individual in family f, we can then obtain the conditional expectation of their missing genotype G_i given their observed phenotype D_i, covariates X_i, and the observed mutation status G_o of other family members, especially if the proband's genotype G_p is conditioned as:

$$\begin{aligned} E_{\theta^{(k)}}[G_i|D_i, X_i, G_p = 1] &= P_{\theta^{(k)}}(G_i|D_i, X_i, G_p = 1) \\ &= \frac{P_{\theta^{(k)}}(D_i|X_i, G_i)P(G_i|G_p = 1)}{P_{\theta^{(k)}}(D_i|X_i, G_i = 1)P(G_i = 1|G_p = 1) + P_{\theta^{(k)}}(D_i|X_i, G_i = 0)P(G_i = 0|G_p = 1)} . \end{aligned}$$

Here $P(G_i|G_p = 1)$ is the conditional probability of the mutation carrier status for family member i, using the family proband's known mutation status. Based on Mendelian transmission probabilities, we can express these as simple constants under an assumed genetic model. Under the model assumptions given above, the phenotype probabilities conditional on genotype status for the ith individual can be expressed in terms of the hazard function h and the corresponding survival function S depending on his/her affection status δ_i as

$$P(D_i|X_i, G_i) = S(t_i; X_i, G_i)h(t_i; X_i, G_i)^{\delta_i} .$$

In the M step of the algorithm, we take the partial derivatives of Q with respect to θ and set to zero, that will maximize Q.

3.2 Robust variance estimator for the EM algorithm

We illustrate the use of robust variance estimators (sandwich estimators) to account for within-family dependencies for disease risk estimates. In the presence of missing genotypes, the variance estimators are modified accordingly upon the use of the EM algorithm (Louis, 1982).

Let $U(\theta)$ and $B(\theta)$ denote the score vector and the negative of the associated matrix of second derivatives for the complete data, respectively, and $U^*(\theta)$ and $B^*(\theta)$ be the corresponding vector and matrix for the incomplete data. Then, the observed information matrix can be expressed as

$$I_o(\theta) = E_\theta[B(\theta)|g_o, d_o] - E_\theta[U(\theta)U^\top(\theta)|g_o, d_o] + U^*(\theta)U^{*\top}(\theta), \tag{3}$$

where g_o and d_o denote the vectors of observed genotypes and phenotypes from data. At the maximum likelihood estimate of θ, because of the convergence of the EM algorithm, U^*

is zero. Thus, the observed information matrix can be obtained as the first two terms on the right hand side of (3) that arise from the complete data log-likelihood analysis. The first term is evaluated as

$$E_\theta[B(\theta)|g_o, d_o] = E_\theta\left[-\frac{\partial^2 \ell(\theta)}{\partial\theta\partial\theta^\top}|g_o, d_o\right].$$

Oakes (1999) explicitly expressed the information matrix in terms of derivatives of the $Q(\theta|\theta^{(k)})$ function in equation (2) invoked by the EM algorithm, as given by

$$I_o(\theta) = \frac{\partial^2 \ell}{\partial\theta\partial\theta^\top} = \left\{\frac{\partial^2 Q(\theta|\theta^{(k)})}{\partial\theta\partial\theta^\top} + \frac{\partial^2 Q(\theta|\theta^{(k)})}{\partial\theta\partial\theta^{(k)\top}}\right\}_{\theta=\theta^{(k)}}, \quad (4)$$

where ℓ represents the observed data log-likelihood and the second term is viewed as the 'missing information.'

To account for familial correlation, as our model assumes the independence of the individuals in the family, we obtain the robust variance estimator for the ascertainment corrected likelihood with missing genotypes in a 'sandwich' form (White, 1982),

$$\text{Var}(\hat{\theta}) = I_o(\theta)^{-1}\left\{\sum_{f=1}^{n} U_f^*(\theta)U_f^*(\theta)^\top\right\} I_o(\theta)^{-1}, \quad (5)$$

where $U_f^*(\theta)$ is the conditional expectation of the complete data score vector for family f given the observed data. Thus, the robust variance of $\hat{\theta}$ can be estimated by replacing θ by $\hat{\theta}$ in equation (5).

4. Simulation study

We carried out simulation studies to investigate the properties of our proposed likelihood methods and the effect of design misspecification. The simulation study aims to (1) assess bias and efficiency in disease risk estimation (relative risk and penetrance) for the retrospective likelihood-based approaches for family data from different study designs, (2) investigate potential bias and efficiency loss in risk estimation when the study designs are misspecified, and (3) evaluate the first two aims using combined data from two different study designs.

4.1 Family data generation

The simulation of family data is based on the method developed by Gauderman (1995) and further extended by Choi et al. (2008). We generated families of three generations: two parents and their two offspring, one of whom is the proband (affected individual from whom the family is selected). Each offspring has a spouse and their children ranged in number from two to five. At the first stage, all family members' ages at examination were obtained using a normal distribution with mean age 65 for the first generation and 45 for the second generation, with variance fixed at 2.5 years for both generations. It resulted in an average of 20 years difference between the parents and offspring. At the next stage, the proband's genotype of a major gene was determined conditioning on the proband's affection status by her/his age at examination, assuming Hardy-Weinberg equilibrium (HWE) with the fixed population allele frequency. Given the proband's genotypes, the genotypes of the other family members were then determined using HWE and Mendelian transmission probabilities calculated with Bayes' formula. Once we simulated the age at examination and genotype information for all family members, then the time-to-onset of individual i was simulated from the proportional hazards model,

$$h(t_i|g_i) = h_0(t_i)\exp(\beta x_i),$$

where x_i indicates a carrier status of disease mutation gene for subject i and the baseline hazard is assumed to follow the Weibull distribution which has a form, $h_0(t) = \lambda\rho\{\lambda(t - 20)\}^{\rho-1}$.

The proband's age at onset was generated conditioning on the fact that the proband was affected before his(her) age at examination, a_p,

$$T_p \sim T|T < a_p\ .$$

For the rest of family members, their times to onset were generated unconditionally. We also assumed the minimum age at onset was 20 years of age and the maximum age for followup was 90 years of age. Finally, the affection status δ_i for the ith individual was determined by comparing the age at onset T_i and age at examination a_i; $\delta_i = 1$ if $T_i < a_i$ and 0 otherwise.

4.2 Simulation study designs

Data were simulated under different configurations. We assumed Weibull baseline hazard functions with scale (λ) and shape (ρ) parameters equal to 0.01 and 3.2, respectively. This leads to a cumulative risk of 10% among mutation non-carriers by age 70. Two penetrances were considered: high and low penetrances corresponding to the log relative risk of a major gene (β) given by 2.4 and 1.8, respectively. The high penetrance represents a lifetime risk of 70% by age 70 among carriers of a major gene, which assumes a rare gene with the allele frequency 0.02 under the dominant model. The low penetrance provides a lifetime risk of 48% by age 70 among carriers.

We designed the simulation studies, first to investigate the effect of design misspecification, and second, to examine the properties of our proposed likelihood for combined family data from different study designs in the estimation of disease risks associated with a mutated gene.

(1) To study the effect of design misspecification, the study designs POP, POP+, CLI, and CLI+ were used to generate family data. For each design, two retrospective likelihood methods were applied to fit the data—one using correct adjustment of the study design and the other using a design with misspecified correction; for example, population-based ascertainment correction was used for the families under CLI+ design and clinic-based ascertainment correction was used for the families under POP+ design as for the misspecified design. We simulated 500 random samples of 200 families for each simulation configuration.

(2) To investigate potential bias and efficiency loss in disease risk estimation for the proposed likelihood approach for combined family data from population-based and clinic-based designs. We considered the combined families either from POP+ and CLI+ designs or POP and CLI designs with three mixing ratios between two designs—50-50, 70-30 and 80-20. For example, with the total 400 families sampled, the ratio 50-50 corresponds to equal numbers of families from POP+ and CLI+ designs, the 70-30 sampling corresponds to 280 POP+ families and 120 CLI+ families and the ratio 80-20 to 320 POP+ and 80 CLI+ families. The same numbers were examined for combining POP and CLI families. For each simulation configuration, 500 random samples were simulated.

4.3 Simulation results

Results of the simulation studies are described based on the empirical summary measures of bias and standard error obtained from the maximum likelihood estimates.

4.3.1 The effect of design misspecification

We first assessed bias and precision in disease risk estimation (relative risk and penetrance) for the retrospective likelihood with correct design adjustment for family data from different study designs. The results are summarized in Table 2.

With the correct design adjustment, the estimates of both the log relative risk and penetrance appeared unbiased; the absolute values of bias were less than 0.05 under both high and low penetrance models regardless of the study design. The magnitude of the bias was much smaller than the standard errors. In the log relative risk estimation, the precision of clinic-based designs was higher (smaller standard errors) than that of population-based designs. The population-based designs provided more accurate and precise estimates of the log relative risk for high penetrance than for low penetrance, whereas the clinic-based designs performed better for low penetrance. However, in the penetrance estimation, all designs provided more precise penetrance estimates (smaller standard errors) for high penetrance than for low penetrance.

We then examined the effect of design misspecification in terms of bias and precision of the log relative risk and penetrance estimates obtained from the retrospective likelihoods when the study design was misspecified. The clinic-based ascertainment correction was applied to the family data under the population-based designs and the population-based ascertainment correction to the clinic-based study. It is worth noting that the clinic-based design with the population-based correction provided relatively large bias in both disease risks, however, the bias in the population-based design with the clinic-based ascertainment correction was not notably large. Especially, under POP+ design (with affected and mutation carrier probands), the clinic-based retrospective likelihood yielded estimates at least as accurate as those from probands-only adjustment (correct design), although their standard errors were larger under the misspecified design.

4.3.2 The likelihood methods for combined family data from different study designs

We evaluated the accuracy and precision of the disease risk (log relative risk and penetrance) estimates based on the three retrospective likelihoods for combined data. Simulation results based on the combined data from CLI+ and POP+ designs are summarized in Table 3, and those from combining CLI and POP families in Table 4 .

Combined data from POP+ and CLI+ designs

In the log relative risk estimation, as expected, the population-based likelihoods for the combined data yielded overestimates because the ascertainment correction was based on only probands, which would not be sufficient for the families from clinic-based designs. However, the clinic-based retrospective likelihood provided slightly negative but less biased estimates in log relative risk but slightly larger standard errors. Although the population-based likelihoods provided smallest standard errors, they were subject to positive bias. Moreover, the log relative risk estimates for low penetrance performed better (less bias and higher precision) than for high penetrance. Our proposed likelihood was almost as efficient as the

Log relative risk (β) estimation

	High Penetrance ($\beta = 2.4$)				Low Penetrance ($\beta = 1.8$)			
	POP	POP+	CLI	CLI+	POP	POP+	CLI	CLI+
Correct Design	-0.002 (0.129)	0.010 (0.236)	0.044 (0.095)	-0.015 (0.171)	-0.006 (0.153)	0.017 (0.256)	0.017 (0.066)	-0.003 (0.136)
Misspecified Design	0.033 (0.159)	-0.022 (0.265)	1.456 (0.201)	0.444 (0.165)	0.041 (0.185)	0.009 (0.272)	0.665 (0.151)	0.475 (0.144)

Penetrance estimation

	High Penetrance (70%)				Low Penetrance (48%)			
	POP	POP+	CLI	CLI+	POP	POP+	CLI	CLI+
Correct Design	0.013 (0.049)	0.015 (0.033)	0.028 (0.078)	0.020 (0.084)	0.008 (0.057)	0.012 (0.040)	0.049 (0.115)	0.037 (0.103)
Misspecified Design	0.034 (0.087)	0.009 (0.098)	0.290 (0.003)	0.282 (0.004)	0.056 (0.140)	0.014 (0.135)	0.501 (0.003)	0.480 (0.006)

Table 2. Effects of the design misspecification: bias and precision in disease risk estimation based on retrospective likelihoods with correct and incorrect design adjustments; standard errors are in parenthesis.

population-based likelihood and as accurate as the clinic-based likelihood, regardless of the mixing rates we considered. Especially, the combined likelihood appeared to perform better for relative risk estimation when more CLI+ families were included in the sample.

In the penetrance estimation, we observed similar patterns as in the log relative risk estimation. The population-based likelihood provided substantially large bias with small standard errors, whereas the clinic-based likelihood yielded less bias with large standard errors. However, our proposed likelihood method offered the least bias and improved precision compared to the clinic-based likelihood. In addition, the penetrance was more precisely estimated with the combined likelihood when fewer CLI+ families were recruited (20% CLI+ families).

Combined data from POP and CLI designs

The patterns of bias and precision of the three likelihood methods were more clear with the combined data from POP and CLI designs, as shown in Table 4. In the log relative risk estimation, our proposed likelihood yielded both the most accurate and precise estimates. It also provided more precise estimates when 50% CLI families were included. Similarly, in penetrance estimation, the population-based likelihood provided heavily biased estimates; however, the combined likelihood performed well in terms of both bias and precision. With fewer CLI families (20%) in the data, more precise estimates were obtained.

Log relative risk (β) estimation

	High Penetrance ($\beta = 2.4$)			Low Penetrance ($\beta = 1.8$)		
POP+ vs. CLI+	50-50	70-30	80-20	50-50	70-30	80-20
POP+ corrected likelihood	0.279 (0.132)	0.196 (0.142)	0.145 (0.149)	0.326 (0.123)	0.240 (0.139)	0.191 (0.145)
CLI+ corrected likelihood	-0.024 (0.140)	-0.024 (0.154)	-0.026 (0.163)	-0.004 (0.124)	-0.010 (0.141)	-0.002 (0.150)
Combined likelihood	-0.025 (0.134)	-0.026 (0.143)	-0.028 (0.149)	-0.005 (0.123)	-0.011 (0.140)	-0.005 (0.147)

Penetrance estimation

	High Penetrance (70%)			Low Penetrance (48%)		
POP+ vs. CLI+	50-50	70-30	80-20	50-50	70-30	80-20
POP+ corrected likelihood	0.209 (0.009)	0.151 (0.015)	0.113 (0.017)	0.348 (0.012)	0.247 (0.017)	0.182 (0.020)
CLI+ corrected likelihood	0.019 (0.060)	0.016 (0.067)	0.015 (0.067)	0.032 (0.079)	0.021 (0.083)	0.024 (0.085)
Combined likelihood	-0.008 (0.031)	-0.011 (0.029)	-0.012 (0.027)	0.002 (0.033)	-0.002 (0.030)	-0.002 (0.028)

Table 3. Bias and precision in disease risk estimation based on three retrospective likelihood approaches for combined data from different family based designs (POP+ and CLI+) with affected and mutation carrier probands; standard errors are in parenthesis.

5. Application to Lynch Syndrome families

Lynch Syndrome, also referred to as hereditary non-polyposis colorectal cancer is an autosomal dominant condition which predisposes carriers to colorectal cancer (CRC). Several DNA mismatch repair (MMR) genes responsible for the majority of Lynch Syndrome cancers have been identified, predominantly MLH1 and MSH2. For the study of CRC, Lynch Syndrome families share a founder mutation in an MMR gene sampled from Newfoundland and Ontario. The Newfoundland data consist of 315 phenotyped individuals (74 affected and 241 not affected) from 12 very large families identified using a high risk criteria. Of them, 261 were genotyped (162 carriers, 99 non-carriers) and 54 were not genotyped. Each family had a carrier proband and other affected relatives, which corresponds to the study design CLI+. The Ontario data were identified through the Ontario Familial Colorectal Cancer Registry (Cotterchio et al., 2000) and consist of 506 phenotyped individuals (126 affected and 380 not affected) from 32 families with MMR mutation carrier probands, which corresponds to the

Log relative risk (β) estimation

	High Penetrance ($\beta = 2.4$)			Low Penetrance ($\beta = 1.8$)		
POP vs. CLI	50-50	70-30	80-20	50-50	70-30	80-20
POP corrected likelihood	0.911 (0.089)	0.644 (0.079)	0.485 (0.078)	0.700 (0.094)	0.609 (0.089)	0.506 (0.089)
CLI corrected likelihood	0.044 (0.079)	0.035 (0.086)	0.038 (0.094)	0.020 (0.063)	0.024 (0.077)	0.029 (0.087)
Combined likelihood	0.014 (0.072)	-0.009 (0.076)	-0.017 (0.080)	0.003 (0.058)	0.000 (0.068)	-0.002 (0.076)

Penetrance estimation

	High Penetrance (70%)			Low Penetrance (48%)		
POP vs. CLI	50-50	70-30	80-20	50-50	70-30	80-20
POP corrected likelihood	0.269 (0.005)	0.237 (0.010)	0.203 (0.013)	0.467 (0.007)	0.413 (0.012)	0.353 (0.018)
CLI corrected likelihood	0.043 (0.055)	0.041 (0.055)	0.042 (0.056)	0.059 (0.081)	0.060 (0.082)	0.062 (0.082)
Combined likelihood	0.006 (0.042)	-0.002 (0.038)	-0.005 (0.036)	0.015 (0.047)	0.008 (0.043)	0.006 (0.042)

Table 4. Bias and precision in disease risk estimation based on three retrospective likelihood approaches for combined data from different family based designs (POP and CLI) with random affected probands; standard errors are in parenthesis.

study design POP+. Of them, 154 individuals were genotyped (92 carriers, 62 non-carriers) and 352 were not genotyped.

The three likelihood methods (POP+ corrected, CLI+ corrected and combined likelihoods) were applied to combined families with Lynch Syndrome identified from Newfoundland (CLI+) and Ontario (POP+). A Weibull model was used to assess the effects of MMR mutation gene and gender on the age at onset of colorectal cancer. The EM algorithm was implemented to infer missing genotypes. The results of fitting these Lynch Syndrome families using different likelihood methods are presented in Table 5, and the age-specific penetrance estimates based on the combined likelihood are graphically illustrated in Figure 1.

In the analysis based on the combined likelihood, the β parameters for the genetic and gender effects were estimated to be 1.13 with robust standard error (se) = 0.18 and -0.51 with se=0.17, respectively, which lead to the hazards ratio of the MMR mutation carriers for the colorectal cancer as 3.10 (se=0.55) and the hazards ratio between female and male as 0.60 (se=0.11).

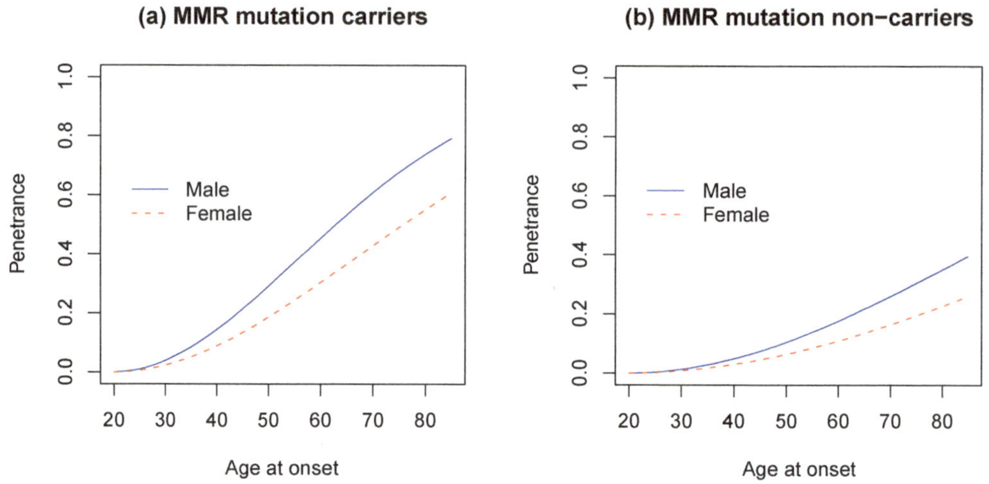

Fig. 1. (a) Estimated cumulative risk of developing colorectal cancer for carriers of any MMR gene mutation for the Lynch Syndrome families from Newfoundland and Ontario. (b) Same as (a) for non-carriers.

Log relative risk estimation in terms of hazards ratio

	MMR mutation		Gender	
POP+ corrected likelihood	1.07	(0.17)	-0.42	(0.16)
CLI+ corrected likelihood	1.15	(0.18)	-0.52	(0.18)
Combined likelihood	1.14	(0.18)	-0.51	(0.17)

Age-specific penetrance estimation among mutation carriers

	Male		Female	
POP+ corrected likelihood	62.4%	(4.08)	47.5%	(4.06)
CLI+ corrected likelihood	58.9%	(4.27)	40.9%	(4.18)
Combined likelihood	60.7%	(4.15)	42.8%	(4.10)

Table 5. Disease risk estimates and their corresponding robust standard errors in parenthesis using different likelihood methods for the Lynch Syndrome families from Newfoundland and Ontario

These relative risks indicated that the MMR mutation carriers were approximately three times more likely to develop the colorectal cancers than non-carriers, whereas among males and females, females showed about one third lower the hazard rate than males. There was very little difference observed between the relative risk estimates obtained by the CLI+ corrected likelihood and the combined likelihood, although their precisions were slightly better with the combined likelihood.

We obtained that the penetrance of colorectal cancer by age 70 was 61% (se=4.15) among male carriers and 43% (se=4.1) among female carriers using the combined likelihood. These estimates were comparable with those obtained using the POP+ and CLI+ corrected retrospective likelihoods. Penetrances were overestimated (62% for male and 48% for female carriers) with higher precision (se=4.08 for male, 4.06 for female) under POP+ correction but slightly underestimated (59% for male carriers and 41% for female carriers) with lower precision (se=4.27 for male and 4.18 for female) under CLI+ correction, as seen in our simulation study.

6. Conclusion

In genetic epidemiology, family studies have been widely used for identifying genes responsible for traits and characterizing their risks in the population and they are often based on various family-based designs to sample families depending on the objectives of the study or their budget. To make population-based inferences, the study design should be properly taken into account, especially when the sampling is not randomly conducted as often is the case with the sampling of families.

In this study, for estimating disease risks—relative risk and penetrance, we have proposed the use of a retrospective likelihood to take the sampling process of families into account, and investigated the effect of sampling design misspecification on disease risk estimation. Our study showed that the misspecification of study design undoubtedly lead to bias; overestimation of risks when the study design adjustment was less than it should be (i.e, the clinic-based designs were analyzed with the correction by probands only), and underestimation with overcorrection by multiple affected family members. However, the magnitudes of bias and precision varied depending on the study design and the size of the penetrance. We found that undercorrection created more bias although it provided smaller standard error. This implies that conditioning more individuals would be safer for obtaining accurate estimates at the price of loss of precision if the study design is not known. The POP+ design with clinic-based correction in fact provided unbiased estimates of relative risk and penetrance. In general, the population-based designs performed better for high penetrance for estimating both disease risks but the clinic-based designs performed differently: penetrance was more efficiently estimated under high penetrance but relative risk was more efficiently estimated under low penetrance. In addition, we have proposed the combined likelihood for families sampled under different study designs and the effect of design misspecification was also investigated for combined data. Our proposed likelihood is applicable even when the study designs of the combined data are not clearly known since we can divide families into two categories—high risk families with at least three affected individuals and low risk families, otherwise. Our proposed combined retrospective likelihood method yielded accurate and precise estimates of both disease risks. Comparatively, the clinic-based likelihoods applied to combined data and provided unbiased estimates less efficiently compared to those from the combined likelihood. It is noteworthy that the EM algorithm we developed for inferring missing genotypes is a novel way to impute the missing genotypes using the observed genotypic and phenotypic information from other family members.

In practice, it might be difficult to collect families with a mutation-carrier proband. However, with the emergence of large international consortiums such as the Breast and Colon Cancer Family Registries, the planning of studies using designs POP+ and CLI+ is now quite feasible. Therefore, the use of 200 families in the CLI+ design, as specified in our simulation study, seems to provide a reasonable sample size; however, the efficiency gains with more families would clearly be greater.

There are potential limitations to our study. First, we assumed the Weibull distribution, chosen to model the penetrance function because of flexible modeling of the baseline hazard function which includes constant, increasing or decreasing hazard functions. There might be potential for model misspecification. Kopciuk et al. (2009) employed the generalized log-Burr model for more flexible modeling as it includes the Weibull model or the log-logistic model as special cases (Lawless, 2003), where the Weibull model has a monotonic functional form of the hazard whereas the log-logistic model does not. The baseline hazard can be also modeled semiparametrically using a step function while assuming proportional hazards. Second, between-family heterogeneity in allele frequencies and baseline hazards can lead to bias in parameter estimates based on the homogeneous models. A random effect model would allow us to take between-family heterogeneity into account while avoiding a great number of family-specific parameters. Finally, familial correlation is a common feature of family data due to the unobserved genetic or environmental risk factors shared within families. We did not explicitly model within-family dependencies, instead, we accommodated a robust variance estimator. However, ignoring familial correlation can lead to biased estimates of the model parameters, and so to biased disease risks (Choi et al., 2008). Relating to other work, several authors have adopted mixed effect models for binary outcomes in family studies (Heagerty, 1999; Pfeiffer et al., 2008; Zheng et al., 2010). Shared frailty models can allow us to model times to onset data from families while explicitly modeling familial correlation. We are planning to develop such frailty models in the context of various family designs.

7. Acknowledgment

This research was supported by the Canadian Institutes of Health Research-Interdisciplinary Health Research Team, Grant no. 43821, the Institutes of Genetics and Population and Public Health of the Canadian Institutes of Health Research, Grant no. 110053 and the Natural Sciences and Engineering Research Council of Canada.

8. References

Carayol, J. & Bonaïti-Pellié, C. (2007). Estimating Penetrance From Family Data Using a Retrospective Likelihood When Ascertainment Depends on Genotype and Age of Onset, *Genetic Epidemiology*, Vol. 27: 109–117, ISSN 1098-2272.

Choi, Y.-H.; Kopciuk, K.A. & Briollais, L. (2008). Estimating disease risk associated with mutated genes in family-based designs, *Human Heredity*, Vol. 66: 238–251, ISSN 0001-5652.

Cotterchio, M.; McKeown-Eyssen, G.; Sutherland, H.; Buchan, G.; Aronson, M.; Easson, A.M.; Macey, J.; Holowaty, E. & Gallinger, S. (2000). Ontario familial colon cancer registry: methods and first year response rates, *Chronic Diseases in Canada*, Vol. 21: 81–86, ISSN 0228-8699.

Dempster, A.P.; Laird, N.M. & Rubin, D.B. (1977). Maximum likelihood from incomplete data via the EM algorithm, *Journal of the Royal Statistical Society. Series B*, Vol. 39:1–38, ISSN 1369-7412.

Gong, G. & Whittemore, A.S. (2003). Optimal designs for estimating penetrance of rare mutations of a disease-susceptibility gene, *Genetic Epidemiology*, Vol. 24:173–180, ISSN 1098-2272.

Green, J.; O'Driscoll, M.; Barnes, A.; Maher, E.R.; Bridge, P.; Shields, K. & Parfrey, P.S. (2002). Impact of gender and parent of origin on the phenotypic expression of hereditary nonpolyposis colorectal cancer in a large Newfoundland kindred with a common MSH2 mutation, *Diseases of the Colon and Rectum*, Vol. 45:1223–1232, ISSN 1530-0358.

Heagerty, P.J. (1999). Marginally specified logistic-normal models for longitudinal binary data, *Biometrics*, Vol. 55: 688–698, ISSN 1541-0420.

Hsu, L. & Gorfine, M. (2006). Multivariate survival analysis for case-control family studies, *Biostatistics*, Vol. 7: 387–398, ISSN 1468-4357.

Kopciuk, K.A.; Choi, Y.-H.; Parkhomenko, E.; Parfrey, P.; McLaughlin, J.; Green, J. & Briollais, L. (2009) Penetrance of HNPCC-related cancers in a retrospective cohort of 12 large Newfoundland families carrying a MSH2 founder mutation: an evaluation using modified segregation models, *Hereditary Cancer in Clinical Practice*, Vol.7: 16, ISSN 1897-4287.

Kraft, P. & Thomas, D.C. (2000). Bias and efficiency in family-based gene-characterization studies: conditional, prospective, retrospective, and joint likelihoods, *The American Journal of Human Genetics*, Vol. 66: 1119–1131, ISSN 1537-6605.

Lawless, J.F. (2003). *Statistical Models and Methods for Lifetime Data*, (Second Ed.), John Wiley and Sons Inc., ISBN 9780471372158, Hoboken.

Le Bihan, C.; Moutou, C.; Brugières, L.; Feunteun, J. & Bonaïti-Pellié, C. (1995). ARCAD: a method for estimating age-dependent disease risk associated with mutation carrier status from family data, *Genetic Epidemiology*, Vol. 12: 13–25, ISSN 1098-2272.

Li, H.; Yang, P. & Schwartz, A.G. (1998). Analysis of age of onset data from case-control family studies, *Biometrics*, Vol. 54: 1030–1039, ISSN 1541-0420.

Oakes, D. (1999). Direct calculation of the information matrix via the EM algorithm, *Journal of Royal Statistical Society, Series B*, Vol. 61, 479–482, ISSN 1369-7412.

Pfeiffer, R. M., Pee, D. & Landi, M.T. (2008). On combining family and case-control studies, *Genetic Epidemiology*, Vol. 32:638–646, ISSN 1098-2272.

Schaid, D.J.; McDonnell, S.K.; Riska, S.M.; Carlson, E.E. & Thibodeau, S.N. (2010). Estimation of genotype relative risks from pedigree data by retrospective likelihoods, *Genetic Epidemiology*, Vol. 34:287–298, ISSN 1098-2272.

Shih, J.H. & Chatterjee, N. (2000). Analysis of survival data from case-control family studies, *Biometrics*, Vol. 58: 502–509, ISSN 1541-0420.

Siegmund, K.D.; Whittemore, A.S. & Thomas, D.C. (1999). Multistage sampling for disease family registries, *Journal of the National Cancer Institute Monographs*, Vol. 26: 43–48, ISSN 1745-6614.

Thomas, D.C. (2004). *Statistical Methods in Genetic Epidemiology*, Oxford University Press, ISBN-13 978-0195159394, New York.

Wacholder, S.; Hartge, P.; Struewing, J.P.; Pee, D.; McAdams, M.; Brody, L. & Tucker, M. (1998). The kin-cohort study for estimating penetrance, *American Journal of Epidemiology*, Vol. 148:623–630, ISSN 1476-6256.

White, H. (1982). Maximum likelihood estimation of misspecified models, *Econometrica*, Vol. 50:1–25, ISSN 1468-0262.

Whittemore, A. S. & Halpern, J. (1997). Multi-stage sampling designs in genetic epidemiology, *Statistics in Medicine*, Vol. 16: 153–167, ISSN 1097-0258.

Zheng, Y.; Heagerty, P.J.; Hsu, L. & Newcomb, P.A. (2010) On combining family-based and population-based case-control data in association studies, *Biometrics*, Vol. 66: 1024–1033, ISSN 1541-0420.

Permissions

The contributors of this book come from diverse backgrounds, making this book a truly international effort. This book will bring forth new frontiers with its revolutionizing research information and detailed analysis of the nascent developments around the world.

We would like to thank Maria de Lourdes Ribeiro de Souza da Cunha, for lending her expertise to make the book truly unique. She has played a crucial role in the development of this book. Without her invaluable contribution this book wouldn't have been possible. She has made vital efforts to compile up to date information on the varied aspects of this subject to make this book a valuable addition to the collection of many professionals and students.

This book was conceptualized with the vision of imparting up-to-date information and advanced data in this field. To ensure the same, a matchless editorial board was set up. Every individual on the board went through rigorous rounds of assessment to prove their worth. After which they invested a large part of their time researching and compiling the most relevant data for our readers. Conferences and sessions were held from time to time between the editorial board and the contributing authors to present the data in the most comprehensible form. The editorial team has worked tirelessly to provide valuable and valid information to help people across the globe.

Every chapter published in this book has been scrutinized by our experts. Their significance has been extensively debated. The topics covered herein carry significant findings which will fuel the growth of the discipline. They may even be implemented as practical applications or may be referred to as a beginning point for another development. Chapters in this book were first published by InTech; hereby published with permission under the Creative Commons Attribution License or equivalent.

The editorial board has been involved in producing this book since its inception. They have spent rigorous hours researching and exploring the diverse topics which have resulted in the successful publishing of this book. They have passed on their knowledge of decades through this book. To expedite this challenging task, the publisher supported the team at every step. A small team of assistant editors was also appointed to further simplify the editing procedure and attain best results for the readers.

Our editorial team has been hand-picked from every corner of the world. Their multi-ethnicity adds dynamic inputs to the discussions which result in innovative outcomes. These outcomes are then further discussed with the researchers and contributors who give their valuable feedback and opinion regarding the same. The feedback is then collaborated with the researches and they are edited in a comprehensive manner to aid the understanding of the subject.

Apart from the editorial board, the designing team has also invested a significant amount of their time in understanding the subject and creating the most relevant covers. They scrutinized every image to scout for the most suitable representation of the subject and create an appropriate cover for the book.

The publishing team has been involved in this book since its early stages. They were actively engaged in every process, be it collecting the data, connecting with the contributors or procuring relevant information. The team has been an ardent support to the editorial, designing and production team. Their endless efforts to recruit the best for this project, has resulted in the accomplishment of this book. They are a veteran in the field of academics and their pool of knowledge is as vast as their experience in printing. Their expertise and guidance has proved useful at every step. Their uncompromising quality standards have made this book an exceptional effort. Their encouragement from time to time has been an inspiration for everyone.

The publisher and the editorial board hope that this book will prove to be a valuable piece of knowledge for researchers, students, practitioners and scholars across the globe.

List of Contributors

R. Cisterna, G. Ezpeleta and O. Tellería
Clinical Microbiology and Infection Control Department, Basurto Hospital, Avenida Montevideo - Bilbao, Spain

Katarzyna Kalinowska
Wroclaw Medical University, Poland

Astrid Helga Paulitsch-Fuchs
Institute of Hygiene, Microbiology and Environmental Medicine, Medical University of Graz, Graz, Austria
Wetsus Centre of Excellence for Sustainable Water Technology, Leeuwarden, The Netherlands

Birgit Willinger
Division of Hygiene and Medical Microbiology, Medical University of Vienna, Vienna, Austria

Bettina Heiling and Walter Buzina
Institute of Hygiene, Microbiology and Environmental Medicine, Medical University of Graz, Graz, Austria

Patrícia Yoshida Faccioli-Martins and Maria de Lourdes Ribeiro de Souza da Cunha
UNESP- Univ. Estadual Paulista, Biosciences Institute, Botucatu, SP, Brazil

Mariana Fávero Bonesso, Adilson de Oliveira and Maria de Lourdes Ribeiro de Souza da Cunha
UNESP- Univ. Estadual Paulista, Department of Microbiology and Immunology, Biosciency Institute, Botucatu-SP, Brazil

André Martins and Maria de Lourdes Ribeiro de Souza da Cunha
UNESP- Univ. Estadual Paulista, Biosciences Institute, Botucatu, SP, Brazil

Kuschel Annett
Humboldt Universität zu Berlin, Germany

Nagafumi Doi
Ibaraki Prefectural Medical Center of Psychiatry, Japan

Yoko Hoshi, Masanari Itokawa and Tomoe Ichikawa
Tokyo Metropolitan Institute of Medical Science, Japan

Takeo Yoshikawa
RIKEN Brain Science Institute, Japan

Blair Ortiz, William Cornejo and Lucía Blazicevich
Universidad de Antioquia, Child Neurology Group, Child and Adolescent Diseases Research Group PEDIACIENCIAS, Colombia

Nese Kocabasoglu and Reha Bayar
Cerrahpasa Medical School, Department of Psychiatry, Turkey

Gul Karacetin
Department of Child and Adolescent Psychiatry, Turkey

Turkay Demir
Cerrahpasa Medical School, Department of Child and Adolescent Psychiatry, Turkey

B. Lapin and M. Chikobava
Research Institute of Medical Primatology of the Russian Academy of Medical Sciences, Sochi, Russia

Maira Aguiar and Nico Stollenwerk
Centro de Matemática e Aplicações Fundamentais, Lisbon University, Portugal

BobW. Kooi
Faculty of Earth and Life Sciences, Department of Theoretical Biology, Vrije Universiteit, The Netherlands

Massimo Mirandola
Azienda Ospedaliera Universitaria Integrata Verona (The Hospital Trust of Verona), Coordinamento Regionale per il Management e la Progettazione Europea (Regional Coordination Centre for European Project Management), Veneto Region, Verona, Italy

Ruth Joanna Davis and Lorenzo Gios
Azienda Ospedaliera Universitaria Integrata Verona (The Hospital Trust of Verona), Coordinamento Regionale per il Management e la Progettazione Europea (Regional Coordination Centre for European Project Management), Veneto Region, Verona, Italy

Jean-Pierre Foschia, Michele Breveglieri, Martina Furegato and Enrica Castellani
ULSS20, Veneto Region, Verona, Italy

Dunia Ramarli
UO immunologia (Department of Pathology, Immunology), Azienda Ospedaliera Universitaria Integrata Verona (The Hospital Trust of Verona), Verona, Italy

Paola Coato
UO immunologia (Department of Pathology, Microbiology), Azienda Ospedaliera Universitaria Integrata Verona (The Hospital Trust of Verona), Verona, Italy

Nuno Santos and Margarida Correia-Neves
Life and Health Sciences Research Institute (ICVS), School of Health Sciences, University of Minho, Campus de Gualtar, Braga, Portugal

Virgílio Almeida
Centro de Investigação Interdisciplinar em Sanidade Animal - Faculdade de Medicina Veterinária (CIISA/FMV), TULisbon, Pólo Universitário do Alto da Ajuda, Lisbon, Portugal

Christian Gortázar
IREC National Wildlife Research Institute (CSIC-UCLM-JCCM), Ciudad Real, Spain

Zelalem Yilma
East Africa Dairy Development (EADD) Program, Addis Ababa, Ethiopia

Zahra Mozaheb
Mashhad University of Medical Science, Iran

Paolo Ruggero Errante and Antonio Condino-Neto
Department of Immunology, Institute of Biomedical Sciences, University of São Paulo, São Paulo, Brazil

Yun-Hee Choi
University of Western Ontario, Canada